Karuna Sachdeva

Pharmaceutical Biotechnology

2nd Edition

Other books of interest

Basic Endocrinology – For Students of Pharmacy and Allied Health Sciences
A. Constantini, R. Bartke and R. Khardori

Immunology – For Pharmacy Students
W.C. Shen and S. Louie

Drug Delivery and Targeting – For Pharmacists and Pharmaceutical Scientists
A.M. Hillery, A.W. Lloyd and J. Swarbrick

Transgenic Animals – Generation and Use
L.M. Houdebine

Pharmaceutical Biotechnology

An Introduction for Pharmacists and Pharmaceutical Scientists

2nd Edition

Edited by
Daan J.A. Crommelin *(Department of Pharmaceutics, Utrecht Institute for Pharmaceutical Sciences, Utrecht University, The Netherlands)*
and
Robert D. Sindelar *(Faculty of Pharmaceutical Sciences, University of British Columbia, Vancouver, Canada, formerly at the Department of Medicinal Chemistry, School of Pharmacy, University of Mississippi, USA)*

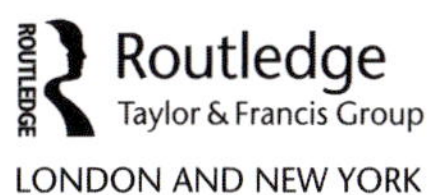
Routledge
Taylor & Francis Group
LONDON AND NEW YORK

First published 1997 by OPA (Overseas Publishers Association)

Second edition first published 2002
by Taylor & Francis
11 New Fetter Lane, London EC4P 4EE

Simultaneously published in the USA and Canada
by Taylor & Francis Inc,
325 Chestnut Street, 8th Floor, Philadelphia, PA 19106, USA

Taylor & Francis is an imprint of the Taylor & Francis Group

Typeset by Graphicraft Limited, Hong Kong
Printed and bound in Malta by
Gutenberg Press

Every effort has been made to ensure that the advice and information in this book is true and accurate at the time of going to press. However, neither the publisher nor the authors can accept any legal responsibility or liability for any errors or omissions that may be made. In the case of drug administration, any medical procedure or the use of technical equipment mentioned within this book, you are strongly advised to consult the manufacturer's guidelines.

British Library Cataloguing in Publication Data
A catalogue record for this book is available from the British Library

Library of Congress Cataloging in Publication Data
A catalog record for this book has been requested

ISBN 0-415-28500-3 (Hbk)
ISBN 0-415-28501-1 (Pbk)

Source acknowledgement for the cover illustration

The cover illustration shows a ribbon representation of the antigen binding fragment of bacterial antibody $MN_{12}H_2$ in complex with a synthetic peptide. The peptide is derived from the top of extracellular loop 4 of outer membrane protein PorA of *Neisseria meningitides* (strain $H_{44}/_{76}$). This model is based on an X-ray crystallography study performed by Jean van den Elsen (Antibody Recognition of *Neisseria meningitides*: a thermodynamic and structural analysis of the interaction between a bacterial monoclonal antibody and a class 1 outer membrane epitope (1996), thesis, Utrecht University.

Table of Contents

Preface to the second edition

The field of pharmaceutical biotechnology is developing rapidly. For those working in the field of pharmacy and pharmaceutical sciences, completely new and novel techniques and products appear at a rapid pace. This is the result of the interplay between a number of different disciplines, among those must be mentioned: molecular biology, molecular genetics, (bio-)engineering, (protein/sugar/nuclear acid) chemistry and, last but not least, the pharmaceutical sciences.

The total worldwide sales of biotechnology-produced pharmaceuticals continue to increase fast. For instance, in 1990 US sales amounted to approximately $2.0 billion. Sales increased to $5.1 billion in 1994 and $7.7 billion in 1995 (compared to $85 billion total US pharmaceutical sales). Estimates predict US biotech pharmaceuticals approaching $16 billion by 2004. Growth in the use of biotech compounds surpasses the growth of conventional pharmaceutical products.

Not only sales figures distinguish biotech compounds. Many of them are indicated for the treatment or prevention of serious life-threatening diseases (e.g. cancer, viral infection, or hereditary deficiencies), or for previously untreatable conditions, dramatically improving the patient's quality of life.

We believe that there is a strong need for an introductory textbook on Pharmaceutical Biotechnology that provides detailed coverage of both the basic science and clinical use of biotechnology-produced pharmaceuticals. Therefore, the goal of this book is to provide the reader with an introductory text to familiarize him or herself with biotechnology-related issues and terms. There is a strong focus on those issues that are related to the pharmaceutical profession and the pharmaceutical sciences. One target group is those pharmacists who wish to update their knowledge of biotechnology. A second target group is the present generation of pharmacy students at our universities. Thirdly, the pharmaceutical scientist who has not been in contact with modern biotechnology and wishes to become acquainted with the principles of this fast moving field. We are hopeful that this book will be used at universities, in life-long learning courses and in the professional environment of the pharmacist and industrial pharmaceutical scientist all over the world.

Chapter topics to be included were discussed at length with a number of academic and industrial experts. It was decided to start with a rather comprehensive introduction to biotechnology with issues relevant to the target groups (Chapter 1). As pharmaceutical biotech products are mainly (glyco)proteins, attention is paid to typically chemical aspects of (glyco)proteins to help the reader to understand the intricacies of the (physico)chemistry of these high molecular weight compounds (Chapter 2).

The advent and development of biotech products has created a number of unique pharmaceutical problems. The production, down stream processing, and characterization of biotech products are, in many ways, very different than the ways in which 'conventional' low molecular weight products are handled. The same applies to the delivery and pharmacokinetic aspects of proteins (Chapters 3, 4 and 5).

Chapter 6 consists of an introduction to a number of additional biotechnology-based methodologies important to pharmacy and the pharmaceutical sciences. These include bioengineered animals, protein engineering, antisense approaches, glycobiology and the immense impact of biotechnology on the drug discovery process.

The exciting field of gene therapy is reviewed in chapter 7. The reader is led through the fascinating world of gene delivery to somatic cells and introduced to the potentials and limitations of the present generation of gene transfection strategies.

In Chapters 8 to 17 presently registered recombinant proteins are discussed. Each chapter covers a therapeutic group of biotech products in terms of their chemistry, pharmacology and therapeutic indications.

In Chapter 18 the issue of how to handle pharmaceutical biotech products in the practice setting is discussed and sources for professional and patient information and education are provided.

A new Chapter 19 was added in this second edition dealing specifically with pharmaco-economic aspects of biotech products.

Chapter 20 gives the reader an insight into the new products that are in the biotech pipeline.

For educational purposes, each chapter concludes with a number of self-assessment questions and several of literature references for further reading. The multi-color printing of the art work in this book should assist the reader in mastering the contents. To help the reader with the many abbreviations and acronyms in the text, a list of abbreviations is added, as well.

We encourage the reader to suggest to us how we can improve coming editions of this book both in terms of topics to be discussed or deleted and in terms of errors that undoubtedly were made in spite of our careful checking.

The marketing of recombinant human insulin in the early 1980s and the development of monoclonal antibody-based kits ushered in a new era pharmacy. Rapidly evolving developments in the techniques and products of biotechnology necessitate a solid understanding by pharmacists, future pharmacists and pharmaceutical scientists. We believe this text will contribute to this necessary understanding.

Daan J.A. Crommelin and Robert D. Sindelar

Contributors

- Arakawa, T., Alliance Protein Laboratories Inc., Camarillo, California
- Beals, J.M., Research Technologies and Product Development, Lilly Research Laboratories, Eli Lilly and Company, Indianapolis, Indiana
- Beuvery, E.C., Laboratory for Product and Process Development, National Institute of Public Health and Environmental Protection (RIVM), Bilthoven, The Netherlands
- Bout, A., Crucell, Leiden, The Netherlands
- Brader, M.L., Research Technologies and Product Development, Lilly Research Laboratories, Eli Lilly and Company, Indianapolis, Indiana
- Braeckman, R., Pan Pacific Pharmaceuticals Inc., Rhode Island
- Combs, D.L., Department of Pharmacokinetics and Metabolism, Genentech Inc., San Francisco, California
- Crommelin, D.J.A., Department of Pharmaceutics, Utrecht Institute for Pharmaceutical Sciences (UIPS), Utrecht University/OctoPlus, Leiden, The Netherlands
- Deckelbaum, L., Centocor, Malvern, Pennsylvania
- DeFilippis, M.R., Research Technologies and Product Development, Lilly Research Laboratories, Eli Lilly and Company, Indianapolis, Indianapolis, Indiana
- Evens, R.P., MAPS 4 Biotec, Inc. Jacksonville, Florida and College of Pharmacy, University of Florida, Gainesville, Florida
- Flynn, J., Professional Services, Amgen Inc., Thousand Oaks, California
- Foote, M.A., Medical Writing Department, Amgen Inc., Thousand Oaks, California.
- Hamers, M., Biosynco, Amsterdam, The Netherlands.
- Hoekstra, W.P.M., Department of Molecular Cell Biology, Utrecht University, the Netherlands
- Jordan, R., Centocor, Malvern, Pennsylvania
- Jiskoot, W., Department of Pharmaceutics, Utrecht Institute for Pharmaceutical Sciences (UIPS), Utrecht University, The Netherlands
- Kadir, F., POA, Institute for Postacademic Education of Pharmacists, Bunnik, The Netherlands
- Kersten, G.F.A., Laboratory for Product and Process Development, National Institute of Public Health and Environmental Protection (RIVM), Bilthoven, The Netherlands
- Kolassa, E.M., Department of Pharmacy Administration, School of Pharmacy, University of Mississippi, Oxford, Mississippi
- Kovach, P.M., Research Technologies and Product Development, Lilly Research Laboratories, Eli Lilly and Company, Indianapolis, Indiana
- Marian, M., Department of Pharmacokinetics and Metabolism, Genentech Inc., San Francisco, California
- Modi, N.B., ALZA Corporation, Mountain View, California
- Nakada, M., Centocor, Malvern, Pennsylvania
- Peters, M., Program Management Reproductive Medicine, NV Organon, Oss, The Netherlands
- Philo, J.S., Alliance Protein Laboratories Inc., Camarillo, California
- Piascik, P., College of Pharmacy, University of Kentucky, Lexington, Kentucky,
- Salvado, A.J., Medical Writing Department, Amgen Inc., Thousand Oaks, California.
- Sam, T., Regulatory Affairs, NV Organon, Oss, The Netherlands
- Sindelar, R.D., Department of Medicinal Chemistry, School of Pharmacy, University of Mississippi, Oxford, Mississippi
- Sinicropi, D., Department of Pharmacokinetics and Metabolism, Genentech Inc., San Francisco, California
- Smeekens, J.C.M., Department of Molecular Cell Biology, Utrecht University, the Netherlands
- Smith, G., Department of Pharmacy Practice and Science, School of Pharmacy, Baltimore, Maryland
- Tami, J., Operations Manager, Drug Development, Isis Pharmaceuticals, California
- Van Dijk, M.A., GenMab A/s, Immunotherapy Laboratory, Utrecht
- Vidarsson, G., Immunotherapy Laboratory, University Medical Center Utrecht, Utrecht; Department of Vaccine Research (LVR), National Institute of Public Health and Environmental Protection (RIVM), Bilthoven, The Netherlands
- Ziska, D.S., School of Pharmacy, University of Mississippi, Jackson, Mississippi

Abbreviations

3-D	Three-dimensional
^{125}I-hGH	iodine labeled human growth hormone
5HT2a	serotonergic receptor subtype
A	(d)ATP(deoxy)adenosine 5′-triphosphate (Chapter 1)
A	adenine
Å	angstroms
AA	amino acid(s)
AAV	adeno-associated virus
Ab	antibody
ABO	blood group antigens
AC	anthracycline plus cyclophosphamide
ACT	activated clotting time
ADA	adenosine deaminase
ADCC	antibody-dependent cellular cytotoxicity
ADME	absorption, distribution, metabolism, excretion
ADP	adenosine diphosphate
Ag	antigen
AG-LCR	asymmetric gap ligation chain reaction
AHF	antihemophiliac factor/factor VIII
AIDS	acquired immune deficiency syndrome
ALS	amyotrophic lateral sclerosis
AMI	acute myocardial infarction
AML	acute myelogenous leukemia
ANC	absolute neutrophil count
AP	alkaline phosphatase
APC	antigen presenting cell
aPCC	activated prothrombin complex concentrate
apoE	apolipoprotein E
APSAC	acylated plasminogen-streptokinase activator
ARDS	adult respiratory distress syndrome
Asn	asparagine
Asp	aspartic acid
ATP	adenosine 5′-triphosphate
ATPase	adenosine triphosphatase
AUC	area under the curve
B	biotin
batching	preparing batches
BCG	bacille Calmette-Guérin
BCGFII	B-cell growth factor
BDNF	brain-derived neurotrophic factor
BHK	baby hamster kidney
BMD	bone mineral density
BMT	bone marrow transplantation
bp	base pairs of DNA
BRCA1	breast cancer genes
BRMs	biological response modifiers
BSA	bovine serum albumin
C	(d)CTP(deoxy)cytidine 5′-triphosphate (Chapter 1)
C	cytosine
C	plasma concentration (Chapter 5)
CAM	cell adhesion molecules
CAR	Coxsackie adenovirus receptor
CCK	cholecystokinin
CD	circular dichroism (Chapter 2)
CD	cluster designation (term to label surface molecules of lymphocytes) (Chapter 9)
CDC	complement-dependent cytotoxicity
CDL	lytic complement pathway
cDNA	copy DNA/complementary deoxyribonucleic acid (sometimes also 'cloned DNA')
CDR	complementarity determining region
C_E	concentration in effect compartment (Chapter 5)
CEA	cost-effectiveness analysis
CETP	cholesterol (cholesteryl) ester transfer protein
CF	cystic fibrosis
CFTR	cystic fibrosis transmembrane conductance regulator
CFU	colony-forming unit
CFU-GM	granulocyte-macrophage progenitor cells
CG	chorionic gonadotropin
CGD	chronic granulomatous disease
C_H(1,2,3)	constant region(s) of heavy chain of IgG

CHO	Chinese hamster ovary
C_L	constant region of light chain of IgG (Chapter 13)
CL	elimination clearance from central compartment (Chapter 5)
CL_d	distributional clearance (Chapter 5)
CL_e	linear clearance for distribution of drug to the effector compartment and elimination from the effector compartment (Chapter 5)
CMI	cell-mediated immunity
CMK	chronic myelogenous leukemia
CML	chronic myelogenous leukemia
CMV	cytomegalovirus
CNS	central nervous system
Con A	concanavalin A
COPD	chronic obstructive pulmonary disease
CRI	chronic renal insufficiency
CRS	cytokine release syndrome
CSF(s)	colony stimulating factor(s)
cSNPs	SNPs occurring in gene coding regions
CT	cholera toxin
CTCL	cutaneous T-cell lymphoma
CTL	cytotoxic T-lymphocyte
CTP	cytidine 5′-triphosphate
CUA	cost utility analysis
D2	dopaminergic D2 receptors
D5W	dextrose 5% in water
DAB_{389} CD4	a fusion protein
DAB_{389} EGF	a fusion protein
DAB_{389} hGM-CSF	fused peptide sequence of human GM-CSF
DAB_{389} IL-2	IL-2 fusion protein
DAB_{389} IL-2	IL-2 fusion protein; also called IL-2 fusion toxin
DAB_{389} IL-4	a fusion protein
DAB_{389} IL-6	a fusion protein
dATP	deoxyadenosine 5′-triphosphate
dCTP	deoxycytidine 5′-triphosphate
DDA	dioctadecyldimethylammoniumbromide
DDBJ	DNA Data Bank of Japan
ddNTP	dideoxyribonucleotide triphosphate
DF	denatured form
DF	diafiltration
dGTP	deoxyguanosine 5′-triphosphate
ΔG_u	free energy
di	supplied diluent (Chapter 18)
DLS	dynamic light scattering
DNA	deoxyribonucleic acid
DNase	deoxyribonuclease (1)
DNF	do not freeze (Chapter 18)
dNTP	deoxyribonucleotide triphosphate
DS	degree of cross-linking
DSC	differential scanning calorimetry
DTP	diphtheria-tetanus-pertussis
dTTP	Deoxythymidine-5′-triphosphate
	deep vein thrombosis
E	effect (Chapter 5)
E	enzyme (Chapter 2)
E_o	baseline effect (Chapter 5)
EBV	Epstein-Barr virus
EC_{50}	concentration that produces 50% of maximum inhibition or stimulation (Chapter 5)
ECD	extracellular domain
EDF	eosinophil differentiation factor
EDTA	ethylenediaminetetraacetic acid
EGF	epidermal growth factor
EGFR	epidermal growth factor receptor
EI	electrospray ionization
ELISA	enzyme-linked immunosorbent assay
E_{max}	maximum inhibition or stimulation (Chapter 5)
EMAX	maximal efficacy (Chapter 14)
EMBL	European Molecular Biology Laboratory
EMEA	European Medicine Evaluation Agency
EPO	erythropoietin (Epoetin alfa)
ERK/MAP	extracellular signal-regulated kinase/mitogen activated protein kinase
ES	embryonic stem cells
EU	endotoxin unit
ex da	see expiration date on package (Chapter 18)
$F(ab')_2$	proteolysis product of IgG (cf. Chapter 13)
Fab	proteolysis product of IgG (cf. Chapter 13) (fragment of antigen binding)
FACS	fluorescence activated cell sorter
Fc	constant fragment (of immunoglobulins)
FcRN	Brambell receptor/F_c salvage receptor
FDA	Food and Drug Administration
FEV_1	mean forced expiratory volume in one second
FGF	fibroblast growth factor
FH	familial hypercholesterolemia
fMLP	formyl-methionyl-leucyl-phenylalanine
FPLC	fast protein liquid chromatography
FSH	follicle-stimulating hormone

FTIR	Fourier transform infrared spectroscopy
F_V	variable domains of light and heavy chains
FVC	forced vital capacity
G	(d)GTP(deoxy)guanosine 5'-triphosphate (Chapter 1)
G	guanine
G-CSF	granulocyte colony-stimulating factor
G-LCR	gap ligation chain reaction
Ga-DF	gallium-desferal
GCV	gancyclovir
GDNF	glial-derived neurotrophic growth factor
GEMM	granulocyte, erythrocyte, monocyte and megakaryocyte
GERD	gastroesophageal reflux disease
GF	growth factor
GFR	glomerular filtration rate
GH	growth hormone
GHBP	growth hormone binding protein
GHD	growth hormone deficiency
GHRH	growth hormone releasing hormone
GIFT	gamete infra-fallopian transfer
GIT/GI tract	gastrointestinal tract
GlcNAc	N-acetyl-glucosamine
GLP	good laboratory practice
GM-CSF	granulocyte-macrophage colony-stimulating factor
GMP	good manufacturing practice
GnRH	gonadotropin releasing hormone
GO	glucose-oxidase
Gp/GP	glycoprotein
GPIIb-IIIa	integrin $\alpha_{IIb}\beta_3$, the fibronectin receptor
GRF	growth hormone releasing factor
GTP	guanosine 5'-triphosphate
GvHD	graft versus host disease
HACA	human anti-chimeric antibody
HAMA	humane anti-mouse antibodies
HB(sAg)	hepatitis B (surface antigen)
Hct	hematocrit
HEPA	high efficiency particulate air filters
HER2	human epidermal growth factor receptor gene
hG-CSF	human granulocyte colony-stimulating factor
HGF	hematopoietic growth factor
hGH	human growth hormone
hGH-N	normal hGH gene
hGH-V	variant hGH gene
HGI	Human Genome Initiative
HGP	Human Genome Project
HIC	hydrophobic interaction chromatography
His	histidine
HIV	human immunodeficiency virus
HLA	humane leukocyte antigen
HMWP	high molecular weight protein
HPLC	high-performance liquid chromatography
HPRT	hypoxanthine phosphoribosyl transferase
HRP	horseradish peroxidase
HSA	human serum albumin
HSCs	hematopoietic stem cells
HSV(-tk)	herpes simplex virus (-thymidine kinase)
HTS	high-throughput screening
IA	intra-arterial
IC	intracoronary
ICAM-1	intracellular adhesion molecule-1
ICSI	intracytoplasmic sperm injection
IEF	iso-electric focusing
iep	iso-electric point
IFN	interferon(s)
IFN-α	interferon α
IFN-β	interferon β
IFN-γ	interferon γ
Ig	immunoglobulin
IgA	immunoglobulin A
IgD	immunoglobulin D
IgE	immunoglobulin E
IGF	insulin-like growth factor
IGF-I	insulin growth factor-I
IGF-II	insulin growth factor-II
IGFBP	IGF binding protein
IgG	immunoglobulin G
IgM	immunoglobulin M
IL	interleukin(s)
IL	intralesional (Chapter 18)
IL-1	interleukin-1
IL-1 ra	IL-1 receptor antagonist
IL-2	interleukin-2
IL-2R	interleukin-2 receptor
IL-3	interleukin-3
IL-10	interleukin-10
IL-11	interleukin-11
IM	inner membrane (Chapter 1)
IM/im	Intramuscular
IO	intra-orbital
IP	intraperitoneal
IPTG	iso-propyl-β-thiogalactoside
IPV	inactivated polio vaccine
ISS	idiopathic short stature
ITP	idiopathic thrombocytopenic purpura

ITR	inverted terminal repeat
IUGR	intrauterine growth retardation
iv/IV	intravenous
IVB	intravenous bolus (Chapter 18)
IVF	*in vitro* fertilization
IVIF	intravenous infusion (Chapter 18)
IVIN	intravenous injection (Chapter 18)
K_{01} and K_{10}	rate constants (Chapter 5)
Kb	thousand base pairs of DNA
K_d	rate constant resembling distribution and transduction delays (Chapter 5)
Kd	dissociation rate constant (Chapter 13)
kDa	kilodalton
K_{out}	first order rate constant for effect disappearance (Chapter 5)
KGF	keratinocyte growth factor
K_m	Michaelis Menten constant
LAF	lymphocyte activating factor
LAK	leucocyte activated killer (cells)
LAtTP	long acting tissue plasminogen activator
LCR	ligation chain reaction
LDL	low-density lipoprotein
LDLR	low-density lipoprotein receptor
LH	luteinizing hormone
LHRH	luteinizing hormone releasing hormone
LIF	leukemia inhibitory factor
LPD	lymphoproliferative disorders
LPS	lipopolysaccharide
LRP	(low-density) lipoprotein receptor-related protein
LTR	long terminal repeat
LYZ	lysozyme
M1	muscarinic receptor subtype
M3	muscarinic receptor subtype
M cells	microfold cells
MAb(s)	monoclonal antibody(s)
MAC	membrane attack complex
MALDI	matrix-assisted laser desorption ionization
MAP	multiple antigen peptide
Mb	million base pairs of DNA
MCB	master cell bank
M-CSF	macrophage colony-stimulating factor
MDR-1	multiple drug resistance
Meg	megakaryocyte
Met-GH	methionine human growth hormone
met-rhGH	methionyl recombinant human growth hormone, contains N-terminal methionine
mfg	contact manufacturer (Chapter 18)
MGDF	megakaryocyte growth and development factor
MHC	major histocompatibility complex
MI	myocardial infarction
MMAD	mean mass aerodynamic diameter
MMR	measles-mumps-rubella
MPS	mononuclear phagocyte system
M_r	relative molecular mass
mRNA	messenger ribonucleic acid/ messenger RNA
MTP-PE	muramyltripeptide-phosphatidylethanolamine
MuLV	murine leukemia virus
mUPA	murine urokinase-type plasminogen activator
M_W	relative molecular mass
NA	not available (Chapter 18)
NBP	non-ionic block copolymers
NCBI	National Center for Biotechnology Information
NCS	neocarzinostatin
NESP	novel erythropoiesis stimulating protein
NF	natural form
NF-κB	transcription factor in B- and T-cells
NFs	neurotrophic factors
NGF	nerve growth factor
NIH	National Institutes of Health
NK	natural killer cell(s)
NMR	nuclear magnetic resonance spectroscopy
NOESY	2-D nuclear Overhauser effect NMR technique
NPH	neutral protamine Hagedorn
NPL	neutral protamine lispro
NS	normal saline (Chapter 18)
NSAIDs	non-steroidal anti-inflammatory drugs
NZS	neocarzinostatin
ODNs	oligodeoxynucleotides
OLA	oligonucleotide ligation assay
OM	outer membrane (Chapter 1)
OMP	outer membrane protein
ON	oligonucleotide
ori	origin of replication
PAGE	polyacrylamide gel electrophoresis
PAI	plasminogen activator inhibitors
PAI-1	plasminogen activator inhibitor type-1
PBPCs	peripheral blood progenitor cells
PCI	percutaneous coronary intervention
PCR	polymerase chain reaction

PCTA	percutaneous transluminal coronary angioplasty
PD	pharmacodynamics
PDGF	platelet-derived growth factor
PEG	polyoxyethylene = polyethyleneglycol
PEG IL-2	PEGylated interleukin-2(polyethylene glycol modified interleukin-2)
PEG-rhMGDF	pegylated-recombinant human megakaryocyte growth and development factor
PEI	polyethylene imines
PG	peptidoglycans (Chapter 1)
pl	iso-electric point, negative logarithm
pit-hGH	pituitary-derived human growth hormone
PIXY-321	fusion protein between GM-CSF/IL-3
PK	pharmacokinetics
PLGA	polylactic-coglycolic acid
PNA	peptide nucleic acid
PP	polypropylene
PT	prothrombin time
PTCA	percutaneous transluminal coronary angioplasty
PTH	parathyroid hormone (recombinant human)
PTO	United States Patent and Trademark Office
PTT	partial thromboplastin time
PVC	polyvinyl chloride
PVDF	polyvinylidine difluoride
QALY	quality-adjusted life year
pwd	powder (Chapter 18)
rAAT	recombinant α1–antitrypsin
RAC	US Recombinant DNA Advisory Committee
rAHF	recombinant anti-hemophilia factor
RB	roller bottle
RBC	red blood cells
rBPI	recombinant bactericial/permeability-increasing protein
rDNA	recombinant deoxyribonucleic acid/recombinant-DNA
Ref	refrigerator (Chapter 18)
rG-CSF	recombinant granulocyte colony-stimulating factor (filgrastim)
RGD	amino acid sequence Arg-Gly-Asp (arginine-glycine-aspartic acid)
rGM-CSF	recombinant granulocyte-macrophage colony-stimulating factor
rhDNase	recombinant human deoxyribonuclease I
rh-EPO	recombinant human erythropoietin
rhG-CSF	recombinant human granulocyte colony-stimulating factor
rhGH	recombinant human growth hormone, natural sequence
rhGm-CSF	recombinant human granulocyte-macrophage colony-stimulating factor
rhIL-11	recombinant human interleukin-11
RIA	radioimmunoassay
rBPI	recombinant bactericidal/permeability increasing protein
rIFN γ	recombinant interferon γ
R_{in}	zero order appearance rate (Chapter 5)
RME	receptor mediated endocytosis
RMS	root mean square
RNA	ribonucleic acid
RNase P	ribonuclease P
Rnase H	ribonuclease H
R_{out}	first order disappearance rate (Chapter 5)
RP-HPLC	reversed-phase high performance liquid chromatography
rRNA	ribosomal RNA
RSV	respiratory syncytial virus
RT	reverse transcriptase
RT	room temperature (only Chapter 18)
rt-PA	recombinant tissue-type plasminogen activator
RT-PCR	reverse transcription polymerase chain reaction
RTU	ready to use solution (Chapter 18)
S	substrate (Chapter 2)
SA	streptavidin
SBS	short bowel syndrome
SBWFI	sterile bacteriostatic water for injection (Chapter 18)
SC	suspension culture (Chapter 14)
sc/SC	subcutaneous
SCF	stem cell factor (also known as c-kit ligand and steel factor)
ScF_V	single chain variable fragments
SCI	subcutaneous infusion
SCN	severe chronic neutropenia
scu PA	single chain urokinase plasminogen activator
SDS-PAGE	sodium dodecyl sulfate polyacrylamide-gel electrophoresis
SEC	size-exclusion chromatography
Ser	serine

sIL2R	soluble interleukin-2 receptor
SLE	systemic lupus erythematosus
SNP(s)	single nucleotide polymorphism(s)
SOD	superoxide dismutase
sol	solution (Chapter 18)
SQ	subcutaneous injection (Chapter 18)
SQI	subcutaneous infusion (Chapter 18)
SSC	large scale suspension culture process
STI	soy bean trypsin inhibitor
SWFI	sterile water for injection (Chapter 18)
T/dTTP	deoxythymidine 5'-triphosphate (Chapter 1)
T	thymine
Tac	CD_{25}
t-PA	tissue plasminogen activator
$t_{1/2\alpha}$,$t_{1/2\beta}$	half lives in α and β phase of two compartment kinetic model (Chapter 5)
T3, T4	thyroid hormones
TAC	T-cell activating antigen
TAS	transcription-based amplification system
TCGF	T-cell growth factor
T_{DTH}	delayed type hypersensitivity T-cells
T_e	eutectic temperature
TFF	tangential flow filtration
TFPI	tissue factor pathway inhibitor
T_g	glass transition temperature
TGF	tissue growth factor
T_h**-cell**	T-helper cell
$TH_{1,2}$	Tyle 1 or 2 T-helper cell
Ti	tumor inducing
TIL	tumor infiltrating lymphocytes
TIMI	thrombolysis in myocardial infraction
TNF-α	tumor necrosis factor α
tPA	tissue-type plasminogen activator
TPMT	thiopurine methyltransferase
TPO	thrombopoietin
TR	terminal repeats
TRAP	thrombin receptor activating peptide
TRF	T cell replacement factor
tRNA	transfer RNA
TSE	transmissible spongiphormous encephalitis
TSH	thyroid-stimulating hormone
TSP	thrombospondin
U	uracil
U	UTP/uridine 5′-triphosphate (Chapter 1)
UF	ultrafiltration
uPA	urokinase-type plasminogen activator
USPC	United States Pharmacopeia Convention
UTP	uridine 5′-triphosphate
UV	ultraviolet
V_β	volume of distribution of peripheral compartment of two-compartment kinetic model (Chapter 5)
V_E	apparent volume of distribution in the effect compartment (Chapter 5)
VEGF	vascular endothelial growth factor
V_H	variable region of heavy chain of IgG
V_L	variable region of light chain of IgG
VLP	virus like particles
VSV	vesicular stomatitis virus
W	weight
WCB	working cell bank
WHO	World Health Organization
WHO-IUIS	World Health Organisation-International Union of Immunologic Societies
X-FEL	x-ray free electron laser

1 Molecular Biotechnology

Wiel P. M. Hoekstra and Sjef C.M. Smeekens

Introduction

Biotechnology has been defined in many different ways, providing many useful terms for the precise functions of pharmaceutical biotechnology. In general, biotechnology implies the use of microorganisms, plants and animals or parts thereof for the production of useful compounds. Consequently, pharmaceutical biotechnology should be considered as the biotechnological manufacturing of pharmaceutical products.

Various forms of biotechnology existed in ancient times. The Bible documents the ancient origin of biotechnology, telling of Noah who apparently knew how to make wine from grapes. Based merely on experience bioproducts were for many ages homemade in a traditional fashion without an understanding of the underlying principles.

An insight into the nature of the traditional processes was achieved in about 1870. Pasteur illustrated that chemical conversions in these processes were performed by living cells, and thus the traditional processes should be considered biochemical conversions. Biotechnology became science! In the decades following Pasteur's discovery, biotechnological knowledge increased when the catalytic role of enzymes for most biochemical conversions became apparent. Based on that knowledge, tools became available for the control and optimization of the traditional processes.

A further and very important breakthrough took place after the development of molecular biology. The notion, brought forward by the pioneers in molecular biology in around 1950, that DNA encodes proteins and in this way controls all cellular processes was the impetus for a new period in biotechnology. The fast evolving DNA technologies, after the development of the recombinant DNA technology in the seventies, allowed biotechnologists to control gene expression in the organisms used for biotechnological manufacturing. Moreover, the developed technologies opened ways for the introduction of foreign DNA into all kinds of organisms. As will be shown later, genetically modified organisms constructed in this way opened up completely new possibilities for biotechnology. The new form of biotechnology, based on thorough knowledge of the DNA molecule and the availability of manipulation technologies of DNA, is frequently described as "molecular biotechnology." The molecular approaches introduced possibilities for the further development of biotechnology, although the expectations were sometimes overestimated. At the same time, biotechnology became the subject of public debate. An important question in the debate deals with potential risks: do genetically modified organisms used in production facilities pose unknown risks for an ecosystem and for the human race itself? Moreover, a profound ethical question was brought forward: is it right to modify the genetic structure of living organisms?

In this chapter we will focus mainly on the new biotechnology by describing its means and goals. Concerning the potential risks of the technology, we will confine ourselves to stating that all sorts of measures are taken to avoid risks while using genetically modified organisms. The ethical aspects, interesting as they are, are beyond the scope of this chapter.

The Cell

Biotechnology uses complete organisms in addition to single cells and cell constituents. Basic understanding of cell biology is therefore required to comprehend biotechnology to its full extent.

Cells from all sorts of organisms are used in biotechnology. Not only are prokaryotic cells used, like simple unicellular bacteria, but also eukaryotic cells, like those of higher microorganisms, plants and animals. Those eukaryotic cell types are not dealt with in detail. The unifying concepts in cell biology and the diversification relevant to pharmaceutical biotechnology will be the main topic of discussion in chapter 1.

The Prokaryotic Cell

The prokaryotes, to which the bacteria belong, represent the simplest cells in nature. A schematic illustration (Figure 1.1) depicts a prokaryotic cell. Such a cell is, in fact, no more than cytoplasm surrounded by some surface layers, generally described as the cell envelope. In the bacterial world one distinguishes two main types of organisms: Gram-positive or Gram-negative, depending on different

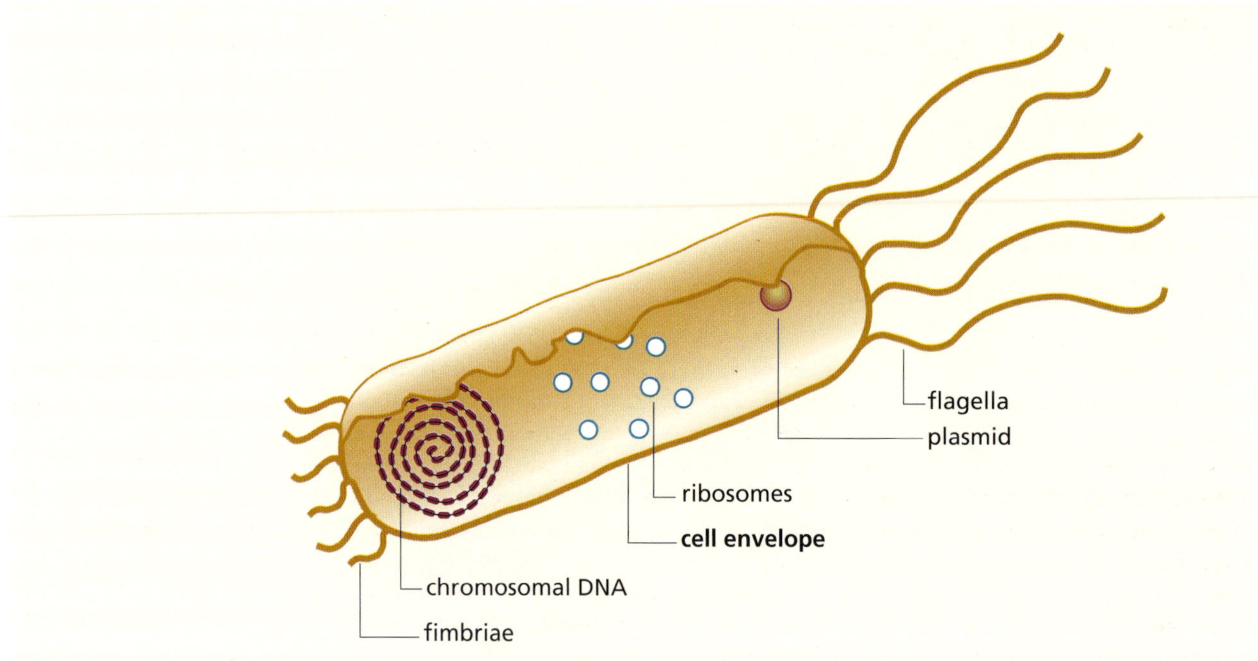

Figure 1.1. Cross section (artificial) through a bacterial cell. The surface structures (fimbrae and flagella) are not essential structures but allow the cells to adhere and to move.

behavior observed in a classical cell staining technique. The fundamental differences between these two prokaryotic types are mainly apparent in the structure of the cell envelope.

The bacterial cell envelope consists of a cytoplasmic membrane and a very characteristic wall structure called the peptidoglycan layer. The cells of Gram-positive organisms are multilayered with peptidoglycan, while only one or two such layers are found in cells of gram-negative organisms. However, the clearest distinction between the two types of bacterial cells is that in gram-negative organisms the cell is surrounded by a very specific extra membrane layer, called outer membrane (OM) (Figure 1.2). Located next to the cytoplasmic membrane, also called

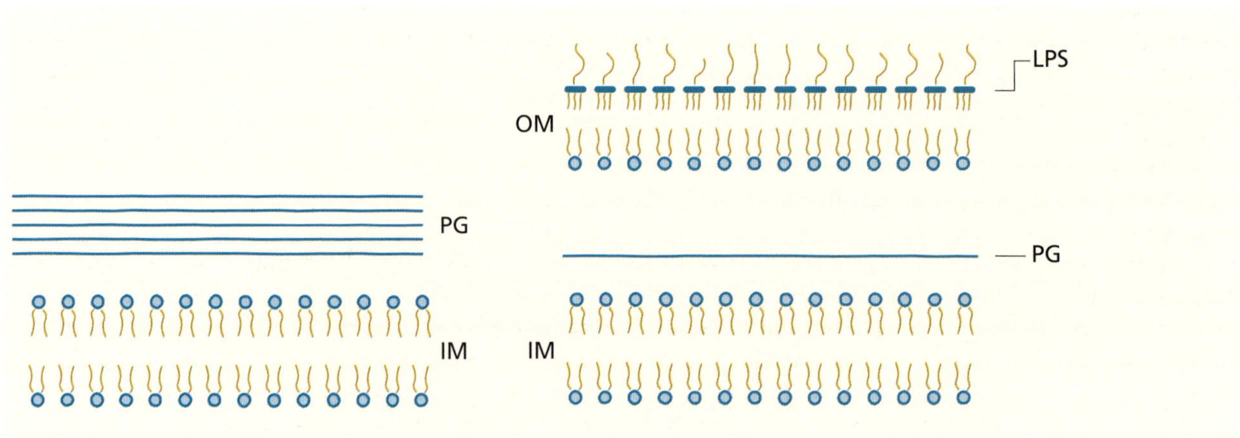

Figure 1.2. Cell envelope G^+ cell (left) and G^- cell (right). G^+ = gram – positive; G^- = gram – negative; PG = peptidoglycans; LPS = lipopolysaccharide; OM = outer membrane; IM = inner membrane.

the inner membrane (IM), the OM acts as a permeation barrier for substances that are transported into and out of the cell.

A prominent and very particular chemical constituent of the OM is the compound named lipopolysaccharide (LPS). Biopharmaceutical products gained from Gram-negative organisms must be extensively purified, especially when they are used as a pharmaceutical for man or animals (Chapters 3, 4), since LPS set free during the isolation of the product has, even in a very low concentration, severe toxic effects to man and animals.

In the bacterial cell DNA is generally organized in one large circular molecule. The bacterial DNA is not surrounded by a nuclear membrane and is not as complex in organization as DNA in eukaryotic cells. One generally refers to bacterial DNA as chromosomal DNA, analogous to the nomenclature in eukaryotic cells. Bacteria may, apart from the chromosomal DNA, harbor autonomously replicating small DNA molecules, called plasmids. Functions that are essential for a bacterial cell are usually encoded by the chromosome, whereas functions encoded by plasmids are generally in no way essential. Nevertheless, plasmids endow the bacterial cell with properties that may be very important for the survival of the bacteria. Antibiotic resistances and the production of toxic proteins, for example, are well known plasmid encoded traits. As we will see later, plasmids are used in biotechnology as important and basic tools for the recombinant DNA technology.

When we refer to plasmids as small DNA molecules, this is of course in comparison to the size of the chromosomal DNA. Besides, one has to realize that plasmids vary in size. Small plasmids, generally the relevant ones for biotechnology, harbor about 6000 DNA building units, called nucleotides. Chromosomal DNA of a bacterium contains at least 1000 times more nucleotides. The DNA content of an animal or plant cell on the other hand exceeds several hundred times that of a bacterial cell. Moreover, the DNA of the former cells is no longer organized in one molecule, but in several linear chromosomes. A popular way to illustrate this fast growing complexity of DNA molecules in nature is by using a metaphor of pages and books. One can easily write on one page the composition of the DNA of a small plasmid by its nucleotide composition using the symbols A, C, G and T for the various nucleotides in the DNA. To do the same for the bacterial chromosome, a book with about 1000 pages is needed. To describe the DNA of an animal cell or a plant cell requires a few hundred books, each containing about 1000 pages.

Bacterial cells, like all cells, harbor ribosomes in their cytoplasm as essential structures for protein synthesis. The cytoplasm also harbors a great variety of enzymes and other (macro)molecules required for the proper physiology of the cell. Most importantly, however, is that, apart from chromosome, ribosomes and sometimes plasmids, generally no other distinct structures are visible in the cytoplasm of the bacterial cell, even when studied with an electron microscope. Furthermore, there are no compartments present in the cytoplasm of the prokaryotic cell.

The Eukaryotic Cell

Figure 1.3 presents a schematic picture of a plant cell as an example of an eukaryotic cell. The eukaryotic cell has a very complex structure, defined not only by the presence of cell organelles like the nucleus, mitochondria and chloroplast (the latter exclusively found in plant cells), but also by the presence of specific internal membranes and of vacuoles. This complex and compartmentalized structure implies complicated functional behavior and is one of the reasons that in the initial phase of modern biotechnology simple bacterial cells, easier to handle and simpler to modify, were prominently used. Nowadays, molecular biotechnologists use all sorts of eukaryotic cells, exploiting the fast growing insights in cell biology.

Gene Expression

Genetic information, chemically determined by the DNA structure, is transferred to daughter cells by DNA replication and is expressed by transcription (conversion of DNA into RNA) followed by translation (conversion of RNA into protein). This set of processes is found in all cells and generally proceeds in similar ways. It is one of the main unifying concepts in cell biology. The pioneers of molecular biology called this series of events the "central dogma" of biology. It was found later that retroviruses, a special class of animal RNA viruses, served to encode an enzyme that catalyses the conversion of RNA into complementary DNA. This enzyme, called reverse transcriptase as it directs the reverse of the transcription, enables an information flow from RNA into DNA. Reverse transcriptase became, as will be shown later, a very important tool for DNA technology.

The various DNA linked processes are schematically depicted below:

$$\text{DNA} \leftrightarrow \text{RNA} \rightarrow \text{protein}$$

The "central dogma" was based on investigations done with bacteria and viruses. Later it was found that in eukaryotic organisms many genes were expressed differently from what was predicted by the dogma in the strict sense. In some cases the RNA derived by transcription of a eukaryotic DNA segment is subject to a process called splicing before it leaves the nucleus. During this process certain parts (the introns) of the nascent RNA molecules

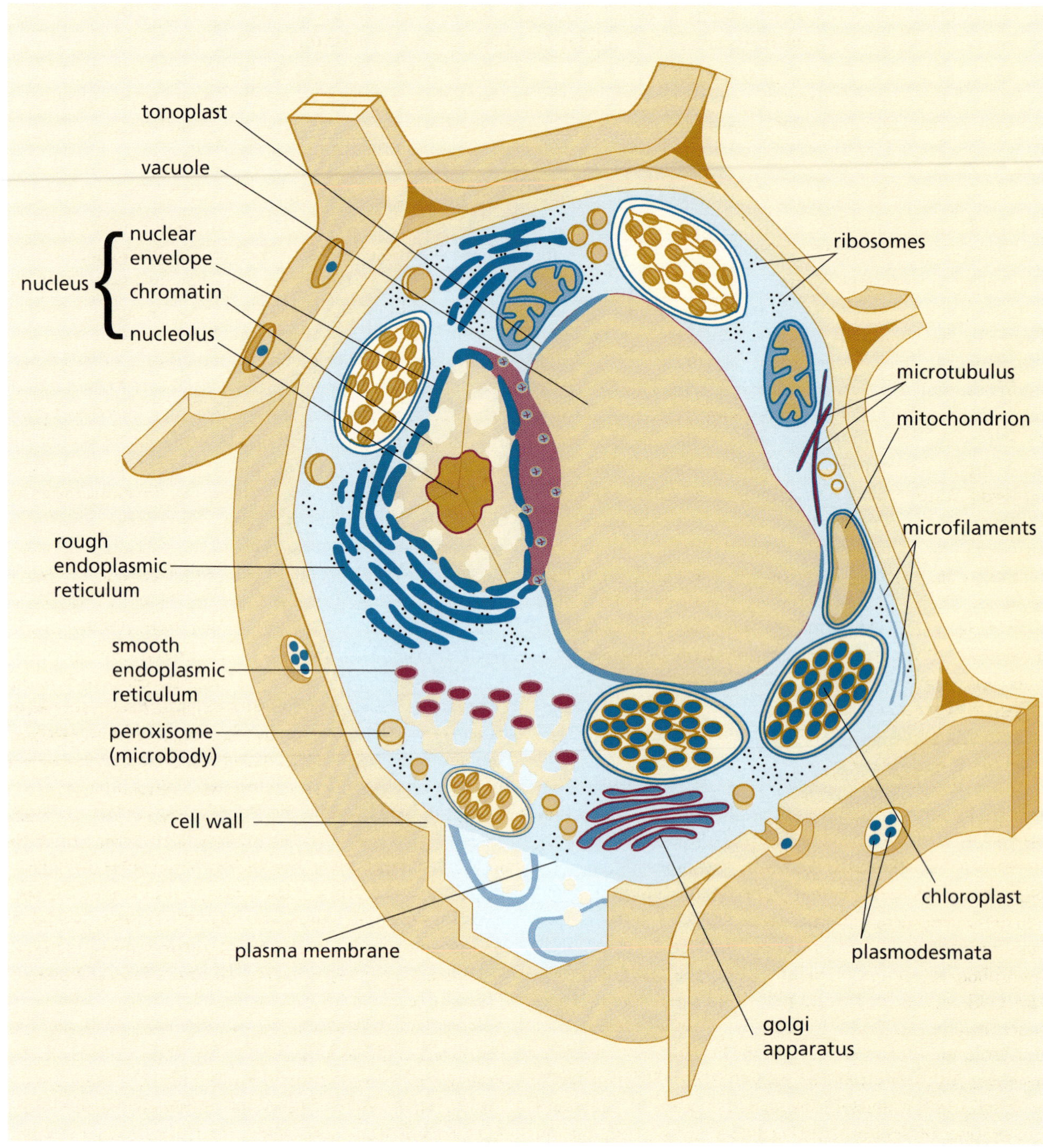

Figure 1.3. Plant cell, schematic view.

are removed, after which the other parts (the exons) link together and form the effective RNA for the protein synthesis (Figure 1.4).

Furthermore, it is important to realize that a nascent protein – the direct result of the translation – is not necessarily identical to the protein that functions in the cell as an enzyme or structural protein. Most proteins as we find them in the cell are modified by post-translational events. Nascent proteins are, for example, trimmed by peptidases; in some cases lipidic groups are linked to the protein, while in eukaryotic cells modification through linking of sugar groups (glycosylation) is a common event. Such post-translational modifications are important features with regard to the specific function of the protein.

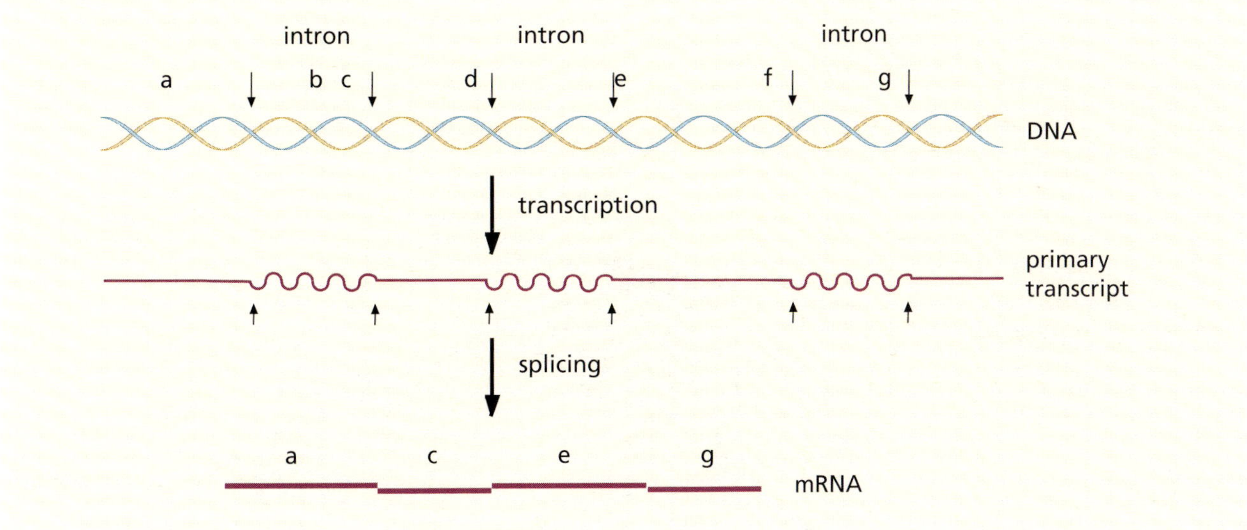

Figure 1.4. RNA splicing.

Precise knowledge of the information flow in the cell is very important for biotechnology, since it offers possibilities for controlling cellular processes at the level of gene expression. Therefore, the essentials of the elements and processes involved in the flow of genetic information are described below.

DNA Replication

Although DNA may be organized differently in various organisms, one or more double-stranded DNA molecules in a helix conformation are the predominant structures. Strands of DNA are composed of four specific building elements: the deoxyribonucleotides dATP, dCTP, dGTP and dTTP (shortly written as A, C, G and T), linked by phosphodiester bonds. The two strands in the DNA helix are held together through hydrogen bonds between the nucleotides in the various strands. The DNA strands in the helix are complementary in their nucleotide composition: an A in one strand is always facing a T in the other one, while a C is always facing a G (Figure 1.5). Moreover, the strands in double-stranded DNA run antiparallel: the 5'-P end of the one strand faces the 3'-OH end of the complementary strand, and vice versa.

During cell division the genetic information in a parental cell is transferred to the daughter cells by DNA replication. Essential in the very complex DNA replication process is the action of DNA polymerases. During replication each DNA strand is copied into a complementary strand that runs antiparallel. The topological constraint for replication imposed by the double-helix structure of the DNA is solved by the unwinding of the helix, a process catalysed by the enzyme helicase. In a set of biochemical events, deoxyribonucleotide monomers are added one by one to the end of a growing DNA strand in the 5' to 3' direction.

DNA replication starts from specific sites, called origins of replication (*ori*). The bacterial chromosome and many plasmids have only one such site. In the much larger eukaryotic genomes there can be hundreds of *oris* present. For circular DNA molecules, like bacterial chromosomes and plasmids, there are two possible methods of the replication (Figure 1.6). Semi-conservative replication proceeding in the closed circle (Figure 1.6b) is one way. The constraint brought forward by the rotation as a consequence of the unwinding (there is no free end) is resolved by the activity of a special class of enzymes, the topoisomerases. Alternatively, replication proceeds via a rolling circle model. In that case, the replication starts by cutting one of the DNA strands in the *ori* region and then proceeds as indicated in Figure 1.6c.

Bacterial plasmids are defined as autonomously replicating DNA molecules. The basis for this statement is the presence of an *ori* site in the plasmids. The autonomous qualification, however, does not imply that a plasmid is independent from host factors for replication and expression. Some plasmids depend on very specific host factors and consequently they can only replicate in specific hosts. Other plasmids are less specific and are able to replicate in a broad set of hosts. As will be demonstrated later, this difference in host range is meaningful when plasmids are exploited in biotechnology.

Transcription

Genetic information located in the genes is formed by discrete segments of the cellular DNA. In a process called

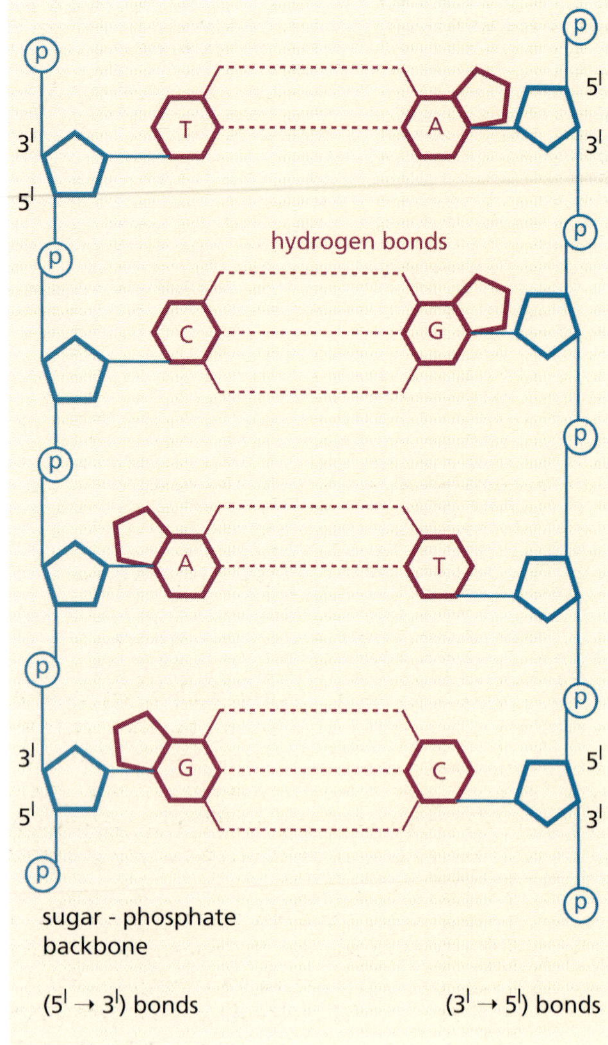

Figure 1.5. Schematic DNA structure showing polarity and complementarity.

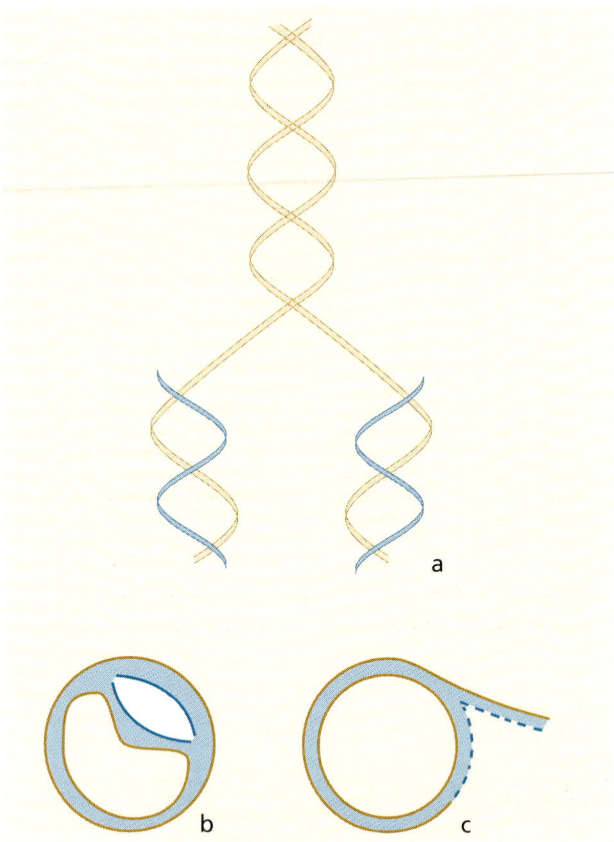

Figure 1.6. a. DNA replication (general picture); b. Closed circle replication; c. Rolling circle model.

transcription (presented schematically in Figure 1.7), genes are copied into a complementary length of ribonucleic acid (RNA) by the enzyme RNA polymerase. Most of the RNA molecules, the messenger RNAs (mRNAs), specify the amino acid composition of the cellular proteins. Other RNA molecules derived by transcription, ribosomal RNA (rRNA) and transfer RNA (tRNA), participate as auxiliary molecules for translation.

The discovery of how the specific arrangement of nucleotides in the gene codes the sequence of amino acids in the protein, tantamount to the unravelling of the genetic code, is one of the milestones of the DNA epoch. It was found that triplets of nucleotides in the DNA, and consequently in the mRNA, code for the amino acid composition of a protein. The most important discovery was finding that the genetic code was (almost) universal in nature. A given triplet of nucleotides, a so-called codon, in mRNA codes for the same amino acid in nearly all organisms.

However, the mRNA molecules contain more information than merely the triplets required for the encoded protein. The protein encoding information is preceded by a piece of RNA that allows binding to the ribosome, while another section of the RNA functions in the termination of the transcription process. Thus, signals are required within the mRNA molecule to ensure a proper start and finish for the protein synthesis. Near the 5'-end of the mRNA a specific triplet – coding for the amino acid methionine – dictates the proper start of the protein synthesis and near the 3'-end a specific triplet (a stop codon) dictates a proper finish. The genetic code, on the basis of the triplets in the mRNA, is presented in Table 1.1. One may see that there are three different stop codons. Moreover, it is clear from Table 1.1 that the code is highly redundant: for certain amino acids there are several codons. Whenever there is a choice between various codons for one amino acid, different organisms tend to show different preferences. Later it will become clear that this organism dependent codon preference has consequences for certain biotechnological processes.

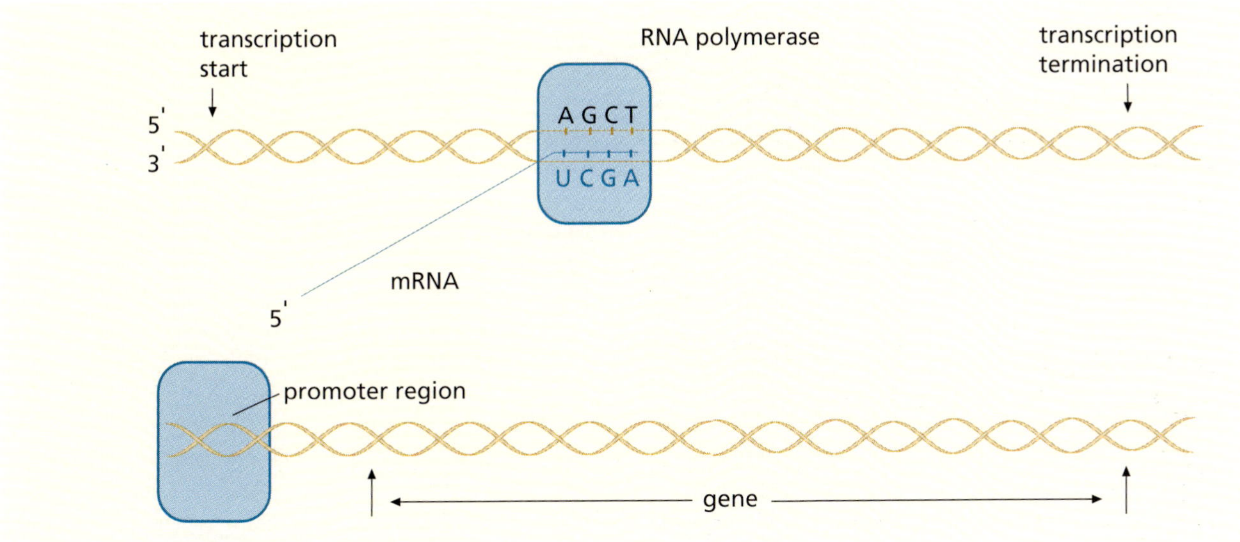

Figure 1.7. Transciption. Upper part shows ongoing transcription. The lower panel depicts the start, involving specific binding of RNA polymerase to the promoter region.

First position (5'-end)	Second position U	C	A	G	Third position (3'-end)
U	Phe	Ser	Tyr	Cys	U
	Phe	Ser	Tyr	Cys	C
	Leu	Ser	Stop	Stop	A
	Leu	Ser	Stop	Trp	G
C	Leu	Pro	His	Arg	U
	Leu	Pro	His	Arg	C
	Leu	Pro	Gln	Arg	A
	Leu	Pro	Gln	Arg	G
A	Ile	Thr	Asn	Ser	U
	Ile	Thr	Asn	Ser	C
	Ile	Thr	Lys	Arg	A
	Met	Thr	Lys	Arg	G
G	Val	Ala	Asp	Gly	U
	Val	Ala	Asp	Gly	C
	Val	Ala	Glu	Gly	A
	Val	Ala	Glu	Gly	G

Table 1.1. The 'universal' genetic code. Note: the bold codons are used for initiation.

Transcription starts with the binding of the enzyme RNA polymerase at a specific site, called promoter, immediately upstream from a gene or from a set of genes transcribed as an operational unit (an operon). Promoters vary in their efficiency to bind RNA polymerase. Some promoters, the strong promoters, are highly efficient, while others are weak and often require additional factors for the effective binding of RNA polymerase. Promoter structures, in prokaryotes as well as in eukaryotes, have been studied in great detail. Based on such studies it is now feasible in biotechnology to fuse very effective promoter structures to any gene that one wishes to be expressed.

After the binding of the RNA polymerase, the DNA helix is partially unwound and the transcription process starts. RNA synthesis then proceeds with the ribonucleotides ATP, GTP, CTP and UTP as building units. One DNA strand in the gene, the so-called template strand, serves as the matrix for this RNA synthesis. Like in the DNA synthesis, the RNA synthesis runs antiparallel in the direction 5' to 3' and proceeds in a complementary way. The latter implies that a G in the matrix DNA leads to C in the RNA, a C leads to a G, a T to an A, yet an A in the DNA shows up as a U in the RNA. The transcription may stop either on the basis of intrinsic structural features of the RNA at the end of the gene or the operon, or by the intervention of a site-specific terminating protein factor.

Transcription can be regulated at various stages in the process. The intrinsic properties of the promoter, in addition to various kinds of proteins that can either repress or stimulate the binding of RNA polymerase, regulate the transcription start. Transcription termination can also be regulated. Termination may, under the influence of physiological factors, occur at a premature stage. Alternatively, the normal termination signal could be ignored (a process called read-through). This may lead to various lengths of transcripts starting from the same promoter. Finally, gene activity can also be regulated at the level of the formed mRNA.

All transcripts are subject to degradation, but rates of degradation can vary widely: some transcripts have a short half-life time while others are very stable. Biotechnologists try to influence the expression of a gene encoding a relevant biotechnological protein at each of these regulation levels in order to achieve optimal production.

Translation

Translation, presented schematically in Figure 1.8, is a complex cellular process where mRNA molecules, ribosomes, tRNA molecules, amino acids, aminoacyl synthetases and a number of translation factors act together in a highly coordinated way. The ribosome, an organelle built from rRNA molecules and proteins, is the cellular structure where the various compounds for the protein synthesis assemble.

The building blocks of the proteins, the amino acids, are used in the protein synthesis in a manner convenient for interaction with the mRNA. The adaptation of the amino acid is achieved by coupling it to a specific tRNA molecule through the catalytic action of specific aminoacyl synthetases. The adapted amino acid links to the 3'-OH terminus of a specific tRNA molecule. Each tRNA molecule contains a specific triplet in a characteristic loop of the molecule. This triplet is complementary and runs antiparallel to the codon for the linked amino acid and is consequently designated the anticodon. Coupling through base pairing of the anticodon in the tRNA to the codon in the mRNA is the process by which the code in the mRNA positions amino acids.

Translation starts with the formation of a specific initiation complex. In a bacterial cell the initiation complex consists of a 30S ribosomal subunit, a tRNA carrying the amino acid methionine, GTP and various initiation factors all positioned at the start codon AUG of the mRNA. The 5'-end region of the bacterial messenger is important to the formation of this initiation complex. This region, which itself is not translated, harbors a specific ribosome binding site. A 50S ribosomal subunit binds to the initiation complex, creating a functional 70S ribosome. Translation then proceeds, with the help of specific elongation factors, in such a way that the 70S ribosomes are transported along the mRNA molecule stepwise over a distance of one triplet. This stepwise transport guarantees that protein synthesis proceeds in a coordinated way dictated by the (triplet) codons. The amino acids, delivered by the specific tRNA molecules, are linked together, one after the other, by peptide bond formation. Meanwhile the tRNA carriers are set free again.

At the end of an mRNA molecule there are one or more stop codons. These triplets do not accept any tRNA-aminoacyl molecules and are therefore terminating signals for protein synthesis. After termination the protein is released from the 70S ribosome. The ribosomes then fall apart in their 30S and 50S subunits which may be used in a further translation cycle.

Although there is a common general picture for translation in prokaryotes and eukaryotes, there are nevertheless variously distinct differences, especially in the nature of initiation and elongation factors. A very clear distinction is a direct consequence of the difference in DNA organization between pro- and eukaryotes. In the prokaryotic cell, mRNA is already available for the ribosomes while it is still in the process of transcription. In the eukaryotic cell, on the other hand, the mRNA is only available for translation after it is completely synthesized and after it is transported through the nuclear membrane. Consequently, transcription and translation are coupled processes in the prokaryotic cell, while these processes occur separately in the eukaryotic cell.

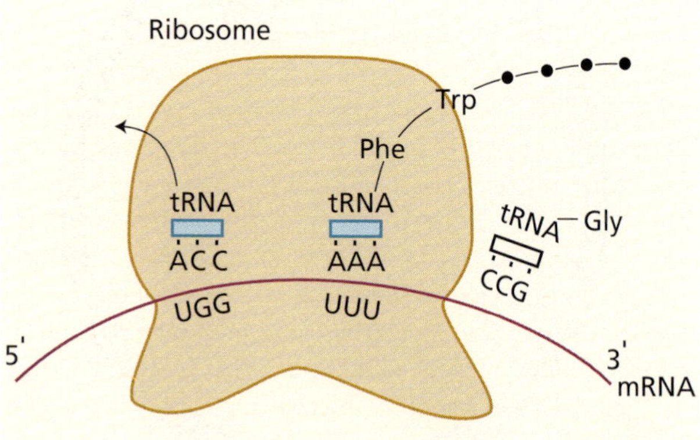

Figure 1.8. Schematic picture of ongoing translation. The amino acid Phe is linked to the growing peptide chain. The tRNA that delivered the previous amino acid Trp is leaving the ribosome complex. The next amino acid to be linked will be Gly, according to the mRNA code.

Recombinant DNA Technology

After it was established that DNA was the chemical constituent for the hereditary properties of the cell and after the discovery that some (bacterial) cells could spontaneously take up DNA, investigators immediately tried to manipulate the genetic properties of all kind of cells. To achieve this, they simply added foreign DNA to microbial cells, plant cells or animal cells. All these attempts failed. There are two reasons for this lack of success. First of all, only a limited number of bacterial species is able to take up DNA spontaneously; most bacteria and certainly animal and plant species are unable to do this. Secondly, foreign DNA, if at all taken up, is generally not maintained in the receptor cell. DNA brought into a cell from outside will only be maintained if it is able to replicate autonomously, or if it is integrated in the recipient genome. In all other cases foreign DNA will not be propagated in the cell culture and will eventually disappear by degradation through the activity of cellular nucleases.

Genetic modification of organisms became feasible later on when recombinant DNA technologies were developed. This development enabled the fusion of any DNA fragment to DNA molecules able to maintain themselves by autonomous replication (such molecules are called replicons). The various techniques developed to introduce recombinant DNA molecules into all sorts of biological cells led to successful genetic modification strategies.

Replicons used as carriers for foreign DNA fragments are termed vectors. The vectors exploited in the DNA technology include mainly plasmids from bacteria or yeast, or DNA from bacterioviruses, animal viruses or plant viruses. Especially small microbial plasmids are very popular as vectors in biotechnology since they can be easily isolated as intact circular double-stranded molecules. Plasmids with a broad host range, mentioned previously, are very attractive since they can be used in various hosts and consequently enable a flexible application of the DNA technology.

For the application of plasmids in biotechnology, one has to fuse foreign DNA to the isolated plasmid in order to create a recombinant DNA molecule. The technology for this, the so-called recombinant DNA technology or DNA cloning technology, became feasible after the discovery of a specific class of nucleases, the so-called restriction endonucleases. Next to nucleases able to cleave any phosphodiester bond in DNA, nucleases which only cleave DNA at very specific sites are present in nature. These enzymes, the restriction enzymes, were discovered in around 1970 in microorganisms. Their function is to discriminate between foreign DNA and self DNA. Microbial cells may in real life be confronted with DNA from an unrelated cell via various genetic transfer systems. Although all DNA is built likewise, DNA can be marked specifically at particular sites by a characteristic pattern of methylated or glucosylated nucleotides. This DNA marking, which does not interfere with the coding and replicating functions, is host specific. Restriction enzymes have the remarkable property of being able to recognize DNA on the basis of the specific host marking. When DNA is transferred and the marking does not fit with the recipient cell, such DNA will be recognized and cut at specific sites by the restriction enzyme. Once the DNA is cut it will be further degraded in the cell. As is the case in many biological systems, things are never absolute: some DNA molecules may escape from the action of the restriction enzymes and by getting a proper marking they can be rescued.

The very selective action of the restriction enzymes is the basis for their application in the recombinant DNA technology. The addition of a restriction enzyme to a plasmid without the proper marking will convert the closed circular molecule to linear fragments, provided that the plasmid harbors recognition sites for the chosen restriction enzyme. In Figure 1.9 the action of a restriction enzyme is

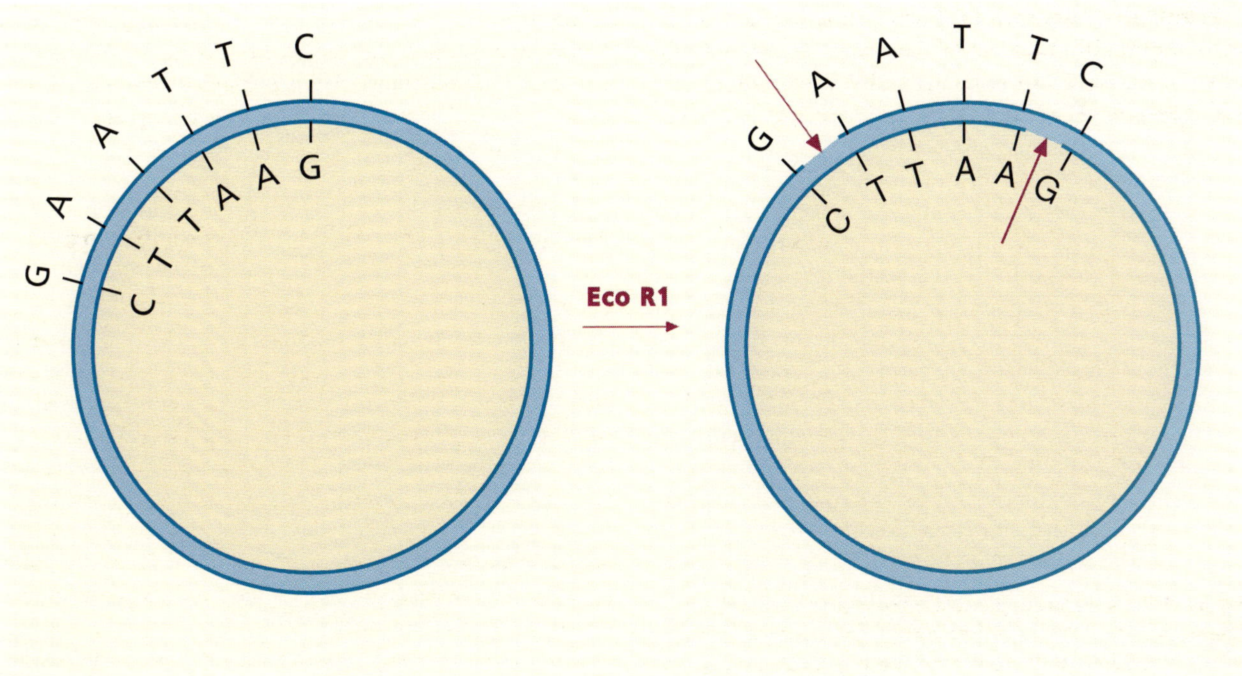

Figure 1.9. Treatment of a plasmid with an unique Eco R1 site. This restriction enzyme will open the plasmid and makes it amenable for manipulation.

depicted for a special, but representative case. A plasmid with only one recognition site for the restriction enzyme *Eco*R I is treated with this enzyme. The double-stranded DNA is then asymmetrically cut at the recognition site, encompassing six bases, namely GAATTC, which leads to linear DNA with typical short single-stranded ends. If foreign DNA – isolated either from microbial, plant or animal cells – with recognition sites for the enzyme *Eco*R I is likewise cut with this enzyme, fragments with single-stranded ends characteristic for *Eco*R I are formed. When the open vector and the foreign DNA fragments are brought together under appropriate physico-chemical conditions, the various single-stranded ends may recombine due to the presence of complementary bases. A possible reaction product could be a plasmid to which a specific foreign DNA fragment, as a passenger, is linked. Although the DNA pieces in such a construct are interlinked by base pairing, they do not form a closed circular molecule. The enzyme DNA ligase, present in all sorts of cells and able to catalyse the formation of phosphodiester bonds, is used to create a closed circular recombinant DNA molecule. Although DNA fragments with complementary single-stranded ends (so-called cohesive ends) are the most favorable ones for linking, DNA ligase is also able to link fragments with blunt ends.

According to the technology presented schematically in Figure 1.10, recombinant DNA molecules consisting of vector and passenger DNA can be created. A great number of restriction enzymes with very specific recognition sites are available to cut DNA at a specific site. Some enzymes, like *Eco*R I, recognize a sequence of six base pairs, while other enzymes recognize just four bases. Some, again like *Eco*R I, cut the DNA asymmetrically while others create blunt ends when cutting DNA. In Table 1.2 some representative restriction enzymes are listed.

Recombinant DNA molecules are of no interest biologically as long as they reside in the reaction tube. The transfer of the construct to a living cell, however, may change the situation drastically. If the vector that served for the construct is able to replicate in the host, all daughter cells will inherit a precise copy (a clone) of the recombinant DNA molecule. Therefore the term "cloning" is frequently used for the technology described above.

The cloning technique is very suitable to obtain large amounts of a specific DNA fragment by fusing such a fragment to an appropriate vector and transferring the construct to a host that can easily be cultivated to high cell densities. The recombinant DNA molecules, which can then be isolated from the cell mass, form an abundant source for the specific DNA fragment. Moreover and most importantly for pharmaceutical biotechnology, if the cloned piece of foreign DNA harbors an intact gene with the appropriate signals for gene expression, the modified host cells may, based on the universal character of gene expression,

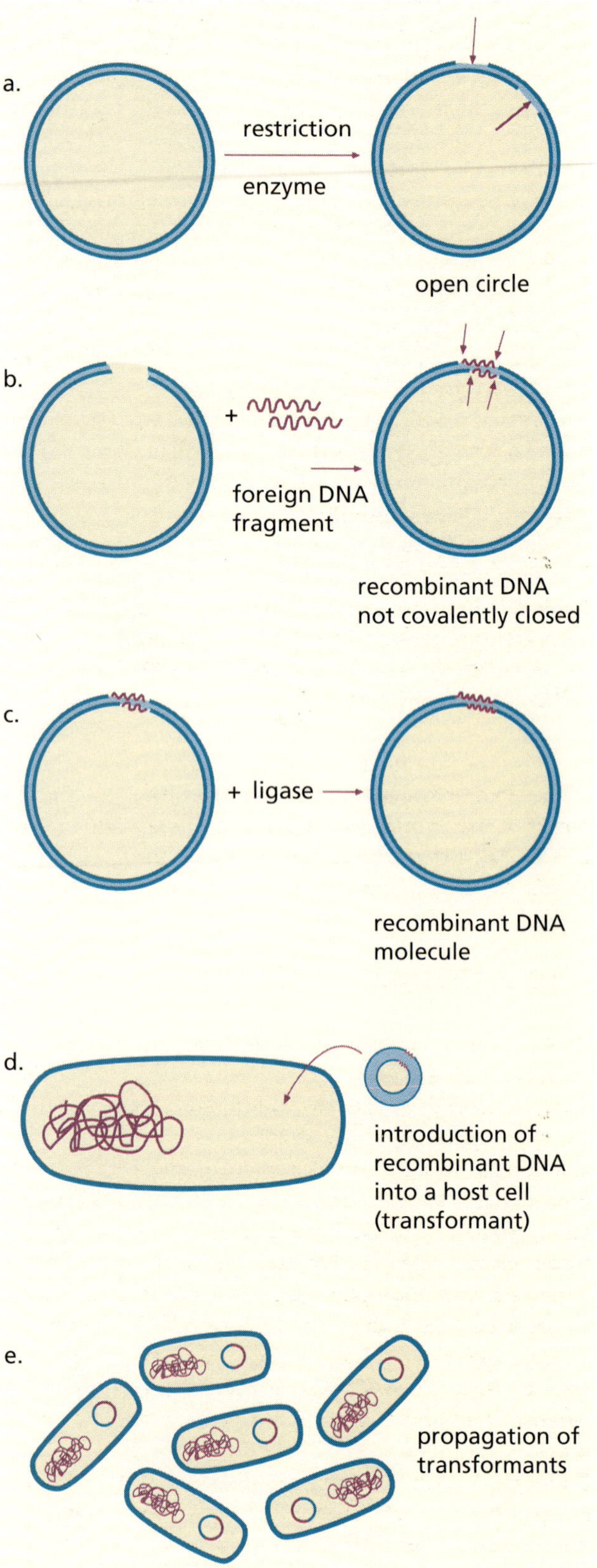

Figure 1.10. Principle of cloning a foreign DNA fragment.

Enzyme	Source	Cutting sequence
EcoR I	*Escherichia coli*	↓ G AATT C C TTAA↑G
Pst I	*Providencia stuartii*	↓ C TGCA G G↑ACGT C
Taq I	*Thermus aquaticus*	↓ T CG A A GC↑T
Hinf I	*Haemophilus influenzae*	↓ * G ANT C C TNA↑G
Msp I	*Moraxella species*	↓ C CG G G GC↑C
Hae III	*Haemophilus aegyptus*	↓ GG CC CC↑GG

Table 1.2. Some restriction enzymes, their origin and their recognition site. Note: open space in the recognition site indicates the endonucleolytic cut by the enzyme.
* N means: no base preference.

produce proteins encoded by the foreign DNA. This is the power of the recombinant DNA technology in a nutshell: it is an efficient way to amplify DNA fragments and a way to gain all sorts of gene products from hosts that one can choose.

DNA Transfer

As stated above, the transfer of a recombinant DNA molecule to a cell is an essential step in the DNA technology. Some bacterial cells, like those of the species *Bacillus subtilis* which are frequently used in industrial biotechnology, are able to take up DNA under physiological conditions. This process is described as natural transformation. In most cases, however, microbial cells have to be forced to take up DNA by an unusual regimen. For example, in the case of microorganisms such non-physiological conditions are created by applying a heat shock to the host cells in the presence of high amounts of Ca^{2+} ions. An alternative technique used to force DNA uptake is electroporation. For that purpose DNA and cells are brought together in a cuvette which is then subjected to a vigorous electrical discharge. Under these artificial conditions the cell envelope is forced to open itself, after which DNA may enter through the 'holes' that are created. The brute force in these techniques kills a large fraction of the cells, but a sufficient number of cells survive, among which are several that take up DNA. The technique of electroporation is widely applicable and frequently used.

Next to the direct transfer of recombinant DNA molecules, there is, at least for transfer to bacterial cells, the possibility of packaging DNA in a bacteriophage capsid and then mimicking the normal bacteriophage infection procedure (Figure 1.11). Transfer to bacterial cells can also be achieved by making use of conjugation. Conjugation is a process where DNA transfer takes place by cell-cell mating. For conjugation a special class of plasmids is required, so-called conjugative plasmids. If a cell with such a plasmid – the donor – meets a cell without such a plasmid – the recipient – they may together form cell aggregates. In the so-called mating aggregate, the plasmid from the donor has the ability to transfer itself to the recipient cell as a consequence of a conjugative replication process according to the rolling circle model. By manipulating the conjugative plasmids one may create donors harboring recombinant DNA molecules which can then be transferred rather efficiently by cell-cell contact.

If an animal virus or a plant virus is used as a vector for the recombinant DNA technology, one may exploit natural virus infection processes to transfer DNA to an animal or a plant cell (cf. Chapter 7). Like the case in microorganisms, DNA transfer to animal cells can be forced by

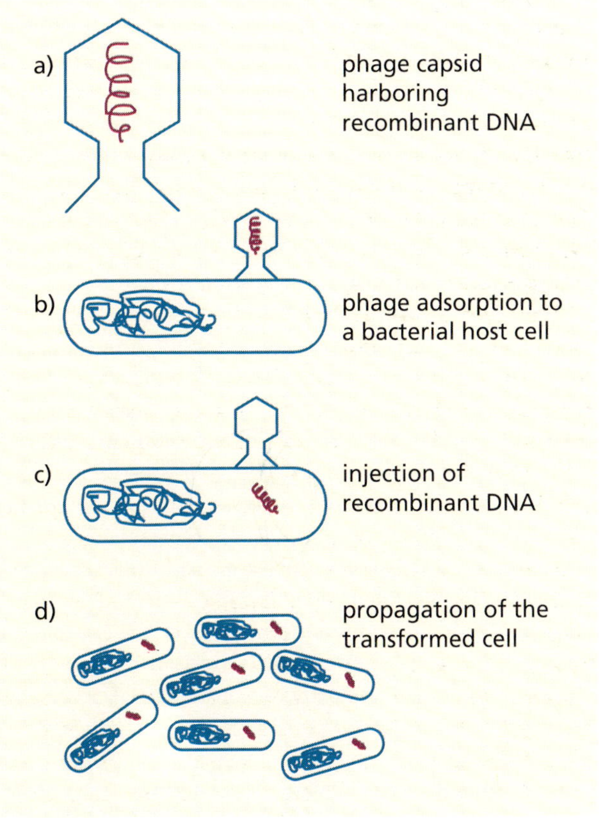

Figure 1.11. Phage as a mediator for transfer of recombinant DNA.

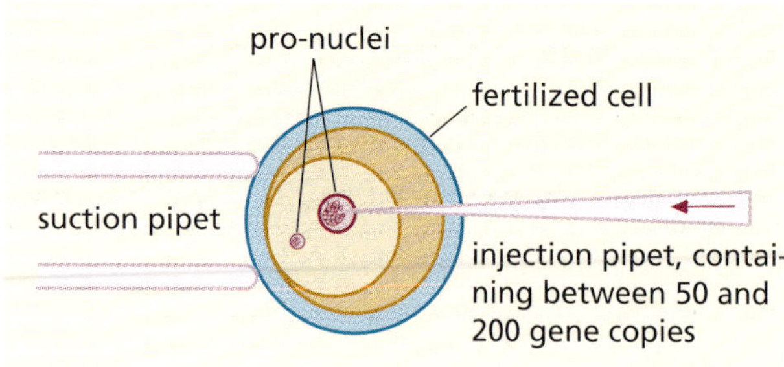

Figure 1.12. Injection of foreign DNA into a fertilized cell.

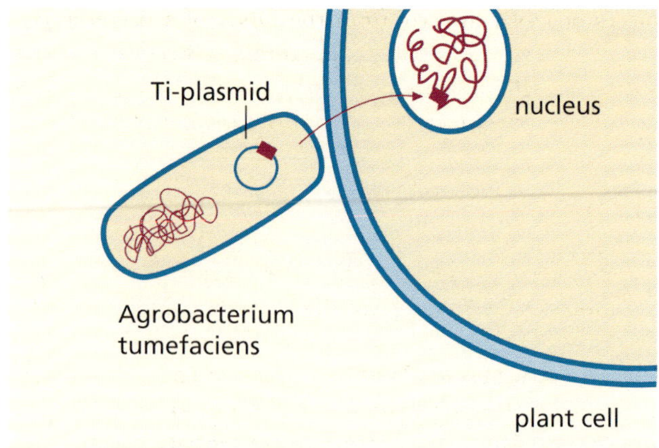

Figure 1.13. Plant cell modification by Ti-plasmid. Part of the Ti-plasmid (marked) is transferred to the plant cell and may be stably integrated in the plant DNA.

a treatment with high amounts of Ca^{2+}-ions or by another chemical treatment. In addition, it is possible to inject DNA with a syringe into the nucleus of the cell. The latter technique (one could speak of a kind of microsurgery) is feasible due to the relatively large dimensions of the animal cells compared to bacteria. This technique is also applied to plant cells and is illustrated in Figure 1.12. The cell is brought on the tip of a thin glass tube and is fixed to the tube by suction at the other end of the tube. By means of a micromanipulator a small syringe filled with DNA is directed to the nucleus of the fixed cell and then the DNA is injected into the nucleus.

A very successful way to transfer DNA into plant systems is based on a very special type of conjugation. The soil bacterium, *Agrobacterium tumefaciens*, harbors a conjugative plasmid called Ti (acronym for tumor inducing). If such a bacterium infects wounded tissues of certain plants, part of the Ti-plasmid is transferred to a plant cell in a conjugation-like process. This transfer is followed by integration of the transferred DNA into the genome of the plant. The infected plant cells lose normal growth control and develop a tumor (a plant disease called crown gall). By manipulating the Ti-plasmid, such that its tumor inducing properties are lost and foreign DNA fragments are linked to it, any DNA can be transferred in a convenient way from the modified *Agrobacterium* donor to a plant cell. Figure 1.13 illustrates this remarkable process, where, in fact, biological kingdom barriers are crossed in a natural fashion.

Since the wall of the plant cell is the main barrier for the uptake of DNA, scientists have exploited protoplasts of plant cells (i.e. plant cells lacking walls) to introduce DNA. Protoplasts can take up DNA quite easily. It is feasible to regenerate intact plant cells from genetically modified protoplasts. Finally, a very artificial method to introduce DNA in plant tissue has been recently developed. Microprojectiles covered with DNA are shot with a gun into plant cells. In fact, many plant species that can not readily be genetically modified with any of the methods mentioned above can be modified using this rather bizarre gun method.

The various techniques used to transfer DNA are generally not very efficient and may cause, as stated before, extensive killing of cells. Moreover, the fate of the transferred DNA is not always predictable. For example, in some cases the introduced DNA is subject to nuclease mediated breakdown, while in animal or plant cells the introduced DNA does not always reach the nucleus, nor is it always integrated in a proper way. All methods to transfer DNA yield, in general, only a few cells that are vital and more or less stably modified. Therefore, effective selection techniques for finding these rare cells are highly desirable. Most selection techniques use a marker on the vector that codes for a selective property. Markers which code for a resistance towards a specific antibiotic substance are frequently used. If the cell that has to be modified is sensitive towards that antibiotic, the few modified cells from the transfer trial can easily be selected by bringing samples of the treated cells (either microbial cells, plant cells or animal cells) in a medium containing the relevant antibiotic. Only the cells that take up DNA and maintain that DNA in their progeny will proliferate; all other cells are killed or, at least, do not grow. An alternative selection method uses recipient cells with specific growth deficiencies and vectors carrying genes which overcome such deficiencies.

DNA Sources

As stated previously, any DNA can be used to construct recombinant DNA molecules. Protein production based on recombinant DNA technology requires very distinct pieces of DNA. Referring to the metaphor described before in this chapter, only a few lines on a specific page in one of the many books are required. Isolation of specific pieces of DNA directly from the DNA of a bacterial cell and, certainly, of a plant or an animal cell requires a very tedious search. How can one find a specific DNA fragment in a more convenient way? There are several strategies.

Synthetic DNA

It is feasible to use synthetic DNA as a source for the desired recombinant DNA sequence. If one seeks DNA that codes for a specific protein, the amino acid sequence of that protein is sometimes known. With the genetic code as a guide, one may synthesize the coding DNA by organic synthesis and use that DNA to construct an appropriate recombinant DNA molecule. Although the technique to unravel the amino acid composition of proteins and the possibilities of the organic DNA synthesis have improved over the past years, the organic DNA synthesis approach is only feasible to clone genes coding small proteins. For example, the synthetic approach has been used successfully for the large-scale production of human insulin.

The synthetic DNA approach allows the triplet used most frequently in the host selected for the production to be chosen whenever there are more triplets available for a certain amino acid. In other words, this technique allows one to master the codon usage problem, mentioned earlier in this chapter.

cDNA

An alternative for the direct isolation of cellular DNA coding for a specific protein is the copy DNA (cDNA) approach. This important development in DNA technology became apparent when the enzyme reverse transcriptase was exploited as a tool.

Genes are not always expressed in the cell, nor are they expressed everywhere in the organism. Some genes are only expressed at a certain stage of cell growth, or under very specific environmental conditions, or expressed only in very specific tissues of an organism. The mRNA molecules in a cell thus represent a minority of all the available genes, namely those that are actually expressed. Knowledge of the cell physiology or knowledge of the specific biological tasks of animal and plant tissues enables the isolation of a particular and characteristic set of mRNA molecules. Conversion of these mRNA molecules by the enzyme reverse transcriptase into DNA leads to the synthesis of the genes that were expressed. These DNA molecules, called c(opy) DNA molecules, to distinguish them from the natural DNA molecules, can then be used for gene cloning. Provided that the search starts with the right kind of cell culture conditions or with the appropriate tissues, the cDNA strategy can be very efficient. It is illustrated in Figure 1.14.

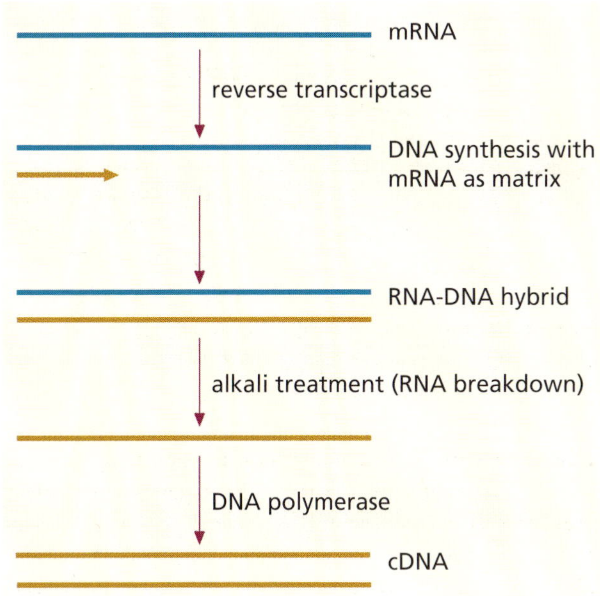

Figure 1.14. Synthesis of cDNA.

cDNA cloning has some obvious consequences. In contrast to a gene that is directly isolated from the chromosome, cDNA lacks a promoter region. Furthermore, in the case of genes harboring exons and introns, cDNA is built only from exons. The lack of the authentic promoter requires that, in the cloning strategy, a promoter should be fused to the cDNA in order to achieve gene expression. Usually a strong promoter that can be switched on and off, depending on environmental or tissue condition, is fused to cDNA.

Control over foreign gene expression by using a suitable promoter is essential. Foreign proteins, as a result of uncontrolled gene expression, may disturb the physiology of the host cell and cause a premature termination of cell development. Therefore, a promoter like the *lac* promoter is frequently used in bacterial cells to direct the synthesis of a foreign protein. This promoter is only switched on when an appropriate inducer like iso-propyl-β-thiogalactoside (IPTG) is added to the medium. Cultivation of the cells in absence of the inducer allows optimal cell growth since the possible deleterious foreign gene product is not produced in all cells. When high cell numbers are present in the culture, the inducer is added and the foreign gene product is produced. Possible negative effects of the foreign protein on the cell are minimal since high cell numbers, often near to the maximum yield, are present when the harmful production starts.

In an animal or a plant a foreign gene should preferably be expressed only in certain tissues to keep the animal or the plant vital or for efficient isolation of the protein. In those biotechnological applications where mammals like sheep, goats or cows are used as hosts for pharmaceutical products (an approach called "pharmaceutical farming"), the mammary gland is frequently used as an expression tissue. The cDNA for an objective protein is therefore fused to a promoter that is only expressed in that tissue. Transferring such a DNA construct into embryos of the host animal may lead to genetically modified animals that exclusively deliver the pharmaceutical product as part of their milk. This production route enables an efficient isolation and allows relatively simple purification strategies (cf. Chapter 6).

The lack of introns in the cDNA has the advantage that cDNA may lead to a functional gene product even in organisms where splicing does not occur (like in prokaryotic cells) or where splicing is ambiguous or unreliable.

DNA Libraries

The mRNA approach is not feasible if precise knowledge of gene expression is lacking and does not allow cloning of DNA that is not expressed. A general approach in mastering very complex DNA molecules for recombinant DNA technology is to create a DNA library. To do so, random DNA fragments from a bacterial, plant or animal cell are fused to a vector and then transferred to an appropriate host. By isolating from a bacterial cell, for example, DNA fragments that on average amount to 1% of the total DNA and linking these fragments individually to a vector, one may create together a few hundred different recombinant DNA molecules which represent the total bacterial chromosome. Using the 'DNA book' metaphor again, the original bacterial 'DNA book' with about 1000 pages maybe divided into about 150 small booklets of 10 pages each. These booklets tell, with some overlap and without an *a priori* ordering, the same story as told in the complete book. The immediate advantage of this approach is that large molecules are split into suitably smaller pieces linked to a replicon.

An individual host with a specific recombinant DNA molecule thus harbors a fragment of the total DNA on a replicating vector. By preselecting from the library the cells carrying gene(s) or DNA of interest, one may obtain a smaller molecule harboring little more than the DNA of interest by trimming the fragment isolated from these cells. By subsequent cloning of such smaller fragments one may achieve the final goal: a recombinant DNA molecule with a very distinct piece of foreign DNA. DNA libraries are available from many organisms, and cDNA libraries exist from many tissues, such as the human brain. By analysis of the various fragments, insight into the genetic structure of all sorts of organisms is rapidly growing. In this respect, the present unravelling of the human genome, a project involving scientists all over the world, is worth mentioning.

Production by Recombinant DNA Technology

Only two of the many examples available of the production of biopharmaceuticals by recombinant DNA technology will be treated here: the production of human insulin and the production of the human growth hormone (hGH). The pharmaceutical aspects of both proteins are discussed in more detail in Chapters 10 and 11, respectively.

The large scale production of human insulin is a good illustration of the synthetic DNA approach. Moreover, this example shows clearly that, besides knowledge of the coding gene, detailed knowledge of the protein to be produced is required.

The structural gene for human insulin is 1430 nucleotides long, while the gene is intervened by intron sequences of 179 and 786 nucleotides. The protein encoded by the gene is 110 amino acids in length. However, the mature protein encompasses a total of 51 amino acids. It consists of two separate chains: an A chain of 21 amino acids and a B chain of 30 amino acids. Chains A and B are held together by S bonds between the amino acid cysteine on the adjacent chains. The human insulin protein is processed extensively after translation. Processing occurs in two steps. The primary product, called preproinsulin, is 110 amino acids long in accordance with the prediction from the DNA sequence. During the membrane translocation of the protein the "pre" part of the protein, a stretch of 24 amino acids serving as the leader sequence for membrane translocation, is cleaved off. The remaining protein, 86 amino acids long, is called proinsulin. This protein is further processed in pancreatic cells, while an internal fragment (called the C or connecting chain) of 33 amino acids, together with a few assorted amino acids, is enzymatically removed. The A and B chains left are associated through S-bonds and form the mature and biologically active insulin.

The strategy for gene cloning according to the detailed knowledge of the mature protein was to clone and produce the chains A and B separately. The information for the fragment A was synthesized by linking a set of appropriate oligonucleotides. This DNA was then fused by ligation to the end of the gene *lacZ*, controlled by the *lac*-promoter, in the plasmid pBR322, a very well known *E. coli* cloning vector. At the fusion point between *lacZ* and the information for chain A a codon for the amino acid methionine was built in, for reasons that will be explained later on. The information for fragment B was (for strategic reasons) synthesized in two steps. Firstly, the N-terminal coding part was synthesized by linking oligonucleotides. This fragment was fused to the plasmid pBR322 and propagated in *E. coli*. Secondly, the C-terminal coding part was synthesized and also propagated after ligating it to pBR322. The two DNA fragments were then isolated from the respective

NA transfer.
natural transfer
electroporation — heat shock / ↑ amts of Ca++.
· of host - bacterial cell
then foreign DNA → bacteriophage → transferred by conjugative replication process - rolling circle model
- of vector - virus - infected by viral infection
· microinjection injection
- host - plant cell
Agrobacterium tumefaciens harbors the Ti plasmid
Role of Ti plasmid
alter the properties of Ti plasmid
marker on ...

...vere linked to- ... in the plasmid ...cid methionine

...d B to the *lacZ* ...peron, has two ...epend for their ...romoter and the ...ve and control- ...d B are synthe- ...nce particularly ...re very vulner- ...strategy is an ...eatment of the ...nogen bromide ...d B. This agent ...ever the amino ...mediately after ...nor B of insulin ...tegy guarantees ...point, the isola- ...mple. The final ...ing the S bonds ...ts the procedure ...nthetic DNA.

...ng hGH shows ..., the production was initiated by making ... a mRNA pool derived from the human pituitary, the tissue where hGH is synthesized. The cDNA molecule coding for the hGH was isolated and, since it contained the information of 24 amino acids that would guarantee transport in the human cell, it was reduced with an appropriate restriction enzyme. However, in this procedure the coding information for some of the amino acids essential for the activity of the mature hormone was lost. This missing part of information lost from the original cDNA molecule was chemically synthesized and fused to the fragmented cDNA molecule in order to get the full information for the mature hGH. Next, the construct was linked to a bacterial vector in such a way that it was fused to a strong promoter. In some constructs, information coding for a bacterial leader sequence was linked to the hGH gene. Then, sequences coding for a bacterial leader peptide (a N-terminal sequence of about 20 amino acids) were added to induce translocation of the protein over the cytoplasmic membrane.

This additional translocation sequence has rather specific physico-chemical properties. The leader peptide signal enables a protein to cross the cytoplasmic membrane barrier, during which the leader peptide is cleaved off. The reason for attaching an additional signal in this case is that in certain production strategies one wishes to obtain products released from the cytoplasm to be able to select a convenient purification strategy afterwards. If the hGH gene is linked to an appropriate leader peptide and expressed in the host *E. coli*, hGH molecules will show up in the space between the IM and the OM, the so-called periplasmic space. It is possible to damage the OM in such a way that the contents of the periplasm are set free. Then, purification of hGH is easier and cheaper than purification of hGH as a product in the cytoplasm of *E. coli*. Cloning strategies that guarantee membrane translocation are frequently selected in order to release a protein from the cytoplasm.

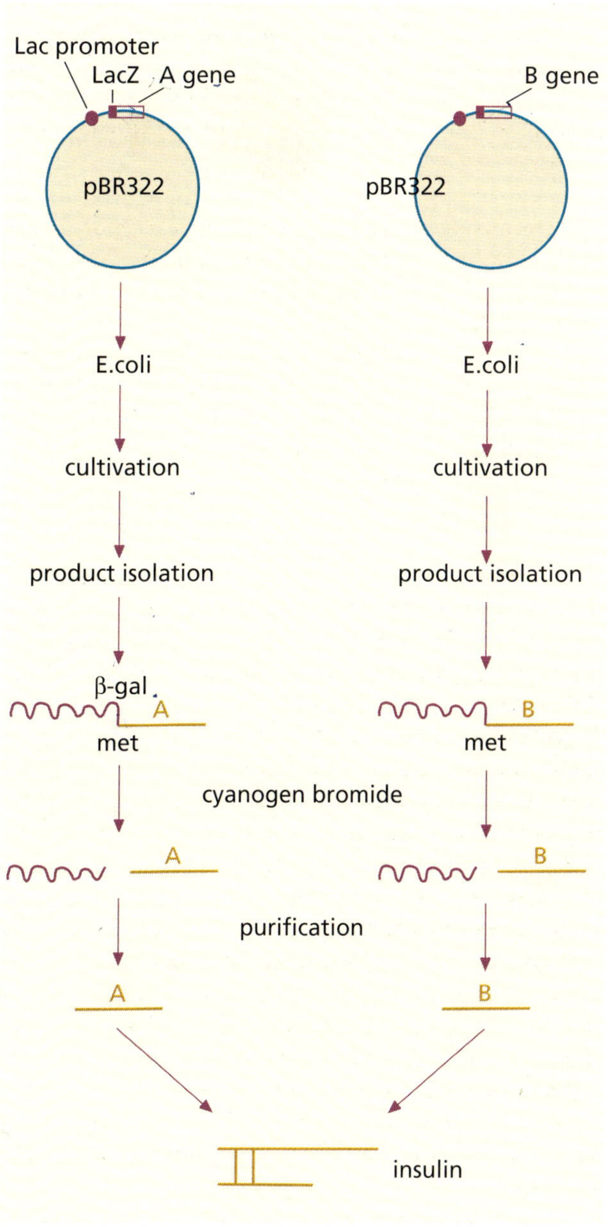

Figure 1.15. Synthesis of insulin by synthetic DNA.

Specific DNA Techniques

DNA Sequencing

The development of technologies for the detailed nucleotide sequence determination of DNA molecules has been of immense importance. This knowledge opens the way for very precise DNA modifications, like changing individual nucleotides in order to change an individual amino acid in a protein, for example (cf. Chapter 6).

In 1977 two different methods were published for DNA sequencing. The Maxam and Gilbert method is based on chemical degradation of DNA, whereas the Sanger method, also called the chain termination method, uses DNA replication enzymology. The Sanger method is the most popular method and is described here. It uses a DNA polymerase enzyme normally involved in DNA replication. DNA polymerases are template dependent, meaning that they need a single-stranded DNA molecule which they will copy according to the A-T and G-C base pairing rules, and are primer dependent, meaning that they need a free 3'-hydroxyl group of an oligonucleotide as a starting point for the incorporation of deoxyribonucleotide triphosphates (dATP, dCTP, dTTP and dGTP). The primer is a short, chemically synthesized molecule, about 20 nucleotides in length which is complementary and antiparallel to a segment in the single-stranded DNA molecule to be sequenced. Under the right conditions it will hybridize and thus provide a specific starting point for the elongation reaction by the polymerase.

The method depends, in essence, on the inclusion of a so-called dideoxyribonucleotide triphosphate (ddNTP) in the reaction mixture. These molecules not only lack the 2' hydroxyl group on the ribose, as is normal in DNA, but also the 3' hydroxyl group; hence the name *di*-deoxy. These ddNTP's can be incorporated into DNA strands by DNA polymerase. However, since the 3'-hydroxyl group required for DNA elongation is lacking, the DNA molecules which have incorporated such a ddNTP are no longer substrate for further chain elongation: the chain terminates with a ddNTP and this principle is used for the sequencing reaction. Four tubes per reaction are set up each containing template, primer and the four dNTPs. To the four tubes ddNTP is added. To the first tube ddATP is added, to the second tube ddCTP, to the third tube ddTTP and to the fourth tube ddGTP. The ratio of dNTP versus ddNTP in each tube is chosen in such a way that a small number of templates in each tube will incorporate the specific ddNTP and will no longer be substrates for elongation (chain termination). Therefore, in each tube a fraction of the strands will terminate with the specific ddNTP present in that particular tube.

The length of the terminated strands is determined by the oligonucleotide primer, which sets a fixed starting point, and the ddNTP is incorporated. In the first reaction tube, for example, fragment lengths are determined by the position of the various A nucleotides in the template. After the synthesis reaction, the contents of the four individual sequencing tubes are applied to a high resolution polyacrylamide gel electrophoresis system which separates individual elongation products based on their length. Tube 1 reveals the positions of A, tube 2 of C, tube 3 of T and tube 4 of G. The reaction products can be visualized either by autoradiography in case a small aliquot of radioactively labeled dNTP has been incorporated in all reactions (usually α^{32}P-dCTP), or by fluorography in case a fluorescent group has been chemically added to the sequencing primer during its synthesis. The latter method is particularly well suited for automation. Currently sequencing machines are commercially available which, in one run, can sequence over 800 nucleotides. In such machines 20–40 runs can be loaded and analyzed simultaneously which tremendously enhances productivity. Needless to say, sequences are handled, analyzed and stored electronically. Three interlinked computer sequence databases are operational in the world which are freely accessible via Internet.

Genome Sequencing

In recent years whole genomes of various organisms have been sequenced, and the sequencing of other organisms is going on all over the world. Such projects started with sequencing the genome of microorganisms, as well as various prokaryotes and eukaryotes. These projects were then extended to higher organisms like the nematode *Caenorhabditis elegans*, the insect *Drosophila melanogaster*, the plant *Arabidopsis thaliana* and finally, considered as the most prominent, the genome of the *Human sapiens*.

The detailed knowledge of genome structures ("genomics") will have a great impact on biotechnology, especially on pharmaceutical biotechnology. Knowing the genome sequence is only a start, but it will enable researchers to approach functional aspects of the genome in a direct manner: when and how are genes expressed, in what way do genes cooperate during their expression, enabling us to understand gene networks, etc.? Such integrative genetic approaches are generally called "functional genomics." Functional genomics, together with the detailed studies on the proteins that the cell produces (called "proteomics"), will give pharmaceutical biotechnology a new outlook.

As an example, the new future for pharmaceutical biotechnology can be illustrated by the development of new antibiotics. Classical antibiotics are isolated from nature as secondary metabolites produced by various microorganisms. Their antibiotic properties are based on the interference with vital processes in pathogenic microorganisms. The number of target molecules in the bacterial cells which are affected by the classical antibiotics are rather limited.

(N.B. the different meaning of 'target' in this context, as compared to 'drug targeting' discussed in Chapter 4.) For example, *Mycobacterium tuberculosis* causes tuberculosis, a disease with a great impact on the world's human population. Detailed knowledge of the genome structure of pathogenic bacteria might reveal a variety of specific vital target molecules in this pathogen. Detailed knowledge of new target molecules will enable the pharmaceutical scientist to synthesize chemical compounds that interfere with (the products of) vital target genes. The problem of the prevalence of pathogenic microorganisms resistant to classical antibiotics is now, in principle, open for a solution by synthesizing new target-directed chemical compounds.

Moreover, the human genome knowledge will be the basis for recognition of the polymorphisms that distinguish individual people. In the near future, insight into the individual genes of a patient opens the way for more effective therapies based on a patient's individual characteristics and needs. This emerging field in the pharmaceutical sciences is called "pharmacogenetics".

The pharmaceutical industry is highly interested in the possibilities arising from more detailed genome knowledge and is investing in functional genomics, proteomics and pharmacogenetics. In Chapter 6 the technological background and implications of functional genomics, proteomics and pharmacogenitics is discussed in more detail.

DNA Hybridization

Sequencing is the final approach for gaining insight into the DNA composition. There is, however, the possibility of acquiring information about DNA structure by hybridization with the help of so-called DNA probes. In essence, the probe is a specific single-stranded DNA fragment. Such a probe forms double-stranded DNA (hybridize) whenever it encounters a single-stranded complementary piece of DNA under appropriate conditions. There are many applications for DNA probes.

For example, to see which recombinant DNA molecule in an extensive DNA library harbors a gene of interest, one might use a DNA probe. DNAs from the library are converted into single-stranded DNA and then confronted with a probe that reflects a characteristic segment of the desired gene. Hybridization will only occur with target DNA molecules that harbor the gene of interest, provided that the probe has the required specificity.

The use of DNA hybridization probes in diagnostic testing in humans can be illustrated by using cystic fibrosis (CF) as an example. The frequency of this heritable and deadly disease is approximately once in 2000 live births, making it the most frequent genetic disorder among Caucasians. The cloning of the gene in 1989, based on its position on the human genetic map, was a *tour de force* involving several laboratories. It enabled the molecular analysis of the genetic defect, revealing that approximately 70% of the diseased genes contain an identical mutation: a three base pair deletion in the protein coding gene, resulting in the loss of a phenylalanine amino acid at position 508 of the 1480 amino acid-long protein. This mutation was named CFdel508 and the knowledge gained was used to design oligonucleotide probes for rapid screening purposes.

These single-stranded DNA probes are complementary to the normal and CFdel508 regions of the CF gene shown below. The symbols L, E, etc. represent various amino acids (see Chapter 2). F, for example, stands for phenylalanine.

Normal:

```
   L    E    N    I    I    F    G    V
5'-AAA GAA AAT ATC ATC TTT GGT GTT-3'
```

Mutant (CFdel508):

```
   L    E    N    I    I         G    V
5'-AAA GAA AAT ATC AT- —T GGT GTT-3'
```

For example, DNA isolated from white blood cells of suspected carriers or from amnion fluid is boiled to make it single-stranded and is then immobilized on filter paper. Next, hybridization with normal and CFdel508 specific probes clarifies whether one has the disease (when both the maternal and the paternal genes are affected) or if one is a carrier of the disease (only one of the two genes is affected).

Variation on this technology allows for the automated and simultaneous screening for many genetic diseases for which the molecular lesions are known. Kits which contain all the reagents necessary for a particular test are commercially available.

PCR Technology

For the detection of DNA or for testing the presence of mutations in DNA the probe method described above is very powerful. For current probe techniques, however, a substantial amount of DNA is required to facilitate detection of target DNA. The PCR (polymerase chain reaction) technology has become very popular in recent years for acquiring large amounts of DNA.

In PCR technology target DNA is amplified by *in vitro* DNA synthesis, occurring in a number of fast repeating steps. The reaction starts with the conversion of the double-stranded target DNA to single-stranded DNA and uses a specific oligonucleotide as a primer to allow DNA polymerase to do its job. The choice of the oligonucleotide primers, hybridizing with both target strands, will determine the left and right limits of the DNA to be amplified.

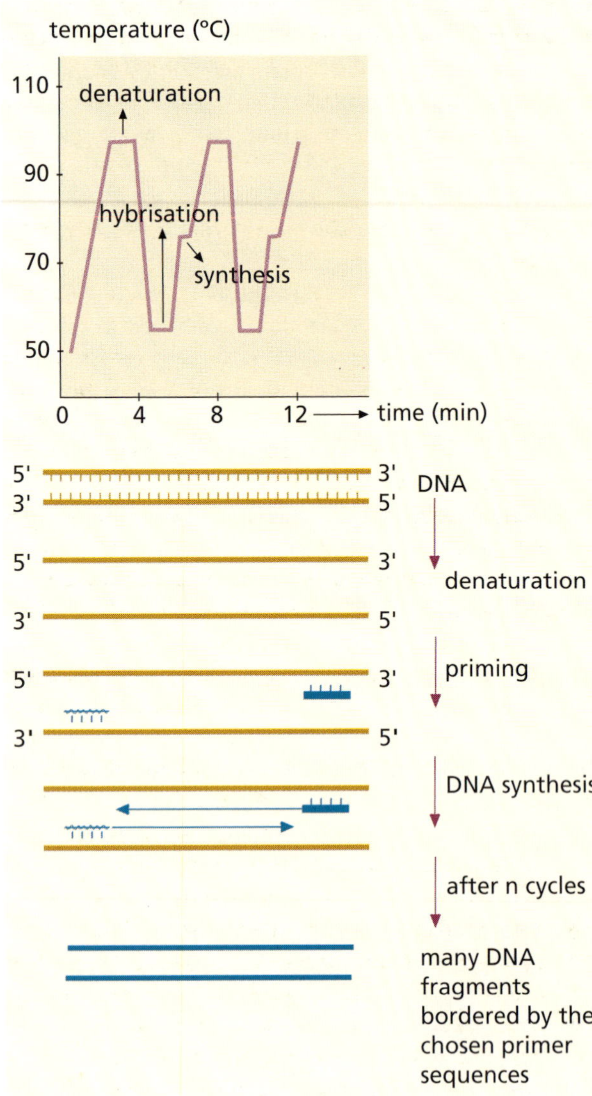

Figure 1.16. PCR-method. Upper panel: sequence of heating, hydridizing, synthesis. Below: synthesis events.

Each PCR cycle (illustrated in Figure 1.16) consists of three steps, each requiring only one to three minutes. In the first step the target DNA must be made single-stranded and this is done by heating the sample to 92 °C. The second step involves the specific hybridization of the two primers to the complementary single-stranded DNA. The optimal temperature for this process is about 35 °C. In the third step DNA polymerase will extend the primer sequence using the single-stranded DNA as a template. The optimal extension temperature is about 72 °C, since the DNA polymerase chosen is derived from a thermophilic bacterium, *Thermus aquaticus*, which normally grows in hot springs at temperatures above 80 °C. This DNA polymerase is extremely resistant to heat denaturing and survives the 92 °C DNA denaturing step. All reagents (target DNA, primers, dNTPs and polymerase) are put in a tube which is sealed and 20–30 PCR cycles are usually performed. The procedure can be automated and PCR machines are available which control the temperature for each of the three separate steps of a PCR cycle. Such machines can process hundreds of tubes simultaneously and produce results within two to four hours.

Ideally each cycle of DNA replication doubles the amount of DNA which is located in between the chosen primers. Thirty PCR cycles will give an amplification of 2^{30} times. This means that minute quantities of DNA can be amplified with specific primers to easily detectable levels. It should be realized that the specificity of the reaction is fully determined by the PCR primers and these primers will also determine the length of the amplified fragment. The tremendous sensitivity of the technique has sparked the development of a great number of applications where such sensitivity is of paramount importance. Also, compared to many other detection methods, the PCR procedure is very fast.

For example, the presence of microbial pathogens in raw and processed food products can be unequivocally determined using this technology. DNA is extracted from this material and the PCR reaction is performed using primers which are specific for the suspected pathogen(s). Detailed knowledge of the DNA sequences of many genes in many organisms allows for the development of such specific primers, which is the main prerequisite for diagnostic PCR technology. Detection of specific amplified DNA products is proof that the pathogen is present in the material. Also in clinical material (blood, urine, etc.) the technique is used extensively as a rapid and sensitive test for the presence of bacterial and viral pathogens. A third area where PCR has become standard technology is in forensic science. At a crime scene often minute quantities of potentially important evidence is found (single hairs, blood drops, semen stains, etc.) and PCR technology can be used to get enough DNA to show the origin of this material. These are but a few examples of the use of PCR technology. PCR is often an essential step in elaborate diagnostic and detection procedures, and novel applications are continuously being developed.

As for the application of the PCR technology for the diagnosis of pathogens, one has to realize that for most purposes the intent is to detect viable pathogens. The PCR technology obviously cannot distinguish DNA from vital or dead material, and in that respect it is not always an adequate technique. The PCR technique is a very sensitive one since minute amounts of DNA are highly amplified. This high sensitivity may limit the discriminative power of the technique when applied for diagnostic purposes. For example, it may detect minor contaminants in the samples. Moreover, DNA contaminants may be introduced during the performance of the tests. It is therefore a major concern in the application of PCR to avoid DNA contaminations that could produce contaminated reactions.

Cell Cultures

Biotechnology depends heavily on techniques to cultivate prokaryotic and eukaryotic cells, since these cells are sources of bioproducts or of mediators of various bioconversions. The scale of culturing is an important issue in biotechnology. Experience gained from the production of small scale cultures is not directly transferable to large scale culturing in manufacturing industries. What can be cultivated in small flasks in a research laboratory cannot always be cultivated efficiently on an industrial scale. Simply enlarging the culture devices from small flasks to tanks containing many thousands of liters is not enough. Cultivation on an industrial level requires very sophisticated and delicate process technologies (cf. Chapter 3).

Cultivation of Microbes

Some microbial species are very popular in biotechnology since they can be cultivated in an easy and safe way. To microbial species with a long lasting tradition in biotechnology belong bacterial species like *Clostridium acetobutyricum*, *Corynebacterium sp.*, *Xanthomonas sp.*, *Bacillus sp.*, *Lactobacillus sp.*, as well as the fungi *Saccharomyces cerevisiae* (baker's yeast), *Penicillium sp.* and *Aspergillus sp.*.

In general, microbes can be cultivated either in vessels or tanks filled with an appropriate liquid growth medium or on plates containing a growth medium solidified with agar (cf. Chapter 3). Culturing in this way implies that the conditions for the growing cells gradually diminish, since nutrients are depleted by the growing cells and growth inhibiting metabolites gradually accumulate. However, there are culture devices like the continuous culture apparatus, which allow indefinite growth of the microorganisms. This indefinite growth is achieved by continuously adding fresh medium to the culture, whilst removing growing cells and metabolites by an overflow device. Under a proper regimen of addition and removal, a 'steady state' situation where cells continuously grow is created. The suggestive name for such cultures is "continuous culture." Most industrial biotechnology, however, is based on culturing in tanks without a supply and overflow device. Such culture devices are called "batch cultures."

Figure 1.17 presents a typical picture of bacterial growth in a batch culture. There are several characteristic phases in the so-called bacterial growth curve. Bacteria generally do not immediately start multiplying when they are inoculated in a fresh medium. A phase, called the lag phase,

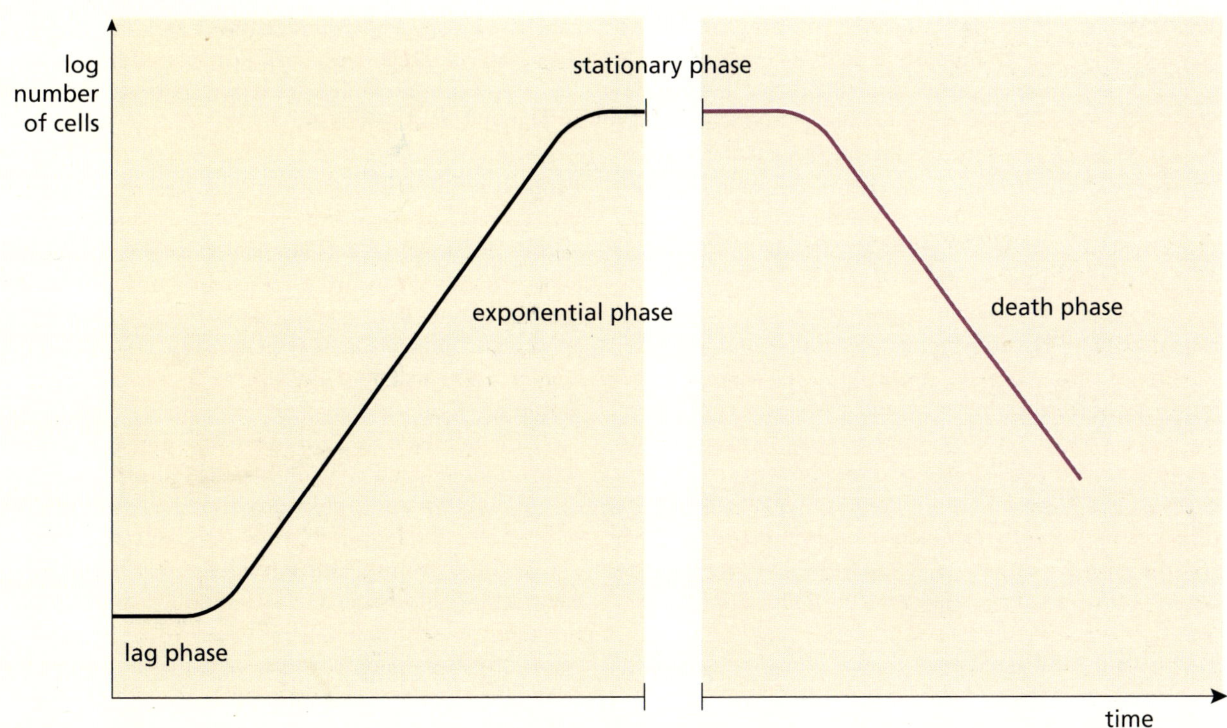

Figure 1.17. Bacterial growth curve.

where cells do not divide but gradually adapt to the specific growth conditions in the medium, precedes the phase where all cells start to divide. This phase, the actual growth phase, is called the logarithmic or exponential phase. The exponential growth phase is relevant for many biotechnological applications since most of the genes are then optimally expressed. The exponential phase is followed by the stationary phase, where active growth comes to an end due to depletion and spoilage of the medium.

The stage when the exponential growth is about to end is of interest for some biotechnological purposes. At this stage, for reasons that are not completely understood, some microorganisms start the synthesis of so-called secondary metabolites. These metabolic products are, according to their name, not essential for the basic cellular metabolism, but may be useful as bioproducts. Secondary metabolites relevant for pharmaceutical biotechnology are antibiotics, as produced by some microorganisms.

After some time the stationary phase is followed by a phase where the bacteria die off. This stage is clearly not of great interest for biotechnology.

The bacterial growth curve is not directly applicable for microbes that do not reproduce by binary fission. However, a lag phase preceding a phase of active growth and followed by a stationary phase is generally found.

Also, in biotechnology time is money and maximum cell yields are therefore essential. Thus, one tries to keep the lag phase as short as possible and to postpone the onset of the stationary phase. The first goal is achieved by inoculating the tank with cells that, by proper preculturing, are optimally adapted to the medium in the tank. The second goal is achieved in various ways. A successful approach, especially when cells are limited in outgrowth by medium depletion, consists of adding fresh medium near the end of the exponential phase. This technique is called "fed batch culture."

To achieve optimal growth of microorganisms, not only is it essential to provide a medium with the proper nutrients, but conditions like pH, oxygen tension and temperature must also be chosen appropriately and should be controlled while cultivating. Finally, infection with other microorganisms should be prevented. This prevention requires strict sterility measures and work protocols.

To give an idea about the impressive performance of fast growing microbial cells, such cells may grow with doubling times of about 30 minutes and cultures can easily reach densities of 10^9 cells per mL. If one cultivates bacterial cells on plates, a colony on such a plate, appearing after one day or so, might easily harbor millions of cells.

Animal Cell Cultures

Animal cells can be isolated out of a particular tissue after a protease (trypsin) treatment. When such cells are transferred to glass or plastic they will adhere and start growing, if supplied with a suitable liquid growth medium. A cell culture of this type is called a "primary" culture. Such cultures die after a while and are thus not very useful for biotechnology.

Some animal cell types, however, become exceptional in their growth characteristics when they are cultivated. The main characteristic is that the cell becomes immortal. Such cells are used to prepare 'continuous' cell lines. They may survive for months or even years, as long as they are diluted and recultured at frequent intervals. Some cells of malignant origin or cells originating from normal cells transformed by a virus like the Epstein Barr virus are immortal and grow to high cell densities. For pharmaceutical biotechnology, the latter cell lines may be of limited value since they are of malignant nature and may release transforming viruses as a contaminant for the pharmaceutical product. Most useful are non-malignant immortalized cell lines, e.g. 3T3 fibroblasts.

Some cell lines depend on solid support for their growth, while others can be cultivated in suspension, which may be advantageous for biotechnology. Successful cultivation of animal cells *in vitro* requires a suitable, very complex growth medium providing not only all nutritional requirements for the cells but also a number of specific growth factors and hormones. The pH must be buffered around 7.0 and proper osmotic conditions isotonic with the cell cytoplasm are required (cf. Chapter 3).

Animal cell cultivation is certainly much more complicated than cultivation of common microorganisms. For pharmaceutical biotechnology there are various safe cell lines available, each with their specific characteristics.

Plant Cell Cultures

Plants have always been an important source of pharmacologically active compounds. The complex structure of many of these compounds preclude their chemical synthesis, certainly on a commercial scale. Many active compounds are extracted from intact plants or plant parts. Such compounds are usually present in very low quantities and this has triggered research into the use of alternative production methods.

Cell biologists have tried to produce high levels of active compounds in plant cell cultures, but this has not been an easy task. Next to the problems associated with large scale cell cultures, a major problem with plant cells is that they can not be kept in the differentiated state. When fully differentiated plant tissues are excised to initiate a cell culture this differentiated state is usually lost. Often the compound of interest is made only in specialized tissues in the intact plants. Use of these tissues for cell culture initiation results in a significant decrease in the production of the compound of interest. The addition of plant hormones (e.g. auxins and cytokinins) may alleviate this problem, but up until now the efficient production of pharmaceutically interesting compounds in plant cell culture systems has been rare. Systems that are available are usually based on procedures involving repeated selection of cell lines with the highest production potential.

Production capacity of cell lines can be further improved by feeding strategically chosen, cheaply available precursors to the culture for the compound of interest. The cells then perform the final and chemically most demanding biosynthetic steps. A better understanding of cellular differentiation processes, combined with genetic modification technology of plant cells, may help in overcoming these problems and allow for a more efficient use of plant cell cultures in pharmaceutical biotechnology. To circumvent the plant culturing problems one might exploit the recombinant DNA technology, described previously. Several of the plant genes which encode enzymes involved in biosynthesis of pharmaceutically active compounds have been cloned. Expression of such genes in heterologous host systems opens an *ex planta* way for enzymatic synthesis of active compounds.

Conclusion

Growing knowledge in the physiology of microbial, animal and plant cells, together with detailed insight into gene structure and function, has opened new ways for pharmaceutical biotechnology. This chapter is merely an introductory illustration of new approaches based on DNA technology. In order to appreciate and exploit the achievements of cell biology and recombinant DNA technology, further reading is required. The books listed below are just a few of a large number of excellent books available. ■

Books for Further Reading

- **Alberts, B., Johnson, A., Lewis, J., Raff, M., Roberts, K. and Walter, P.** (2002). Molecular biology of the cell 4th ed. Garland Publ. Inc., New York.
- **Alcamo, I.E.** (1999). DNA technology. The awesome skill. 2nd edition. Harcourt Acad. Press.
- **Bourgaize, D., Jewell, Th.R. and Buiser, R.G.** (2000). Biotechnology. Demystifying the concepts. 2000. Addison Wesley Longman Inc.
- **Brown, T.A.** (1999). Genomes. Bios Scientific Publishers Ltd., Oxford.
- [illegible] **and Zolle, M.** (1992). Recombinant DNA 2nd ed. Freeman and Company, New York.

Self-Assessment Questions

Question 1: *A bacterial strain carrying a foreign structural gene with its own promoter on an appropriate plasmid does not yield a substantial amount of the encoded gene product. What factors could explain this failure?*

Question 2: *What kind of bacterial plasmid is needed in order to function as an optimal vector for DNA cloning in a particular bacterial host?*

Question 3: *Potential hosts for the biotechnological production by the recombinant-DNA technology of a human protein, lacking functional post-translational modifications, and to be used as a biopharmaceutical are:*

a. Escherichia coli K-12
b. Bacillus subtilis
c. Saccharomyces cerevisiae (a yeast)
d. Aspergillus nidulans (a fungus)
e. plant cells
f. animal cells

Which one(s) would you prefer? Why?

Question 4: *Same question as above but now the biological activity of the protein is dependent on specific post-translational modifications.*

Question 5: *To gain microbial products in biotechnology one may use batch cultures or continuous cultures. What are the differences between these culture methods and what are the practical consequences of these differences?*

Question 6: *If one uses a batch culture for production, what kind of measures have to be taken in order to achieve an efficient production yield?*

Question 7: *If one wants to isolate an animal gene for the purpose of isolating the gene product in a bacterial host, what would be the most appropriate isolation procedure?*

Question 8: *A foreign product, encoded by a recombinant plasmid, appears harmful for the bacterial host which should produce that product. What kind of measures should be taken in order to still gain substantial amounts of that product?*

Question 9: *The PCR technology, using specific primers for Salmonella typhimurium, reveals a clear signal in: i) a food product, or ii) in a pharmaceutical product produced through biotechnology. What conclusions can be drawn as to the safety of the food product, or of the pharmaceutical product?*

Question 10: *DNA probes may reveal genetic diseases. Is this feasible with all genetic diseases?*

Answers

Answers 1. There are various possible explanations, at each stage of the gene expression something may go wrong or occur with low efficiency. For example:

a) it might be that the authentic promoter of the foreign does not (optimally) function in the specific host.
b) it might be that the foreign gene contains introns. Since the bacterial host is not able to cope with introns, a functional gene product is not feasible.
c) the construct may yield a mRNA without appropriate translational signals, e.g. a ribosome binding signal. Fusion of the gene towards a leading fragment of a functional bacterial gene might at least overcome the translational start problem. In that case a fused gene product may be produced in substantial amounts.
d) the mRNA molecule may appear very unstable. In that case the gene expression is doomed to be low.
e) the foreign gene product is produced in the bacterial host, but appears very unstable as it is degraded by one or more of the bacterial proteases. Therefore, one frequently uses bacterial strains with minimal proteolytic activity as production hosts.

Answers 2. The crucial demands are that the plasmid is able to replicate (preferably as a multicopy plasmid) in the specific host and that it is maintained in a stable fashion in the host. Advantages for the optimal application are the presence on the plasmid of selective markers (mostly antibiotic resistance determinants) and a range of restriction sites. A relatively small size of the plasmid will allow rather simple experimental procedures.

Answers 3. The product should be produced in a safe and economic way. Since the product is not depending on post translational modifications, prokaryotic hosts like *E. coli* K-12 or *B. subtilis* are attractive (from the point of safety and economics, based on long lasting biotechnological experience). The fact that *E. coli* is a Gram-negative host causes extra efforts when it comes to purification of the product. A safe biopharmaceutical should be completely free of LPS. Taking this into consideration *B. subtilis* is preferable. The eukaryotic micro-organisms *S. cereviseae* and *A. nidulans* could be options in companies with a lot of experience with these organisms (and most likely with specific patents around the application of such organisms). Plant and animal cells are, *a priori*, not specifically required and are not appropriate, since plant and animal cell cultures are production-wise very demanding.

Answers 4. In this case the prokaryotic organisms can not be used, since they have only a very limited post-translational modification activity. Animal cells could fulfil the post-translational modifications, as can the human cells responsible for the protein production. They are therefore, despite high costs, most desirable. However, it is known that the *Aspergillus* species are remarkably active in post-translational modification, and it is certainly worthwhile to consider these organisms since they can be cultivated in an economic way.

Answers 5. In the batch culture device the medium is gradually depleted and various (unwanted) metabolites of the growing cells appear, while in the continuous culture device there is a continuous nutrient supply and a simultaneous removal of cells and growth inhibiting metabolites. The practical consequence for cultivation in a batch device is that the production inevitably comes to an end and regular restarts (time and money consuming) of the culture are required. Continuous cultures on the other hand do not need restarts and have the outlook to be more economic. However, the control and handling of a (large scale) continuous culture is complicated.

Answers 6. Prevent an extensive lag phase. This is achieved by using an inoculum for the culture that is optimally adapted to the conditions in the batch device. In addition, one may try to postpone an early onset of the stationary phase, by adding extra nutrients after a while, for example.

Answers 7. If the gene encodes a rather small protein with a known amino acid sequence, one may chemically synthesize the gene. If the gene product is a large protein this is not feasible. Since one has to keep in mind that the gene might be endowed with introns, it seems most appropriate to start by isolating mRNA from appropriate sources. mRNA should then be converted into cDNA.

Answers 8. In that case the foreign gene should be controlled by a bacterial promoter that can be switched "on" and "off" at will. Cultivation of the cells under conditions where the promoter is "off" allows cells to grow. When cells are present in high amounts and still metabolically active, the promoter is switched "on," for example by the addition of a specific inducing agent to the medium.

Answers 9. The signal achieved by PCR specifically reveals the presence of DNA. This DNA might be present as such or set free from *Salmonella* cells, either alive or dead. The safety of a food product depends on the presence of harmful bacterial cells that are alive or, in some instances, on the presence of a toxin produced by the bacterium. PCR technology analyses does not therefore conclusively answer the question whether the food is safe or not. As to the biopharmaceutical, the safety regulations are more stringent as drug safety may be jeopardized by the presence of bacterial constituents (e.g. endo- or exotoxins). Therefore, PCR revealing Salmonella *typhimurium* DNA in a biopharmaceutical is very alarming.

Answers 10. No, a probe can be developed and used as a detection tool only for genetic diseases with a well known and well defined genetic basis. So far, most genetic diseases are not known at the level of the DNA. Some diseases are known to be the result of rather complex DNA changes and their detection will, therefore, not be amenable for straightforward DNA probing.

2 Biophysical and Biochemical Analysis of Recombinant Proteins

structure and analysis of proteins

Tsutomu Arakawa and John S. Philo

Introduction

For a recombinant protein to become a human therapeutic, its biophysical and biochemical characteristics must be well understood. These properties serve as a basis for comparison of lot-to-lot reproducibility, for establishing the range of conditions to stabilize the protein during production, storage and shipping, and for identifying characteristics useful for monitoring stability during long-term storage.

A number of techniques can be used to determine the biophysical properties of proteins and to examine their biochemical and biological integrity. Where possible, the results of these experiments are compared with those obtained using naturally occurring proteins in order to be confident that the recombinant protein has the desired characteristics of the naturally occurring one.

Protein Structure

Primary Structure

Most proteins which are developed for therapy perform specific functions by interacting with other small and large molecules, e.g. cell surface receptors, binding proteins, nucleic acids, carbohydrates and lipids. The functional properties of proteins are derived from their folding into distinct three-dimensional structures. Each protein fold is based on its specific polypeptide sequence in which different amino acids are connected through peptide bonds in a specific way. This alignment of the twenty amino acids, called a primary sequence, has in general all the information necessary for folding into a distinct tertiary structure comprising different secondary structures such as α-helices and β-sheets (see below). Because the twenty amino acids possess different side chains, polypeptides with widely diverse properties are obtained.

All of the twenty amino acids consist of a C_α carbon to which an amino group, a carboxyl group, a hydrogen, and a side chain bind in L configuration (Figure 2.1). These amino acids are joined by condensation to yield a peptide bond consisting of a carboxyl group of an amino acid joined with the amino group of the next amino acid (Figure 2.2). The condensation gives an amide group, NH, at the N-terminal side of C_α, and a carbonyl group, C=O, at the C-terminal side. These groups, as well as the amino acyl side chains, play important roles in protein folding. Due to their ability to form hydrogen bonds, they make major energetic contributions to the formation of two important secondary structures, α-helix and β-sheet. The peptide bonds between various amino acids are very much equivalent, however, so that they do not determine which part of a sequence should form an α-helix or β-sheet. Sequence-dependent secondary structure formation is determined by the side chains.

The twenty amino acids commonly found in proteins are shown in Figure 2.3. They are described by their full names and three- and one-letter codes. Their side chains are structurally different in such a way that at neutral pH,

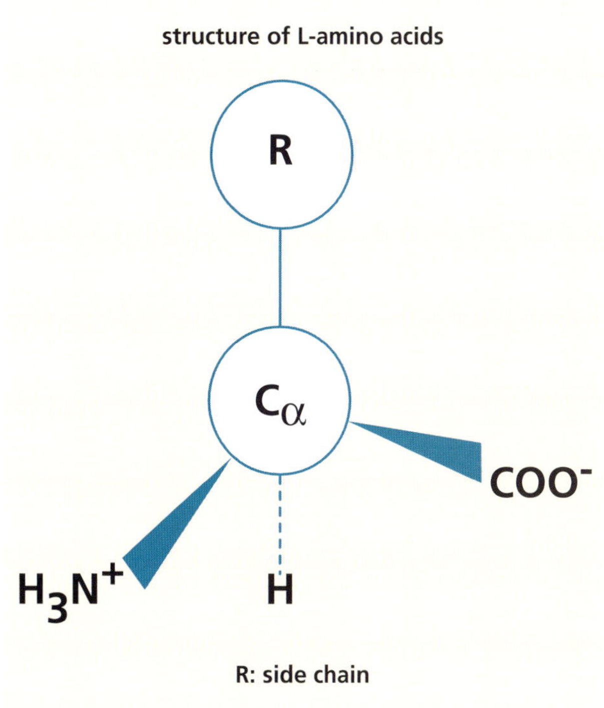

Figure 2.1. Structure of L-amino acids.

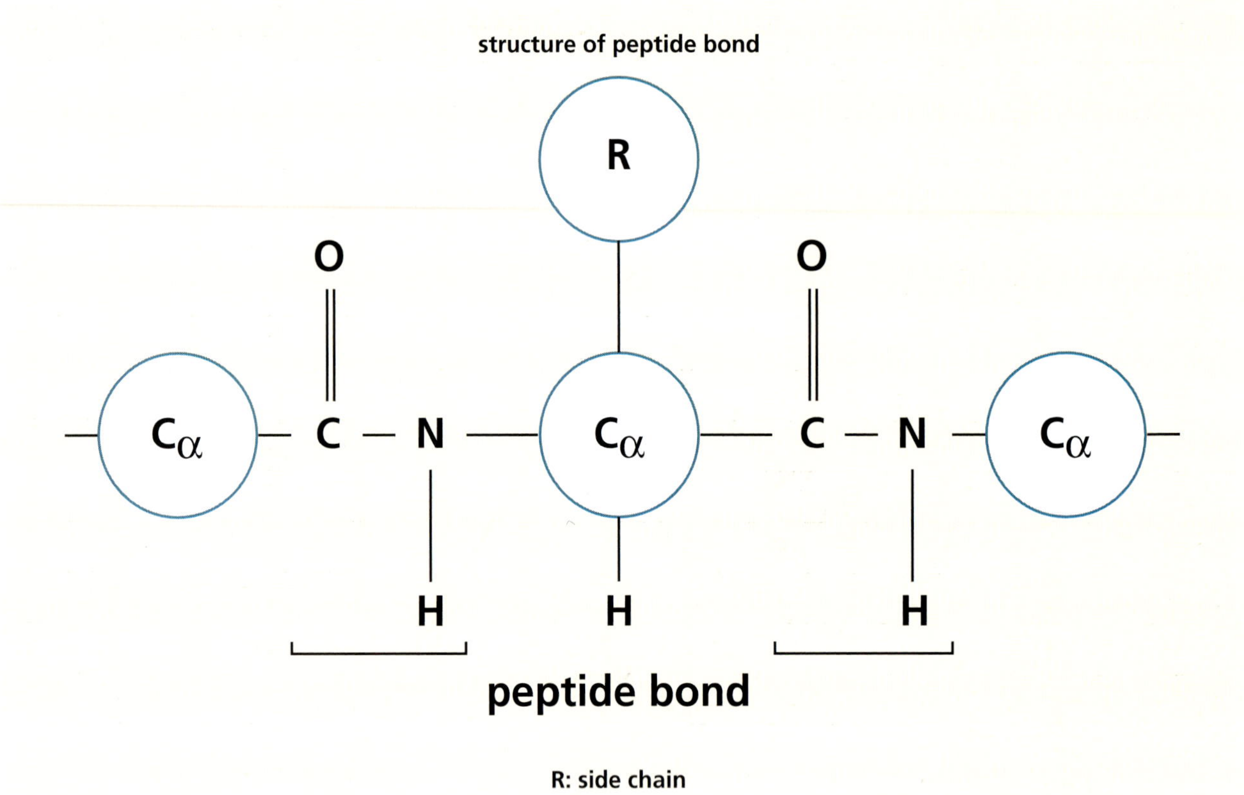

Figure 2.2. Structure of peptide bond.

aspartic and glutamic acid are negatively charged and lysine and arginine are positively charged. Histidine is positively charged to an extent that depends on the pH. At pH 7.0, on average about half of the histidine side chains are positively charged. Tyrosine and cysteine are protonated and uncharged at neutral pH, but become negatively charged above pH 10 and 8, respectively.

Polar amino acids consist of serine, threonine, asparagine, and glutamine, as well as cysteine, while non-polar amino acids consist of alanine, valine, phenylalanine, proline, methionine, leucine, and isoleucine. Glycine behaves neutrally while cystine, the oxidized form of cysteine, is characterized as hydrophobic. Although tyrosine and tryptophan often enter into polar interactions, they are better characterized as non-polar, or hydrophobic, as described later.

These twenty amino acids are incorporated into a unique sequence based on the genetic code, as the example in Figure 2.4 shows. This is an amino acid sequence of granulocyte-colony stimulating factor (G-CSF), which selectively regulates proliferation and maturation of neutrophils. Although the exact properties of this protein depend on the location of each amino acid and hence the location of each side chain in the three-dimensional structure, the average properties can be estimated simply from the amino acid composition, as shown in Table 2.1; i.e. a list of the total number of each type of amino acid contained in this protein molecule.

Parameter	Value
Molecular weight	18673
Total number of amino acids	174
1 microgram	53.5 picomoles
Molar extinction coefficient	15820
1 A(280)	1.18 mg/ml
Isoelectric point	5.86
Charge at pH 7	- 3.39

Table 2.1a. Amino acid composition and structural parameters of granulocyte colony stimulating factor.

Amino acid	Number	% by weight	% by frequency
A Ala	19	7.23	10.92
C Cys	5	2.76	2.87
D Asp	4	2.47	2.30
E Glu	9	6.22	5.17
F Phe	6	4.73	3.45
G Gly	14	4.28	8.05
H His	5	3.67	2.87
I Ile	4	2.42	2.30
K Lys	4	2.75	2.30
L Leu	33	20.00	18.97
M Met	3	2.11	1.72
N Asn	0	0.00	0.00
P Pro	13	6.76	7.47
Q Gln	17	11.66	9.77
R Arg	5	4.18	2.87
S Ser	14	6.53	8.05
T Thr	7	3.79	4.02
V Val	7	3.71	4.02
W Trp	2	1.99	1.15
Y Tyr	3	2.62	1.72

Table 2.1b. Amino acid composition and structural parameters of granulocyte colony stimulating factor.

Using the pK_a values of these side chains and one amino and carboxyl terminus, one can calculate total charges (positive plus negative charges) and net charges (positive minus negative charges) of a protein as a function of pH, i.e. a titration curve. Since cysteine can be oxidized to form a disulfide bond or can be in a free form, accurate calculation above pH 8 requires knowledge of the status of cysteinyl residues in the protein. The titration curve thus obtained is only an approximation, since some charged residues may be buried and the effective pKa values depend on the local environment of each residue. Nevertheless, the calculated titration curve gives a first approximation of the overall charged state of a protein at a given pH and hence its solution property. Other molecular parameters, such as isoelectric point (pI where the net charge of a protein becomes zero), molecular weight, extinction coefficient, partial specific volume and hydrophobicity, can also be estimated from the amino acid composition, as shown in Table 2.1.

The primary structure of a protein, i.e. the sequence of the twenty amino acids, can lead to the three-dimensional structure because the amino acids have diverse physical properties. First, each type of amino acid has the tendency to be more preferentially incorporated into certain secondary structures. The frequencies with which each amino acid is found in α-helix, β-sheet and β-turn, secondary structures that are discussed later in this chapter, can be calculated as an average over a number of proteins whose three-dimensional structures have been solved. These frequencies are listed in Table 2.2. The β-turn has a distinct

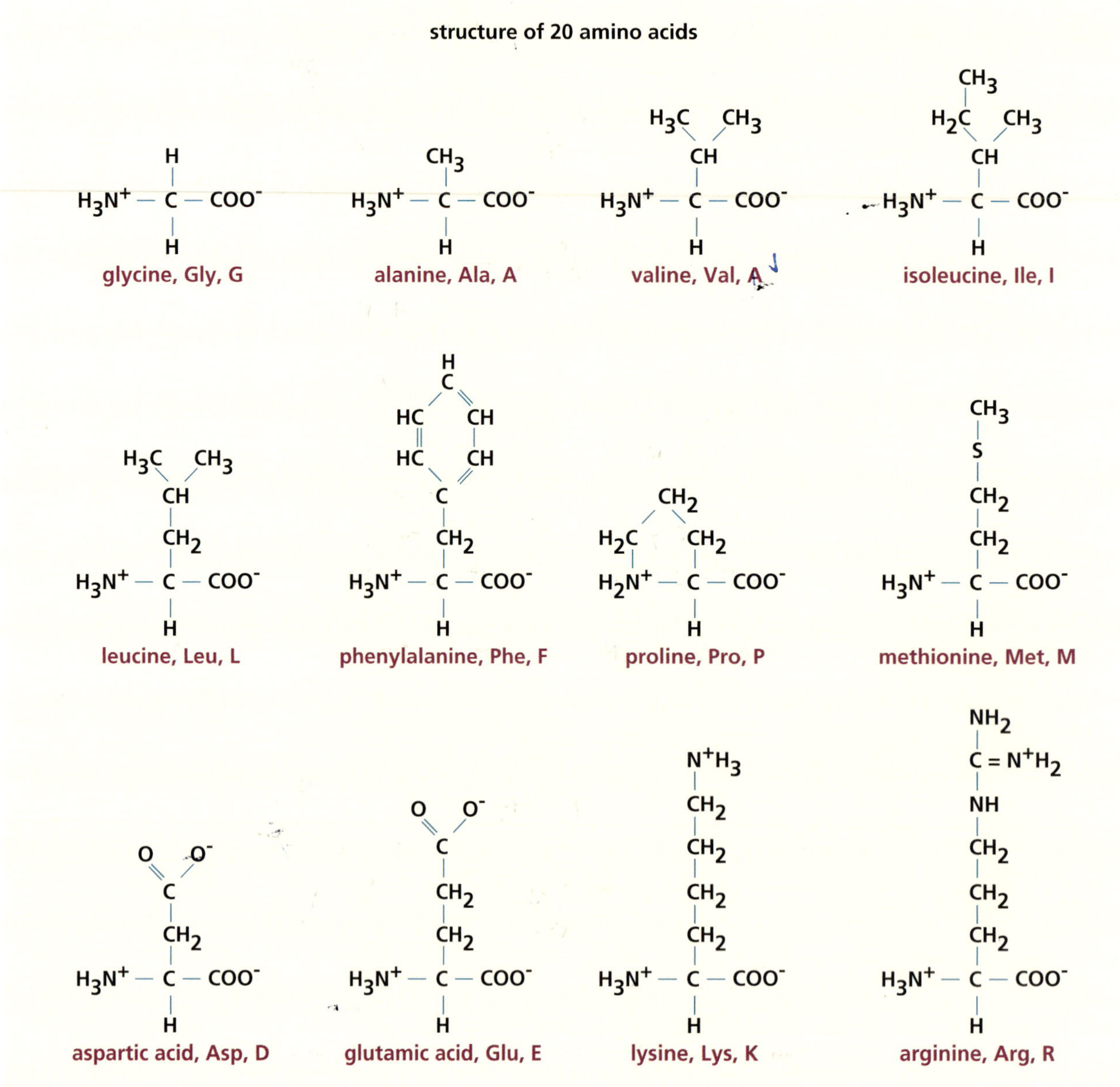

Figure 2.3a. Structure of 20 amino acids.

configuration consisting of four sequential amino acids and there is a strong preference for specific amino acids in these four positions. For example, asparagine has an overall high frequency of occurrence in a β-turn and is most frequently observed in the first and third position of a β-turn. This characteristic of asparagine is consistent with its side chain being a potential site of N-linked glycosylation. Effects of glycosylation on the biological and physicochemical properties of proteins are extremely important; however, their contribution to structure is not readily predictable based on the amino acid composition.

Based on these frequencies, one can predict for particular polypeptide segments which type of secondary structure they are likely to form. As shown in Figure 2.5a, there are a number of methods developed to predict the secondary structure from the primary sequence of the proteins. Using G-CSF (Figure 2.5b) as an example, regions of α-helix, β-sheets, turns, hydrophilicity, and antigen sites can be suggested.

Another property of amino acids, which impacts on protein folding, is the hydrophobicity of their side chains. Although non-polar amino acids are basically hydrophobic,

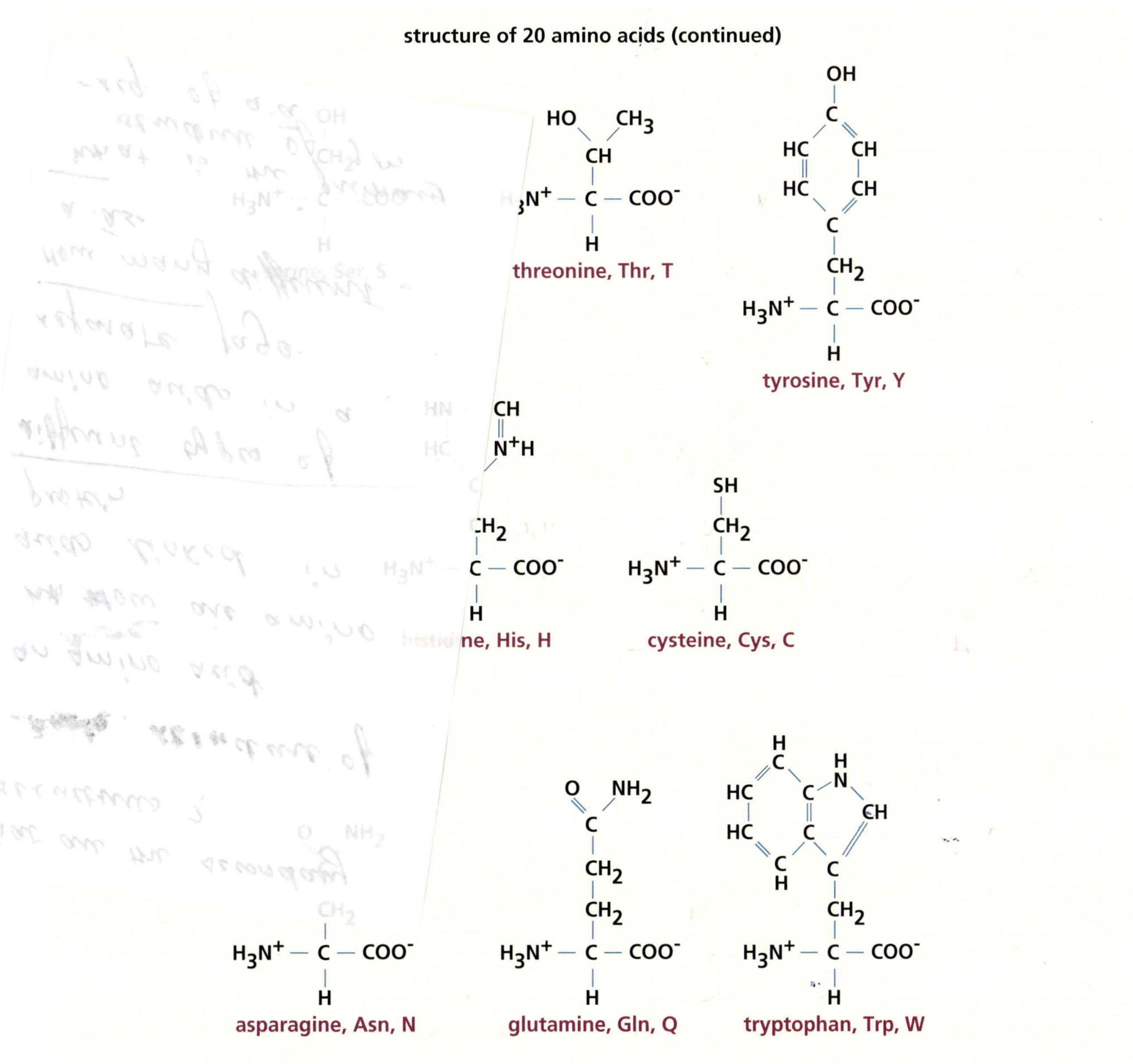

Figure 2.3b. Structure of 20 amino acids.

it is important to know how hydrophobic they are. This property has been determined by measuring the partition coefficient or solubility of amino acids in water and organic solvents and normalizing such parameters relative to glycine. Relative to the side chain of glycine, H, such normalization shows how strongly the side chains of non-polar amino acids prefer the organic phase to the aqueous phase. A representation of such measurements is shown in Table 2.3. The values indicate that the free energy increases as the side chain of tryptophan and tyrosine are transferred from an organic solvent to water and that such transfer is thermodynamically unfavorable. Although it is unclear how

TPLGPASSLPQSFLLKCLEQVRKIQGDGAALQEKLCATYK 40
LCHPEELVLLGHSLGIPWAPLSSCPSQALQLAGCLSQLHS 80
GLFLYQGLLQALEGISPELGPTLDTLQLDVADFATTIWQQ 120
MEELGMAPALQPTQGAMPAFASAFQRRAGGVLVASHLQSF 160
LEVSYRVLRHLAQP

Figure 2.4. Amino acid sequence of granulocyte-colony stimulating factor.

α-helix		β-sheet		β-turn		β-turn position 1		β-turn position 2		β-turn position 3		β-turn position 4	
Glu	1.51	Val	1.70	Asn	1.56	Asn	0.161	Pro	0.301	Asn	0.191	Trp	0.167
Met	1.45	Ile	1.60	Gly	1.56	Cys	0.149	Ser	0.139	Gly	0.190	Gly	0.152
Ala	1.42	Tyr	1.47	Pro	1.52	Asp	0.147	Lys	0.115	Asp	0.179	Cys	0.128
Leu	1.21	Phe	1.38	Asp	1.46	His	0.140	Asp	0.110	Ser	0.125	Tyr	0.125
Lys	1.16	Trp	1.37	Ser	1.43	Ser	0.120	Thr	0.108	Cys	0.117	Ser	0.106
Phe	1.13	Leu	1.30	Cys	1.19	Pro	0.102	Arg	0.106	Tyr	0.114	Gln	0.098
Gln	1.11	Cys	1.19	Tyr	1.14	Gly	0.102	Gln	0.098	Arg	0.099	Lys	0.095
Trp	1.08	Thr	1.19	Lys	1.01	Thr	0.086	Gly	0.085	His	0.093	Asn	0.091
Ile	1.08	Gln	1.10	Gln	0.98	Tyr	0.082	Asn	0.083	Glu	0.077	Arg	0.085
Val	1.06	Met	1.05	Thr	0.96	Trp	0.077	Met	0.082	Lys	0.072	Asp	0.081
Asp	1.01	Arg	0.93	Trp	0.96	Gln	0.074	Ala	0.076	Tyr	0.065	Thr	0.079
His	1.00	Asn	0.89	Arg	0.95	Arg	0.070	Tyr	0.065	Phe	0.065	Leu	0.070
Arg	0.98	His	0.87	His	0.95	Met	0.068	Glu	0.060	Trp	0.064	Pro	0.068
Thr	0.83	Ala	0.83	Glu	0.74	Val	0.062	Cys	0.053	Gln	0.037	Phe	0.065
Ser	0.77	Ser	0.75	Ala	0.66	Leu	0.061	Val	0.048	Leu	0.036	Glu	0.064
Cys	0.70	Gly	0.75	Met	0.60	Ala	0.060	His	0.047	Ala	0.035	Ala	0.058
Tyr	0.69	Lys	0.74	Phe	0.60	Phe	0.059	Phe	0.041	Pro	0.034	Ile	0.056
Asn	0.67	Pro	0.55	Leu	0.59	Glu	0.056	Ile	0.034	Val	0.028	Met	0.055
Pro	0.57	Asp	0.54	Val	0.50	Lys	0.055	Leu	0.025	Met	0.014	His	0.054
Gly	0.57	Glu	0.37	Ile	0.47	Ile	0.043	Trp	0.013	Ile	0.013	Val	0.053

Table 2.2. Frequency of occurrence of 20 Amino acids in α-helix, β-sheet and β-turn. Taken and edited from Chou, P.Y. and Fasman, G.D., 1978, Ann. Rev. Biochem. 47, 251–276 with permission from Annual Reviews, Inc.

comparable the hydrophobic property is between an organic solvent and the interior of protein molecules, the hydrophobic side chains favor clustering together, resulting in a core structure with properties similar to an organic solvent. These hydrophobic characteristics of non-polar amino acids and hydrophilic characteristics of polar amino acids generate a partition of amino acyl residues into a hydrophobic core and hydrophilic surface, resulting in overall folding.

Secondary Structure

α-HELIX

Immediately evident in the primary structure of a protein is that each amino acid is linked by a peptide bond. The amide, NH, is a hydrogen donor and the carbonyl, C=O, is a hydrogen acceptor, and they can form a stable

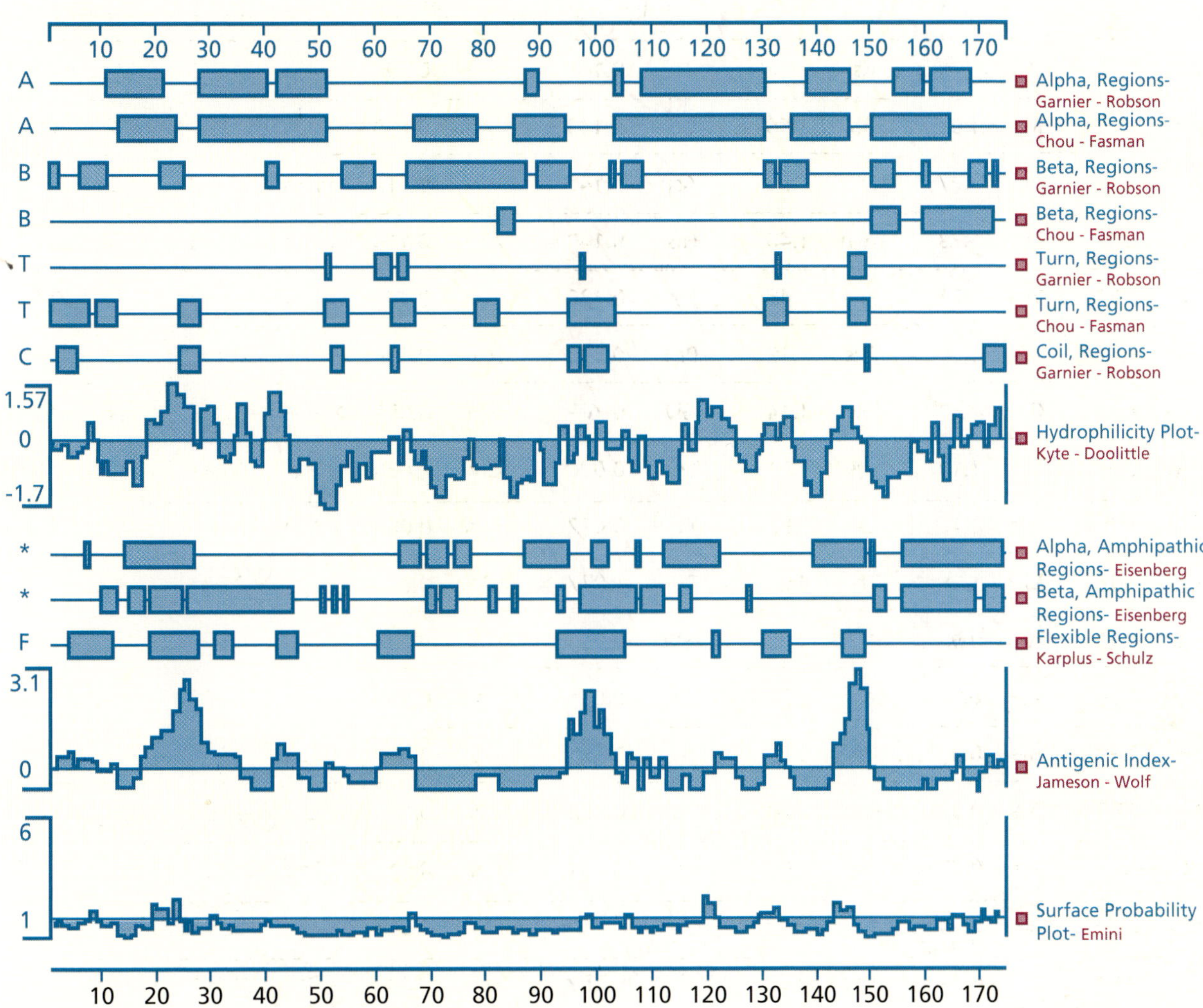

Figure 2.5a. Predicted secondary structure of granulocyte-colony stimulating factor. Obtained using a program "DNA Star" (DNASTAR Inc., Madison, WI).

hydrogen bond when they are positioned in an appropriate configuration of the polypeptide chain. Such structures of the polypeptide chain are called secondary structure. Two main structures, α-helix and β-sheet, accommodate such stable hydrogen bonds. The main chain forms a right-handed helix, because only the L-form of amino acids are in proteins, and makes one turn per 3.6 residues. The overall length of α-helices can vary widely. Figure 2.6 shows an example of a short α-helix. In this case, the C=O group of residue 1 forms a hydrogen bond to the NH group of residue 5 and C=O group of residue 2 forms a hydrogen bond with the NH group of residue 6. Thus, at the start of an α-helix, four amide groups are always free and at the end of an α-helix four carboxyl groups are also free. As a result, both ends of an α-helix are highly polar.

Moreover, all the hydrogen bonds are aligned along the helical axis. Since both peptide NH and C=O groups have electric dipole moments pointing in the same direction, they will add to a substantial dipole moment throughout the entire α-helix, with the negative partial charge at the C-terminal side and the positive partial charge at the N-terminal side.

The side chains project outward from the α-helix. This projection means that all the side chains surround the outer surface of an α-helix and interact both with each other and with side chains of other regions which come in contact with these side chains. These interactions, so-called

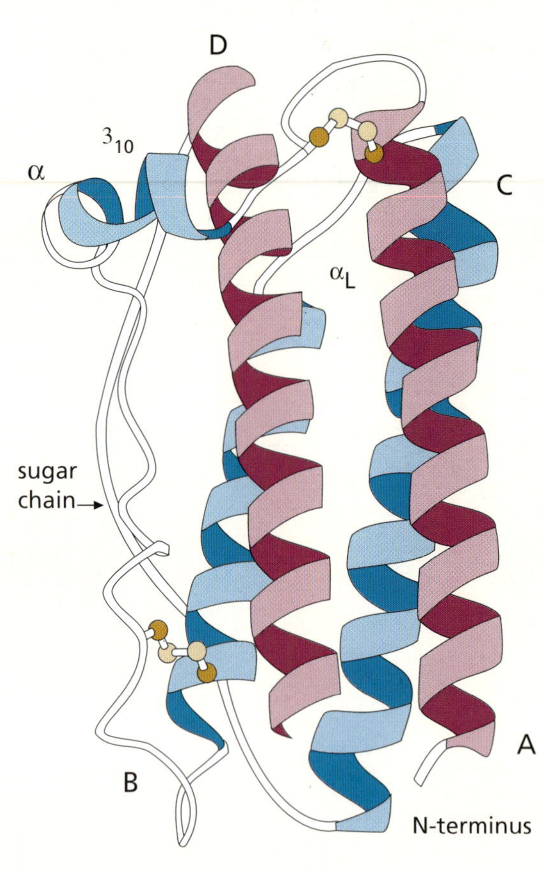

Figure 2.5b. Secondary structure of Filgrastim (recombinant G-CSF). Filgrastim is a 175-amino acid polypeptide. Its four anti-parallel alpha helices (A, B, C and D) and short 3-to-10 type helix (3_{10}) form a helical bundle. The two biologically active sites (α and α_L) are remote from modifications at the N terminus of the A helix and the sugar chain attached to loop C-D.
Note: Filgrastim is not glycosylated; the sugar chain is included to illustrate its location in endogenous G-CSF.

Amino acid side chain	cal/mole
Tryptophan	3400
Norleucine	2600
Phenylalanine	2500
Tyrosine	2300
Dihydroxyphenylalanine	1800
Leucine	1800
Valine	1500
Methionine	1300
Histidine	500
Alanine	500
Threonine	400
Serine	–300

Table 2.3. Hydrophobicity scale: transfer free energies of amino acid side chains from organic solvent to water. Taken from Nozaki, Y. and Tanford, C., 1971, J. Biol. Chem. 246, 2211–2217 with permission from American Society of Biological Chemists.

long-range interactions, can stabilize the α-helical structure and help it to act as a folding unit. Often an α-helix serves as a building block for the three-dimensional structure of globular proteins by bringing hydrophobic side chains to one side of a helix and hydrophilic side chains to the opposite side of the same helix. Distribution of side chains along the α-helical axis can be viewed using the helical wheel. Since one turn in an α-helix is 3.6 residues long, each residue can be plotted every 360°/3.6 = 100° around a circle (viewed from the top of α-helix), as shown in Figure 2.7. Such a plot shows the projection of the position of the residues onto a plane perpendicular to the helical axis. One of the predicted helices in erythropoietin is shown in Figure 2.7, using an open circle for hydrophobic side chains and an open rectangle for hydrophilic side chains. It becomes immediately obvious that one side of the α-helix is highly hydrophobic, suggesting that this side forms an internal core, while the other side is relatively hydrophilic and is hence most likely exposed to the surface. Since many biologically important proteins function by interacting with other macromolecules, the information obtained from the helical wheel is extremely useful. For example, mutations of amino acids in the solvent-exposed side may lead to identification of regions responsible for biological activity, while mutations in the internal core may lead to altered protein stability.

β-SHEET

The second major secondary structural element found in proteins is the β-sheet. In contrast to the α-helix, which is built up from a continuous region with a peptide hydrogen bond linking every fourth amino acid, the β-sheet is comprised of peptide hydrogen bonds between

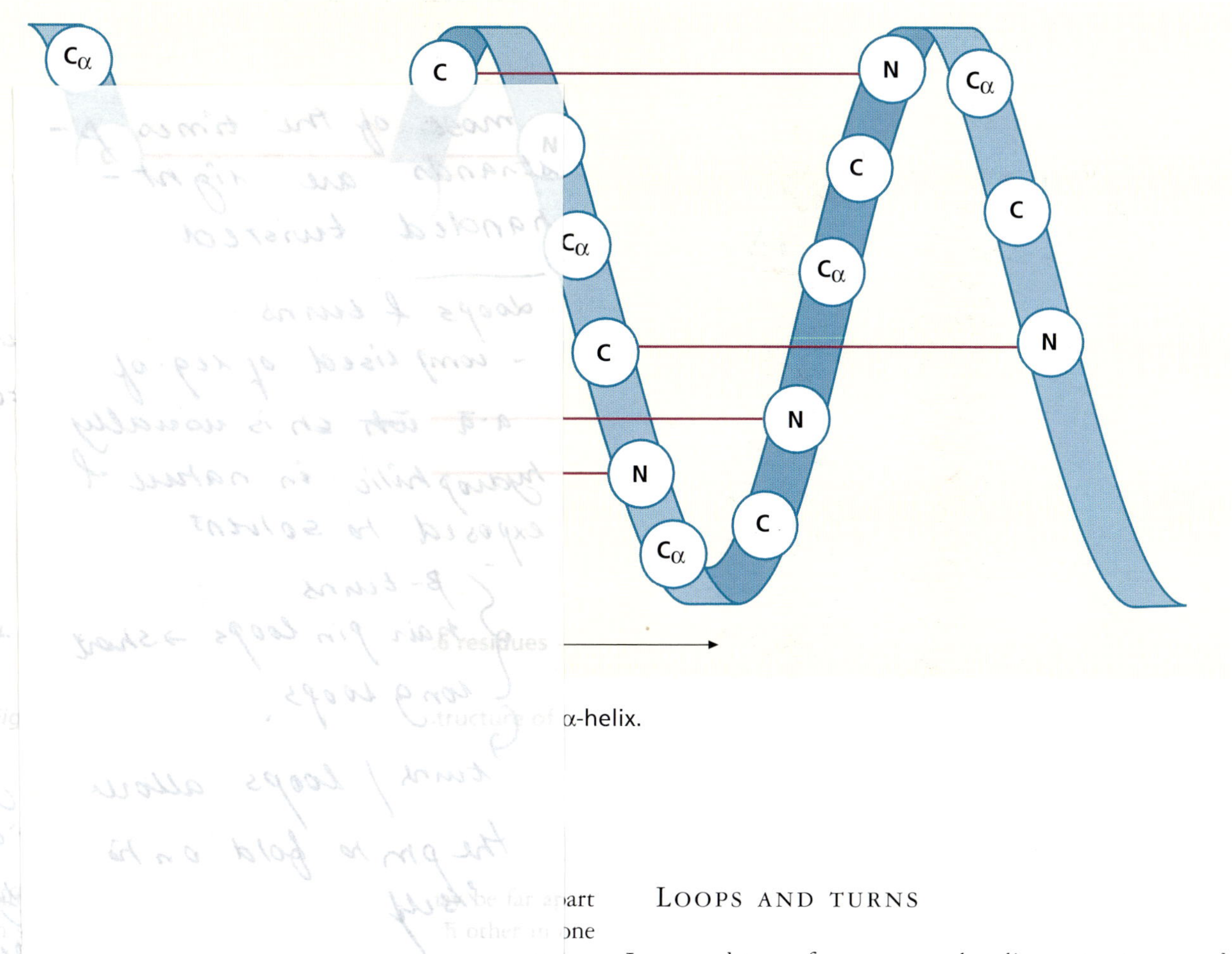

[illegible] α-helix.

[illegible] be far apart [illegible] other in one [illegible] other parallel or [illegible] is oriented in [illegible] bonds formed between the strands, while in antiparallel β-sheets, the polypeptide sequences are oriented in the opposite direction. In both structures, the C=O and NH groups project into opposite sides of the polypeptide chain, and hence a β-strand can interact from either side of that particular chain to form peptide hydrogen bonds with adjacent strands. Thus, more than two β-strands can contact each other either in a parallel or in an antiparallel manner, or even in combination. Such clustering can result in all the β-strands lying in a plane as a sheet. The β-strands which are at the edges of the sheet have unpaired alternating C=O and NH groups.

Side chains project perpendicularly to this plane in opposite directions and can interact with other side chains within the same β-sheet or with other regions of the molecule, or may be exposed to the solvent.

In almost all known protein structures, β-strands are right-handed twisted. This way, the β-strands adapt into widely different conformations. Depending on how they are twisted, all the side chains in the same strand or in different strands do not necessarily project in the same direction.

LOOPS AND TURNS

Loops and turns form more or less linear structures, and interact with each other to form a folded three-dimensional structure. They are comprised of an amino acid sequence which is usually hydrophilic and exposed to the solvent. These regions consist of β-turns (reverse turns), short hairpin loops, and long loops. Many hairpin loops are formed to connect two antiparallel β-strands.

As shown in Figure 2.5a, the amino acid sequences which form β-turns are relatively easy to predict, since turns must be present periodically to fold a linear sequence into a globular structure. Amino acids found most frequently in the β-turn are usually not found in α-helical or β-sheet structures. Thus, proline and glycine represent the least observed amino acids in these typical secondary structures. However, proline has an extremely high frequency of occurrence at the second position in the β-turn while glycine has a high preference at the third and fourth position of a β-turn.

Although loops are not as predictable as β-turns, amino acids with high frequency for β-turns also can form a long loop. Even though difficult to predict, loops are an important secondary structure, since they form a highly solvent exposed region of the protein molecules and allow the protein to fold onto itself.

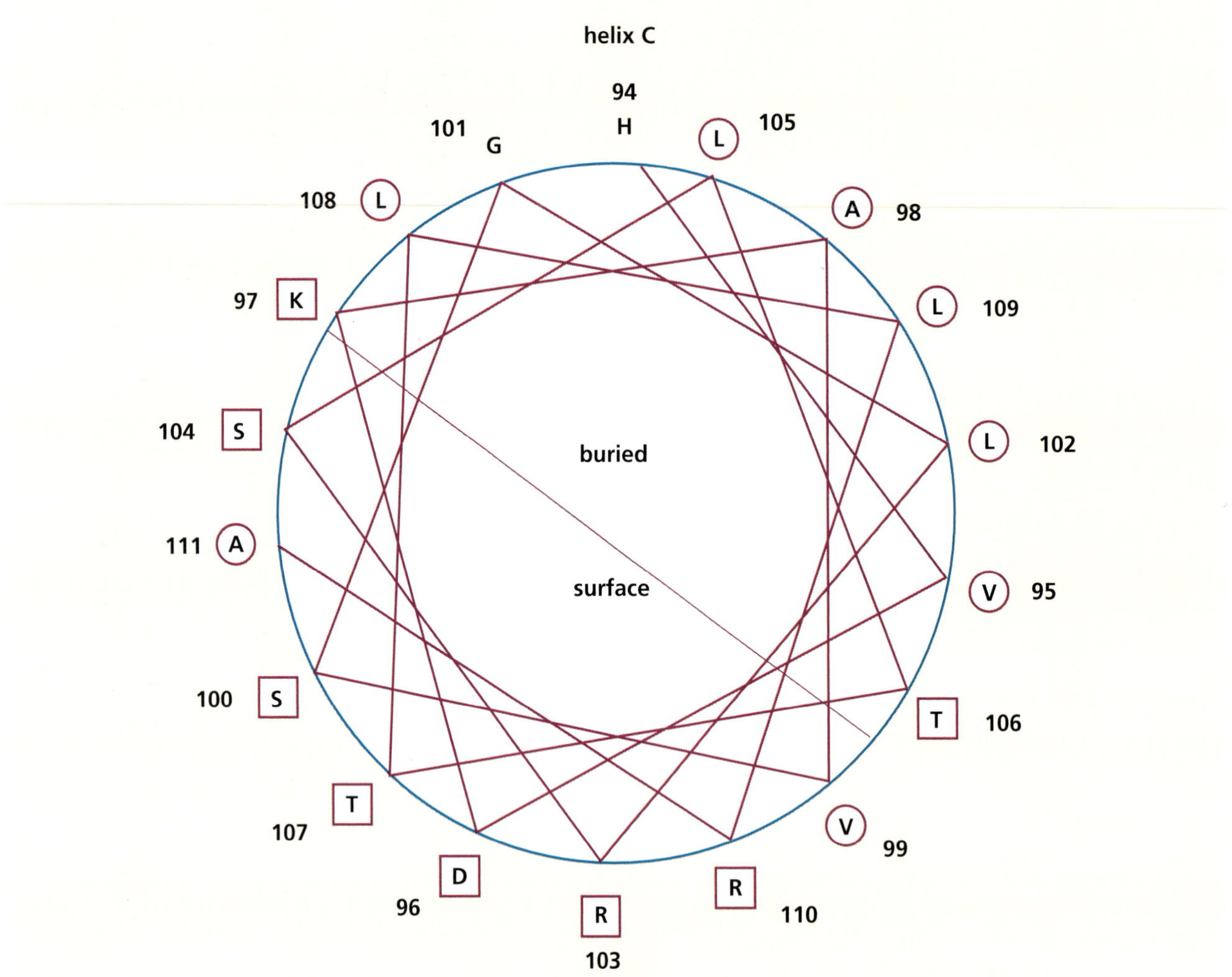

Figure 2.7. Helical wheel analysis of erythropoietin sequence, from His94 to Ala111 (Elliott, S., personal communication).

Tertiary Structure

Combination of the various secondary structures in a protein results in its three-dimensional structure. Many proteins fold into a fairly compact, globular structure.

The folding of a protein molecule into a distinct three-dimensional structure determines its function. Enzyme activity requires the exact coordination of catalytically important residues in the three-dimensional space. Binding of antibody to antigen and binding of growth factors and cytokines to their receptors all require a distinct, specific surface for high affinity binding. These interactions do not occur if the tertiary structures of antibodies, growth factors and cytokines are altered.

A unique tertiary structure of a protein can often result in the assembly of the protein into a distinct quaternary structure consisting of a fixed stoichiometry of protein chains within the complex. Assembly can occur between the same proteins or between different polypeptide chains. Each molecule in the complex is called a subunit. Actin and tubulin self-associate into F-actin and microtubule, while hemoglobin is a tetramer consisting of two α and two β subunits. Among the cytokines and growth factors, interferon-γ is a homodimer, while platelet-derived growth factor is a homodimer of either A or B chains or a heterodimer of the A and B chain. The formation of a quaternary structure occurs via non-covalent interactions or through disulfide bonds between the subunits.

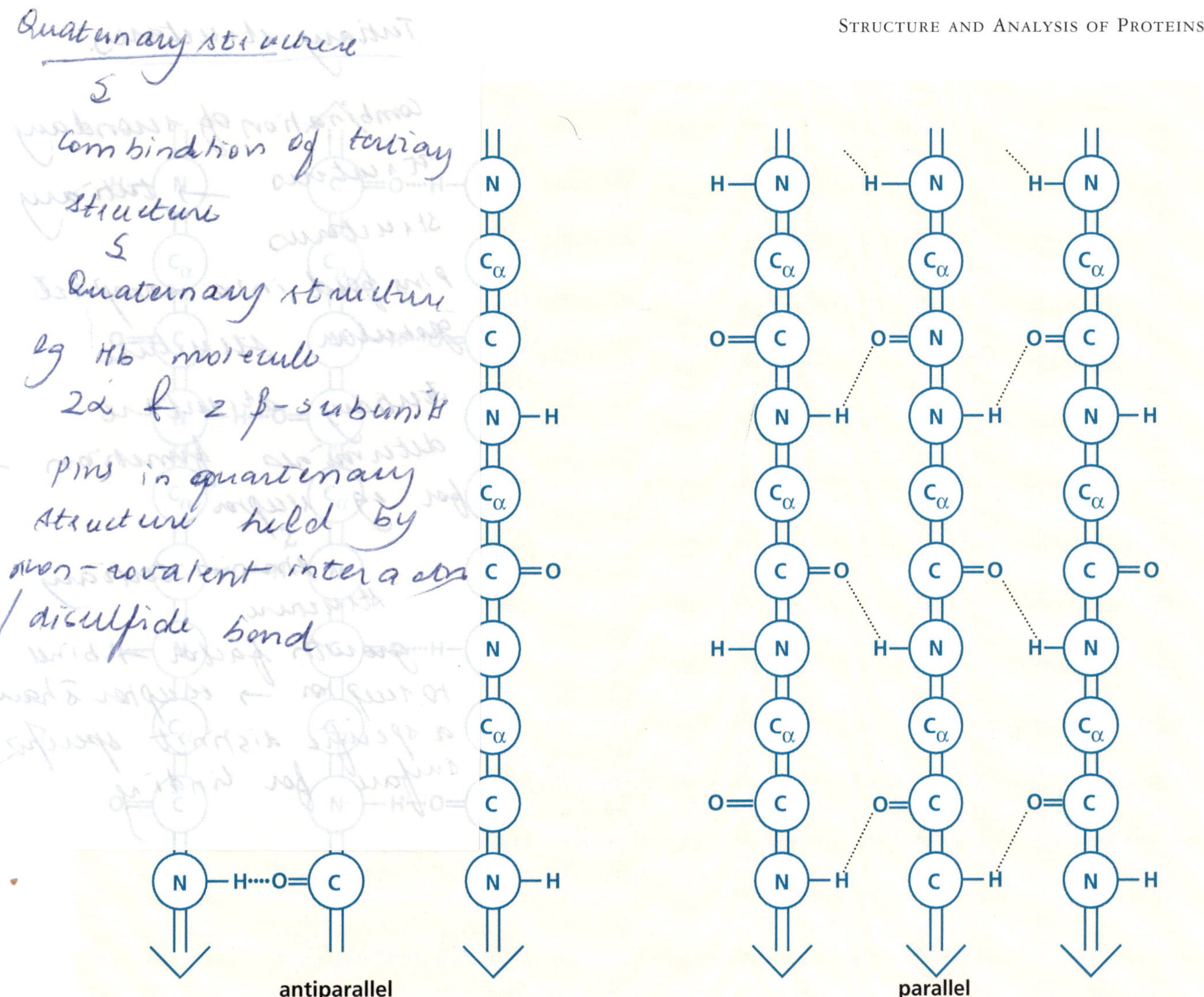

Figure 2.8. Schematic illustration of the structure of antiparallel (left side) and parallel (right side) β-sheet. Arrow indicates the direction of amino acid sequence from the N-terminus to C-terminus.

Forces

Interactions occurring between chemical groups in proteins are responsible for formation of their specific secondary, tertiary and quaternary structures. Either repulsive or attractive interactions can occur between different groups. Repulsive interactions consist of steric hindrance and electrostatic effects. Like-charges repel each other and bulky side chains, although they do not repel each other, cannot occupy the same space. Folding is also against the natural tendency to move toward randomness, i.e. increasing entropy. Folding leads to a fixed position of each atom and hence a decrease in entropy. For folding to occur this decrease in entropy, as well as the repulsive interactions, must be overcome by attractive interactions, i.e. hydrophobic interactions, hydrogen bonds, electrostatic attraction and van der Waals interactions. Hydration of proteins, discussed in the next section, also plays an important role in protein folding.

These interactions are all relatively weak and can be easily broken and formed. Hence, each folded protein structure arises from a fine balance between these repulsive and attractive interactions. The stability of the folded structure is a fundamental concern in developing protein therapeutics.

Hydrophobic interactions

The hydrophobic interaction reflects a summation of the van der Waals attractive forces among non-polar groups in the protein interior, which change the surrounding water structure necessary to accommodate these groups if they become exposed. The transfer of non-polar groups from the interior to the surface requires a large decrease in entropy so that hydrophobic interactions are essentially entropically driven. The resulting large positive free energy change prevents the transfer of non-polar groups from the largely sheltered interior to the more solvent exposed exterior of the protein molecule. Thus, non-polar groups preferentially reside in the protein interior while the more polar groups are exposed to the surface and surrounding environment. The partitioning of different amino acyl residues between the inside and outside of a protein correlates well with the hydration energy of their side chains, that is, their relative affinity for water.

Hydrogen bonds

The hydrogen bond is ionic in character since it depends strongly on the sharing of a proton between two electronegative atoms (generally oxygen and nitrogen atoms). Hydrogen bonds may form either between a protein atom and a water molecule or exclusively as protein intramolecular hydrogen bonds. Intramolecular interactions can have significantly more favorable free energies (because of entropic considerations) than intermolecular hydrogen bonds, so the contribution of all hydrogen bonds in the protein molecule to the stability of protein structures can be substantial. In addition, when the hydrogen bonds occur in the interior of protein molecules, the bonds become stronger due to the hydrophobic environment.

Electrostatic interactions

Electrostatic interactions occur between any two charged groups. According to Coulomb's law, if the charges are of the same sign, the interaction is repulsive with an increase in energy, but if they are opposite in sign it is attractive, with a lowering of energy. Electrostatic interactions are strongly dependent upon distance, according to Coulomb's law, and inversely related to the dielectric constant of the medium. Electrostatic interactions are much stronger in the interior of the protein molecule because of a lower dielectric constant. The numerous charged groups present on protein molecules can provide overall stability by the electrostatic attraction of opposite charges, for example, between negatively charged carboxyl groups and positively charged amino groups. However, the net effects of all possible pairs of charged groups must be considered. Thus, the free energy derived from electrostatic interactions is actually a property of the whole structure, not just of any single amino acid residue or cluster.

Van der Waals interactions

Weak van der Waals interactions exist between atoms (except the bare proton), whether they are polar or non-polar. They arise from net attractive interactions between permanent dipoles and/or induced (temporary and fluctuating) dipoles. However, when two atoms approach each other too closely, the repulsion between their electron clouds becomes strong and counterbalances the attractive forces. The repulsive force is even more sensitive to the distance between two atoms.

Hydration

Water molecules are bound to proteins internally and externally. Some water molecules occasionally occupy small internal cavities in the protein structure, and are hydrogen-bonded to peptide bonds and side chains of the protein and often to a prosthetic group, or cofactor, within the protein. The protein surface is large and consists of a mosaic of polar and non-polar amino acids, and it binds a large number of water molecules, i.e. it is hydrated, from the surrounding environment. As described in the previous section, water molecules trapped in the interior of protein molecules are bound more tightly to hydrogen-bonding donors and acceptors because of a lower dielectric constant.

Solvent around the protein surface clearly has a general role in hydrating peptide and side chains but might be expected to be rather mobile and non-specific in its interactions. Well-ordered water molecules can make significant contributions to protein stability. One water molecule can hydrogen-bond to two groups distant in the primary structure on a protein molecule, acting as a bridge between these groups. Such a water molecule may be highly restricted in motion, and can contribute to the stability, at least locally, of the protein, since such tight binding may exist only when these groups assume the proper configuration to accommodate a water molecule that is present only in the native state of the protein. Such hydration can also decrease the flexibility of the groups involved.

There is also evidence for solvation over hydrophobic groups on the protein surface. So-called hydrophobic hydration occurs because of the unfavorable nature of the interaction between water molecules and hydrophobic surfaces, resulting in the clustering of water molecules. Since this clustering is energetically unfavorable, such hydrophobic hydration does not contribute to the protein stability. However, this hydrophobic hydration facilitates hydrophobic interaction. This unfavorable hydration is diminished as the various hydrophobic groups come in contact either intramolecularly or intermolecularly, leading to the folding of intrachain structures or to protein-protein interactions.

Both the loosely and strongly bound water molecules can have an important impact, not only on protein stability but also on protein function. For example, certain enzymes function in non-aqueous solvent provided that a small amount of water, just enough to cover the protein surface, is present. Bound water can modulate the dynamics of surface groups, and such dynamics may be critical for enzyme function. Dried enzymes are, in general, inactive and become active after they absorb 0.2 g water per g protein. This amount of water is only sufficient to cover surface polar groups, yet may give sufficient flexibility for function.

Evidence that water bound to protein molecules has a different property from bulk water can be demonstrated by the presence of non-freezable water. Thus, when a protein solution is cooled below – 40 °C, a fraction of water, ~0.3 g water/g protein, does not freeze and can be detected by high resolution NMR. Several other techniques also detect a similar amount of bound water. This unfreezable water reflects the unique property of bound water that prevents it from adopting an ice structure.

Protein folding

Proteins become functional only when they assume a distinct tertiary structure. Many physiologically and therapeutically important proteins present their surface for recognition by interacting with molecules such as substrates, receptors, signaling proteins and cell-surface adhesion macromolecules. When recombinant proteins are produced in *Escherichia coli*, they often form inclusion bodies into which they are deposited as insoluble proteins. Formation of such insoluble states does not naturally occur in cells where they are normally synthesized and transported. Therefore, an *in vitro* process is required to refold insoluble recombinant proteins into their native, physiologically active state. This is usually accomplished by solubilizing the insoluble proteins with detergents or denaturants, followed by the purification and removal of these reagents concurrent with refolding the proteins (cf. Chapter 3).

Unfolded states of proteins are usually highly stable and soluble in the presence of denaturing agents. Once the proteins are folded correctly, they are also relatively stable. During the transition from the unfolded form to the native state, the protein must go through a multitude of other transition states in which it is not fully folded and denaturants or solubilizing agents are at low concentrations or even absent.

The refolding of proteins can be achieved in various ways. The dilution of proteins at high denaturant concentration into aqueous buffer will decrease both denaturant and protein concentration simultaneously. The addition of an aqueous buffer to a protein-denaturant solution also causes a decrease in concentrations of both denaturant and protein. The difference in these procedures is that, in the first case, both denaturant and protein concentrations are the lowest at the beginning of dilution and gradually increase as the process continues. In the second case, both denaturant and protein concentrations are highest at the beginning of dilution and gradually decrease as the dilution proceeds. Dialysis or the diafiltration of protein in the denaturant against an aqueous buffer resembles the second case, since the denaturant concentration decreases as the procedure continues. In this case, however, the protein concentration remains unchanged. Refolding can also be achieved by first binding the protein in denaturants to a solid phase, i.e. to a column matrix, and then equilibrating it with an aqueous buffer. In this case, protein concentrations are not well-defined. Each procedure has advantages and disadvantages and may be applicable for one protein, but not to another.

If proteins in the native state have disulfide bonds, cysteines must be correctly oxidized. Such oxidation may be done in various ways, e.g. air oxidation, glutathione catalyzed disulfide exchange, or adduct formation followed by reduction and oxidation or by disulfide reshuffling.

Protein folding has been a topic of intensive research since Anfinsen's demonstration that ribonuclease can be refolded from the fully reduced and denatured state in *in vitro* experiments. This folding can be achieved only if the amino acid sequence itself contains all information necessary for folding into the native structure. This is the case, at least partially, for many proteins. However, a lot of other proteins do not refold in a simple one-step process. Rather, they refold via various intermediates which are relatively compact and possess varying degrees of secondary structures, but which lack a rigid tertiary structure. Intrachain interactions of these preformed secondary structures eventually lead to the native state. However, the absence of a rigid structure in these preformed secondary structures can also expose a cluster of hydrophobic groups to those of other polypeptide chains, rather than to their own polypeptide segments, resulting in intermolecular aggregation. High efficiency in the recovery of native protein depends to a large extent on how this aggregation of intermediate forms is minimized. The use of chaperones or polyethylene glycol has been found quite effective for this purpose. The former are proteins which aid in the proper folding of other proteins by stabilizing intermediates in the folding process and the latter serves to solvate the protein during folding and diminishes interchain aggregation events.

When recombinant proteins are expressed in eukaryotic cells and secreted into media, the proteins are generally folded into the native conformation. If the proteins have sites for N-linked or O-linked glycosylation, they undergo varying degrees of glycosylation depending on the host cells used and level of expression. For many glycoproteins, glycosylation is not essential for folding, since they can be refolded into the native conformation without carbohydrates, nor is glycosylation often necessary for receptor binding and hence biological activity. However, glycosylation can alter important biological and physicochemical properties of proteins, such as pharmacokinetics, solubility, and stability.

Techniques Specifically Suitable for Characterizing Protein Folding

Conventional spectroscopic techniques used to obtain information on the folded structure of proteins are circular dichroism (CD), fluorescence, and Fourier transform infrared spectroscopies (FTIR). CD and FTIR are widely used to estimate the secondary structure of proteins. The α-helical content of a protein can be readily estimated by CD in the far UV region (180–260 nm) and by FTIR. FTIR signals from loop structures, however, occasionally overlap with those arising from an α-helix. The β-sheet gives weak CD signals, which are variable in peak positions and intensities due to twists of interacting β-strands, making far UV CD unreliable for evaluation of these structures. On the other hand, FTIR can reliably estimate the β-structure content as well as distinguish between parallel and antiparallel forms.

CD in the near UV region (250–340 nm) reflects the environment of aromatic amino acids, i.e. tryptophan, tyrosine and phenylalanine, as well as that of disulfide structures. Fluorescence spectroscopy yields information on the environment of tyrosine and tryptophan residues. CD and fluorescence signals in many cases are drastically altered upon refolding and hence can be used to follow the formation of the tertiary structure of a protein.

None of these techniques can give the folded structure at the atomic level, i.e. they give no information on the exact location of each amino acyl residue in the three-dimensional structure of the protein. This information can only be determined by X-ray crystallography or NMR. However, CD, FTIR, and fluorescence spectroscopic methods are fast and require lower protein concentrations than either NMR or X-ray crystallography, and are amenable for the examination of the protein under widely different conditions. When a naturally occurring form of the protein is available, these techniques, in particular near UV CD and fluorescence spectroscopies, can quickly address whether the refolded protein assumes the native folded structure.

Temperature dependence of these spectroscopic properties also provides information about protein folding. Since the folded structures of proteins are built upon cooperative interactions of many side chains and peptide bonds in a protein molecule, elimination of one interaction by heat can cause cooperative elimination of other interactions, leading to the unfolding of protein molecules. Thus, many proteins undergo a cooperative thermal transition over a narrow temperature range. Conversely, if the proteins are not fully folded, they may undergo non-cooperative thermal transitions as observed by a gradual signal change over a wider range of temperature.

Such a cooperative structure transition can also be examined by differential scanning calorimetry. When the structure unfolds, it requires heat. Such heat absorption can be determined using this highly sensitive calorimetry technique.

Hydrodynamic properties of proteins change greatly upon folding, going from elongated and expanded structures to compact globular ones. Sedimentation velocity and size exclusion chromatography (see under Analytical Techniques) are two frequently used techniques for the evaluation of hydrodynamic properties, although the latter is much more accessible. The sedimentation coefficient (how fast a molecule migrates in a centrifugal field) is a function of both the molecular weight and hydrodynamic size of the proteins, while elution position in size exclusion chromatography (how fast it migrates through pores) depends only on the hydrodynamic size (cf. Chapter 3). In both methods, comparison of the sedimentation coefficient or elution position with that of a globular protein with an identical molecular weight (or upon appropriate molecular weight normalization) gives information on how compactly the protein is folded.

For oligomeric proteins, the determination of molecular weight of the associated states and acquisition of the quaternary structure can be used to assess the folded structure. For strong interactions, specific protein association requires that intersubunit contact surfaces perfectly match each other. Such an associated structure, if obtained by covalent bonding, may be determined simply by sodium dodecylsulfate polyacrylamide gel electrophoresis. If protein association involves non-covalent interactions, sedimentation equilibrium or light scattering experiments can assess this phenomenon. Although these techniques have been used for many decades with some difficulty, emerging technologies in analytical ultracentrifugation and laser light scattering, and appropriate software for analyzing the results, have greatly facilitated their general use, as described in detail below.

Two fundamentally different light scattering techniques can be used in characterizing recombinant proteins. "Static" light scattering measures the intensity of the scattered light. "Dynamic" light scattering measures the fluctuations in the scattered light intensity as molecules diffuse in and out of a very small scattering region (Brownian motion).

Static light scattering is often used on-line in conjunction with size-exclusion chromatography (SEC). The scattering signal is proportional to the product of molecular mass times weight concentration. Dividing this signal by one proportional to the concentration, such as obtained from an UV absorbance or refractive index detector, then gives a direct and absolute measure of the mass of each peak eluting from the column, independent of molecular conformation and elution position. This SEC-static scattering combination allows rapid identification of whether the native state of a protein is a monomer or an oligomer and the stoichiometry of multi-protein complexes. It is also very useful in identifying the mass of aggregates which may be present, and thus is useful for evaluating protein stability.

Dynamic light scattering (DLS) measures the diffusion rate of the molecules, which can be translated into the Stokes radius, a measure of hydrodynamic size. Although the Stokes radius is strongly correlated with molecular mass, it is also strongly influenced by molecular shape (conformation) and thus DLS is far less accurate than static scattering for measuring molecular mass. The great strength of DLS is its ability to cover a very wide size range in one measurement, and to detect very small amounts of large aggregates (< 0.01% by weight). Other important advantages over static scattering with SEC are a wide choice of buffer conditions and no potential loss of species through sticking to a column.

An analytical ultracentrifuge incorporates an optical system and special rotors and cells in a high speed centrifuge to permit measurement of the concentration of a sample versus position within a spinning centrifuge cell. There are two primary strategies: analyzing either the sedimentation velocity or the sedimentation equilibrium. When analyzing the sedimentation velocity the rotor is spun at very high speed, so the protein sample will completely sediment and form a pellet. The rate at which the protein pellets is measured by the optical system to derive the sedimentation coefficient, which depends on both mass and molecular conformation. When more than one species is present (e.g. a monomer plus a covalent dimer degradation product), a separation is achieved based on the relative sedimentation coefficient of each species.

Because the sedimentation coefficient is sensitive to molecular conformation, and can be measured with high precision (~0.5 %), sedimentation velocity can detect even fairly subtle differences in conformation. This ability can be used, for example, to confirm that a recombinant protein has the same conformation as the natural wild-type protein, or to detect small changes in [illegible] cture with changes in the pH or salt [illegible] ay be too subtle [illegible]) or differential [illegible]

[illegible] er rotor speed [illegible] dimentation [illegible] the outside [illegible] centration [illegible] by diffusion [illegible] n. After [illegible] n equi[illegible] on are [illegible] anges [illegible] concentra[illegible] molecular mass and [illegible] Thus, self-association for the formation of dimers or higher oligomers (whether reversible or irreversible) is readily detected, as are binding interactions between different proteins. For reversible association, it is possible to determine the strength of the binding interaction by measuring samples over a wide range of protein concentrations.

In biotechnology applications, sedimentation equilibrium is often used as the "gold standard" for confirming that a recombinant protein has the expected molecular mass and biologically active state of oligomerization in solution. It can also be used to determine the average amount of glycosylation or conjugation of moieties such as polyethylene glycol. The measurement of binding affinities for receptor-cytokine, antigen-antibody, or other interaction can also sometimes serve as a functional characterization of recombinant proteins (although some such interactions are too strong to be measured by this method).

Site specific chemical modification and proteolytic digestion are also powerful techniques for studying the folding of proteins. The extent of chemical modification or proteolytic digestion depends on whether the specific sites are exposed to the solvent or are buried in the interior of the protein molecules and are thus inaccessible to these modifications. For example, trypsin cleaves peptide bonds on the C-terminal side of basic residues. Although most proteins contain several basic residues, brief exposure of the native protein to trypsin usually generates only a few peptides, as cleavage occurs only at the accessible basic residues, whereas the same treatment can generate many more peptides when done on the denatured (unfolded) protein, since all the basic residues are now accessible, cf. peptide mapping.

Protein stability

Although freshly isolated proteins may be folded into a distinct three-dimensional structure, this folded structure is not necessarily retained indefinitely in aqueous solution. The reason is that proteins are neither chemically nor physically stable. The protein surface is chemically highly heterogeneous and contains reactive groups. Long term exposure of these groups to environmental stresses causes various chemical alterations. Many proteins, including growth factors and cytokines, have cysteine residues. If some of them are in a free or sulfhydryl form, they may undergo oxidation and disulfide exchange. Oxidation can also occur on methionyl residues. Hydrolysis can occur on peptide bonds and on amides of asparagine and glutamine residues. Other chemical modifications can occur on peptide bonds, tryptophan, tyrosine, and amino and carboxyl groups. Table 2.4 lists both a number of reactions that can occur during purification and storage of proteins and methods that can be used to detect such changes.

	Physical property effected	Method of analysis
Oxidation Cys Disulfide intrachain interchain Met, Trp, Tyr	hydrophobicity size hydrophobicity	RP-HPLC, SDS-PAGE size exclusion chromatography mass spectrometry
Peptide bond Hydrolysis	size	size exclusion chromatography SDS-PAGE
N to O migration Ser, Thr	hydrophobicity chemistry	RP-HPLC inactive in Edman reaction
α-Carboxy to β-Carboxy migration Asp, Asn	hydrophobicity chemistry	RP-HPLC inactive in Edman reaction
Deamidation Asn, Gln	charge	ion exchange chromatography
Acylation α-amino group, ε-amino group	charge	ion exchange chromatography mass spectrometry
Esterification/Carboxylation Glu, Asp, C-terminal	charge	ion exchange chromatography mass spectrometry
Secondary structure changes	hydrophobicity size sec/tert structure sec/tert structure aggregation sec/tert structure, aggregation	RP-HPLC size exclusion chromatography CD FTIR light scattering analytical ultracentrifugation

Table 2.4. Common reactions affecting stability of proteins.

Physical stability of a protein is expressed as the difference in free energy, ΔG_u, between the native and denatured states. Thus, protein molecules are in equilibrium between the above two states. As long as this unfolding is reversible and ΔG_u is positive, it does not matter how small the ΔG_u is. In many cases, this reversibility does not hold. This is often seen when ΔG_u is decreased by heating. Most proteins denature upon heating and subsequent aggregation of the denatured molecules results in irreversible denaturation. Thus, unfolding is made irreversible by aggregation:

$$\text{Native state} \underset{\Delta G_u}{\Leftrightarrow} \text{Denatured state} \underset{k}{\Rightarrow} \text{Aggregated state}$$

Therefore, any stresses that decrease ΔG_u and increase k will cause the accumulation of irreversibly inactivated forms of the protein. Such stresses may include chemical modifications as described above and physical parameters, such as pH, ionic strength, protein concentration, and temperature. Development of a suitable formulation that prolongs the shelf-life of a recombinant protein is essential when it is to be used as a human therapeutic.

The use of protein stabilizing agents to enhance storage stability of proteins has become customary. These compounds affect protein stability by increasing ΔG_u. These compounds, however, may also increase k and hence their net effect on long-term storage of proteins may vary among proteins, as well as on the storage conditions.

When unfolding is irreversible due to aggregation, minimizing the irreversible step should increase the stability, and often this may be attained by the addition of mild detergents. Prior to selecting the proper detergent concentration and type, however, their effects on ΔG_u must be carefully evaluated.

Another approach for enhancing storage stability of proteins is to lyophilize, or freeze-dry, the proteins (cf. Chapter 4). Lyophilization can minimize the aggregation step during storage, since both chemical modification and aggregation is reduced in the absence of water. The effects of a lyophilization process itself on ΔG_u and k are not fully understood and hence such a process must be optimized for each protein therapeutic.

Analytical Techniques

In one of the previous sections on 'Techniques Specifically Suitable for Characterizing Folding' a number of (spectroscopic) techniques were mentioned that can be specifically used to monitor protein folding. These were: CD, FTIR, fluorescence, and DSC. Moreover, analytical ultracentrifugation and light scattering techniques were discussed in more detail. In this section other techniques will be discussed.

Blotting Techniques

Blotting methods form an important niche in biotechnology. They are used to detect very low levels of unique molecules in a milieu of proteins, nucleic acids, and other cellular components. They can detect aggregates or breakdown products occurring during long-term storage and they can be used to detect components from the host cells used in producing recombinant proteins.

Biomolecules are transferred to a membrane ('blotting'), and this membrane is then probed with specific reagents to identify the molecule of interest. Membranes used in protein blots are made of a variety of material including nitrocellulose, nylon, and polyvinylidine difluoride (PVDF), all of which avidly bind protein.

Liquid samples can be analyzed by methods called dot blots or slot blots. A solution containing the biomolecule of interest is filtered through a membrane which captures the biomolecule. The difference between a dot blot and a slot blot is that the former uses a circular or disk format, while the latter is a rectangular configuration. The latter method allows for a more precise quantification of the desired biomolecule by scanning methods and relating the integrated results to that obtained with known amounts of material.

Often the sample is subjected to some type of fractionation, such as polyacrylamide gel electrophoresis, prior to the blotting step. An early technique, Southern blotting, named after the discoverer, E.M. Southern, is used to detect DNA fragments. When this procedure was adapted to RNA fragments and to proteins, other compass coordinates were chosen as labels for these procedures, i.e. northern blots for RNA and western blots for proteins. Western blots involve the use of labeled antibodies to detect specific proteins.

Transfer of proteins

Following polyacrylamide gel electrophoresis, the transfer of proteins from the gel to the membrane can be accomplished in a number of ways. Originally, blotting was achieved by capillary action. In this commonly used method, the membrane is placed between the gel and absorbent paper. Fluid from the gel is drawn toward the absorbent paper and the protein is captured by the intervening membrane. A blot, or impression, of the protein within the gel is thus made.

The transfer of proteins to the membrane can occur under the influence of an electric field, as well. The electric field is applied perpendicularly to the original field used in separation so that the maximum distance the protein needs to migrate is only the thickness of the gel, and hence the transfer of proteins can occur very rapidly. This latter method is called electroblotting.

Detection systems

Once the transfer has occurred, the next step is to identify the presence of the desired protein. In addition to various colorimetric staining methods, the blots can be probed with reagents specific for certain proteins, as for example, antibodies to a protein of interest. This technique is called immunoblotting. In the biotechnology field, immunoblotting is used as an identity test for the product of interest. An antibody that recognizes the desired protein is used in this instance. Secondly, immunoblotting is sometimes used to show the absence of host proteins. In this instance, the antibodies are raised against proteins of the organism in which the recombinant protein has been expressed. This latter method can attest to the purity of the desired protein.

Table 2.5 lists major steps needed for the blotting procedure to be successful. Once the transfer of proteins is completed, residual protein binding sites on the membrane need to be blocked so that antibodies used for detection react only at the location of the target molecule, or antigen, and not at some non-specific location. After blocking, the specific antibody is incubated with the membrane.

The antibody reacts with a specific protein on the membrane only at the location of that protein because of its specific interaction with its antigen. When immunoblotting techniques are used, methods are still needed to recognize the location of the interaction of the antibody with its specific protein. A number of procedures can be used to detect this complex (see Table 2.6).

The antibody itself can be labeled with a radioactive marker such as ^{125}I and placed in direct contact with X-ray film. After exposure of the membrane to the film for a suitable period, the film is developed and a photographic negative is made of the location of radioactivity on the membrane. Alternatively, the antibody can be linked to an enzyme which, upon the addition of appropriate reagents,

1. Transfer protein to membrane e.g. by electroblotting.
2. Block residual protein binding sites on membrane with extraneous proteins such as milk proteins.
3. Treat membrane with antibody which recognizes the protein of interest. If this antibody is labeled with a detecting group then go to step 5.
4. Incubate membrane with secondary antibody which recognizes primary antibody used in step 3. This antibody is labeled with a detecting group.
5. Treat the membrane with suitable reagents to locate the site of membrane attachment of the labeled antibody in step 4 or step 5.

Table 2.5. Major steps in blotting proteins to membranes.

catalyzes a color or light reaction at the site of the antibody. These procedures entail purification of the antibody and specifically label it. More often, "secondary" antibodies are used. The primary antibody is the one which recognizes the protein of interest. The secondary antibody is then an antibody that specifically recognizes the primary antibody. Quite commonly, the primary antibody is raised in rabbits. The secondary antibody may then be an antibody raised in another animal, such as goat, which recognizes rabbit antibodies. Since this secondary antibody recognizes rabbit antibodies in general, it can be used as a generic reagent to detect rabbit antibodies in a number of different proteins of interest that have been raised in rabbits. Thus, the primary antibody specifically recognizes and complexes a unique protein, and the secondary antibody, suitably labeled, is used for detection (cf. ELISA and Figure 2.10).

The secondary antibody can be labeled with a radioactive or enzymatic marker group and used to detect several different primary antibodies. Thus, rather than purifying a number of different primary antibodies, only one secondary antibody needs to be purified and labeled for recognition of all the primary antibodies. Because of their wide use, many common secondary antibodies are commercially available in kits containing the detection system and follow routine, straightforward procedures.

In addition to antibodies raised against the amino acyl constituents of proteins, specific antibodies can be used which recognize unique post-translational components in proteins, such as phosphotyrosyl residues, which are important during signal transduction, and carbohydrate moieties of glycoproteins.

Figure 2.9 illustrates a number of detection methods that can be used on immunoblots. The primary antibody, or if convenient, the secondary antibody, can have an appropriate label for detection. They may be labeled with a radioactive tag as mentioned previously. Secondly, these antibodies can be coupled with an enzyme such as horseradish peroxidase (HRP) or alkaline phosphatase (AP). Substrate is added and is converted to an insoluble, colored product at the site of the protein-primary antibody-secondary antibody-HRP product. An alternative substrate can be used which yields a chemiluminescent product. A chemical reaction leads to the production of light which can expose photographic or X-ray film. The chromogenic and chemiluminescent detection systems have comparable sensitivities to radioactive methods. The former detection methods are displacing the latter method, since problems associated with handling radioactive material and radioactive waste solutions are eliminated.

As illustrated in Figure 2.9, streptavidin, or alternatively avidin, and biotin can play an important role in detecting proteins on immunoblots. This is because biotin forms very tight complexes with streptavidin and avidin. Secondly, these proteins are multimeric and contain four binding sites for biotin. When biotin is covalently linked to proteins such as antibodies and enzymes, streptavidin binds to the covalently bound biotin, thus recognizing the site on the membrane where the protein of interest is located.

1. Antibodies are labeled with radioactive markers such as ^{125}I.
2. Antibodies are linked to an enzyme such as horseradish peroxidase (HRP) or alkaline phosphatase (AP). On incubation with substrate an insoluble colored product is formed at the location of the antibody. Alternatively, the location of the antibody can be detected using a substrate which yields a chemiluminescent product, an image of which is made on photographic film.
3. Antibody is labeled with biotin. Streptavidin or avidin is added to strongly bind to the biotin. Each streptavidin molecule has four binding sites. The remaining binding sites can combine with other biotin molecules which are covalently linked to HRP or to AP.

Table 2.6. Detection methods used in blotting techniques.

Immunoassays

ELISA

Enzyme-linked immunosorbent assay (ELISA) provides a means to quantitatively measure extremely small amounts of

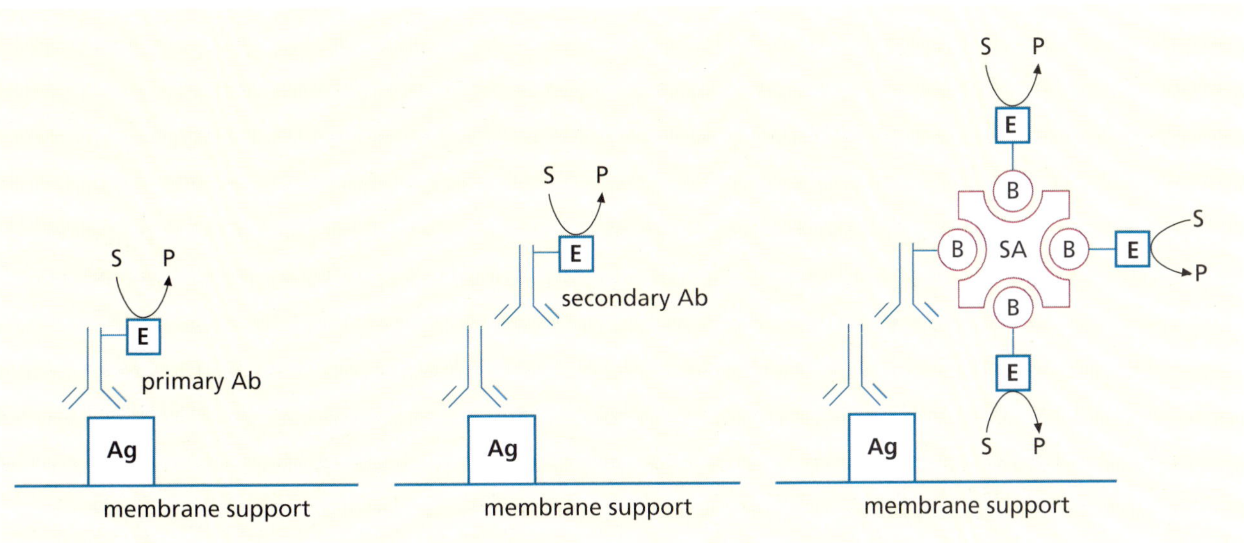

Figure 2.9. Common immunoblotting detection systems used to detect antigens, Ag, on membranes. Abbreviations used: Ab, antibody; E, enzyme, such as horseradish peroxidase or alkaline phosphatase; S, substrate; P, product, either colored and insoluble or chemiluminescent; B, biotin; Sa, streptavidin.

proteins in biological fluids and serves as a tool for analyzing specific proteins during purification. This procedure takes advantage of the observation that plastic surfaces are able to adsorb low but detectable amounts of proteins. This is a solid phase assay. Therefore, antibodies against a certain desired protein are allowed to adsorb to the surface of microtitration plates. Each plate may contain up to 96 wells so that multiple samples can be assayed. After incubating the antibodies in the wells of the plate for a specific period of time, excess antibody is removed and residual protein binding sites on the plastic are blocked by incubation with an inert protein. Several microtitration plates can be prepared at one time since the antibodies coating the plates retain their binding capacity for an extended period. During the ELISA, sample solution containing the protein of interest is incubated in the wells and the protein (Ag) is captured by the antibodies coating the well surface. Excess sample is removed and other antibodies which now have an enzyme (E) linked to them are added to react with the bound antigen.

The format described above is called a sandwich assay since the antigen of interest is located between the antibody on the titer well surface and the antibody containing the linked enzyme. Figure 2.10 illustrates a number of formats that can be used in an ELISA. A suitable substrate is added and the enzyme linked to the antibody-antigen-antibody well complex converts this compound to a colored product. The amount of product obtained is proportional to the enzyme adsorbed in the well of the plate. A standard curve can be prepared if known concentrations of antigen are tested in this system, and the amount of antigen in unknown samples can be estimated from this standard curve. A number of enzymes can be used in ELISAs. However, the most common ones are horseradish peroxidase and alkaline phosphatase. A variety of substrates for each enzyme are available which yield colored products when catalyzed by the linked enzyme. Absorbance of the colored product solutions is measured on plate readers, instruments which rapidly measure the absorbance in all 96 wells of the microtitration plate, and data processing can be automated for rapid throughput of information. Note that detection approaches partly parallel those discussed in the section on 'Blotting.' The above ELISA format is only one of many different methods. For example, the microtitration wells may be coated directly with the antigen rather than having a specific antibody attached to the surface. Quantitation is made by comparison with known quantities of antigen used to coat individual wells.

Another approach, this time subsequent to the binding of antigen either directly to the surface or to an antibody on the surface, is to use an antibody specific to the antibody binding the protein antigen, that is, a secondary antibody. This latter, secondary, antibody contains the linked enzyme used for detection. As already discussed in the section on blotting, the advantage to this approach is that such antibodies can be obtained in high purity and with the desired enzyme linked to them from commercial sources. Thus, a single source of enzyme-linked antibody can be used in assays for different protein antigens. Should a sandwich assay be used, then antibodies from different species need to be used for each side of the sandwich. A possible scenario is that rabbit antibodies are used to coat the microtitration

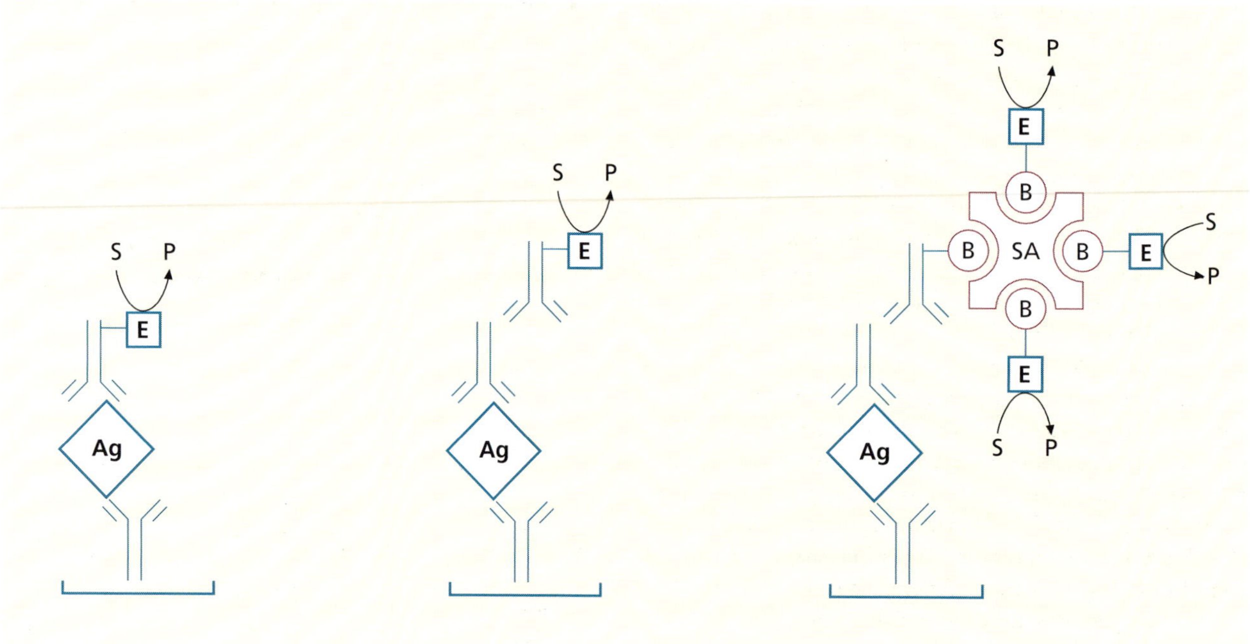

Figure 2.10. Examples of several formats for ELISA in which the specific antibody is adsorbed to the surface of a microtitration plate. See figure 9 for abbreviations used. The antibody is represented by the Y type structure. The product, P, is colored and the amount generated is measured with a spectrometer or plate reader.

wells; mouse antibodies, possibly a monoclonal antibody, are used to complex with the antigen and then a goat anti-mouse immunoglobulin containing linked HRP or AP is used for detection purposes.

As with immunoblots discussed above, streptavidin or avidin can be used in these assays if biotin is covalently linked to the antibodies and enzymes (Figure 2.10).

If a radioactive label is used in place of the enzyme in the above procedure, then the assay is a solid phase radioimmunoassay (RIA). Assays are moving away from the use of radioisotopes, because of problems with safety and disposal of radioactive waste and since non-radioactive assays have comparable sensitivities.

Electrophoresis

Analytical methodologies for measuring protein properties stem from those used in their purification. The major difference is that systems used for analysis have a higher resolving power and detection limit than those used in purification. The two major methods for analysis have their bases in chromatographic or electrophoretic techniques.

Polyacrylamide gel electrophoresis

One of the earliest methods for analysis of proteins is polyacrylamide gel electrophoresis (PAGE). In this assay, proteins, being amphoteric molecules with both positive and negative charge groups in their primary structure, are separated according to their net electrical charge. A second factor which is responsible for the separation is the mass of the protein. Thus, one can consider more precisely that the charge to mass ratio of proteins determines how they are separated in an electrical field. The charge of the protein can be controlled by the pH of the solution in which the protein is separated. The farther away the protein is from its pI value, that is, the pH at which it has a net charge of zero, the greater is the net charge and hence the greater is its charge to mass ratio. Therefore, the direction and speed of migration of the protein depend on the pH of the gel. If the pH of the gel is above its pI value, then the protein is negatively charged and hence migrates toward the anode. The higher the pH of the gel the faster the migration. This type of electrophoresis is called native gel electrophoresis.

The major component of polyacrylamide gels is water. However, they provide a flexible support so that after a protein has been subjected to an electrical field for an appropriate period of time, it provides a matrix to hold the proteins in place until they can be detected with suitable reagents. By adjusting the amount of acrylamide that is used in these gels, one can control the migration of material within the gel. The more acrylamide, the more hindrance for the protein to migrate in an electrical field.

The addition of a detergent, sodium dodecyl sulfate (SDS), to the electrophoretic separation system allows for the separation to take place primarily as a function of the size of the protein. Dodecyl sulfate ions form complexes with proteins, resulting in an unfolding of the proteins, and the amount of detergent that is complexed is proportional to the mass of the protein. The larger the protein, the more detergent that is complexed. Dodecyl sulfate is a negatively charged ion. When proteins are in a solution of SDS, the net effect is that the own charge of the protein is overwhelmed by that of the dodecyl sulfate complexed with it, so that the proteins take on net negative charge proportional to their mass.

Polyacrylamide gel electrophoresis in the presence of sodium dodecyl sulfates is commonly known as SDS-PAGE. All the proteins take on a net negative charge, with larger proteins binding more SDS but with the charge to mass ratio being fairly constant among the proteins. An example of SDS-PAGE is shown in Figure 2.11. Here, SDS-PAGE are used to monitor expression of G-CSF receptor and of G-CSF (panel B) in different culture media.

Since all proteins have essentially the same charge to mass ratio, how can separation occur? This is done by controlling the concentration of acrylamide in the path of proteins migrating in an electrical field. The greater the acrylamide concentration, the more difficult it is for large protein molecules to migrate relative to smaller protein molecules. This is sometimes thought of as a sieving effect, since the greater the acrylamide concentration, the smaller the pore size within the polyacrylamide gel. Indeed, if the acrylamide concentration is sufficiently high, some high molecular weight proteins may not migrate at all within the gel. Since in SDS-PAGE the proteins are denatured, their hydrodynamic size, and hence the degree of retardation by the sieving effects, is directly related to their mass. Proteins containing disulfide bonds will have a much more compact structure and higher mobility for their mass unless the disulfides are reduced prior to electrophoresis.

As described above, native gel electrophoresis and SDS-PAGE are quite different in terms of the mechanism of protein separation. In native gel electrophoresis, the proteins are in the native state and migrate on their own charges. Thus, this electrophoresis can be used to characterize proteins in the native state. In SDS-PAGE, proteins are unfolded and migrate based on their molecular mass. As an intermediate case, Blue native electrophoresis is developed, in which proteins are bound by a dye, Coomassie blue, used to stain protein bands. This dye is believed to bind to the hydrophobic surface of the proteins and to add negative charges to the proteins. The dye-bound proteins are still in the native state and migrate based on the net charges, which depend on the intrinsic charges of the proteins and the amounts of the negatively charged dye. This is particularly useful for analyzing membrane proteins, which tend to aggregate in the absence of detergents. The dye prevents the proteins from aggregation by binding to their hydrophobic surface.

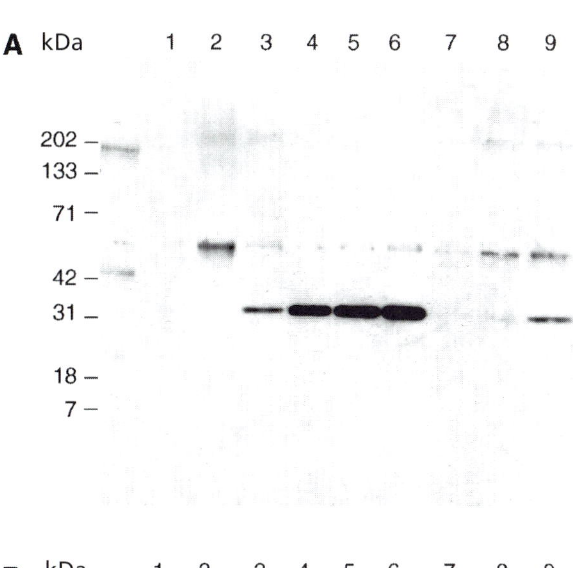

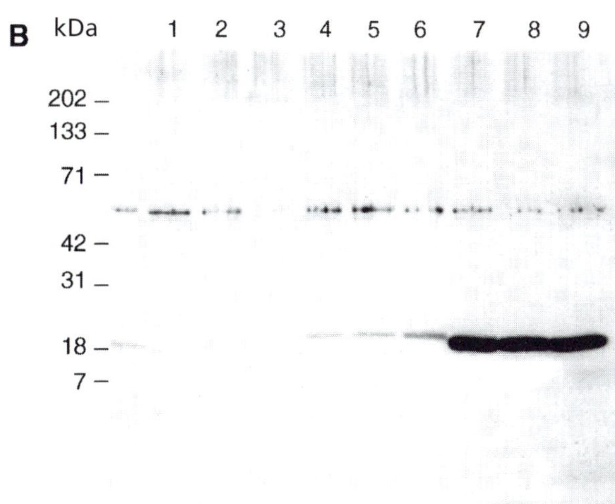

Figure 2.11. SDS-PAGE of G-CSF receptor, about 35 kDa (panel A) and G-CSF, about 20 kDa (panel B). These proteins are expressed in different culture media (lane 1–9). Positions of molecular weight standards are given on the left side. The bands are developed with antibody against G-CSF receptor (panel A) or G-CSF (panel B) after blotting.

Isoelectric focusing (IEF)

Another method to separate proteins based on their electrophoretic properties is to take advantage of their iso-electric point. In a first run a pH gradient is established within the gel using a mixture of small molecular weight ampholytes with varying pI values. The high pH conditions are established at the site of the cathode. Then, the protein is brought on the gel, e.g. at the site where the pH is 7. In the electrical field the protein will migrate until it reaches the pH on the gel where its net charge is zero. If the protein were to migrate away from this pH value it could gain a charge and migrate toward its pI value again, leading to a focusing effect.

2-Dimensional gel electrophoresis

The above methods can be combined into a procedure called 2-D gel electrophoresis. Proteins are first fractionated by isoelectric focusing based upon their pI values. They are then subjected to SDS-PAGE perpendicular to the first dimension and fractionated based on the molecular weights of proteins. SDS-PAGE cannot be performed before isoelectric focusing, since once SDS binds to and denatures the proteins they no longer migrate based on their pI values.

Detection of proteins within polyacrylamide gels

Although the polyacrylamide gels provide a flexible support for the proteins, with time the proteins will diffuse and spread within the gel. Consequently, the usual practice is to fix the proteins or trap them at the location where they migrated to. This is accomplished by placing the gels in a fixing solution in which the proteins become insoluble.

There are many methods for staining proteins in gels, but the two most common and well-studied methods are either staining with Coomassie blue or by a method using silver. The latter method is used if increased sensitivity is required. The principle of developing the Coomassie blue stain is the hydrophobic interaction of a dye with the protein. Thus, the gel takes on a color wherever a protein is located. Using standard amounts of proteins, the amount of protein or contaminant may be estimated. Quantification using the silver staining method is less precise. However, due to the increased sensitivity of this method, very low levels of contaminants can be detected. These fixing and staining procedures denature the proteins. Hence, proteins separated under native conditions, as in native or Blue native gel electrophoresis, will be denatured. To maintain the native state, the gels can be stained with copper or other metal ions.

Capillary electrophoresis

With recent advances in instrumentation and technology, capillary electrophoresis has gained an increased presence in the analysis of recombinant proteins. Rather than having a matrix, as in polyacrylamide gel electrophoresis through which the proteins migrate, they are free in solution in an electric field within the confines of a capillary tube with a diameter of 25–50 micrometers. The capillary tube passes through an ultraviolet light or fluorescence detector that measures the presence of proteins migrating in the electric field. The movement of one protein relative to another is a function of the molecular mass and the net charge on the protein. The latter can be influenced by pH and analytes in the solution. This technique has only partially gained acceptance for routine analysis, because of difficulties in reproducibility of the capillaries and in validating this system. Nevertheless, it is a powerful analytical tool for the characterization of recombinant proteins during process development and in stability studies.

Chromatography

Chromatography techniques are used extensively in biotechnology not only in protein purification procedures (cf. Chapter 3), but also in assessing the integrity of the product. Routine procedures are highly automated so that comparisons of similar samples can be made. An analytical system consists of an autosampler which will take a known amount (usually a known volume) of material for analysis and automatically places it in the solution stream headed toward a separation column used to fractionate the sample. Another part of this system is a pump module which provides a reproducible flow rate. In addition, the pumping system can provide a gradient which changes properties of the solution such as pH, ionic strength, and hydrophobicity. A detection system (or possibly multiple detectors in series) is located at the outlet of the column. This measures the relative amount of protein exiting the column. Coupled to the detector is a data acquisition system which takes the signal from the detector and integrates it into a value related to the amount of material (see Figure 2.12). When the protein appears, the signal begins to increase, and as the protein passes through the detector, the signal subsequently decreases. The area under the peak of the signal is proportional to the amount of material which has passed through the detector. By analyzing known amounts of protein, an area versus amount of protein plot can be generated and this may be used to estimate the amount of this protein in the sample under other circumstances. Another benefit of this integrated chromatography system is that low levels of components which appear over time can be estimated relative to the major desired protein being analyzed. This is a particularly useful function when the long-term stability of the product is under evaluation.

Chromatographic systems offer a multitude of different strategies for successfully separating protein mixtures and for quantifying individual protein components (cf. Chapter 3). The following describes some of these strategies.

Size exclusion chromatography

As the name implies, this procedure separates proteins based on their size or molecular weight or shape. The matrix consists of very fine beads containing cavities and pores accessible to molecules of a certain size or smaller, but inaccessible to larger molecules. The principle of this technique is the distribution of molecules between the volume of solution within the beads versus the volume of solution surrounding the beads. Small molecules have access to a

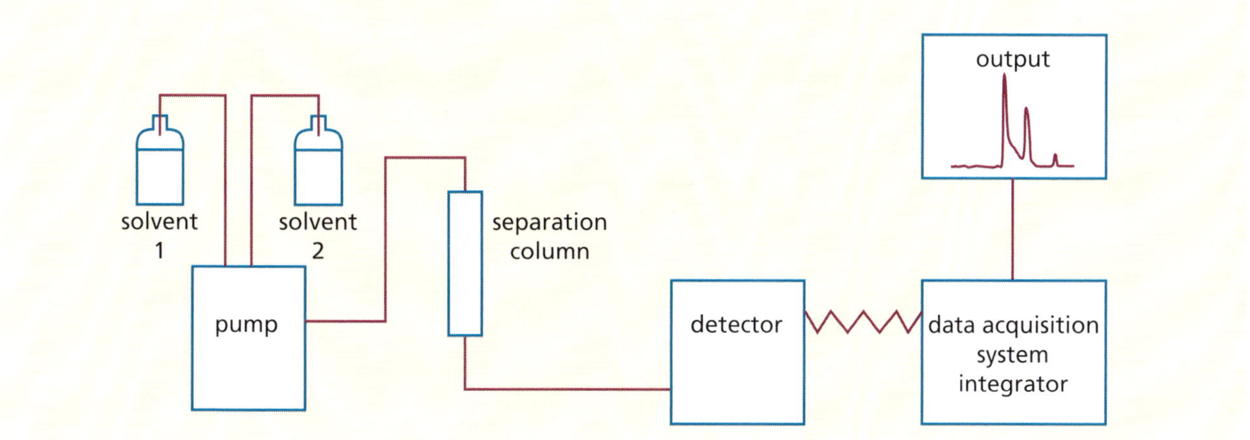

Figure 2.12. Components of a typical chromatography station. The pump combines solvents one and two in appropriate ratios to generate a pH, salt concentration, or hydrophobic gradient. Proteins that are fractioned on the column pass through a detector which measures their occurrence. Information from the detector is used to generate chromatograms and the relative amount of each component.

larger volume than do large molecules. As solution flows through the column, molecules can diffuse back and forth, depending upon their size, in and out of the pores of the beads. Smaller molecules can reside within the pores for a finite period of time whereas larger molecules, unable to enter these spaces, continue along in the fluid stream. Intermediate-sized molecules spend an intermediate amount of time within the pores. They can be fractionated from large molecules that cannot access the matrix space at all and from small molecules that have free access to this volume and spend most of the time within the beads. Protein molecules can distribute between the volume within these beads and the excluded volume based on the mass and shape of the molecule. This distribution is based on the relative concentration of the protein in the beads versus the excluded volume.

Size exclusion chromatography can be used to estimate the mass of proteins by calibrating the column with a series of globular proteins of known mass. However, the separation depends on molecular shape (conformation) as well as mass, and highly elongated proteins–proteins containing flexible, disordered regions– and glycoproteins will often appear to have masses as much as two to three times the true value. Other proteins may interact weakly with the column matrix and be retarded, thereby appearing to have a smaller mass. Thus, sedimentation or light scattering methods are preferred for accurate mass measurement. Over time, proteins can undergo a number of changes that affect their mass. A peptide bond within the protein can hydrolyze, yielding two smaller polypeptide chains. More commonly, size exclusion chromatography is used to assess aggregated forms of the protein. Figure 2.13 shows an example of this. The peak at 22 minutes represents the native protein. The peak at 15 minutes is aggregated protein and that at 28 minutes depicts degraded protein yielding smaller polypeptide chains. Aggregation can occur when a protein molecule unfolds to a slight extent and exposes surfaces that are attracted to complementary surfaces on adjacent molecules. This interaction can lead to dimerization or doubling of molecular weight or to higher molecular weight oligomers. From the chromatographic profile, the mechanism of aggregation can often be implicated. If dimers, trimers, tetramers, etc. are observed, then aggregation occurs by stepwise interaction of a monomer with a dimer, trimer,

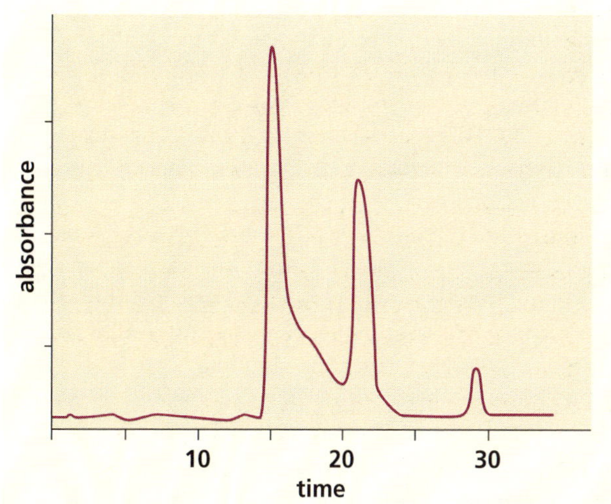

Figure 2.13. Size exclusion chromatography of a recombinant protein which on storage yields aggregates and smaller peptides.

etc. If dimers, tetramers, octamers, etc. are observed, then aggregates can interact with each other. Sometimes, only monomers and high molecular weight aggregates are observed, suggesting that intermediate species are kinetically of short duration and protein molecules susceptible to aggregation combine into very large molecular weight complexes.

Reversed-phase high performance liquid chromatography

This method takes advantage of the hydrophobic properties of proteins. The functional groups on the column matrix contain from one to up to eighteen carbon atoms in a hydrocarbon chain. The longer this chain, the more hydrophobic is the matrix. The hydrophobic patches of proteins interact with the hydrophobic chromatographic matrix. Proteins are then eluted from the matrix by increasing the hydrophobic nature of the solvent passing through the column. Acetonitrile is a common solvent used, although other organic solvents such as ethanol also may be employed. The solvent is made acidic by the addition of trifluoroacetic acid, since proteins have increased solubility at pH values further removed from their pI. A gradient with increasing concentration of hydrophobic solvent is passed through the column. Different proteins have different hydrophobicities and are eluted from the column depending on the 'hydrophobic potential' of the solvent.

This technique can be very powerful. It may detect the addition of a single oxygen atom to the protein, as when a methionyl residue is oxidized, or when the hydrolysis of an amide moiety on a glutamyl or asparginyl residue occurs. Disulfide bond formation or shuffling also changes the hydrophobic characteristic of the protein. Hence, RP-HPLC can be used not only to assess the homogeneity of the protein, but also to follow degradation pathways occurring during long term storage.

Reversed-phase chromatography of proteolytic digests of recombinant proteins may serve to identify this protein. Enzymatic digestion yields unique peptides that elute at different retention times or at different organic solvent concentrations. Moreover, the map, or chromatogram, of peptides arising from enzymatic digestion of one protein is quite different from the map obtained from another protein. Several different proteases, such as trypsin, chymotrypsin and other endoproteinases, are used for these identity tests (cf. below under "Mass Spectrometry").

Hydrophobic interaction chromatography

A companion to RP-HPLC is hydrophobic interaction chromatography (HIC), although in principle this latter method is normal-phase chromatography, i.e. here an aqueous solvent system rather than an organic one is used to fractionate proteins. The hydrophobic characteristics of the solution are modulated by inorganic salt concentrations. Ammonium sulfate and sodium chloride are often used since these compounds are highly soluble in water. In the presence of high salt concentrations (up to several molar), proteins are attracted to hydrophobic surfaces on the matrix of resins used in this technique. As the salt concentration decreases, proteins have less affinity for the matrix and eventually elute from the column. This method lacks the resolving power of RP-HPLC, but is a more gentle method, since low pH values or organic solvents as used in RP-HPLC can be detrimental to some proteins.

Ion exchange chromatography

This technique takes advantage of the electronic charge properties of proteins. Some of the amino acyl residues are negatively charged and others are positively charged. The net charge of the protein can be modulated by the pH of its environment relative to the pI value of the protein. At a pH value lower than the pI, the protein has a net positive charge, whereas at a pH value greater than the pI, the protein has a net negative charge. Opposites attract in ion-exchange chromatography. The resins in this procedure can contain functional groups with positive or negative charges. Thus, positively charged proteins bind to negatively charged matrices and negatively charged proteins bind to positively charged matrices. Proteins are displaced from the resin by increasing salt, e.g. sodium chloride, concentrations. Proteins with different net charges can be separated from one another during elution with an increasing salt gradient. The choice of charged resin and elution conditions are dependent upon the protein of interest.

In lieu of changing the ionic strength of the solution, proteins can be eluted by changing the pH of the medium, i.e. with the use of a pH gradient. This method is called chromatofocusing and proteins are separated based on their pI values. When the solvent pH reaches the pI value of a specific protein, the protein has a zero net charge and is no longer attracted to the charged matrix and hence is eluted.

Other chromatographic techniques

Other functional groups may be attached to chromatographic matrices to take advantage of unique properties of certain proteins. These affinity methodologies, however, are more often used in the manufacturing process than in analytical techniques (cf. Chapter 3). For example, conventional affinity purification schemes of antibodies use Protein-A or -G columns. Protein-A or -G specifically binds antibodies. Antibodies consist of variable regions and constant regions (cf. Chapter 4). The variable regions are antigen-specific and hence vary in sequence from one antibody to another, while the constant regions are common to each sub-group of antibodies. The constant region binds to Protein-A or -G.

Bioassays

Paramount to the development of a protein therapeutic is to have an assay that identifies its biological function. Chromatographic and electrophoretic methodologies can address the homogeneity of a biotherapeutic and be useful in investigating stability parameters. However, it is also necessary to ascertain whether the protein has acceptable bioactivity. Bioactivity can be determined either *in vivo*, i.e. by administering the protein to an animal and ascertaining some change within its body (function), or *in vitro*. Bioassays *in vitro* monitor the response of a specific receptor or microbiological or tissue cell line when the therapeutic protein is added to the system. An example of an *in vitro* bioassay is the increase in DNA synthesis in the presence of the therapeutic protein as measured by the incorporation of radioactively labeled thymidine. The protein factor binds to receptors on the cell surface that triggers secondary messengers to send signals to the cell nucleus to synthesize DNA. The binding of the protein factor to the cell surface is dependent upon the amount of factor present. Figure 2.14 presents a dose response curve of thymidine

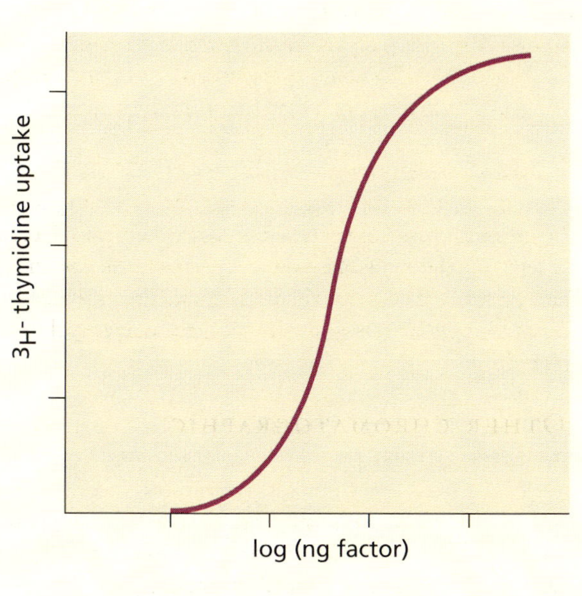

Figure 2.14. An *in vitro* bioassay showing a mitogenic response in which radioactive thymidine is incorporated into DNA in the presence of an increasing amount of a protein factor.

incorporation as a function of concentration of the factor. At low concentrations, the factor is too low to trigger a response. As the concentration increases, the incorporation of thymidine occurs, and at higher concentrations the amount of thymidine incorporation ceases to increase as DNA synthesis is occurring at the maximum rate. A standard curve can be obtained using known quantities of the protein factor. Comparison of other solutions containing unknown amounts of the factor with this standard curve will then yield quantitative estimates of the factor concentration. Through experience during the development of the protein therapeutic, a value is obtained for a fully functional protein. Subsequent comparisons to this value can be used to ascertain any loss in activity during stability studies, or changes in activity when amino acyl residues of the protein are modified.

Other *in vitro* bioassays can measure changes in cell number or production of another protein factor in response to the stimulation of cells by the protein therapeutic. The amount of the secondary protein produced can be estimated by using an ELISA.

Mass Spectrometry

Recent advances in the measurement of the molecular masses of proteins have made this technique an important analytical tool. While this method was used in the past to analyze small volatile molecules, the molecular weights of highly charged proteins with masses of over 100 kilodaltons (kDa) can now be accurately determined.

Because of the precision of this method, post-translational modifications such as acetylation or glycosylation can be predicted. The masses of new protein forms that arise during stability studies provide information on the nature of this form. For example, an increase in mass of 16 Dalton suggests that an oxygen atom has been added to the protein as happens when a methionyl residue is oxidized to a methionyl sulfoxide residue. The molecular mass of peptides obtained after proteolytic digestion and separation by HPLC indicate from which region of the primary structure they are derived. Such HPLC chromatogram is called a "peptide map." An example is shown in Figure 2.15. This is obtained by digesting a protein with pepsin and by subsequently separating the digested peptides by reverse HPLC. This highly characteristic pattern for a protein is called a "protein fingerprint." Peaks are identified by elution times on HPLC. If peptides have molecular masses differing from those expected from the primary sequence, the nature of the modification to that peptide can be implicated. Moreover, molecular mass estimates can be made for peptides obtained from unfractionated proteolytic digests. Molecular masses that differ from expected values indicate that a part of the protein molecules has been altered, that glycosylation or another modification has been altered,

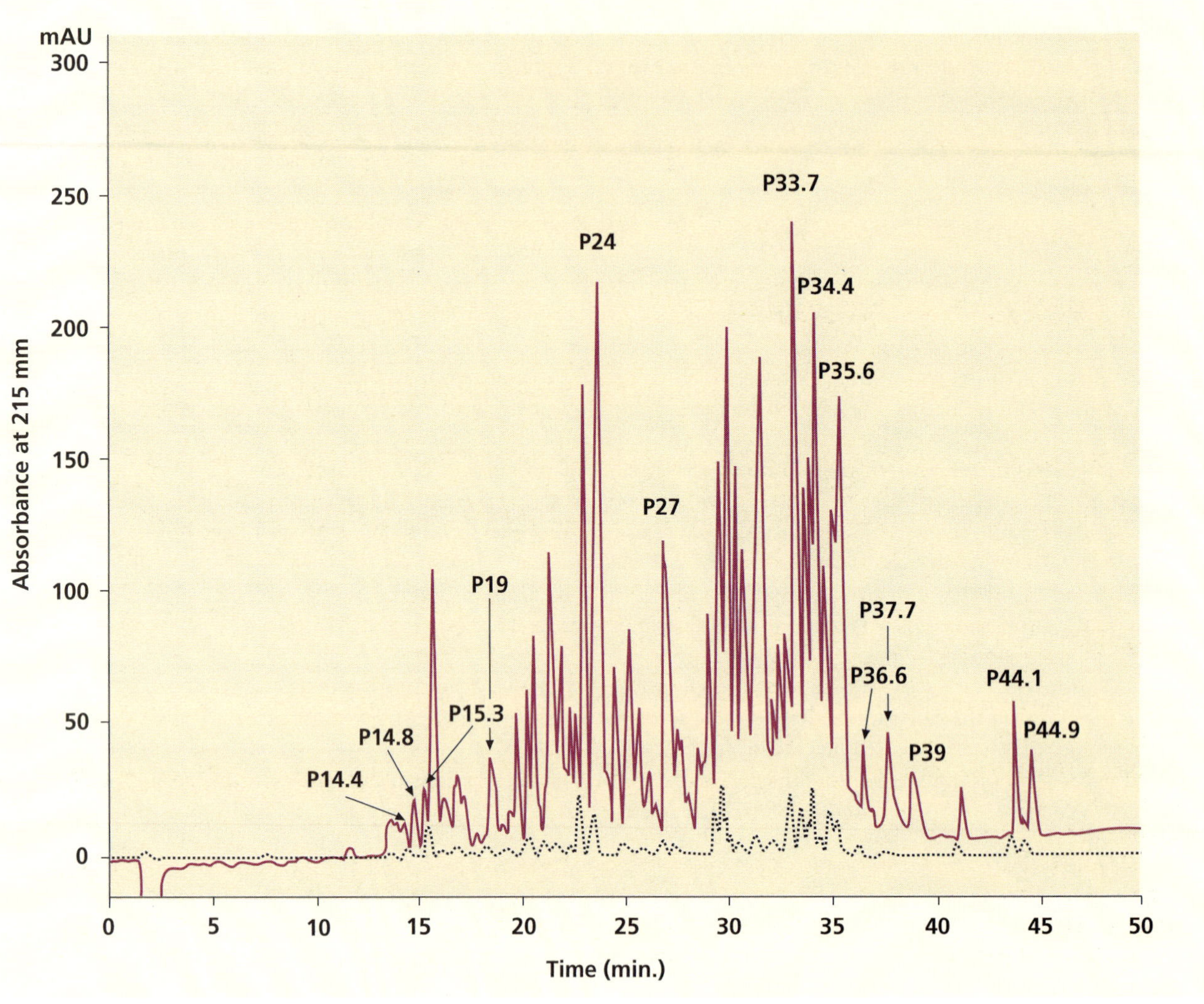

Figure 2.15. Peptide map of pepsin digest of recombinant human β-secretase. Each peptide is labelled by elution time in HPLC.

or that the protein under investigation still contains contaminants.

Another way that mass spectrometry can be used as an analytical tool is in the sequencing of peptides. A recurring structure, the peptide bond, in peptides tends to yield fragments of the mature peptide which differ stepwise by an amino acyl residue. The difference in mass between two fragments indicates the amino acid removed from one fragment to generate the other. Except for leucine and isoleucine, each amino acid has a different mass and hence a sequence can be read from the mass spectrograph. Stepwise removal can occur from either the amino terminus or carboxy terminus.

By changing three basic components of the mass spectrometer, the ion source, the analyzer and the detector, different types of measurement may be undertaken. Typical ion sources which volatilize the proteins are electrospray ionization, fast atom bombardment and liquid secondary ion. Common analyzers include quadrupole, magnetic sector, and time of flight instruments. The function of the analyzer is to separate the ionized biomolecules based on their mass to charge ratio. The detector measures a current whenever impinged upon by charged particles. Electrospray ionization (EI) and matrix-assisted laser desorption (MALDI) are two sources that can generate high molecular weight volatile proteins. In the former method, droplets are generated by spraying or nebulizing the protein solution into the source of the mass spectrometer. As the solvent evaporates, the protein remains behind in the gas phase and passes through the analyzer to the detector. In MALDI, proteins are mixed with a matrix which vaporizes when exposed to laser light, thus carrying the protein into the gas phase. An example of MALDI-mass analysis is shown in Figure 2.16, indicating the singly charged ion (116118 Dalton) and the doubly charged ion (58036.2) for a purified protein. Since proteins are multi-charge compounds, a number

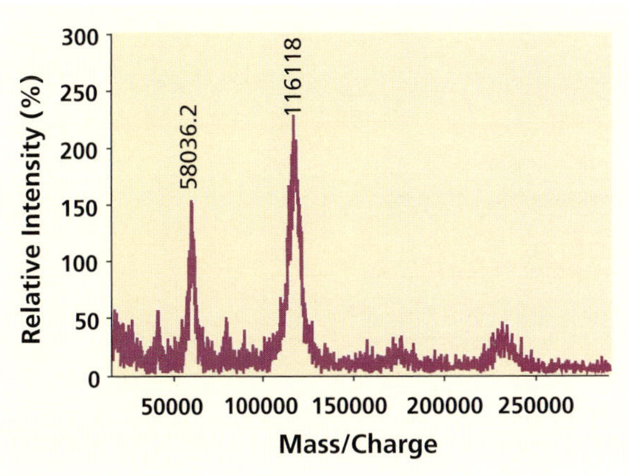

Figure 2.16. MALDI mass analysis of a purified recombinant human β-secretase. Numbers correspond to the singly charged and doubly charged ions.

of components are observed representing mass to charge forms, each differing from the next by one charge. By imputing various charges to the mass to charge values, a molecular mass of the protein can be estimated. The latter step is empirical since only the mass to charge ratio is detected and not the net charge for that particular particle.

Concluding Remarks

With the advent of recombinant proteins as human therapeutics, the need for methods to evaluate their structure, function, and homogeneity has become paramount. Various analytical techniques are used to characterize the primary, secondary, and tertiary structure of the protein and to determine the quality, purity and stability of the recombinant product. Bioassays establish its activity. ■

Further Reading

- **Butler, J.E., ed.** (1991) *Immunochemistry of Solid-Phase Immunoassay,* CRC Press, Boca Raton, Fla.
- **Crabb, J.W., ed.** (1995) *Techniques in Protein Chemistry VI,* Academic Press, San Diego, Calif.
- **Coligan, J., Dunn, B., Ploegh, H., Speicher, D., and Wingfield, P., eds.** (1995) *Current Protocols in Protein Science,* J. Wiley & Sons, New York, N.Y.
- **Creighton, T.E., ed.** (1989) *Protein Structure: A Practical Approach,* IRL Press, Oxford, England.
- **Crowther, J.R.** (1995) *ELISA, Theory and Practice,* Humana Press, Totowa, N.J.
- **Dunbar, B.S.** (1994) *Protein Blotting: A Practical Approach,* Oxford University Press, New York, N.Y.
- **Gregory, R.B., ed.** (1994) *Protein-Solvent Interactions,* Marcel Dekker, New York, N.Y.
- **Hames, B.D. and Rickwood, D., eds.** (1990) *Gel Electrophoresis of Proteins : A Practical Approach,* 2nd ed., IRL Press, New York, N.Y.
- **Landus, J.P., ed.** (1994) *Handbook of Capillary Electrophoresis,* CRC Press, Boca Raton, Fla.
- **McEwen, C.N. and Larsen, B.S., eds.** (1990) *Mass Spectrometry of Biological Materials,* Dekker, New York, N.Y.
- **Price, C.P. and Newman, D.J., eds.** (1991) *Principles and Practice of Immunoassay,* Stockton Press, New York, N.Y.
- **Schulz, G.E. Schulz and Schirmer, R.H., eds.** (1979) *Principles of Protein Structure,* Springer-Verlag, New York, N.Y.
- **Shirley, B.A., ed.** (1995) *Protein Stability and Folding,* Humana Press, Totowa, N.J.

Self-Assessment Questions

Question 1: *What is the net charge of granulocyte-colony stimulating factor at pH 2.0, assuming that all the carboxyl groups are protonated?*

Question 2: *Based on the above calculation, do you expect the protein to unfold at pH 2.0?*

Question 3: *Design an experiment using blotting techniques to ascertain the presence of a ligand to a particular receptor.*

Question 4: *What is the transfer of proteins to a membrane such as nitrocellulose or PDVF called?*

Question 5: *What is the assay in which the antibody is adsorbed to a plastic microtitration plate and then is used to quantify the amount of a protein using a secondary antibody conjugated with horseradish peroxidase named?*

Question 6: *In 2-dimensional electrophoresis, what is the first method of separation?*

Question 7: *What is the method for separating proteins in solution based on molecular size called?*

Answers

Answer 1: Based on the assumption that glutamyl and aspartyl residues are uncharged at this pH, all the charges come from protonated histidyl, lysyl, arginyl residues, and the amino terminus, i.e. 5 His + 4 Lys + 5 Arg + N-terminal = 15.

Answer 2: Whether a protein unfolds or remains folded depends on the balance between the stabilizing and destabilizing forces. At pH 2.0, extensive positive charges destabilize the protein, but whether such destabilization is sufficient or insufficient to unfold the protein depends on how stable the protein is in the native state. The charged state alone cannot predict whether a protein will unfold.

Answer 3: A solution containing the putative ligand is subjected to SDS-PAGE. After blotting the proteins in the gel to a membrane, it is probed with a solution containing the receptor. The receptor, which binds the ligand, may be labeled with agents suitable for detection or, alternatively, the complex can subsequently be probed with an antibody to the receptor and developed as for an immunoblot. Note that the reciprocal of this can be done as well, in which the receptor is subjected to SDS-PAGE and the blot is probed with the ligand.

Answer 4: This method is called blotting. If an electric current is used then the method is called electroblotting.

Answer 5: This assay is called an ELISA, enzyme-linked immunosorbent assay.

Answer 6: Either isoelectric focusing or native polyacrylamide electrophoresis. The second dimension is performed in the presence of the detergent sodium dodecyl sulfate.

Answer 7: Size exclusion chromatography.

3 Production and Downstream Processing of Biotech Compounds

Farida Kadir and Mic Hamers

Introduction

The growing therapeutic use of proteins has created an increasing need for practical and economical processing techniques. As a result, biotechnological production methods have advanced tremendously in recent years. When producing proteins for therapeutic use, a number of issues must be considered relating to the manufacturing, purification and characterization of the products. Biotechnological products for therapeutic use have to meet strict specifications, especially when used via the parenteral route (Walter and Werner, 1993).

In this chapter several aspects of production and purification will be addressed briefly. For further details the reader is referred to the literature mentioned in the References.

Production

Expression systems:

General considerations

Expression systems for proteins of therapeutic interest include both pro- and eukaryotic cells (bacteria, yeast, fungi, plants, insect cells, mammalian cells, and transgenic animals). The choice of a particular system will be determined, to a large extent, by the nature and origin of the desired protein, the intended use of the product, the amount needed, and the cost.

In principle, any protein can be produced using genetically engineered organisms, but not every type of protein can be produced by every type of cell. In the majority of cases, the protein is foreign to the host cells that have to produce it and, although the translation of the genetic code can be performed by the cells, the post-translation modifications of the protein might be different when compared to the original product. At present, over 60 different post-translation modifications of proteins are known and these modifications are species and/or cell type specific. The metabolic pathways that lead to these modifications are genetically determined by the host cell. Thus, even if the cells are capable of producing the desired post-translation modification, like glycosylation, the resulting glycosylation pattern might still be different from that of the native protein. Prokaryotic cells, like bacteria, are not capable of producing glycoproteins at all because they lack this post-translation modification capacity. A possible solution to these glycosylation problems is to use cell types that are as closely related to the original protein-producing cell type as possible. Therefore, for human derived proteins, mammalian cells or transgenic animals are often a better choice than bacteria or yeast. Generalized features of proteins expressed in different biological systems are listed in Table 3.1 (Walter *et al.*, 1992). However, it should be kept in mind that there are exceptions to this table for specific product/expression systems.

Transgenic Animals

Foreign genes can be introduced into animals like mice, rabbits, pigs, sheep, goats and cows through nuclear transfer and cloning techniques. The desired protein is expressed in the milk of the female offspring. During lactation the milk is collected, the milk fats are removed and the skimmed milk is used as the starting material for the purification of the protein.

The advantage of this technology is the relatively cheap method for producing the desired proteins in vast quantities. A disadvantage is the concern about the animal's health. Some proteins expressed in the mammary gland leak back into the circulation and cause serious negative health effects. An example is the expression of erythropoetin in cows. Although the protein was well expressed in the milk, it caused severe health effects and these experiments were stopped.

The purification strategies and purity requirements for proteins from milk are not different from those proteins derived from bacterial or mammalian cell systems, with the possible exception of proteins for oral use when expressed in milk that is otherwise consumed by humans. In the latter case, the 'contaminants' are known to be safe for consumption.

The transgenic animal technology for the production of pharmaceutical proteins is still under development. No products have reached the market yet. More details about this technology are presented in Chapter 6.

	Prokaryotic	Eukaryotic	Eukaryotic
Protein feature	Bacteria	Yeast	Mammalian cells
Concentration	high	high	low
Molecular weight	low	high	high
S-S bridges	limitation	no limitation	no limitation
Secretion	no	yes/no	yes
Aggregation state	inclusion body	singular, native	singular, native
Folding	misfolding	correct folding	correct folding
Glycosylation	no	possible	possible
Retrovirus	no	no	possible
Pyrogen	possible	no	no

Table 3.1. Generalized features of proteins of different biological origin.

Plants

Therapeutic proteins can also be expressed in plants and plant cell cultures (see also Chapter 1). For instance, human albumin has been expressed in potatoes and tobacco. Whether these production vehicles are economically feasible has yet to be established. The lack of genetic stability of plants is sometimes a drawback. Furthermore, most plants contain phenolic oxidases that can damage the expressed protein upon extraction from the plant material. A better route is the expression of the protein in edible seeds. For instance, rice and barley can be harvested and easily kept for a prolonged period of time as raw material sources. Particularly for oral therapeutics or vaccines this harvest and storage technique might be the ideal solution for the production of large amounts of cheap therapeutics, because the 'contaminants' are known to be safe for consumption (cf. Chapter 12).

The use of plant systems for the production of pharmaceutical proteins is still in an experimental phase. More details about this technology are presented in Chapter 6.

Cultivation systems

In general, cells can be cultivated in vessels containing an appropriate liquid growth medium. In this medium the cells are either attached to microspheres, are free in suspension or in an immobilized state such as monolayers, or entrapped in matrices (usually solidified with agar). The culture method will determine the scale of the separation and purification methods. Production-scale cultivation is commonly performed in fermentors or bioreactors. Bioreactor systems can be classified into four different types: stirred-tank, airlift, microcarrier (e.g. fixed bed bioreactors) and membrane bioreactors (e.g. hollow fiber perfusion bioreactors) (see Figure 3.1a–d). Due to its reliability and experience with the design and scaling up potential, the stirred tank is still the most commonly used bioreactor.

The kinetics of cell growth and product formation will not only dictate the type of bioreactor used, but also how the growth process is run. Three types of fermentation protocols are commonly employed: (1) batch, (2) fed-batch and (3) continuous production protocols. In all cases the cells go through four distinctive phases: lag, exponential growth, stationary and death phase. (See Chapter 1). The cell culture has to be free from undesired microorganisms that may destroy the cells or present hazards to the patient. This requires strict measures for both the procedures and materials used (WHOI, 1998; Berthold and Walter, 1994).

Examples of animal cells that are most commonly used for the production of proteins of clinical interest are Chinese Hamster Ovary cells (CHO), Baby Hamster Kidney cells (BHK), lymphoblastoid tumor cells (interferon production), melanoma cells (plasminogen activator) and hybridized tumor cells (monoclonal antibodies).

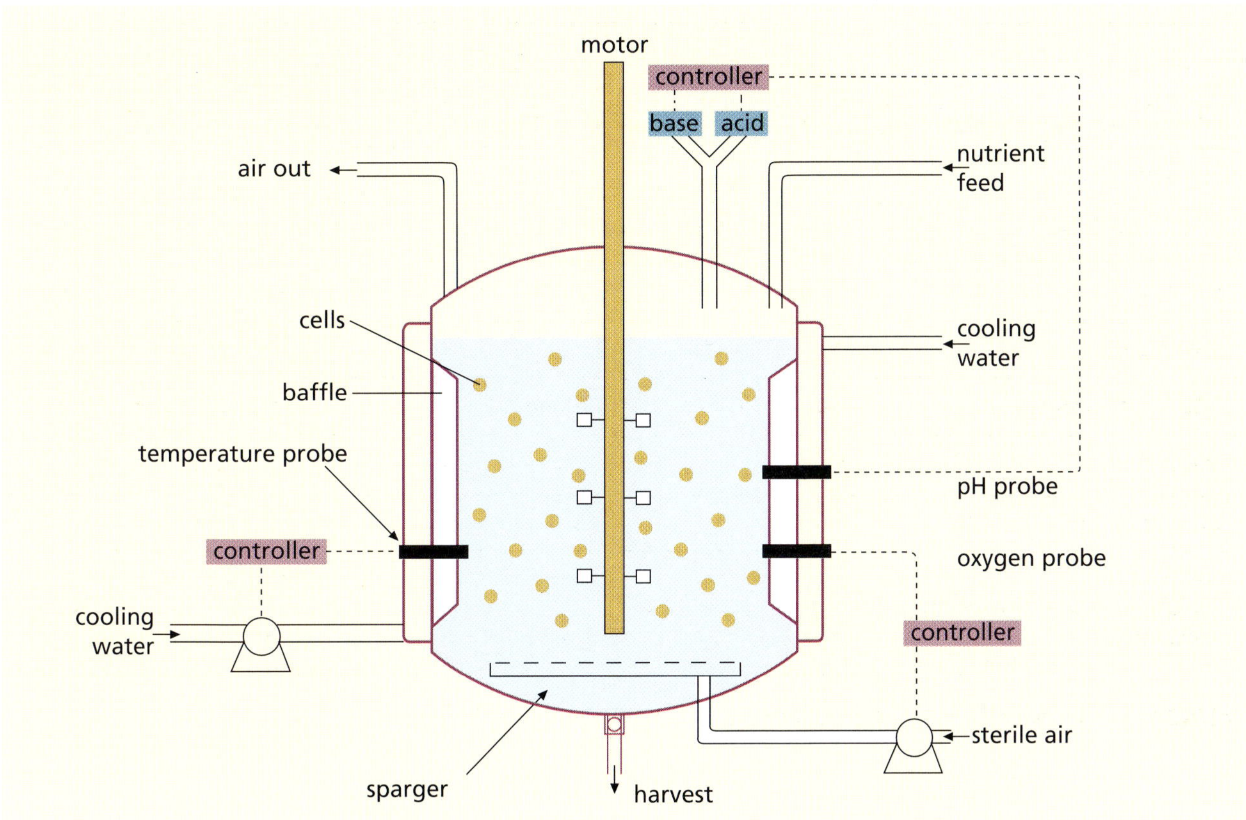

Figure 3.1a. Schematic representation of stirred-tank bioreactor (adapted from Klegerman and Groves, Igg2).

Cultivation Medium

In order to achieve the optimal growth of cells it is of great importance that not only conditions such as pH, oxygen tension and temperature are chosen and controlled appropriately, but also that a medium with the proper nutrients is provided. The media used for mammalian cell culture are complex and consist of a mixture of diverse components, such as sugars, amino acids, electrolytes, vitamins, fetal calf serum and a mixture of peptones, growth factors, hormones and other proteins (see Table 3.2). Many of these ingredients are preblended either as diluted or as homogeneous mixtures of powders. To prepare the final medium, components are dissolved in purified water before sterile filtration. Some supplements, especially fetal calf serum, considerably contribute to the presence of contaminating proteins and may seriously complicate purification procedures. Additionally, the composition of serum is variable; it depends on the individual animal, season of the year, suppliers' treatment, etc. The use of serum may introduce adventitious material such as viruses, mycoplasmas, bacteria and fungi into the culture system (Berthold and Walter, 1994). Furthermore, the possible presence of prions that may cause transmissible spongiphormous encephalitis (TSE) practically eliminates the use of bovine, sheep or goat material. However, if use of this material is inevitable, one must follow the relevant guidelines in which selective sourcing of the material is still the key measure of safety (EMEA, 1999[a]). These problems have been recognized by the customers of media and have directed the manufacturers to meet the customers' need. They offer a range of serum-free media. Completely serum-free media have been shown to give satisfactory results in industrial scale production settings in certain cases, such as in monoclonal antibody production, for example.

Contaminants

Quality is usually measured in terms of product purity and product consistency (reproducibility). An important consideration in the development process of the purification scheme is the ultimate purity required. For pharmaceutical

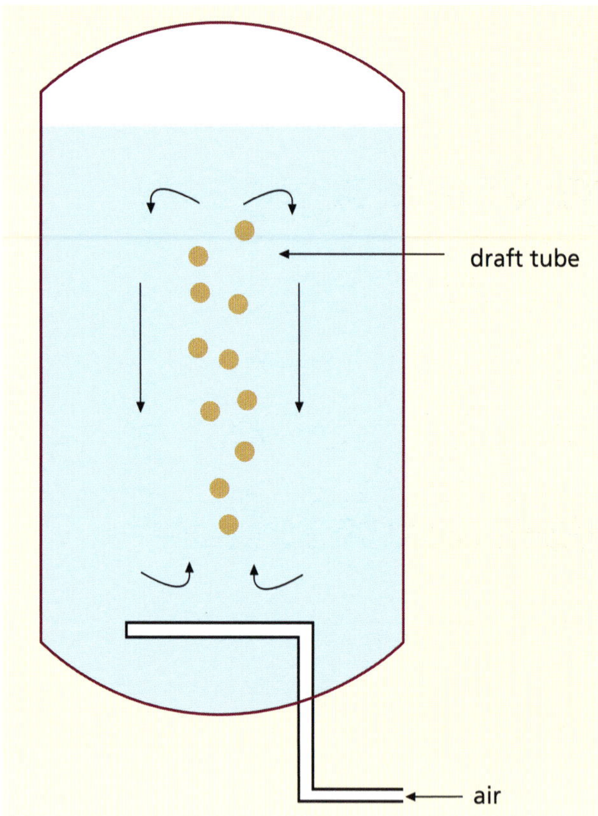

Figure 3.1b. Schematic representation of airlift bioreactor (adapted from Klegerman and Groves, Igg2).

Type of nutrient	Example(s)
Sugars	glucose, lactose, sucrose, maltose, dextrins
Fat	fatty acids, triglycerides
Water (high quality, sterilized)	water for injection
Amino acids	glutamine
Electrolytes	calcium, sodium, potassium, phosphate
Vitamins	ascorbic acid, α-tocopherol, thiamine, riboflavine, folic acid, pyridoxin
Serum (fetal calf serum, synthetic serum)	albumin, transferrin
Trace minerals	iron, manganese, copper, cobalt, zinc
Hormones	growth factors

Table 3.2. Major components of growth media for mammalian cell structures.

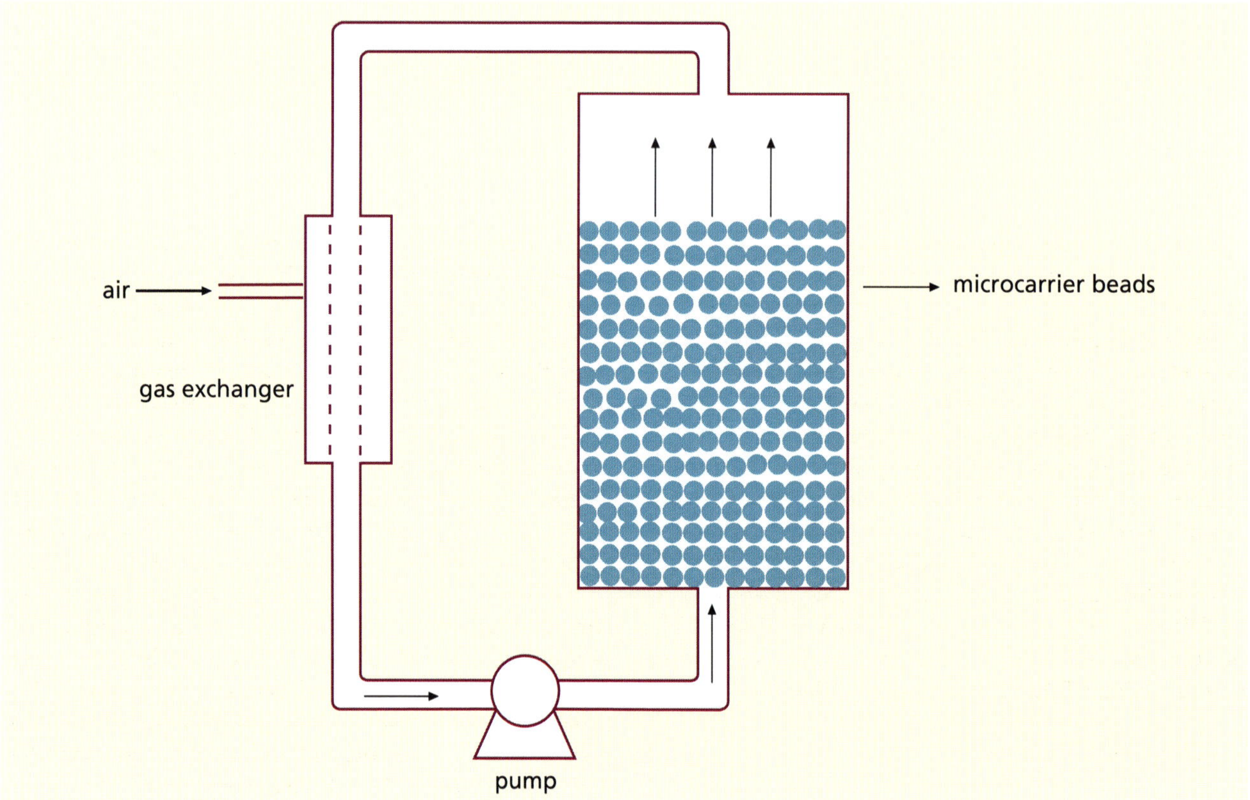

Figure 3.1c. Schematic representation of fixed bed bioreactor (adapted from Klegerman and Groves, Igg2).

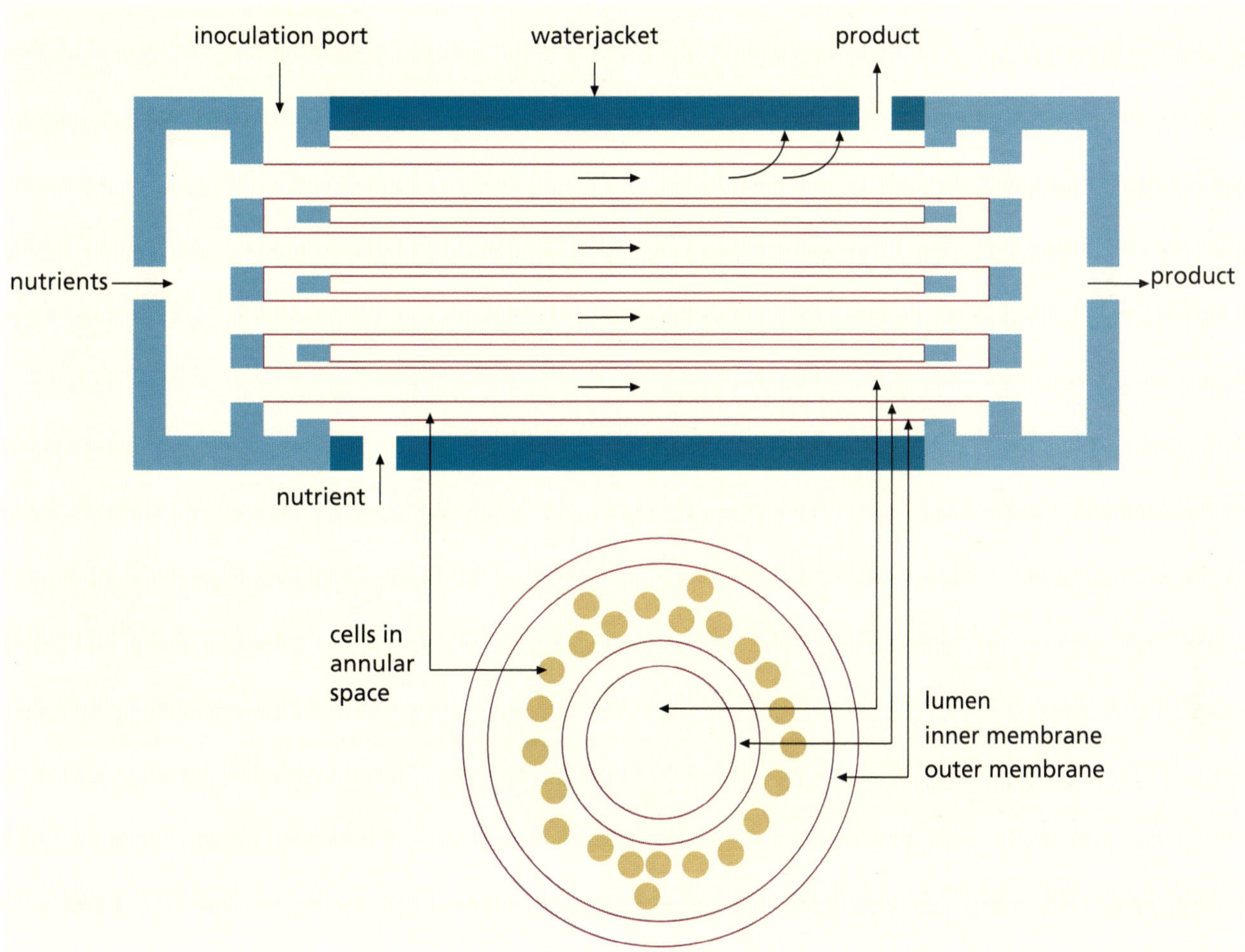

Figure 3.1d. Schematic representation of hollow fiber perfusion bioreactor (adapted from Klegerman and Groves, 1992).

applications, product purity is mostly ≥ 99% when used as a parenteral (Berthold and Walter, 1994; EMEA, 1999[b]).

Purification processes should yield potent proteins with well-defined characteristics for human use from which 'all' contaminants have been removed. The purity of the drug protein in the final product will therefore largely depend upon the purification technology applied.

Table 3.3 lists potential contaminants that may be present in recombinant protein products from bacterial and non-bacterial sources. These contaminants can be either host-related, process-related or product-related. In the following sections special attention is paid to the detection and elimination of contamination by viruses, bacteria, cellular DNA and undesired proteins.

Viruses

Viruses, which require the presence of living cells to propagate, are potential contaminants of animal cell cultures and, therefore, of the final product produced by the cells (Arathoon and Birch, 1986). If present, their concentration in the purified product will be very low and it will be difficult to detect them. Although viruses such as retrovirus (type B) can be visualized under an electron microscope, a highly sensitive *in vitro* assay for their detection is lacking (Liptrot and Gull, 1991). The risks of some viruses (e.g. hepatitis virus) are known (Walter *et al.*, 1991; Marcus-Sekura, 1991), but there are other viruses whose risks can not be properly judged because of the lack of solid experimental data. Some virus infections, such as those caused by parvovirus, can have long latent periods before their clinical effects show up. Long-term effects of introducing viruses into a patient treated with a recombinant protein should not be overlooked. Therefore, it is required that parenterals are free from viruses. The specific virus testing regime required will depend on the cell type used for production (Löwer, 1990; Minor, 1994).

Viruses can be introduced by nutrients or are generated by an infected production cell line. The most frequent

Origin	Contaminant
Host-related	viruses
	host-derived proteins and DNA
	glycosylation variants
	N- and C-terminal variants
	endotoxins (from gram negative bacterial hosts)
Product-related	amino acids substitution and deletion
	denatured protein
	conformational isomers
	dimers and aggregates
	disulfide pairing variants
	deamidated species
	protein fragments
Process-related	growth medium components
	purification reagents
	metals
	column materials

Table 3.3. Potential contaminants in recombinant protein products derived from bacterial and non-bacterial hosts.

source of virus introduction is animal serum. In addition, animal serum can introduce other unwanted agents such as bacteria, mycoplasmas, prions, fungi and endotoxins. It should be clear that appropriate screening of cell banks and growth medium constituents for viruses and other adventitious agents should be strictly regulated and supervised (Walter *et al.*, 1991; FDA, 1993; EMEA, 1997; WHO Technical Report Series 823). There has been a trend toward using more defined growth media in which serum levels are significantly reduced. A validated method to remove possible viral contaminants is mandatory for licensing of all therapeutics derived from mammalian cells or transgenic animals (White *et al.*, 1991; Minor, 1994). Viruses can be inactivated by physical and chemical treatment of the product. Heat, irradiation, sonication, extreme pH, detergents, solvents, and certain disinfectants can inactivate viruses. These procedures can be harmful to the product as well and should therefore be carefully evaluated and validated (Walter *et al.*, 1992; White *et al.*, 1991; Minor, 1994; EMEA, 1997). Removal of viruses by nanofiltration is an elegant and effective technique. Filtration through 15 nm membranes can remove even the smallest non-enveloped viruses such as bovine parvoviruses (Burnouf-Radosevich *et al.*, 1994; Maerz *et al.*, 1996). A number of methods for reducing or inactivating viral contaminants are mentioned in Table 3.4 (Burnouf *et al.*, 1989; Horowitz *et al.*, 1991; Perret *et al.*, 1991; Horowitz *et al.*, 1994).

Bacteria

Unwanted bacterial contamination may be a problem for cells in culture. Usually the size of bacteria allows simple sterile filtration for adequate removal. In order to further prevent bacterial contamination during production, the raw materials used have to be sterilized and the products are manufactured under strict aseptic conditions. Additionally, antibiotic agents can be added to the culture media in some cases, but have to be removed further downstream in the purification process. Because of the persistence of antibiotic residues, which are difficult to eliminate from the product, appropriately designed production plants and extensive quality control systems for added reagents (medium, serum, enzymes, etc.) enabling antibiotic-free operation are preferable.

Pyrogens (usually endotoxins of gram-negative bacteria) are potentially hazardous substances (cf. Chapter 4). Humans are sensitive to pyrogen contamination at very low concentrations (picograms per mL). Pyrogens may elicit a strong fever response and can even be fatal. Simple sterile filtration does not remove pyrogens. Removal is complicated further because pyrogens vary in size and chemical composition. However, sensitive tests to detect and quantify pyrogens are commercially available. Purification schemes usually contain at least one step of ion-exchange chromatography (anionic exchange material) to remove the negatively charged endotoxins (Berthold and Walter, 1994; Nolan, 1975).

Cellular DNA

The application of continuous mammalian cell lines for the production of recombinant proteins might result in the presence of oncogene-bearing DNA-fragments in the final protein product (Walter and Werner, 1993; Löwer, 1990). A stringent purification protocol that is capable of reducing the DNA content to a safe level is therefore necessary (Berthold and Walter, 1994). There are a number of approaches available to validate that the purification method removes cellular DNA and RNA. One such approach involves

Category	type	example
Inactivation	heat treatment	pasteurization
	radiation	UV-light
	dehydration	lyophilization
	cross linking agents, denaturating or disrupting agents	β-propiolactone, formaldehyde, NaOH, organic solvents (e.g., chloroform), detergents (e.g., Na-cholate)
	neutralization	specific, neutralizing antibodies
Removal	chromatography	ion-exchange, immuno-affinity, chromatography
	filtration	nanofiltration
	precipitation	cryoprecipitation

Table 3.4. Methods for reducing or inactivating viral contaminants.

incubating the cell line with radiolabeled nucleotides and determining radioactivity in the purified product obtained through the purification protocol. Another method is dye-binding fluorescence-enhancement assay for nucleotides. If the presence of nucleic acids persists in a final preparation, then additional steps must be introduced in the purification process. The question about a safe level of nucleic acids in biotech products is difficult to answer, because of the lack of relevant know-how. Transfection with so-called naked DNA is very difficult and a high concentration of DNA is needed. Nevertheless, for safety reasons the final product contamination by nucleic acids should not exceed 100 pg – 10 ng per daily dose, depending on the kind of culture system (WHO, 1998; Eur Pharm III, 1997; Kung *et al.*, 1990).

PROTEIN CONTAMINANTS

As previously mentioned, trace amounts of "foreign" proteins may appear in biotech products. These types of contaminants are a potential health hazard because, if present, they may be recognized as antigens by the patient receiving the recombinant protein product. On repeated use the patient may show an immune reaction caused by the contaminant while the protein of interest is performing its beneficial function. In such cases the immunogenicity may be misinterpreted as being due to the recombinant protein itself. Therefore, one must be very cautious in interpreting safety data of a given recombinant therapeutic protein.

Generally, main sources of protein contaminants are the growth medium used or the proteins of the host cells. Among the host derived contaminants, the host species' version of the recombinant protein could be present (WHO, 1998). As these proteins are similar in structure, it is possible that undesired proteins are co-purified with the desired product. For example, urokinase is known to be present in many continuous cell lines. The synthesis of highly active biological molecules, such as cytokines by hybridoma cells, might be another concern (FDA, 1990; Schindler and Dinarello, 1990). Depending upon their nature and concentration these cytokines might enhance the antigenicity of the product.

"Known" or expected contaminants should be monitored at the successive stages in a purification process by suitable in-process controls, e.g. sensitive immunoassay(s). Tracing of the many "unknown" cell-derived proteins is more difficult. When developing a purification process other, less specific analyses such as SDS-PAGE are usually used in combination with various staining techniques.

Downstream Processing

Introduction

Recovering a biological reagent from a cell culture supernatant is one of the critical parts of the manufacturing procedure for biotech products. Usually, the product is available in a very dilute form, e.g. 10–200 mg/L. However, concentration of up to 500–800 mg/L can sometimes be reached (Berthold and Walter, 1994; Garnick *et al.*, 1988). A concentration step is often required to reduce handling volumes for further purification. Usually, the product subsequently undergoes a series of purification steps. Traditionally, the first step captures and initially purifies the product; the subsequent steps remove the bulk of the contaminants, and a final step removes all trace contaminants and variant forms of the molecule. Alternatively, the reverse strategy, where the main contaminants are captured and the product is purified in subsequent steps, might result in a more economic process, especially if the product is not excreted from the cells. In the former case the product will not represent more than 1% to 5% of total cellular protein and aspecific binding of the bulk of the protein in a product specific capture step will ruin its efficiency. If the bulk contaminants can be removed first, the specific capture step will be more efficient and smaller in size, thus cheaper, and chromatographic columns could be used. After purification, additional steps, such as formulation and sterilization, are performed on the bulk product in order to obtain the required stable final product. Formulation aspects will be dealt with in Chapter 4.

When designing a purification protocol, the possibility of scaling up should be considered carefully. For both technical and economic reasons, a process that has been designed for small quantities is most often not suitable for large quantities. Developing a downstream process (i.e. the isolation and purification of the desired product) to recover a biological protein in large quantities occurs in two stages: *design* and *scale-up*.

Separating the impurities from the product protein requires a series of purification steps (*process design*), each removing some of the impurities and bringing the product closer to its final specification. In general, the starting feed stream contains cell debris and/or whole-cell particulate material that must be removed. Defining the major contaminants in the starting material is helpful in the downstream process design. This includes detailed information on the source of the material (e.g. bacterial or mammalian cell culture) and major contaminants (e.g. albumin or product analogs). Moreover, the physical characteristics of the product versus the known contaminants (thermal stability, isoelectric point, molecular weight, hydrophobicity, density, specific binding properties) largely determine the process design. Processes used for production of therapeutics should be reproducible and reliable. Methods used for recovery may expose the protein molecules to high physical stress (e.g. to high temperatures and extreme pH) which may alter the protein properties, leading to appreciable loss in protein activity.

Any substance that is used for injection must be sterile and free from pyrogens below a certain level, depending on the product (limits are stated in the individual monographs which are to be consulted, such as European Pharmacopoeia). This requirement necessitates aseptic techniques and procedures throughout with clean air and microbial control of all materials and equipment. During validation of the purification process it must also be demonstrated that potential viral contaminants can be removed (Walter *et al.*, 1992). The purification matrices should be at least sanitizable or, if possible, steam-sterilizable. For depyrogenation, the purification material must withstand either extended dry heat at 180 °C or treatment with 1–2 M sodium hydroxide (for further information see section on Formulation Aspects). If any material in contact with the product inadvertently releases compounds, these leachables must be analyzed and their removal by subsequent purification steps must be demonstrated during process validation. This problem especially hampers the use of affinity chromatography (see below) in the production of pharmaceuticals for human use. On the laboratory scale affinity chromatography is an important tool for purification and the resulting product might be used for toxicity studies, but for human use the removal of any leached ligands has to be demonstrated. Because free affinity ligands will bind to the product, the removal might be very cumbersome.

Scale-up is the term used to describe a number of processes employed in converting a laboratory procedure into an economical, industrial process. During scale-up phase, the process moves from the laboratory scale to the pilot plant and finally to the production plant. The objective of scale-up is to produce a product of high quality at a competitive price. Since costs of downstream processing can be as high as 50 to 80% of the total cost of a product, practical and economical ways of purifying the product should be used. Superior protein purification methods hold the key to a strong market position (Wheelwright, 1993).

Basic operations required for a downstream purification process used for macromolecules from biological sources are shown in Figure 3.2.

As previously mentioned, the design of downstream processing is highly product dependent. Therefore, each product requires a specific multistage purification procedure (Sadana, 1989). The basic scheme as represented in Figure 3.2 becomes complex. A typical example of a process flow for the downstream processing is shown in Figure 3.3. This scheme represents the processing of a glycosylated recombinant interferon (about 28 kDa) produced in mammalian cells. The aims of the individual unit operations are described.

Once the volume and concentration of the product can be managed, the main purification phase can start. A number of purification methods are available to separate proteins on the basis of a wide variety of different physicochemical criteria, such as size, charge, hydrophobicity and solubility. Detailed information about some separation and purification methods commonly used in purification schemes follows below.

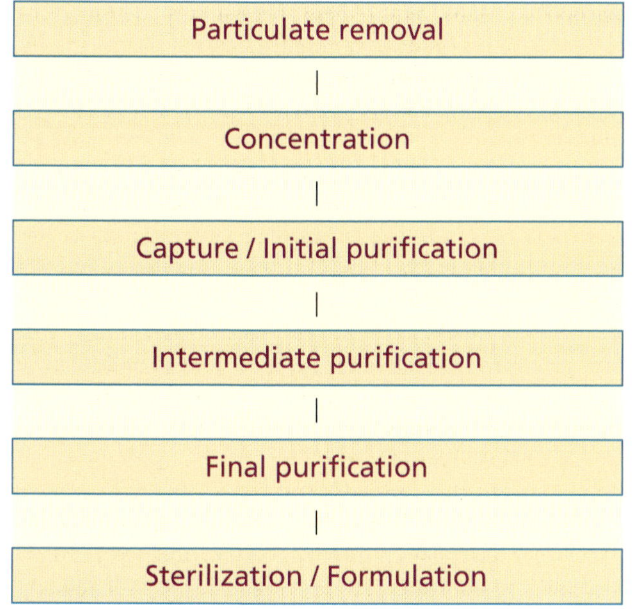

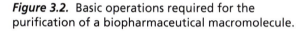

Figure 3.2. Basic operations required for the purification of a biopharmaceutical macromolecule.

Filtration/Centrifugation

Products from the biotechnological industry must be separated from biological systems that contain suspended particulate material, including whole cells, lysed cell material, and fragments of broken cells generated when cell breakage has been necessary to release intracellular products. Most downstream processing flow sheets will, therefore, include at least one unit-operation for the removal (clarification) or concentration – just the opposite – of particulates. The most frequently used methods are centrifugation and filtration techniques (e.g. ultrafiltration, diafiltration and microfiltration). However, the expense and effectiveness of such methods is highly dependent on the physical nature of the particulate material and of the product.

FILTRATION

Filtration can concentrate the biomass prior to further purification. Several filtration systems have been developed for the separation of cells from media, the most successful being tangential flow systems (also referred to as "cross flow"), where high shear across the membrane surface limits fouling, gel layer formation and concentration polarization. In ultrafiltration, mixtures of molecules of different molecular dimensions are separated by the passage of a dispersion under pressure across a membrane with a defined pore size (Minton, 1990). In general, ultrafiltration achieves little purification, because of the relatively large pore size distribution of the membranes. However, this technique is widely used to concentrate macromolecules, and also to change the aqueous phase in which the particles are dispersed or in which molecules are dissolved (diafiltration) to one required for the subsequent purification step.

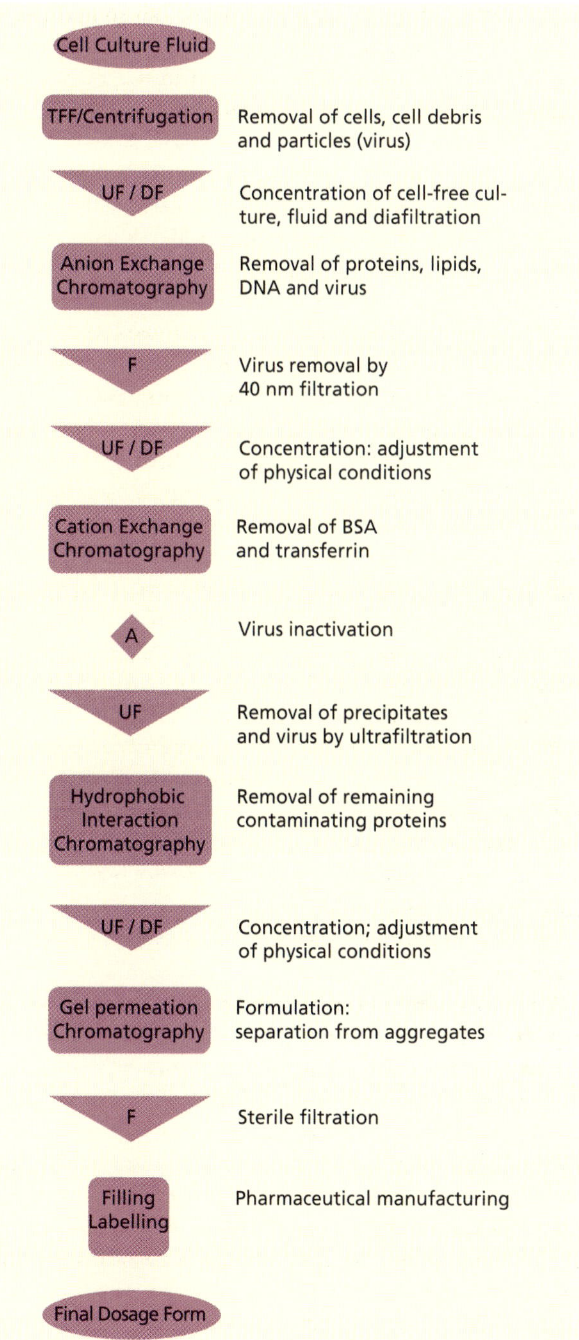

Figure 3.3. Downstream processing of a glycosylated recombinant interferon, describing the purpose of the inclusion of the individual unit operations. (F = Filtration, TFF: Tangential Flow Filtration, UF: Ultrafiltration, DF: Diafiltration, A: Adsorption; adapted from Berthold and Walter, 1994).

Centrifugation

Subcellular particles and organelles, suspended in a viscous liquid (for example the particles produced when cells are disrupted by mechanical procedures) are difficult to separate either by using one fixed centrifugation step or by filtration. But, they can be isolated efficiently by centrifugation at different speeds. For instance, nuclei can be obtained at 400 x g for 20 minutes, while plasma membrane vesicles are pelleted at higher centrifugation rates and longer centrifugation times (fractional centrifugation). In many cases, however, total biomass can easily be separated from the medium by centrifugation (e.g. continuous disc-stack centrifuge). Buoyant density centrifugation can be useful for the separation of particles, as well. This technique uses a viscous fluid with a continuous gradient of density in a centrifuge tube. Particles and molecules of various densities within the density range in the tube will cease to move when the isopycnic region has been reached. Both techniques of continuous (fluid densities within a range) and discontinuous (blocks of fluid with different density) density gradient centrifugation are used in buoyant density centrifugation on a laboratory scale.

However, for application on the industrial scale continuous centrifuges (e.g. tubular bowl centrifuges) are only used for discontinuous buoyant density centrifugation. This type of industrial centrifuge is mainly applied to recover precipitated proteins or contaminants.

Precipitation

The solubility of a particular protein depends on the physico-chemical environment, e.g. pH, ionic species and ionic strength of the solution (cf. Formulation Aspects). A slow, continuous increase of the ionic strength (of a protein mixture) will selectively drive proteins out of solution. This phenomenon is known as "salting-out." A wide variety of agents with different "salting out" potencies are available. Chaotropic series with increasing "salting out" effects of negatively (I) and positively (II) charged molecules are given below (von Hippel *et al.*, 1964):

I - SCN^-, I^-, CLO_4^-, NO_3^-, Br^-, Cl^-, CH_3COO^-, PO_4^{3-}, SO_4^{2-}
II - Ba^{2+}, Ca^{2+}, Mg^{2+}, Li^+, Cs^+, Na^+, K^+, Rb^+, NH_4^+

Ammonium sulfate is highly soluble in cold aqueous solutions and is frequently used in "salting-out" purification.

Another method for the precipitation of proteins is to use water-miscible organic solvents (change in the dielectric constant). Examples of precipitating agents are polyethylene glycol and trichloracetic acid. Under certain conditions, chitosan and non-ionic polyoxyethylene detergents also induce precipitation (Cartwright, 1987; Homma *et al.*, 1993; Terstappen *et al.*, 1993). Precipitation is a scalable, simple and a relatively economical procedure for the recovery of a product from a dilute feed stream. It has been widely used for the isolation of proteins from culture supernatants. Unfortunately, with most bulk precipitation methods the gain in purity is generally limited. Moreover, extraneous components are introduced which must be eliminated later. Finally, large quantities of precipitates may be difficult to handle. Despite these limitations, recovery by precipitation has been used with considerable success for some products.

Chromatography

Introduction

In preparative chromatography systems the molecular species are primarily separated according to differences in distribution between two phases; one which is the stationary phase (mostly a solid phase) and the other which moves. This mobile phase may be liquid or gaseous (cf. Chapter 2). Nowadays, almost all stationary phases (fine particles providing a large surface area) are packed into a column. The mobile phase is passed through by pumps. Downstream purification protocols usually have at least two to three chromatography steps. Chromatographic methods used in the purification procedures of biotech products are listed in Table 3.5 and are briefly discussed in the following sections.

Chromatographic stationary phases

Chromatographic procedures often represent the rate-limiting step in the overall downstream processing. An important primary factor governing the rate of operation is the mass transport into the pores of conventional packing materials. Adsorbents employed include inorganic materials, such as silica gels, glass beads, hydroxyapatite, various metal oxides (alumina) and organic polymers (cross-linked dextrans, cellulose, agarose). Separation occurs by differential interaction of sample components with the chromatographic medium. Ionic groups, such as amines and carboxylic acids, dipolar groups, such as carbonyl functional groups, and hydrogen bond-donating and accepting groups control the interaction of the sample components in conjunction with the stationary phase and these functional groups slow down the elution rate if interaction occurs.

Chromatographic stationary phases for use on a large-scale have improved considerably over the last decades. Hjerten *et al.* (1993) reported on the use of compressed acrylamide-based polymer structures. These materials allow relatively fast separations with good chromatographic

Separation technique	Mode/Principle	Separation based on
Membrane separation	microfiltration ultrafiltration dialysis	size size size
Centrifugation	isopycnic banding non-equilibrium settling	density density
Extraction	fluid extraction liquid/liquid extraction	solubility partition, change in solubility
Precipitation	fractional precipitation	change in solubility
Chromatography	ion-exchange gel filtration affinity hydrophobic interaction adsorption	charge size specific ligand-substrate interaction hydrophobicity covalent/noncovalent binding

Table 3.5. Frequently used separation processes and their physical basis.

performance. Another approach to the problems associated with mass transport in conventional systems is the use of chromatographic particles that contain some large 'through pores' in addition to conventional pores (see Figure 3.4). These flow-through, or "perfusion chromatography," media enable faster convective mass transport into particles and allow operation at much higher speeds, without loss in resolution or binding capacity (Afeyan *et al.*, 1989; Fulton, 1994). Another development is the design of spirally wrapped columns containing the adsorption medium. This configuration permits high throughput, high capacity and good capture efficiency (Cartwright, 1987).

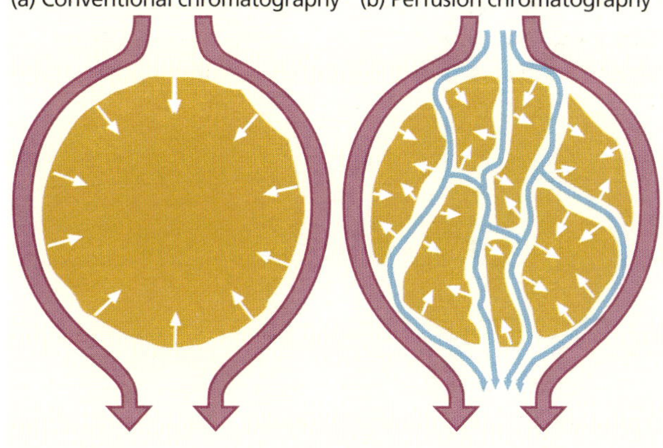

Figure 3.4. The structure of conventional chromatographic particles (a) and perfusion or flow-through chromatographic particles (b) (from Fulton, 1994).

The ideal stationary phase for protein separation should possess a number of characteristics, among which are high mechanical strength, high porosity, no non-specific interaction between protein and the support phase, high capacity, biocompatibility and high stability of the matrix in a variety of solvents. The final characteristic is especially true for columns used for the production of clinical materials that need to be cleaned, depyrogenized, disinfected and sterilized at regular intervals. High-Performance Liquid Chromatography (HPLC) systems fulfil many of these criteria. Liquid phases should be carefully chosen to minimize the loss of biological activity resulting from the use of some organic solvents. In HPLC, small pore size stationary phases that are incompressible are used. These particles are small, rigid and regularly sized (to provide a high surface area). The mobile liquid phase is forced under high pressure through the column material. Reversed-phase HPLC systems, using less polar stationary phases than the mobile phases can be effectively integrated into large-scale purification schemes of proteins and can serve both as a means of concentration and purification (Benedek and Swadesh, 1991).

In production environments, columns which operate at relatively low back pressure are often used. They have the advantage that they can be used in equipment constructed from plastics which, unlike conventional stainless steel equipment, resists all buffers likely to be employed in the separation of biomolecules. These columns are commercially available and permit the efficient separation of proteins in a single run. Results can be obtained rapidly and with high resolution. A new development is the use of stainless steel equipment that resists almost all chemicals used in protein purification, including disinfection and sterilization media.

Unfortunately, HPLC equipment costs are high and this technology finds only limited application in large-scale purification schemes (Strickler and Gemski, 1987; Jungbauer and Wenisch, 1989).

Adsorption Chromatography

In adsorption chromatography (also called "normal phase" chromatography) the stationary phase is more polar than the mobile phase. The protein of interest selectively binds to a static matrix under one condition and is released under a different condition (Chase, 1988). Adsorption chromatography methods enable high ratios of product load to stationary phase volume, thus making this principle economically scalable.

Ion-exchange chromatography

Ion-exchange chromatography can be a powerful step at the beginning of a purification scheme. It can be easily scaled up. Ion-exchange chromatography can be used in a negative mode, i.e. the product flows through the column under conditions that favor the adsorption of contaminants to the matrix, while the protein of interest does not bind (Tennikova and Svec, 1993). The type of the column needed is determined by the protein's properties (e.g. isoelectric point and charge density) to be purified. Anion exchangers bind negatively charged molecules and cation exchangers bind positively charged molecules. In salt-gradient ion-exchange chromatography, the salt concentration in the perfusing elution buffer is continuously or gradually increased. The stronger the binding of an individual protein to the ion exchanger the later it will appear in the elution buffer. Likewise, in pH-gradient chromatography, the pH is changed continuously or in steps. Here, the protein binds at one pH and is released at a different pH. As a result of the heterogeneity in glycosylation, glycosylated proteins may elute in a relatively broad pH range (up to 2 pH units).

In order to simplify purification, a specific amino acid tail can be added to the protein at the gene level to create a 'purification handle'. For example, a short tail consisting of arginine residues allows a protein to bind to a cation exchanger under conditions where almost no other cell proteins bind. However, this technique is only useful for laboratory scale isolation of the product and cannot be used for production scale due to regulatory problems related to the removal of the arginine or other specific tag from the protein.

(Immuno)affinity chromatography

Affinity chromatography is based on highly specific interactions between an immobilized ligand and the protein of interest. Affinity chromatography is a very powerful method for the purification of proteins. Under physiological conditions the protein binds to the ligand. Extensive washing of this matrix will remove contaminants and the purified protein can be recovered either by the addition of ligands competing for the stationary phase binding sites or by changes in physical conditions (such as low or high pH of the eluent) which greatly reduce the affinity. Examples of affinity chromatography include the purification of glycoproteins, which bind to immobilized lectins and the purification of serine proteases with lysine binding sites, which bind to immobilized lysine. In these cases a soluble ligand (sugar or lysine, respectively) can be used to elute the required product under relatively mild conditions. Another example is the use of the affinity of protein A and protein G for antibodies. Protein A and protein G have a high affinity for the Fc portions of many immunoglobulins from various animals. Protein A and G matrices are commercially obtained with a high degree of purity. For the purification of e.g. hormones or growth factors, the receptors or short peptide sequence that mimic the binding site of the receptor molecule can be used as affinity ligands. Some proteins show highly selective affinity for certain dyes commercially available as immobilized ligands on purification matrices. When considering the selection of these ligands for pharmaceutical production, one must realize that some of these dyes are carcinogenic and that a fraction may leach out during the process.

An interesting approach for optimizing purification is to use a gene that codes not only for the desired protein, but also for an additional sequence that facilitates recovery by affinity chromatography. At a later stage the additional sequence is removed by a specific cleavage reaction. As mentioned before, this is a complex process that needs additional purification steps.

In general, use of affinity chromatography in the production process for therapeutics leads to complications during validation of the removal of free ligands or protein extensions. Consequently, this technology is rarely used in the industry. The specific binding of antibodies to their epitopes is used in immunoaffinity chromatography (Chase, 1993; Kamihira *et al.*, 1993). These techniques can be applied for purification of either the antigen or the antibody. The antibody can be covalently coupled to the stationary phase and can act as the 'receptor' for the antigen to be purified. Alternatively, the antigens, or parts thereof, can be attached to the stationary phase for the purification of the antibodies. Advantages of immunoaffinity chromatography are its high specificity and the combination of concentration and purification in one step.

A disadvantage associated with immunoaffinity methods is the sometimes very strong antibody-antigen binding. This binding requires harsh conditions during elution of the ligand. Under such conditions, sensitive ligands could be harmed (for example, by denaturation of the protein to be purified). There harmful conditions can be alleviated by, for example, the selection of antibodies and environmental conditions with high specificity and sufficient affinity to induce an antibody ligand interaction, while the antigen can be released under mild conditions (Jones, 1990).

Another concern is the disruption of the covalent bond linking the 'receptor' to the matrix. This disruption would result in elution of the entire complex. Therefore, in practice, a further purification step after affinity chromatography as well as an appropriate detection assay (e.g. ELISA) is almost always necessary. On the other hand, improved coupling chemistry that is less susceptible to hydrolysis has been developed to prevent leaching (Knight, 1990).

Scale-up of immunoaffinity chromatography is often hampered by the relatively large quantity of the specific 'receptor' (either the antigen or the antibody) that is required and the lack of commercially available, ready-to-use matrices.

Examples of proteins of potential therapeutic value that have been purified using immunoaffinity chromatography are: interferons, urokinase, Factor VIII:c, erythropoietin, interleukin-2, human Factor X, and recombinant tissue plasminogen activator.

Hydrophobic Interaction Chromatography

Under physiological conditions most hydrophobic amino acid residues are located inside the protein core and only a small fraction of hydrophobic amino acids is exposed on the 'surface' of a protein. Their exposure is suppressed because of the presence of hydrophilic amino acids that attract large clusters of water molecules and form a 'shield.' High salt concentrations reduce the hydration of a protein and the surface-exposed hydrophobic amino acid residues become more accessible. Hydrophobic Interaction Chromatography (HIC) is based on non-covalent and non-electrostatic interactions between proteins and the stationary phase. HIC is a mild technique, usually yielding high recoveries of proteins that are not damaged, are folded correctly and are separated from contaminants that are structurally related. HIC is ideally placed in the purification scheme after ion-exchange chromatography, where the protein is usually released in high ionic strength elution media (Heng and Glatz, 1993).

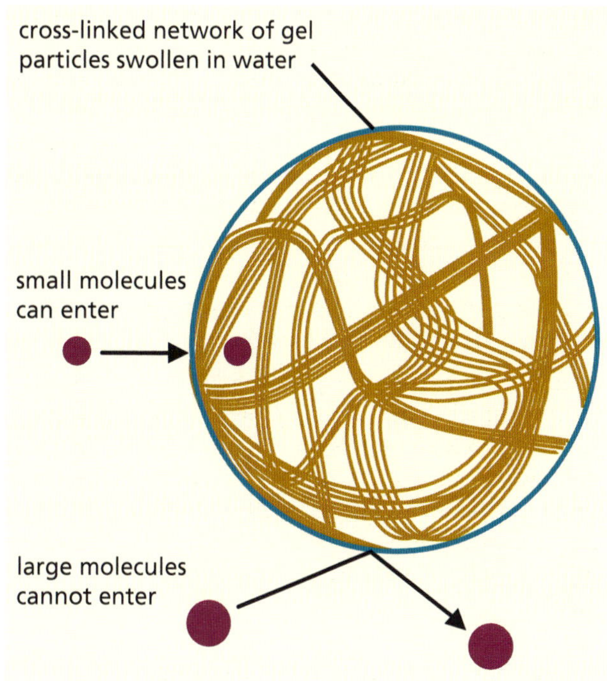

Figure 3.5. Schematic representation of the principle of gel filtration (from James, 1992).

Gel Permeation Chromatography

Gel-permeation or size-exclusion chromatography, also known as gel filtration, separates proteins according to their shape and size (see Figure 3.5). Inert gels with narrow pore-size distributions in the size range of proteins are available. These gels are packed into a column and the protein mixture is then loaded on top of the column and the proteins diffuse into the gel. The smaller the protein, the more volume it will have available in which to disperse. Molecules that are larger than the largest pores are not able to penetrate the gel beads and will, therefore, stay in the void volume of the column. When a continuous flow of buffer passes through the column, the larger proteins will elute first and the smallest molecules last. Gel permeation chromatography is a good alternative to diafiltration for buffer exchange at almost any purification stage, and it is often used in laboratory design. At production scale, the use of this technique is usually limited, because it requires relatively small sample volumes on a large column (up to one-third of the column volume in the case of "buffer exchange"). It is, therefore, best avoided or used late in the purification process when the protein is available in a highly concentrated form. Gel filtration is very commonly used as the final step in the purification to bring proteins in the appropriate buffer used in the final formulation.

Expanded Beds

As previously mentioned, purification schemes are based on multistep protocols. This not only adds greatly to the overall production costs, but can also result in a significant loss of product. Therefore, there is still an interest in the development of new methods for simplifying the purification process. Adsorption techniques are popular methods for the recovery of proteins, and the conventional operating format for preparative separations is a packed column (or fixed bed) of adsorbent. Particulate material, however, can be trapped near the bed, which results in an increase in the pressure drop across the bed and eventually in the clogging of the column. These problems can be avoided by the use of pre-column filters (0.2 μm) which preserve the column integrity. Another solution to this problem may be the use of expanded beds (Chase and Draeger, 1993; Fulton, 1994), also called fluidized beds (see Figure 3.6). In principle, the use of expanded beds enables clarification, concentration and purification to be achieved in a single step. The concept is to employ a particulate solid-phase adsorbent in an open bed with upward liquid flow. The hydrodynamic drag around the particles tends to lift them upwards, which is counteracted by gravity because of a density difference between the particles and the liquid phase. The particles remain suspended if particle diameter, particle density, liquid viscosity and liquid density are properly balanced by choosing the correct flow rate. The expanded bed allows particles (cells) to pass through, whereas molecules in solution are selectively retained (for example, by the use of ion-exchange or affinity adsorbents) on the adsorbent particles. Feedstocks can be applied to the bed without prior removal of particulate material by centrifugation or filtration. Fluidized beds have been previously used for the industrial scale recovery of antibiotics such as streptomycin and novobiocin (Fulton, 1994; Chase, 1994). Stable, expanded beds can be obtained using simple equipment adapted from that used for conventional, packed bed adsorption and chromatography processes. Ion-exchange adsorbents are likely to be chosen for such separations.

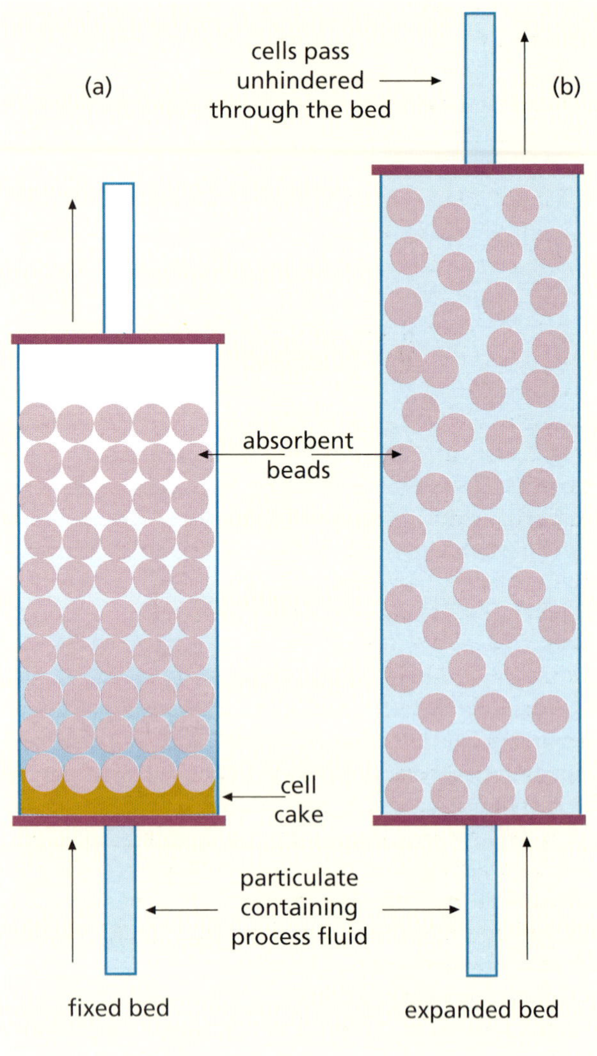

Figure 3.6. Comparison between (a) a packed bed and (b) an expanded bed (adapted from Chase and Draeger, 1993).

Issues to consider in Production and Purification of Proteins

N- and C-terminal heterogeneity

A major difficulty associated with the production of biotech products is the problem associated with the amino (NH_2)-terminus of the protein e.g. in *E. coli* systems, where protein synthesis always starts with f-methyl-methionine. Obviously, it has been of great interest to develop methods (Christensen *et al.*, 1990) that generate proteins with an NH_2-terminus, as found in the authentic protein. When the proteins are not produced in the correct way, the final product may contain several methionyl variants of the protein in question or even contain proteins lacking one or more residues from the amino terminus. This result is called the amino terminal heterogeneity. This heterogeneity can also occur with recombinant proteins (e.g. α-interferon) susceptible to proteases that are either secreted by the host or introduced by serum-containing media. These proteases can clip off amino acids from the C-terminal and/or N-terminal of the desired product (amino- and/or carboxy-terminal heterogeneity) (Garnick *et al.* 1988).

Amino- and/or carboxy-terminal heterogeneity is not desirable since it may cause difficulties in purification and characterization of the proteins. In case of the presence of an additional methionine at the N-terminal end of the protein, its secondary and tertiary structure can be altered. This could affect the biological activity and stability and may make it immunogenic. Moreover, N-terminal methionine and/or internal methionine are sensitive to oxidation (Sharma, 1990).

Chemical modification/conformational changes

Although mammalian cells are able to produce proteins structurally equal to endogenous proteins, some caution is advisable. Transcripts containing the full-length coding sequence could result in conformational isomers of the protein due to unexpected secondary structures that affect translational fidelity (Sharma, 1990). Another factor to be taken into account is the possible existence of equilibria between the desired form and other forms such as dimers. The correct folding of proteins after biosynthesis is important, because it determines the specific activity of the protein (Berthold and Walter, 1994). Therefore, it is important to determine if all molecules of a given recombinant protein secreted by a mammalian expression system are folded in their native conformation. In some cases it may be relatively easy to detect misfolded structures, in other cases it may be extremely difficult. Sometimes selection and purification of the native protein may require the development of novel preparative and analytical technologies for process development and quality assurance.

Apart from conformational changes, proteins can undergo chemical alterations, such as proteolysis, deamidation, hydroxyl and sulfhydryl oxidations during the purification process. These alterations can result in (partial) denaturation of the protein. Vice versa, denaturation of the protein may cause chemical modifications, as well (e.g. as a result of exposure of sensitive groups) (Ptitsyn, 1987).

Glycosylation

Many therapeutic proteins produced by recombinant DNA technology are glycoproteins (Sharma, 1990). The presence and nature of oligosaccharide side chains in proteins affect a number of important characteristics, such as the protein serum half-life, solubility, stability and sometimes even the pharmacological function (Cumming, 1991). As a result, the therapeutic profile may be 'glycosylation' dependent. As previously mentioned, protein glycosylation is not determined by the DNA sequence. It is an enzymatic modification of the protein after translation, and can depend on the environment in the cell. Although mammalian cells can efficiently glycosylate proteins, it is hard to fully control glycosylation. Carbohydrate heterogeneity is detected by variations in the size of the chain, type of oligosaccharide, and sequence of the carbohydrates. This has been demonstrated for a number of recombinant products, including interleukin-4, chorionic gonadotropin, erythropoietin and tissue plasminogen activator. Carbohydrate structure and composition in recombinant proteins may differ from their native counterparts, because the enzymes required for synthesis and processing vary in different expression systems (for example, glycoproteins in insect cells are frequently smaller than the same glycoproteins expressed in mammalian cells) or even from one mammalian system to another.

Proteolytic processing

Proteases play an important role in the processing, maturation, modification, or isolation of recombinant proteins (Sharma and Hopkins, 1981). Proteases from mammalian cells are involved in secreting proteins into the cultivation medium. If secretion of the recombinant protein occurs co-translationally, then the intracellular proteolytic system of the mammalian cell should not be harmful to the recombinant protein. Proteases are released if cells die or break (e.g. during cell break at cell harvest) and undergo lysis. It is, therefore, important to control growth and harvest conditions in order to minimize this effect. Another source of proteolytic attack is found in the components of the medium in which the cells are grown. For example, serum contains a number of proteases and protease zymogens that may affect the secreted recombinant protein. If present in small amounts, and if the nature of the proteolytic attack on the desired protein is identified, appropriate protease inhibitors to control proteolysis could be used. It is best to document the integrity of the recombinant protein after each purification step.

Proteins become much more susceptible to proteases at elevated temperatures. Purification strategies should be designed to carry out all the steps at 4 °C (Sharma, 1990) or proteolytic degradation will occur. Alternatively, Ca^{24} complexing agents (e.g. citrate) can be added, as many proteases depend on Ca^{24} for their activity.

Protein inclusion body formation

In bacteria soluble proteins can from dense, finely granular inclusions within the cytoptasm. These 'inclusion bodies' often occur in bacterial cells that overproduce proteins by plasmid expression. The protein inclusions appear in electron micrographs as large, dense bodies often spanning the entire diameter of the cell. Protein inclusions are probably formed by a build-up of amorphous protein aggregates held together by covalent and non-covalent bonds.

The inability to measure inclusion body proteins directly may lead to the inaccurate assessment of recovery and yield and may cause problems if protein solubility is essential for efficient, large-scale purification (Berthold and Walter, 1994). Several schemes for the recovery of proteins from inclusion bodies have been described (Krueger *et al.*, 1989). The recovery of proteins from inclusion bodies requires cell breakage and inclusion body recovery. Dissolution of inclusion proteins is the next step in the purification scheme. Generally, inclusion proteins dissolve in denaturing agents such as sodium dodecylsulfate (SDS), urea, or guanidine hydrochloride. As bacterial systems are generally incapable of forming disulfide bonds, a protein containing these bonds has to be re-folded under oxidizing conditions to restore these bonds and to generate the biologically active protein. This so-called renaturation step is increasingly difficult if more S-S bridges are present in the molecule, and the yield of renatured product could be as low as only a few percent. Once the protein is solubilized, conventional chromatographic separations can be used for further purification of the protein.

Aggregate formation may seem undesirable at first sight, but there may also be advantages as long as the protein of interest will unfold and refold properly. Inclusion body proteins can easily be recovered to yield proteins with > 50 % purity, a substantial improvement over the purity of soluble proteins (sometimes below 1% of the total cell protein). Furthermore, the aggregated forms of the proteins are more resistant to proteolysis (Krueger *et al.*, 1989), because most molecules of an aggregated form are not accessible to proteolytic enzymes. Thus, the high yield and relatively cheap production system can offset a low yield renaturation process. For a non-glycosylated, simple molecule this is still the production system of choice. ■

References

- **Afeyan, N., Gordon, N., Mazsaroff, I., Varady, L., Fulton, S., Yang, Y., Regnier, F.** (1989) Flow-through particles of the high-performance liquid chromatographic separation of biomolecules, perfusion chromatography. *J. Chromatogr.*, **519**, 1–29.
- **Arathoon, W.R., Birch, J.R.** (1986) Large-scale cell culture in biotechnology. *Science*, **232**, 1390–1395.
- **Benedek, K., Swadesh, J.K.** (1991) HPLC of proteins and peptides in the pharmaceutical industry, In G.W. Fong, S.K. Lam, (eds.), *HPLC in the Pharmaceutical Industry*, Dekker, New York, pp. 241–302.
- **Berthold, W., Walter, J.** (1994) Protein purification: Aspects of processes for pharmaceutical products. *Biologicals*, **22**, 135–150.
- **Burnouf, T., Dernis, D., Michalski, C., Goudemand, M., Huart, J.J.** (1989) Therapeutic advantages of a high purity plasma factor IX concentrate produced by conventional chromatography. *Colloque Inserm.* **175**, 25–334.
- **Burnouf-Radosevich, M., Appourchaux P., Huart J.J., Burnouf T.** (1994) Nanofiltration, a New specific virus elimination method applied to high-purity Factor IX and Factor XI concentrates. *Vox Sang*, **67**, 132–8.
- **Cartwright, T.** (1987) Isolation and purification of products from animal cells, *Trends in Biotechnology.*, **5**, 25–30.
- **Chase, H., Draeger, N.** (1993) Affinity purification of proteins using expanded beds. *J. Chromatogr.*, **597**, 129–145.
- **Chase, H.A.** (1988) Adsorption preparation processes for protein purification. In A. Mizrahi (ed.), *Downstream processes: Equipment and techniques*, A.R. Liss, New York., **Vol. 8**, pp. 163–312.
- **Chase, H.A.** (1994) Purification of proteins by adsorption chromatography in expanded beds. *Tibtech.*, **12**, 296–303.
- **Christensen, T., Dalboge, H., Snel, L.** (1990) Postbiosynthesis modification: human growth hormone and insulin precursors, In: *Drug Manufacture Part IV.*
- **Cumming D.A.** (1991), Glycosylation of recombinant protein therapeutics: control and functional implications. Glycobiology, **1 (2)**, 115–30.
- **European Agency for the Evaluation of Medicinal Products** (EMEA, 1999a), Note for Guidance on minimising the risk of transmission of animal/spongiform encephalopathy agents.
- **European Agency for the Evaluation of Medicinal Products** (EMEA, 1999b), Human Medicines Evaluation Unit. ICH Topic Q6B. Specifications test procedures and acceptance criteria for biotechnology/biological products.
- **European Agency for the Evaluation of Medicinal Products** (EMEA, 1997), Human Medicines Evaluation Unit. ICH Topic Q5D. Quality of biotechnological products: Derivation and characterisation of cell substrates used for production of biotechnological/biological products.
- **European Pharmacopoeia Third Edition**. Strasbourg: Council of Europe, 1997.
- **FDA, Center for Biologics Evaluation and Research** (1990) *Cytokine and growth factor pre-Ppivotal Ttrial information Ppackage with special emphasis on products identified for consideration under 21 CFR 312 Subpart E.*, Bethesda, MD, USA.
- **FDA, Office of Biologicals Research and Review** (1993) *Points to consider in the characterization of cell lines used to produce biologicals*, Rockville Rike, Bethesda MD, USA.
- **Fulton, S.P.** (1994) Large scale processing of macromolecules. *Current Opinion in Biotechnology*, **5**, 201–205.
- **Garnick, R.L., Solli, N.J., Papa, P.A.** (1988) The role of quality control in biotechnology: an analytical perspective. *Anal. Chem.*, **60**, 2546–2557.

- **Heng, M., Glatz, C.** (1993) Charged fusions for selective recovery of β-galactosidase from cell extract using hollow fiber ion-exchange membrane adsorption. *Biotechnol. Bioeng.*, **42**, 333–338.
- **Hippel, von, P.H., Wong, K.-Y.** (1964) Neutral salts: the generality of their effects on the stability of macromolecular conformations, Science, **145**, 577–580.
- **Hjerten, S., Mohammed, J., Nakazato, K.** (1993) Improvement in flow properties and pH stability of compressed, continuous polymer beds for high-performance liquid chromatography. *J. Chromatogr.*, **646**, 121–128.
- **Homma, T., Fuji M., Mori J., Kawakami T., Kuroda K., Taniguchi M.** (1993) Production of cellobiose by enzymatic hydrolysis: removal of β-glucosidae from cellulase by affinity precipitation using chitosan. *Biotechnol. Bioeng.*, **41**, 405–410.
- **Horowitz, M.S., Bolmer, S.D., Horowitz. B.** (1991) Elimination of disease-transmitting enveloped viruses from human blood plasma and mammalian cell culture products. *Bioseperation*, **1**, 409–417.
- **Horowitz, B., Prince, A.M., Hamman, J., Watklevicz, C.** (1994) Viral safety of solvent/detergent-treated blood products. *Blood Coagulation and Fibrinolysis*, **5**, S21–S28.
- **James, A.M.** (1992) Introduction fundamental techniques. In A.M. James (ed.) *Analysis of Amino Acids and Nucleic Acids*, Butterworth-Heinemann, Oxford, pp. 1–28.
- **Jones, K.** (1990) Affinity chromatography, A technology up-date, *Am. Biotechnol. Lab.*, **8**, 26–30.
- **Jungbauer, A., Wenisch, E.** (1989) High Performance Liquid Chromatography and related methods in purification of monoclonal antibodies. In A.R. Liss, (ed.), *Advances in biotechnological processes*, New York, pp. 161–192.
- **Kamihira, M., Kaul, R., Mattiasson, B.** (1993) Purification of recombinant protein A by aqueous two-phase extraction integrated with affinity precipitation. *Biotechnol. Bioeng.*, **40**, 1381–1387.
- **Klegerman, M.E., Groves, M.J.** (1992) *Pharmaceutical Biotechnology*, Interpharm Press, Inc., USA.
- **Knight, P.** (1990) Bioseparations: media and modes. *Biotechnology*, **8**, 200.
- **Krueger, J.K., Kulke, M.H., Schutt, C., Stock, J.** (1989) Protein inclusion body formation and purification. *Pharmaceutical Technology International*, 48–51.
- **Kung, V.T., Panfili, P.R., Sheldon, E.L., King, R.S., Nagainis, P.A., Gomez, B., Ross, D.A., Briggs, J., Zuk, R.F.** (1990) Picogram quantification of total DNA using DNA-binding proteins in a silicon sensor based system. *Anal. Biochem.*, **187**, 220–227.
- **Liptrot, C., Gull, K.** (1991) Detection of viruses in recombinant cells by electron microscopy. In R.E., Spier, J.B. Griffiths, C. MacDonald, (eds.) *Animal Cell Technology, Developments, Processes and Products*, Butterworth-Heinemann Ltd., Oxford, 653–656.
- **Löwer, J.** (1990) Risk of tumor induction in vivo by residual cellular DNA: Quantitative Considerations. *J. Med. Virol.*, **31**, 50–53.
- **Marcus-Sekura, C.J.** (1991) *Validation and Removal of Human Retroviruses.* Center for Biologics Evaluation and Research, FDA, Bethesda, MD, USA.
- **Maerz, H., Hahn, S.O., Maassen, A., Meisel, H., Roggenbuck, D., Sato, T., Tanzmann, H., Emmrich, F., Marx, U.** (1996). Improved removal of viruslike particles from purified monoclonal antibody IgM preparation via virus filtration. Nat Biotechnol, **14**, 651–2.
- **Minton, A.P.** (1990) Quantitative characterization of reversible molecular associations via analytical centrifugation. *Anal. Biochem.*, **190**, 1–6.
- **Minor P.D.** (1994) Ensuring safety and consistency in cell culture production processes: viral screening and inactivation. TIB TECH, **12**, 257–61.
- **Nolan, J.G., McDevitt, J.J., Goldmann, G.S.** (1975) Endotoxin binding by charged and uncharged resin. *Proc. Soc. Exp. Biol. Med.*, **149**, 766–770.
- **Note for Guidance** (1991) *Validation of Virus Removal and Inactivation Procedure*, Ad Hoc Working Party on Biotechnology/ Pharmacy, European Community, DG III/8115/89-EN.
- **Perret, B.A., Poorbeik, M., Morell, A.** (1991) Klinische prüfung von Premogfil M SRK, einem mit monoklonalen antikörpern hochgereinigten gerinningsfaktor VIII-Konzentrat aus humanplasma. *Schweiz. Med. Wochenschr.*, **121**, 1624–1627.
- **Ptitsyn, O.B.** (1987) Protein folding: Hypothesis and experiments. *J. Protein Chem.* **6**, 273–293.
- **Sadana, A.** (1989) Protein inactivation during downstream separation, part I: The Processes, *Biopharm.*, **2**, 14–25.
- **Schindler, R., Dinarello, C.A.** (1990) Ultrafiltration to Remove Endotoxins and other Cytokine-Inducing Materials from Tissue Culture Media and Parenteral Fluids. *Bio. Techniques*, **8**, 408–413.
- **Sharma, S.K., Hopkins, T.R.** (1981) Recent developments in the activation process of bovine chymotrypsinogen A. *Bioorganic Chem.* **10**, 357–374.
- **Sharma, S.K.** (1990) Key issues in the purification and characterization of recombinant proteins for therapeutic use. *Advanced Drug Delivery Reviews*, **4**, 87–111.
- **Strickler, M.P., Gemski, M.J.** (1987) *Commercial Production of Monoclonal Antibodies*, Marcel Dekker, New York, pp 217–245.
- **Tennikova, T., Svec, F.** (1993) High Performance Membrane Chromatography: Highly efficient separation method for proteins in ion-exchange, hydrophobic interaction and reversed phase modes. *J. Chromatogr.*, **646**, 279–288.
- **Terstappen, G., Ramelmeier, R., Kula, M.** (1993) Protein partitioning in detergent-based aqueous two-phase systems. *J. Biotechnol.*, **28**, 263–275.
- **Walter, J., Werner, R.G.** (1993) Regulatory requirements and economic aspects in downstream processing of biotechnically engineered proteins for parenteral application as pharmaceuticals. In K.H. Kroner, N. Papamichael, H. Schütte (eds.), *Downstream Processing, Recovery and Purification of Proteins*, A Handbook of Principles and Practice, John Wiley Publishers Inc., New York.

- **Walter, J., Werz, W., McGoff, P., Werner, R.G., Berthold, W.** (1991) Virus removal/inactivation in downstream processing. In R.E. Spier, J.B. Griffiths, C. MacDonald (eds.), *Animal cell Technology: Development, Processes and Products*, Butterworth-Heinemann Ltd. Linacre House, Oxford, pp. 624–634.
- **Walter, K., Werz, W., Berthold, W.** (1992) Virus removal and inactivation, Concept and data for Pprocess validation of downstream processing, *Biotech. Forum Europe*, **9**, 560–564.
- **Wheelwright, S.M.** (1993) Designing downstream processing for large scale protein purification, *Biotechnology*, **5**, 789–793.
- **White, E.M., Grun, J.B., Sun C-S., Sito, F.** (1991) Process validation for virus removal and inactivation. *BioPharm* 34–9.
- **World Health Organization** (1998), Requirements for the use of animal cells as in vitro substrates for the production of biologicals (Requirements for Biological Substances No. 50). *Technical Report Series* **878**, Biologicals, 26: 175–93.
- **World Health Organization**, Guidelines for assuring the quality of pharmaceutical and biological products prepared by recombinant DNA technology, *Technical Report Series* **823**, 105–115.

Self-Assessment Questions

Question 1: *Name four types of different bioreactors.*

Question 2: *Chromatography is an essential step in the purification of biotech products. Name at least 5 different chromatographic purification methods.*

Question 3: *What are the major safety concerns in the purification of cell-expressed proteins?*

Question 4: *What are the critical issues in production and purification that must be addressed in process validation?*

Question 5: *Mention at least 5 issues to consider in the cultivation and purification of proteins.*

Statement: true or not true *Glycosylation is an important post-translational change of pharmaceutical proteins. Glycosylation is only possible in mammalian cells.*

Question 6: *Glycosylation may affect several properties of the protein. Mention at three possible changes in case of glycosylation.*

Question 7: *Pharmacologically active biotech protein products have complex three dimensional structures. Mention two or more important factors that affect these structures.*

Answers

Answer 1 Stirred-tank, Airlift, Microcarrier and Membrane bioreactors.

Answer 2 Adsorption chromatography, Ion-exchange chromatography, Affinity chromatography, Hydrophobic Interaction Chromatography, Gel permeation or Size-exclusion chromatography.

Answer 3 Removal of viruses, bacteria, protein contaminants and cellular DNA.

Answer 4 Production: scaling up and design. Purification: procedures should be reliable in potency and quality of the product and in the removal of viral, bacterial and protein contaminants.

Answer 5 Grade of purity, pyrogenicity, N- and C-terminal heterogeneity, chemical modification/ conformational changes, glycosylation and proteolytic processing.

not true; glycosylation is also possible in yeast cells.

Answer 6 solubility, pK_a, charge, stability and biological activity.

Answer 7 amino-acid structure, hydrogen and sulfide bridging, post-translational changes and chemical modification of the amino acid rest groups.

4 Formulation of Biotech Products, Including Biopharmaceutical Considerations

Daan J.A. Crommelin

Introduction

This Chapter discusses formulation aspects of pharmaceutical proteins. Both technological questions and biopharmaceutical issues, such as the choice of the delivery systems, the route of administration and possibilities for the site specific delivery of proteins are considered.

Microbiological Considerations

Sterility

Most proteins are administered parenterally and have to be sterile. In general, proteins are sensitive to heat and other regularly used sterilization treatments; they cannot withstand autoclaving, gas sterilization, or sterilization by ionizing radiation. Consequently, sterilization of the end product is not possible. Therefore, protein pharmaceuticals have to be assembled under aseptic conditions, following the established and evolving rules in the pharmaceutical industry for aseptic manufacture. The reader is referred to standard textbooks for details (Halls, 1994; Groves, 1988; Klegerman and Groves, 1992).

Equipment and excipients are treated separately and autoclaved, or sterilized by dry heat (> 160 °C), chemical treatment or gamma radiation to minimize the bioburden. Filtration techniques are used for the removal of microbacterial contaminants. Prefilters remove the bulk of the bioburden and other particulate materials. The final 'sterilizing' step is filtration through 0.2 or 0.22 µm membrane filters. Assembly of the product is done in class 100 (maximum 100 particles > 0.5 µm per cubic foot) rooms with laminar air flow that is filtered through HEPA (high efficiency particulate air) filters. Additionally, the 'human factor' is a major source of contamination, and well-trained operators wearing protective cloths (face masks, hats, gowns, gloves, or head-to-toe overall garments) should operate the facility. The regular exchange of filters, regular validation of HEPA equipment and the thorough cleaning of the room and equipment are critical factors for success.

Viral decontamination

As recombinant DNA products are grown in microorganisms, these organisms should be tested for viral contaminants and appropriate measures should be taken if viral contamination occurs. No (unwanted) viral material should be introduced during the manufacturing process. Excipients with a certain risk factor, such as blood derived human serum albumin, should be carefully tested before use and their presence in the formulation process should be minimized (see Chapter 3).

Pyrogen removal

Pyrogens are compounds that induce fever. Exogenous pyrogens (pyrogens introduced into the body, not generated by the body itself) can be derived from bacterial, viral or fungal sources. Bacterial pyrogens are mainly endotoxins shed from gram negative bacteria. They are lipopolysaccharides. A general structure is shown in Figure 4.1. The basic, conserved structure in the full array of thousands of different endotoxins is the lipid A-moiety. Another general property shared by endotoxins is their high, negative electrical charge. Their tendency to aggregate and to form large units with M_w of over 10^6 in water, in addition to their tendency to adsorb to surfaces, indicates that these compounds are amphipatic in nature. They are stable under standard autoclaving conditions, but break down when heated in the dry state. For this reason equipment and containers are treated at temperatures above 160 °C for prolonged periods (e.g. 30 minutes dry heat at 250 °C).

Pyrogen removal of recombinant products derived from bacterial sources should be an integral part of the preparation process. Ion exchange chromatographic procedures (utilizing its negative charge) can effectively reduce endotoxin levels in solution (cf. Chapter 3).

Excipients used in the protein formulation should be essentially endotoxin-free. For solutions, Water for Injection (compendial standards) is (freshly) distilled or produced by reverse osmosis. The aggregated endotoxins can not pass through the reverse osmosis membrane. Removal of endotoxins immediately prior to the filling of the final

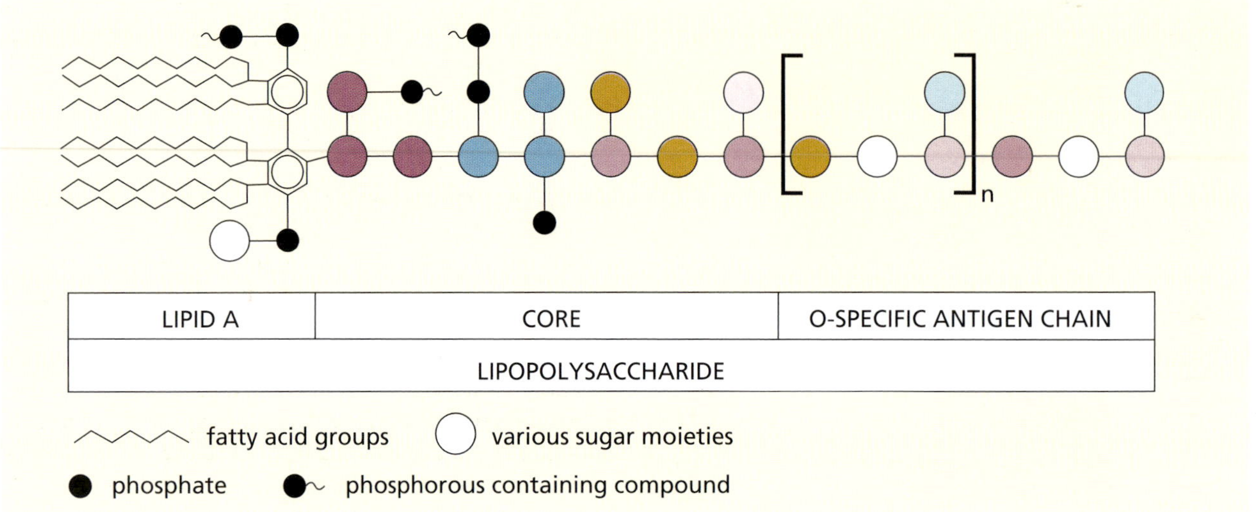

Figure 4.1. Generalized structure of endotoxins. Most properties of endotoxins are accounted for by the active, insoluble 'Lipid A' fraction being solubilized by the various sugar moieties (circles with different colors). Although the general structure is similar, individual endotoxins vary according to their source and are characterized by the O-specific antigenic chain. Adapted from Groves 1988.

container can be accomplished by using activated charcoal or other materials with large surfaces offering hydrophobic interactions. Endotoxins can also be inactivated on utensil surfaces by oxidation (e.g. peroxide) or dry heating (e.g. 30 minutes dry heat at 250 °C).

Excipients Used in Parenteral Formulations of Biotech Products

In a protein formulation one finds, apart from the active substance, a number of excipients selected to serve different purposes. This process of formulation design should be carried out with great care to ensure therapeutically effective and safe products. The nature of the protein (e.g. lability) and its therapeutic use (e.g. multiple injection systems) can make these formulations quite complex in terms of excipient profile and technology (freeze-drying, aseptic preparation). Table 4.1 lists components that can be found in the presently marketed formulations. In the following sections this list is discussed in more detail.

Solubility Enhancers

Proteins, in particular those that are non-glycosylated, may have a tendency to aggregate and precipitate. Approaches that can be used to enhance solubility include the selection of the proper pH and ionic strength conditions the addition of amino acids, such as lysine or arginine (used to solubilize tissue plasminogen activator, t-PA), or surfactants, such as sodium dodecylsulfate, to solubilize non-glucosylated IL-2 can also help to increase the solubility. The mechanism of action of these solubility enhancers depends on the type of enhancer and the protein involved and is not always fully understood.

Figure 4.2 shows the effect of arginine concentration on the solubility of t-PA (alteplase) at pH 7.2 and 25 °C. This Figure clearly indicates the dramatic effect of this basic amino acid on the apparent solubility of t-PA.

In the above examples aggregation is physical in nature, i.e. based on hydrophobic and/or electrostatic interactions between molecules. However, aggregation based on the formation of covalent bridges between molecules through disulfide bonds, and ester or amide linkages has been described, as well (cf. Table 2.4). In these cases proper conditions should be found to avoid these chemical reactions.

- active ingredient
- solubility enhancers
- anti-adsorption and anti-aggregation agents
- buffer components
- preservatives and anti-oxidants
- lyoprotectants/cake formers
- osmotic agents
- carrier system (see later on in this section)

Table 4.1. Components found in parenteral formulations of biotech products.
Not necessarily all of the above • are present in one particular protein formulation.

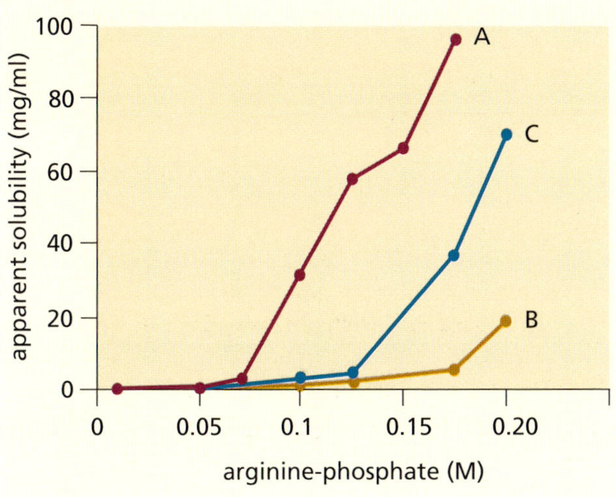

Figure 4.2. Effect of arginine on type I and type II alteplase at pH 7.2 and 25 °C. A, type I alteplase; B, type II alteplase; C, 50:50 mixture of type I and type II alteplase. From Nguyen and Ward, 1993.

Anti-adsorption and Anti-aggregation agents

Anti-adsorption agents are added to reduce adsorption of the active protein to interfaces. Some proteins tend to expose hydrophobic sites, normally present in the core of the native protein structure when an interface is present. These interfaces can be water/air, water/container wall or interfaces formed between the aqueous phase and utensils used to administer the drug (e.g. catheter, needle). These adsorbed, partially unfolded protein molecules form aggregates, leave the surface, return to the aqueous phase, form larger aggregates and precipitate. As an example, the proposed mechanism for aggregation of insulin in aqueous media through contact with a hydrophobic surface (or water-air interface) is presented in Figure 4.3 (Thurow and Geisen, 1984).

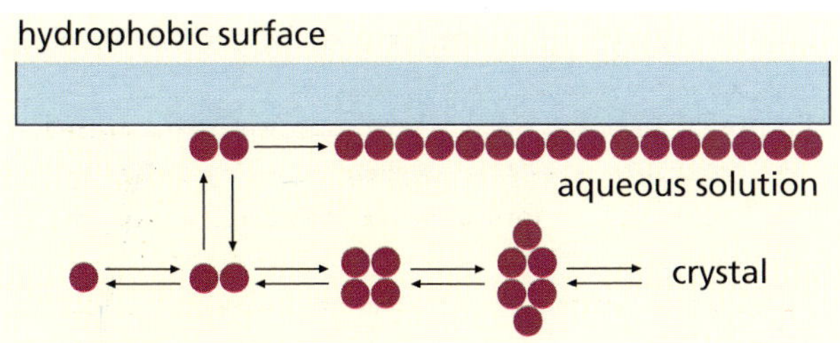

Figure 4.3. Reversible self-association of insulin, its adsorption to the hydrophobic interface and irreversible aggregation in the adsorbed protein film: ● represents a monomeric insulin molecule. Adapted from Thurow and Geisen, 1984.

Native insulin in solution is in an equilibrium state between monomeric, dimeric, tetrameric and hexameric forms (cf. Chapter 10). The relative abundance of the different aggregation states depends on the pH, insulin concentration, ionic strength and specific excipients (e.g. Zn^{2+} and phenol). It has been suggested that the dimeric form of insulin adsorbs to hydrophobic interfaces and subsequently forms larger aggregates at the interface. This adsorption explains why anti-adhesion agents can also act as anti-aggregation agents. Albumin has a strong tendency to adsorb to surfaces and is therefore added in relatively high concentrations (e.g. 1%) to protein formulations as an anti-adhesion agent. Albumin competes with the therapeutic protein for binding sites and supposedly prevents adhesion of the therapeutically active agent by a combination of its binding tendency and abundant presence.

Insulin is one of the many proteins that can form fibrillar precipitates (long rod-shaped structures with diameters in the 0.1 μm range). Low concentrations of phospholipids and surfactants have been shown to exert a fibrillation-inhibitory effect. The selection of the proper pH can also help to prevent this unwanted phenomenon (Brange and Langkjaer, 1993).

Apart from albumin, surfactants can also prevent adhesion to interfaces and precipitation. These molecules readily adsorb to hydrophobic interfaces with their own hydrophobic groups and render this interface hydrophilic by exposing their hydrophilic groups to the aqueous phase.

Buffer Components

Buffer selection is an important part of the formulation process, because of the pH dependence of protein solubility and physical and chemical stability. Buffer systems regularly encountered in biotech formulations are phosphate, citrate and acetate. A good example of the importance of the i.e.p. (iso-electric point, negative logarithm = pI) is the solubility profile of human growth hormone (hGH, pI around 5) as presented in Figure 4.4.

Even short, temporary pH changes can cause aggregation. These conditions can occur, for example, during the freezing step in the freeze-drying process, when one of the buffer components is crystallizing and the other is not. In a phosphate buffer, Na_2HPO_4 crystallizes faster than NaH_2PO_4. This causes a pronounced drop in pH during the freezing step. Other buffer components do not crystallize, but form amorphous systems and then pH changes are minimized.

Preservatives and Anti-oxidants

Methionine, cysteine, tryptophan, tyrosine and histidine are amino acids that are readily oxidized (cf. Table 2.4). Proteins rich in these amino acids are susceptible to

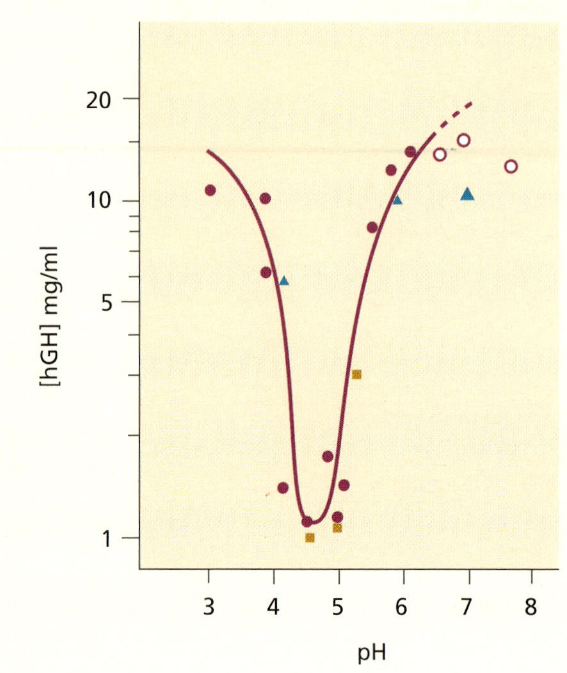

Figure 4.4. A plot of the solubility of various forms of hGH as a function of pH. Samples of hGH were either recombinant hGH (circles), Met-hGH (triangles) or pituitary hGH (squares). Solubility was determined by dialysing an approximately 11 mg/ml solution of each protein into an appropriate buffer for each pH. Buffers were citrate, pH 3-7, and borate, pH 8-9, all at 10 mM buffer concentrations. Concentrations of hGH were measured by UV absorbance as well as by RP-HPLC, relative to an external standard. The closed symbols indicate that precipitate was present in the dialysis tube after equilibration, whereas open symbols mean that no solid material was present, and thus the solubility is at least this amount. From Pearlman and Bewley 1993.

oxidative degradation. The replacement of oxygen by inert gases in the vials helps to reduce oxidative stress. Moreover, the addition of anti-oxidants, such as ascorbic acid or sodium formaldehyde sulfoxylate, can be considered (Groves, 1988). Interestingly, destabilizing effects on proteins have been described for anti-oxidants, as well (Vemuri *et al.*, 1993b); e.g. ascorbic acid can act as an oxidant in the presence of a number of heavy metals.

Certain proteins are formulated in containers designed for multiple injection schemes. After administering the first dose, contamination with microorganisms may occur and preservatives are needed to minimize growth. Usually, these preservatives are present in concentrations that are bacteriostatic rather than bactericide in nature. Antimicrobial agents mentioned in the USP XXIV are the mercury-containing phenylmercuric nitrate and thimerosal and p-hydroxybenzoic acids, phenol, benzyl alcohol and chlorobutanol (XXIV/NF 19, 2000; Groves, 1988; Pearlman and Bewley, 1993).

Osmotic Agents

For proteins, the regular rules apply for adjusting the tonicity of parenteral products. Saline and mono- or disaccharide solutions are commonly used. These excipients may not be inert; they may influence protein structural stability. For example, sugars and polyhydric alcohols can stabilize the protein structure through the principle of "preferential exclusion" (Arakawa *et al.*, 1991). These additives enhance the interaction of the solvent (water structure promoters) with the protein and are themselves excluded from the protein surface layer; the protein is preferentially hydrated. This phenomenon can be monitored through an increased thermal stability of the protein. Unfortunately, a strong "preferential exclusion" effect enhances the tendency of proteins to self-associate.

Shelf Life of Protein Based Pharmaceuticals

Proteins can be stored (1) as an aqueous solution, (2) in freeze-dried form, and (3) in dried form in a compacted state (tablet) (cf. Table 18.3). Some mechanisms behind

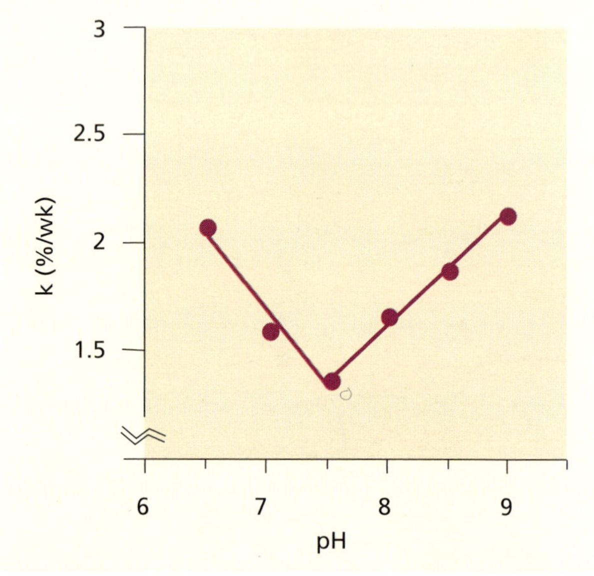

Figure 4.5. pH stability profile (at 25 °C) of monomeric recombinant α_1-antitrypsin (rAAT) by size exclusion-HPLC assay. k = degradation rate constant. Monomeric rAAT decreased rapidly in concentration both under acidic and basic conditions. Optimal stability occurred at pH 7.5. Adjusted from Vemuri *et al.*, 1993.

chemical and physical degradation processes have been briefly discussed in Chapter 2.

The stability of protein solutions strongly depends on factors such as pH, ionic strength, temperature, and the presence of stabilizers. For example, Figure 4.5 shows the pH dependence of α1-antitrypsin and clearly demonstrates the critical importance of pH on the shelf-life of proteins.

Freeze-Drying of Proteins

Proteins in solution often do not meet the preferred stability requirements for industrially produced pharmaceutical products (> 2 years), even when kept permanently under refrigerator conditions (cold chain). The abundant presence of water promotes chemical and physical degradation processes.

Freeze-drying may provide the desired stability. During freeze-drying water is removed via sublimation and not by evaporation. Three stages can be discerned in the freeze-drying process: (1) a freezing step, (2) the primary drying step, and (3) the secondary drying step (Figure 4.6). Table 4.2 explains what happens during these stages.

The freeze-drying of a protein solution without the proper excipients causes, as a rule, irreversible damage to the protein. Table 4.3 lists excipients typically encountered in successfully freeze-dried protein products.

Freezing The temperature of the product is reduced from ambient temperature to a temperature below the eutectic temperature (T_e), or below the glass transition temperature (T_g) of the system. A T_g is encountered if amorphous phases are present.
Primary drying Crystallized and water not bound to protein/excipient is removed by sublimation. The temperature is below the T_e or T_g; the temperature is for example -40 °C and reduced pressures are used.
Secondary drying Removal of water interacting with the protein and excipients. The temperature in the chamber is kept below T_g and rises gradually, e.g., from -40 °C to 20 °C.

Table 4.2. Three stages in the freeze drying process of protein formulations.

Freezing

In the freezing step (cf. Figure 4.6) the temperature of the aqueous system in the vials is lowered. Ice crystal formation does not start right at the thermodynamic or equilibrium freezing point, but supercooling occurs. That means that crystallization often only occurs when temperatures of −15 °C or lower have been reached. During the crystallization step the temperature may temporarily rise in the vial, because of the generation of crystallization heat. During the cooling stage, concentration of the protein and excipients occurs because of the growing ice crystal mass at the expense of the aqueous water phase. The formation of ice crystals can cause precipitation of one or more of the excipients,

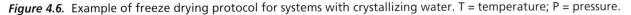

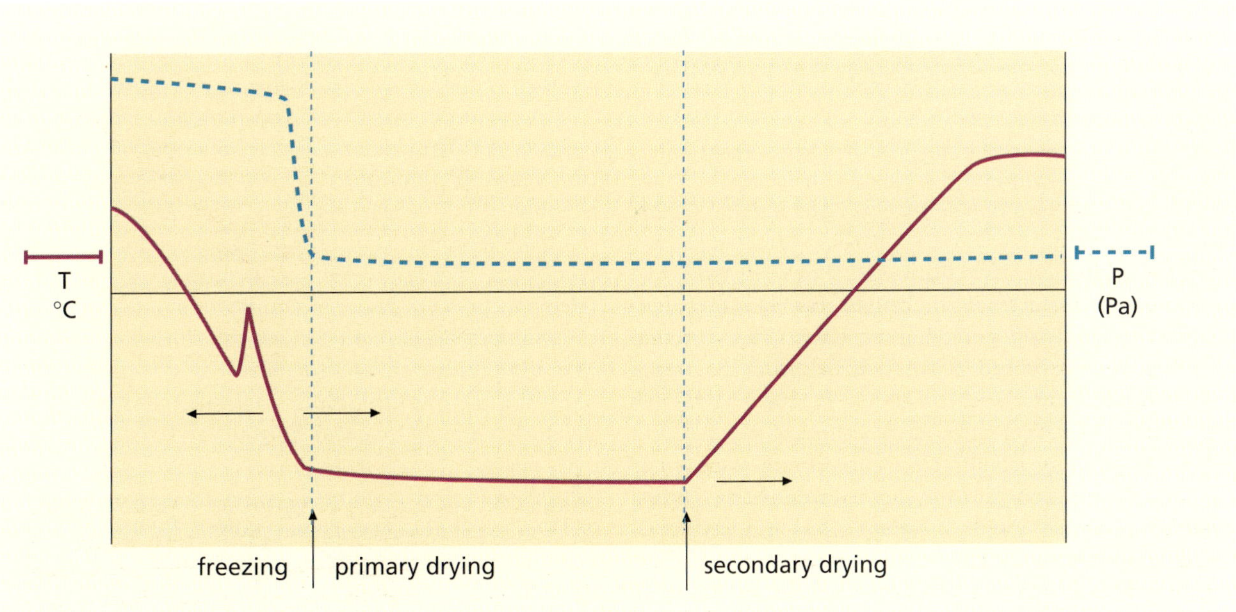

Figure 4.6. Example of freeze drying protocol for systems with crystallizing water. T = temperature; P = pressure.

• bulking agents: mannitol/glycine	reason: elegance/blowout prevention*
• collapse temperature modifier: dextran, albumin/gelatine	reason: increase collapse temperature
• lyoprotectant: sugars, albumin	reason: protection of the physical structure of the protein**

* Blowout is the loss of material taken away by the water vapor that leaves the vial. It occurs when little solid material is present in the vial.

** Mechanism of action of lyoprotectants is not fully understood. Factors that might play a role are:

(1) lyoprotectants replace water as stabilizing agent (water replacement theory),
(2) lyoprotectants increase the Tg of the cake/frozen system
(3) lyoprotectants will absorb moisture from the stoppers
(4) lyoprotectants slow down the secondary drying process and minimize the chances for overdrying of the protein. Overdrying might occur when residual water levels after secondary drying become too low. Pikal (Pikal, 1990b) considers the chance for overdrying 'in real life' small.

Table 4.3. Typical excipients in a freeze-dried protein formulation.

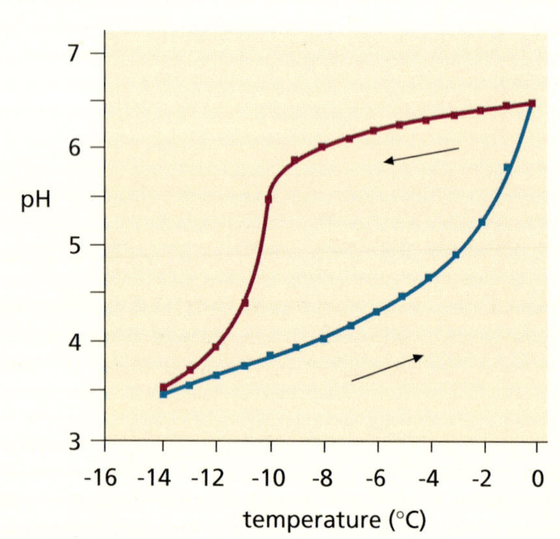

Figure 4.7. Thawing/cooling; ▪ = thawing ▪ = cooling. The effect of freezing on the pH of a citric acid-disodium phosphate buffer system. Cited in Pikal, 1990a.

which may consequently result in pH shifts (see above and Figure 4.7) or ionic strength changes. It may also induce protein denaturation. Cooling of the vials is done through lowering the temperature of the shelf. Selecting the proper cooling scheme for the shelf -and, consequently, for the vial- is important as it dictates the degree of supercooling and ice crystal size. Small crystals are formed during fast cooling; large crystals form by lower cooling rates. Small ice crystals are requested for porous solids and fast sublimation rates (Pikal, 1990a).

If the system does not (fully) crystallize but forms an amorphous mass upon cooling, the temperature during the 'freezing stage' should drop below T_g, the glass transition temperature. In amorphous systems the viscosity changes dramatically in the temperature range around the T_g: a 'rubbery' state exists above and a glass state below the T_g.

At the start of the primary drying stage no 'free and fluid' water should be present in the vials. Minus forty degrees Celsius is a typical freezing temperature before sublimation is initiated through pressure reduction.

Primary Drying

In the primary drying stage (cf. Figure 4.6.) sublimation of the water mass in the vial is initiated by lowering the pressure. The water vapor is collected on a condenser, with a (substantially) lower temperature than the shelf with the vials. Sublimation costs energy (about 2500 kJ/gram ice). Temperature drops are avoided by the supply of heat from the shelf to the vial, so the shelf is heated during this stage.

Heat is transferred to the vial through (1) direct shelf-vial contact (conductance), (2) radiation, and (3) gas-conduction (Figure 4.8). Gas conduction depends on the pressure: if one selects relatively high gas pressures, heat transport is promoted because of a high conductivity. However, mass transfer is reduced because of a low driving force: the pressure between equilibrium vapor pressure at the interface between the frozen mass/dried cake and the chamber pressure (Pikal, 1990a).

During the primary drying stage one transfers heat from the shelf through the vial bottom, and from the frozen mass to the interface frozen mass/dry powder, to keep the sublimation process going. During this drying stage the vial content should never reach or exceed the eutectic temperature or glass transition temperature range. Typically a safety margin of 2–5 °C is used, otherwise the cake will collapse. Collapse causes a strong reduction in sublimation rate and poor cake formation. Heat transfer resistance

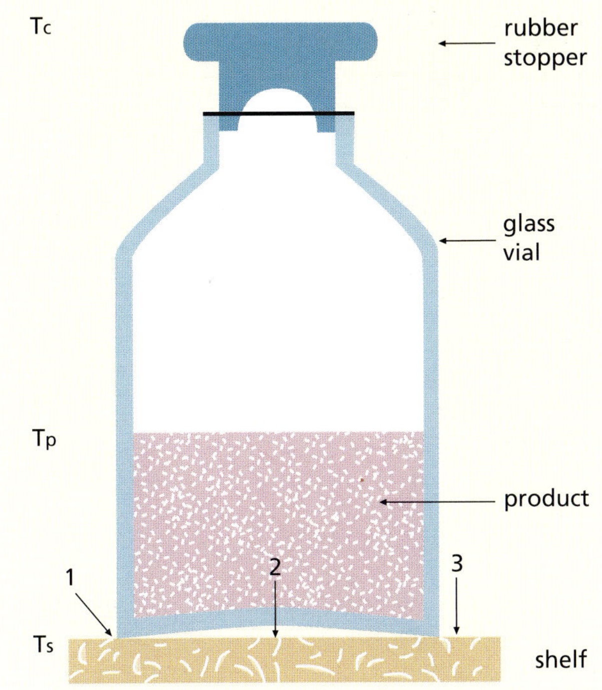

Figure 4.8. Heat transfer mechanisms during the freeze drying process:
1. direct conduction via shelf and glass at points of actual contact,
2. gas conduction: contribution heat transfer via conduction through gas between shelf and vial bottom,
3. radiation heat transfer. Ts = shelf temperature, Tp = temperature sublimating product, Tc = temperature condensor. Ts > Tp > Tc.

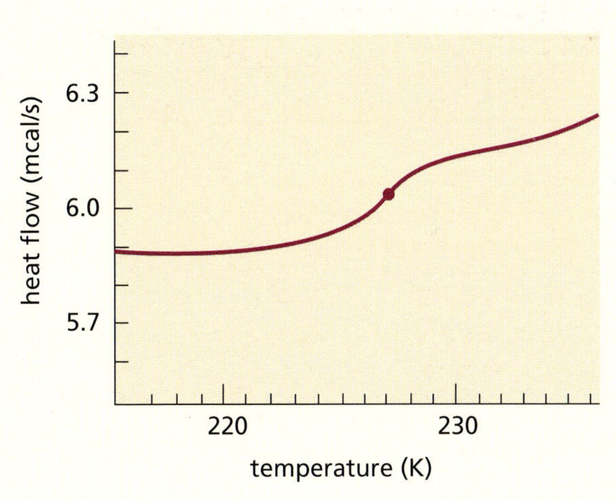

Figure 4.9. Differential scanning calorimetry heating trace for a frozen solution of sucrose and sodium chloride, showing the glass transition temperature of the freeze concentrate at 227 K. For pure freeze-concentrated sucrose, T_g = 241 K (1 cal = 4.2 J). From Franks *et al.*, 1991.

decreases during the drying process as the transport distance is reduced by the retreating interface. With the mass transfer resistance (transport of water vapor), however, the opposite occurs. Mass transfer resistance increases during the drying process as the dry cake becomes thicker.

This situation makes it clear that parameters such as chamber pressure and shelf heating are not necessarily constant during the primary drying process. They should be carefully chosen and adjusted as the drying process proceeds.

The eutectic temperature or glass transition temperature are parameters of great importance for the development of a rationally designed freeze-drying protocol. Information about these parameters can be obtained by microscopic observation of the freeze-drying process, differential scanning calorimetry (DSC), or electrical resistance measurements.

An example of a DSC scan providing information on the T_g is presented in Figure 4.9 (Franks *et al.*, 1991). The T_g heavily depends on the composition of the system: excipients and water content. Lowering the water content of an amorphous system causes the T_g to shift to higher temperatures.

Secondary drying

When all frozen or amorphous water that is non-protein and non-excipient bound is removed, the secondary drying step starts (Figure 4.6). The end of the primary drying stage is reached when product temperature and shelf temperature become equal, or when the partial water pressure drops (Pikal, 1990a). As long as the 'non-bound' water is being removed, the partial water pressure almost equals the total pressure. In the secondary drying stage the temperature is slowly increased to remove 'bound' water; the chamber pressure is still reduced. The temperature should continually stay below the collapse/eutectic temperature, which continues to rise when residual water contents drop. Typically, the secondary drying step ends when the product has been kept at 20 °C for some time. The residual water content is a critical endpoint indicating parameter. Values as low as 1% residual water in the cake have been recommended. Figure 4.10 (Pristoupil, 1985; Pikal 1990a) exemplifies the decreasing stability of freeze-dried hemoglobin with increasing residual water content.

The stability of freeze-dried proteins in the presence of reducing lyoprotectants, such as glucose and lactose, can be affected by the occurrence of the Maillard reaction: amino groups of the proteins react with the lyoprotectant in the dry state and the cake color turns yellow-brown. The use of non-reducing sugars such as sucrose may solve this problem

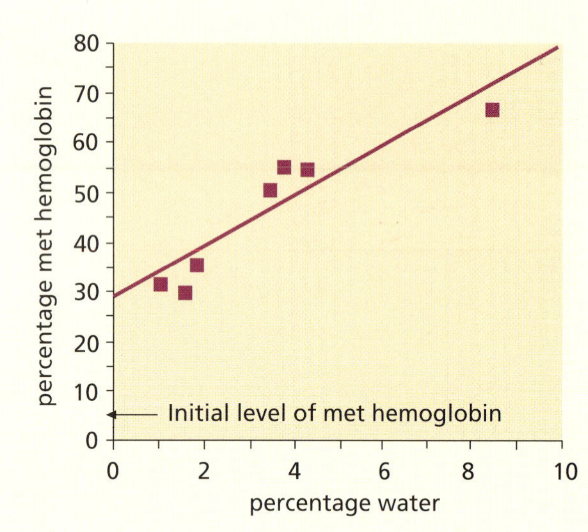

Figure 4.10. The effect of residual moisture on the stability of freeze-dried hemoglobin (~6%) formulated with 0.2 M sucrose; decomposition to met hemoglobin during storage at 23 °C for 4 years. From Pikal, 1990a. Data reported by Pritoupil, *et al.*, 1985.

Other Approaches for Stabilizing Proteins

Compacted forms of proteins are being used for certain veterinary applications, such as for the sustained release of growth hormones. The pellets should contain as few additives as possible. They can be applied subdermally or intramuscularly when the compact pellets are introduced by compressed air-powered rifles into the animals (Klegerman and Groves, 1992).

Delivery of Proteins: Routes of Administration and Absorption Enhancement

The Parenteral Route of Administration

Parenteral administration is defined as administration via those routes where one uses a needle, including intravenous, intramuscular, subcutaneous and intraperitoneal injections. More information on the pharmacokinetic behavior of recombinant proteins is provided in Chapter 5. It suffices here to state that the blood half-life of biotech products can vary considerably. For example, the circulation half-life of tissue plasminogen activator (t-PA) is a few minutes, while monoclonal antibodies reportedly have half-lives of a few days. Obviously, one reason to develop modified proteins through site directed mutagenesis is to enhance circulation half-life. A simple way to expand the mean residence time for short half-life proteins is to switch from intravenous to intramuscular or subcutaneous administration. One should realize that by performing this switch, changes in disposition may occur which have a significant impact on the therapeutic performance of the drug. These changes are related to: (1) the prolonged residence time at the i.m. or s.c. site of injection compared to i.v. administration and the enhanced exposure to degradation reactions (peptidases), and (2) differences in disposition.

Regarding point 1: Prolonged residence time at the i.m. or s.c. site of injection and the enhanced exposure to degradation reactions. For instance, diabetics can become 'insulin resistant' through high tissue peptidase activity (Maberly *et al.*, 1982). Other factors that can contribute to absorption variation are related to differences in exercise level of the muscle at the injection site and also massage and heat at the injection site. The state of the tissue and the occurrence of pathological conditions may be important as well.

Regarding point 2: Differences in disposition. Upon administration, a major fraction of the protein may be transported to the blood through the lymphatics and enter the blood circulation through the capillary wall at the site of injection (Figures 4.11, 4.12). The fraction taking this lymphatic route is dependent on molecular weight (Supersaxo *et al.*, 1990). Lymphatic transport takes time (hours) and uptake in the blood circulation is highly dependent on the injection site. On its way to the blood, the lymph passes through draining lymph nodes in which contact is possible between macrophages, B and T-lymphocytes residing in the lymph nodes.

The Oral Route

Oral delivery of protein drugs would be preferable, because it is patient friendly and no medical professional intervention is necessary to administer the drug. Oral bioavailability, however, is usually very low. Two main reasons for this failure of uptake have been discerned: (1) protein degradation in the GI-tract, and (2) poor permeability of the wall of the GI tract in case of a passive transport process (Lee *et al.*, 1991).

Regarding point 1: Protein degradation in the GI-tract. The human body has developed a very efficient system for breaking down proteins in our food to amino acids, or di- or tri-peptides. These building blocks for body proteins are actively absorbed for use wherever necessary in the body. In the stomach pepsins, a family of aspartic proteases are secreted. They are particularly active between pH 3 and 5 and lose activity at higher pH values. Pepsins are endopeptidases (capable of cleaving peptide bonds distant from the ends of the peptide chain) and they preferentially cleave peptide bonds between two hydrophobic amino acids. Other endopeptidases are active in the gastro-intestinal

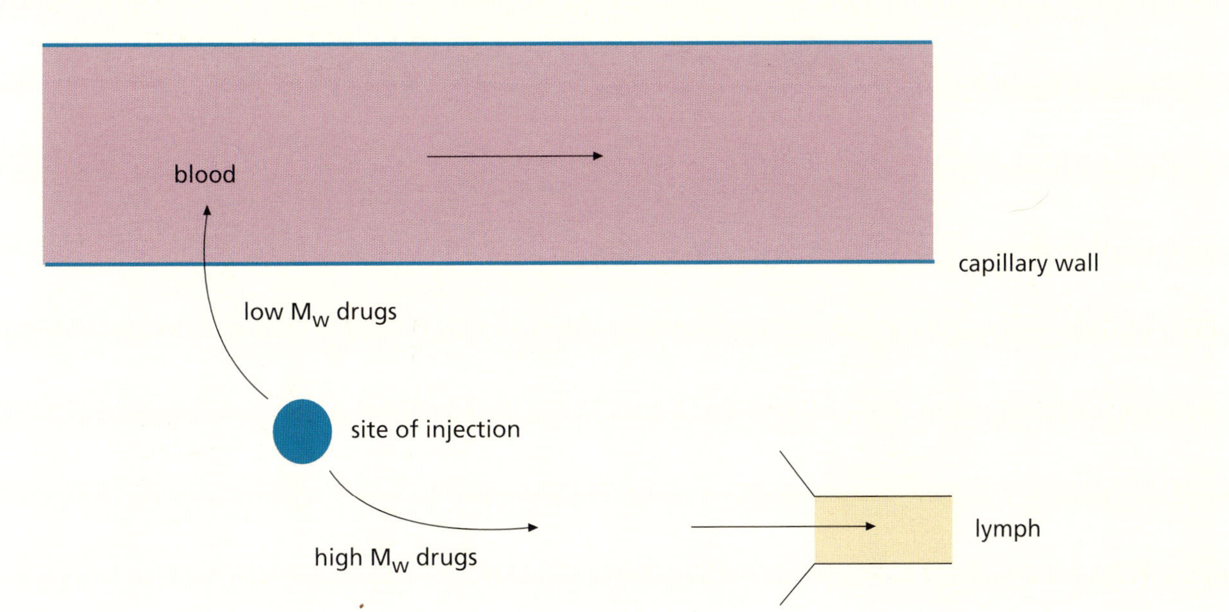

Figure 4.11. Routes of uptake of s.c. or i.m. injected drugs.

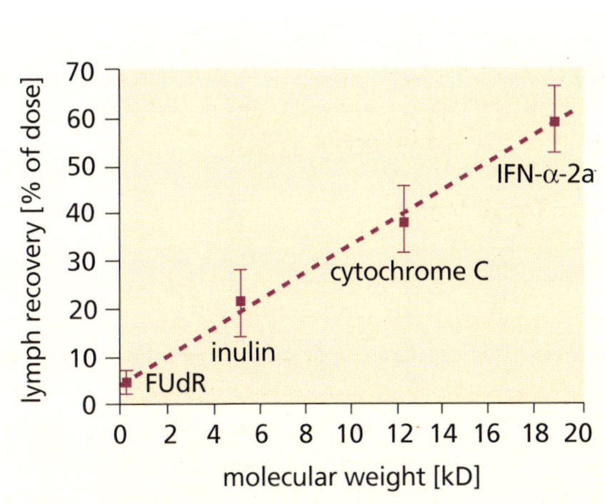

Figure 4.12. Correlation between the molecular weight and the cumulative recovery of rIFN alpha-2a (M_W 19 kDa), cytochrome *c* (M_W 12.3 kDa), inulin (M_W 5.2 kDa), and FUDR (M_W 256.2 kDa) in the efferent lymph from the right popliteal lymph node following s.c. administration into the lower part of the right hind leg of sheep. Each point and bar show the mean and standard deviation of three experiments performed in separate sheep. The line drawn is the best fit by linear regression analysis calculated with the four mean values. The points have a correlation coefficient r of 0.998 ($p < 0.01$). From Supersaxo *et al.*, 1990.

tract at neutral pH values, e.g. trypsin, chymotrypsin and elastase. They have different peptide bond cleavage characteristics that more or less complement each other. Exopeptidases (proteases degrading peptide chains from their ends), are present as well. Examples are carboxypeptidase A and B. In the lumen the proteins are cut into fragments that further break down into amino acids, and di- and tri-peptides by brush border and cytoplasmic proteases of the enterocytes.

Regarding point 2: Permeability. High molecular weight molecules do not readily penetrate the intact and mature epithelial barrier if diffusion is the sole driving force for mass transfer. Their diffusion coefficient goes down with increasing molecule size. Proteins are no exception to this rule. The active transport of intact therapeutic recombinant proteins over the GI-epithelium has not yet been described.

The above analysis leads to the conclusion that nature, unfortunately, does not allow us to use the oral route of administration for therapeutic proteins, if high (or at least constant) bioavailability is required.

However, for the category of oral vaccines the above-mentioned hurdles of degradation and permeation are not necessarily prohibitive. For oral immunization only a (small) fraction of the antigen (protein) has to reach its target site to elicit an immune response. The target cells are lymphocytes and antigen presenting accessory cells located in Peyer's patches (Figure 4.13). The B lymphocyte population includes cells that produce secretory IgA antibodies.

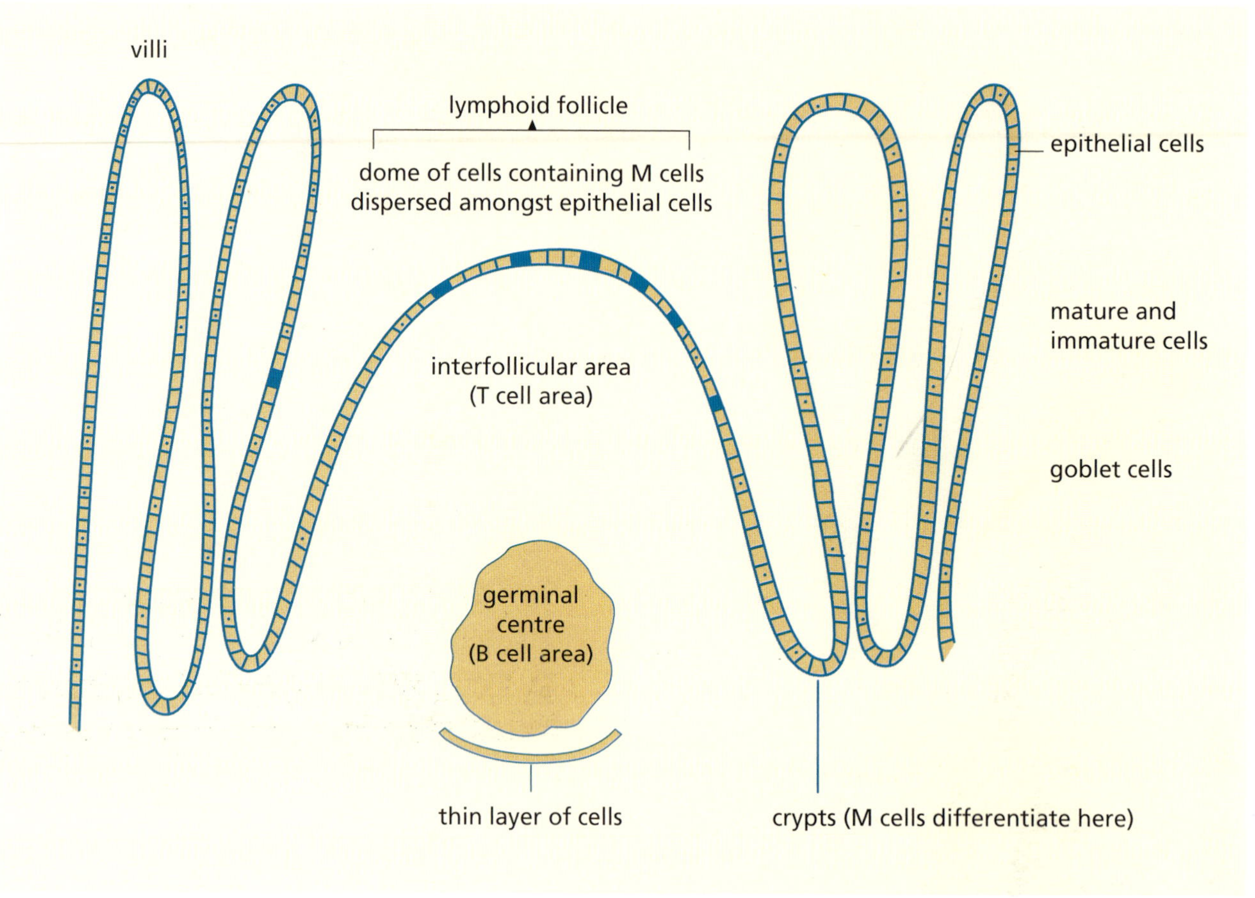

Figure 4.13. Schematic diagram of the structure of intestinal Peyer's patches. M-cells within the follicle-associated epithelium are enlarged for emphasis. From O'Hagan, 1990.

These Peyer's patches are macroscopically identifiable follicular structures located in the wall of the gastrointestinal tract. Peyer's patches are overlaid with microfold (M) cells that separate the luminal contents from the lymphocytes. These M cells have little lysosomal degradation capacity and allow for antigen sampling by the underlying lymphocytes. Moreover, mucus producing goblet cell density is reduced over Peyer's patches. This reduces mucus production and facilitates access to the M cell surface for luminal contents (Jani *et al.*, 1992; Roitt *et al.*, 1993). Attempts to improve antigen delivery via Peyer's patches and to enhance the immune response are made by using microspheres, liposomes or modified live vectors, such as attenuated bacteria and viruses (Eldridge *et al.*, 1990; Holmgren *et al.*, 1989).

Alternative Routes of Administration

Parenteral administration has disadvantages (needles, sterility, injection skills) compared to other possible routes. Therefore, systemic delivery of recombinant proteins by alternative routes of administration for the parenteral route has been studied extensively. The nose, lungs, rectum, oral cavity and skin have been selected as potential sites of application. The potential pros and cons for the different relevant routes have been listed in Table 4.4. (Zhou and Li Wan Po, 1991a; Zhou and Li Wan Po, 1991b).

The nasal, buccal, rectal and transdermal routes have all been shown to be of little clinical relevance if systemic action is required and if simple protein formulations without an absorption enhancing technology are to be used. In general, bioavailability is too low and varies too much. The pulmonary route may be the exception to this rule. In Table 4.5 (from Patton *et al.*, 1994) the bioavailability in rats of intratracheally administered protein solutions with a wide range of molecular weights is presented. Absorption was strongly protein dependent, with no clear relationship to its molecular weight.

In humans the drug should be inhaled instead of intratracheally administered. The delivery of insulin to Type I (juvenile onset) and II (adult onset) diabetics has been extensively studied and clinical phase III trials evaluating

Route + = relative advantage, – = relative disadvantage

Nasal (Edman and Björk, 1992)

+ easily accessible, fast uptake, proven track record with a number of 'conventional' drugs, probably lower proteolytic activity than in the GI tract, avoidance of first pass effect, spatial containment of absorption enhancers is possible

- reproducibility (in particular under pathological conditions), safety (e.g., ciliary movement), low bioavailability for proteins

Pulmonary (Patton and Platz, 1992)

+ relatively easy to access, fast uptake, proven track record with 'conventional' drugs, substantial fractions of insulin are absorbed, lower proteolytic activity than in the GI tract, avoidance of hepatic first pass effect, spatial containment of absorption enhancers (?)

– reproducibility (in particular under pathological conditions, smokers/non-smokers), safety (e.g., immunogenicity), presence of macrophages in the lung with high affinity for particulates

Rectal (Zhou and Li Wan Po, 1991b)

+ easily accessible, partial avoidance of hepatic first pass, probably lower proteolytic activity than in the upper parts of the GI tract, spatial containment of absorption enhancers is possible, proven track record with a number of 'conventional' drugs

– low bioavailability for proteins

Buccal (Zhou and Li Wan Po, 1991b) (Ho et al., 1992)

+ easily accessible, avoidance of hepatic first pass, probably lower proteolytic activity than in the lower parts of the GI tract, spatial containment of absorption enhancers is possible, option to remove formulation if necessary

– low bioavailability of proteins, no proven track record yet (?)

Transdermal (Cullander and Guy, 1992)

+ easily accessible, avoidance of hepatic first pass effect, removal of formulation if necessary is possible, spatial containment of absorption enhancers, proven track record with 'conventional' drugs, sustained/controlled release possible

– low bioavailability of proteins

Table 4.4. Alternative routes of administration to the oral route for biopharmaceuticals.

Molecule	Mw kDa	#AA	absolute bioavailability (%)
α-interferon	20	165	> 56
PTH-84	9	84	> 20
PTH-34	4.2	34	40
calcitonin (human)	3.4	32	17
calcitonin (salmon)	3.4	32	17
glucagon	3.4	29	< 1
somatostatin	3.1	28	< 1

PTH = recombinant human parathyroid hormone
# AA = number of amino acids

Table 4.5. Absolute bioavailability of a number of proteins (intratracheal vs intravenous) in rats (adapted from Patton *et al.*, 1994).

efficacy and safety are ongoing (Patton *et al.*, 1999). Pulmonary inhalation of insulin is specifically tested for meal time glucose control. Uptake of insulin is faster than after a regular s.c. insulin injection (peak 5–60 minutes versus 60–180 minutes). The reproducibility of the blood glucose response to inhaled insulin was equivalent to s.c. injected insulin, but patients preferred inhalation over s.c. injection. Inhalation technology plays a critical role when considering the prospects of the pulmonary route for the systemic delivery of therapeutic proteins. Dry powder inhalers and nebulizers are being tested. The fraction of insulin that is ultimately absorbed depends on: 1) the fraction of the inhaled/nebulized dose that is actually leaving the device, 2) the fraction that is actually deposited in the lung, and 3) the fraction that is being absorbed, i.e. total relative uptake (TO %) = % uptake from device x % deposited in the lungs x % actually absorbed from the

Classified according to proposed mechanism of action
-increase the permeability of the absorption barrier:
* addition of fatty acids/phospholipids, bile salts, enamine derivatives of phenylglycine, ester and ether type (non)-ionic detergents, saponins, salicylate derivatives, derivatives of fusidic acid or glycyrrhizinic acid, or methylated β cyclodextrins
* through iontophoresis,
* by using liposomes
- decrease peptidase activity at the site of absorption and along the 'absorption route': aprotinin, bacitracin, soybean tyrosine inhibitor, boroleucin, borovaline
- enhance resistance against degradation by modification of the molecular structure
- prolongation of exposure time (e.g., bio-adhesion technologies)

Table 4.6. Approaches to enhance bioavailability of proteins (adapted from Zhou and Li Wan Po, 1991a).

Molecule	# AA	Bioavailability (%)	
		without	*with glycocholate*
glucagon	29	< 1	70–90
calcitonin	32	< 1	15–20
insulin	51	< 1	10–30
met-hGH*	191	< 1	7–8

* *cf. chapter 5, Growth Hormones*

Table 4.7. Effect of glycocholate (absorption enhancer) on nasal bioavailability and molecular weights of some proteins and peptides (adapted from Zhou and Li Wan Po, 1991b).

lungs. TO % for insulin is estimated to be between 1 – 8%. The fraction of insulin that is absorbed from the lung is estimated to be around 20%. These figures demonstrate that at present insulin absorption via the lung may be a promising route, but the fraction absorbed is small.

Therefore, different approaches have been evaluated to increase the bioavailability of the pulmonary and other non-parenteral routes of administration. The goal is to develop a system that temporarily decreases the absorption barrier resistance with minimum and acceptable safety concerns. The mechanistic background of these approaches has been given in Table 4.6. Until now no products utilizing one of these approaches have successfully passed clinical test programs. Safety concerns are an important hurdle. Questions center around the specificity and reversibility of the protein permeation enhancing effect and the toxicity.

Examples of Absorption Enhancing Effects

The following section deals with the 'state of the art' of this important issue: absorption enhancement and non-parenteral administration of recombinant proteins. A number of typical examples are provided.

Table 4.7 presents an example of the relationship between nasal bioavailability of some peptide and protein drugs, their molecular weight and the presence of the absorption enhancer glycocholate (Zhou and Li Wan Po, 1991b).

Figure 4.14 (Björk and Edman, 1988) illustrates another case where degradable starch microspheres loaded with insulin were used and where changes in glucose levels were monitored after nasal administration to rats.

In these examples, the effect of the presence of the absorption enhancers is clear. Major issues now being addressed are reproducibility, effect of pathological conditions (e.g. rhinitis) on absorption and safety aspects of chronic use.

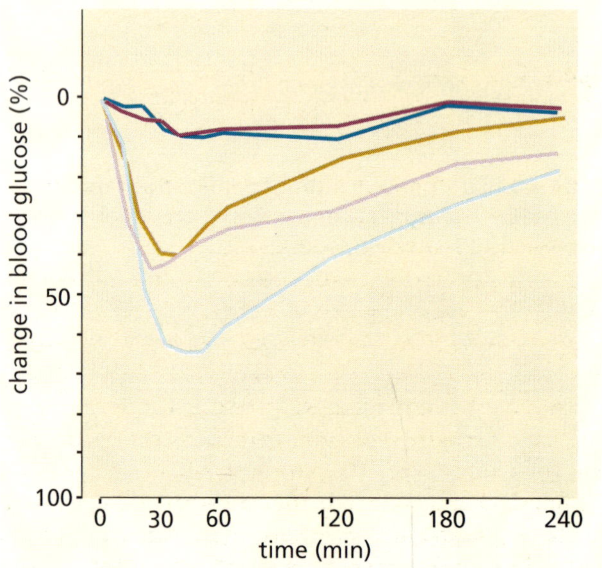

Figure 4.14. Change in blood glucose in rats after intranasal administration of insulin.
— Soluble insulin 2.0 IU/kg i.n.
— Soluble insulin 0.25 IU/kg i.v.
— Degradable starch microspheres-insulin 0.75 IU/kg i.n.
— Degradable starch microspheres-insulin 1.70 IU/kg i.n.
— Empty degradable starch microspheres 0.5 mg/kg i.n.
Discussed by Edman and Björk (Edman and Björk, 1992).

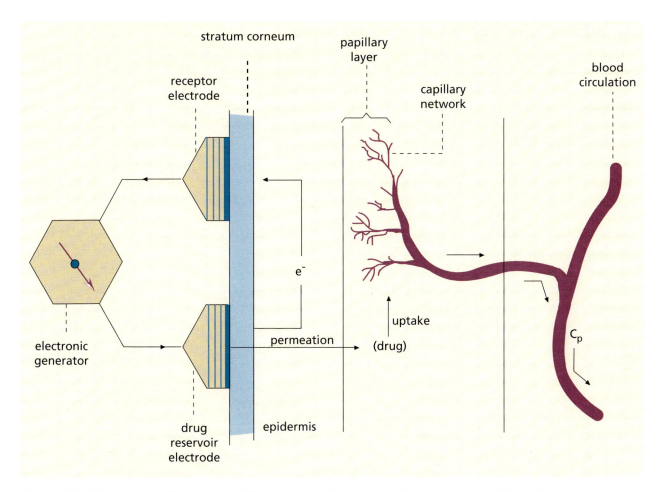

Figure 4.15. Diagrammatic illustration of the transdermal iontophoretic delivery of peptide and protein drugs across the skin. Adapted from Chien, 1991.

Interestingly, absorption enhancing effects were shown to be species dependent. Pronounced differences in effect were observed, as between rats and rabbits.

With iontophoresis, a transdermal electrical current is induced by positioning two electrodes on different places on the skin (Figure 4.15). This current induces a migration of (ionized) molecules through the skin. Delivery depends on the current (on/off, pulsed/direct, wave shape), pH, ionic strength, molecular weight, charge on the protein and temperature. The protein should be charged over the full thickness of the skin (pH of hydrated skin depends on the depth and varies between pH 4 (surface) and pH 7.3), which makes proteins with pI values outside this range prime candidates for iontophoretic transport. It is not clear whether there are size restrictions (protein Mw) for iontophoretic transport. However, only potent proteins will be successful candidates. With the present technology the protein flux through the skin is in the 10 μg/cm²/hr range (Sage *et al.*, 1995).

In Figure 4.16 the plasma profile of growth hormone releasing factor, GRF (44 amino acids), Mw 5 kDa after

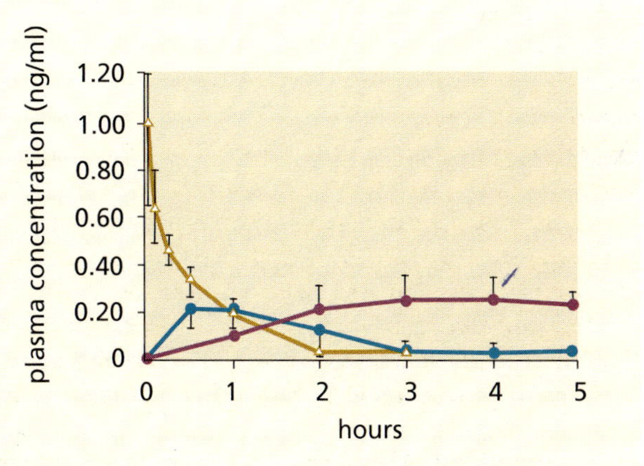

Figure 4.16. Plasma concentration versus time profiles after subcutaneous, intravenous and iontophoretic transdermal administration of GRF (1-44) to hairless guinea pigs. ● – ●: Iontophoresis (1 mg/g; 0.17 mA/cm²; 5 cm² patch). ● – ●: Subcutaneous (10 μg/kg; 0.025 mg/ml). △ – △: Intravenous (10 μg/kg; 0.025 mg/ml). From Kumar *et al.*, 1992.

s.c., i.v. and iontophoretic transdermal delivery to hairless guinea pigs is presented. With iontophoresis a prolonged appearance in the plasma can be observed. Iontophoretic delivery offers interesting opportunities, if pulsed delivery of the protein is required. The device can be worn permanently and only switched on for the desired periods of time, simulating the pulsatile secretion of endogenous hormones, such as growth hormone and insulin.

Delivery of Proteins: Approaches for Rate Controlled and Target Site Specific Delivery by the Parenteral Route

Current therapeutic proteins differ widely in their pharmacokinetic characteristics (cf. Chapter 5). If they are endogenous active agents, such as insulin, tissue plasminogen activator, growth hormone, erythropoetin, interleukins or factor VIII, it is important to realize why, when and where they are secreted. There are three different ways in which cells can communicate with each other: the endocrine, paracrine and autocrine ways (Table 4.8).

The dose-response relationship of these mediators is often not S-shaped, but, for instance, bell-shaped: at high doses the therapeutic effect disappears (cf. Chapter 5). Moreover, the presence of these mediators may activate a complex cascade of events that needs to be carefully controlled. Therefore, key issues for their therapeutic success are: (1) access to target cells, (2) retention at the target site, and (3) proper timing of delivery (Tomlinson, 1987).

In particular, for the paracrine and autocrine acting proteins, site specific delivery can be highly desirable, because otherwise side-effects will occur outside the target area. Severe side-effects were reported with cytokines, such as tumor necrosis factor and interleukin-2 upon parenteral (iv or sc) administration (cf. Chapter 9). The occurrence of these side-effects limits the therapeutic potential of these compounds. Therefore, the delivery of these proteins at the proper site, and the proper rate and dose are crucial aspects in the process of the design and development of these compounds as a pharmaceutical entity. The following sections discuss first concepts developed to control the release kinetics and later concepts for site directed drug delivery.

Endocrine hormones:
a hormone secreted by a distant cell to regulate cell functions distributed widely through the body. The blood stream plays an important role in the transport process
Paracrine acting mediators:
the mediator is secreted by a cell to influence surrounding cells, short range influence
Autocrine acting mediators:
the agent is secreted by a cell and affects the cell by which it is generated, (very) short range influence.

Table 4.8. Communication between cells: chemical messengers.

Approaches for Rate Controlled Delivery

Rate control can be achieved by several different technologies similar to those used for 'conventional' drugs. Insulin is an excellent example. A number of options are available and accepted, and different types of suspensions and continuous infusion systems are marketed (see Chapter 10). Moreover, chemical approaches can be used to change protein characteristics. Polyethyleneglycol-attachment to proteins changes their circulation half-life in the blood dramatically. Figure 4.17 shows an example of this approach. Chemical modification of proteins for pharmacokinetic purposes is dealt with in more detail in Chapter 5.

As a rule, proteins are administered as an aqueous solution. Only recombinant vaccines and most insulin formulations are delivered as (colloidal) dispersions. At the present

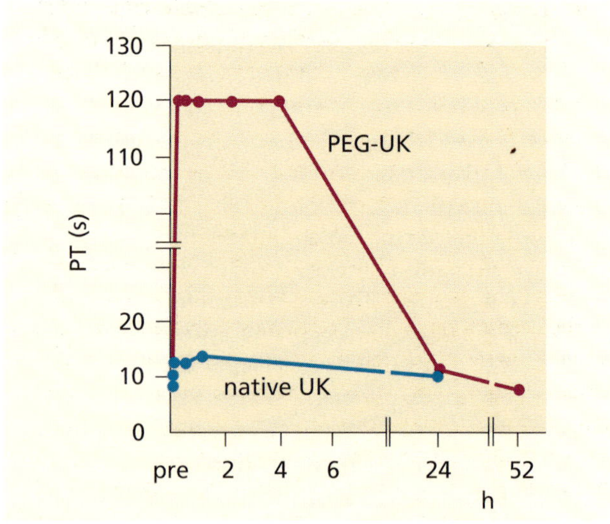

Figure 4.17. Influence of chemical grafting of polyethyleneglycol (PEG) on the ability of urokinase (UK) to affect the prothrombin time (PT) in vivo in beagles with time. Through Tomlinson, 1987.

Rate control through open loop type approach
– continuous infusion with pumps: mechanically or osmotically driven input: constant/pulsatile/wave form – implants: biodegradable polymers, lipids input: limited control
Rate control through closed loop approach/feed back system
– biosensor-pump combination – self regulating system – encapsulated secretory cells

Table 4.9. Controlled release systems for parenteral delivery.

The pump must deliver the drug at the prescribed rate(s) for extended periods of time. It should
– have a wide range of delivery rates – ensure accurate, precise and stable delivery – contain reliable pump and electrical components – contain drugs compatible with pump internals – provide simple means to monitor the status and performance of the pump
The pump must be safe. It should
– have a biocompatible exterior if implanted – have overdose protection – show no leakage – have a fail-safe mechanism – have sterilizable interiors and exteriors (if implantable)
The pump must be convenient. It should
– be reasonably small in size and inconspicuous – have a long reservoir life – be easy to program

Table 4.10. Listing the characteristics of the ideal pump (Banerjee et al., 1991).

time, insulin is routinely and clinically applied through some form of controlled release system (cf. Chapter 10). As experience with biotech drugs grows, more advanced technologies will definitely be introduced to optimize the therapeutic benefit of the drug. Table 4.9 lists some of the technologically feasible options. They are briefly touched upon below. Recently, a new polymer-based controlled release delivery system for hGH received a marketing authorization by the FDA. This technology is dealt with in more detail as it is clear that there is a growing need for such systems.

Open loop systems: mechanical pumps

Mechanically driven pumps are common tools for administering drugs intravenously in hospitals (continuous infusion, open loop type). Pumps are available in different kinds of sizes/prices, portability, location (inside/outside the body), etc. Table 4.10 presents a checklist with issues to be considered when selecting the proper pump.

Controlled administration of a drug does not necessarily imply a constant input rate. Pulsatile or variable-rate delivery is the desired mode of input for a number of protein drugs, and for these drugs pumps should provide flexible input rate characteristics. Insulin is a prime example of a protein drug, where there is a need to adjust the input rate to the needs of the body. Today most experience with pump systems in an ambulatory setting has been gained with insulin. The pump system may fail because of energy-failure, problems with the syringe, accidental needle withdrawal, leakage of the catheter and problems at the injection or implantation site (Banerjee *et al.*, 1991). Moreover, long-term drug stability may become a problem. The protein should be stable at 37 °C or ambient temperature (internal and external device, respectively) between two refills. Finally, even with high tech pump systems, the patient still has to collect data to adjust the pump rate. This implies invasive sampling from body fluids on a regular basis, followed by a calculation of the required input rate. This problem will solved when the concept of closed loop systems is realized (feed back systems, see below).

Open loop systems: osmotically driven systems

The subcutaneously implantable, osmotic mini-pump developed by ALZA (Alzet minipump, Figure 4.18 [Banerjee *et al.*, 1991] has proven to be useful in animal experiments where continuous, constant infusion is required over prolonged periods of time. The rate determining process is the influx of water through the rigid, external semi-permeable membrane. The incoming water empties the drug-containing reservoir (solution or dispersion) surrounded by a flexible impermeable membrane. The release rate depends on the characteristics of this semi-permeable membrane and on osmotic pressure differences over this membrane (osmotic agents inside the pump). Zero-order kinetics exist as long as the osmotic pressure difference over the semi-permeable membrane is constant.

The protein solution (or dispersion) must be physically and chemically stable at body temperature over the full term of the experiment. Moreover, the protein solution must be compatible with the pump parts to which it is exposed. A limitation of the system is the fixed release rate, which is not always desired (see above). These devices are not currently used on a regular basis in the clinic.

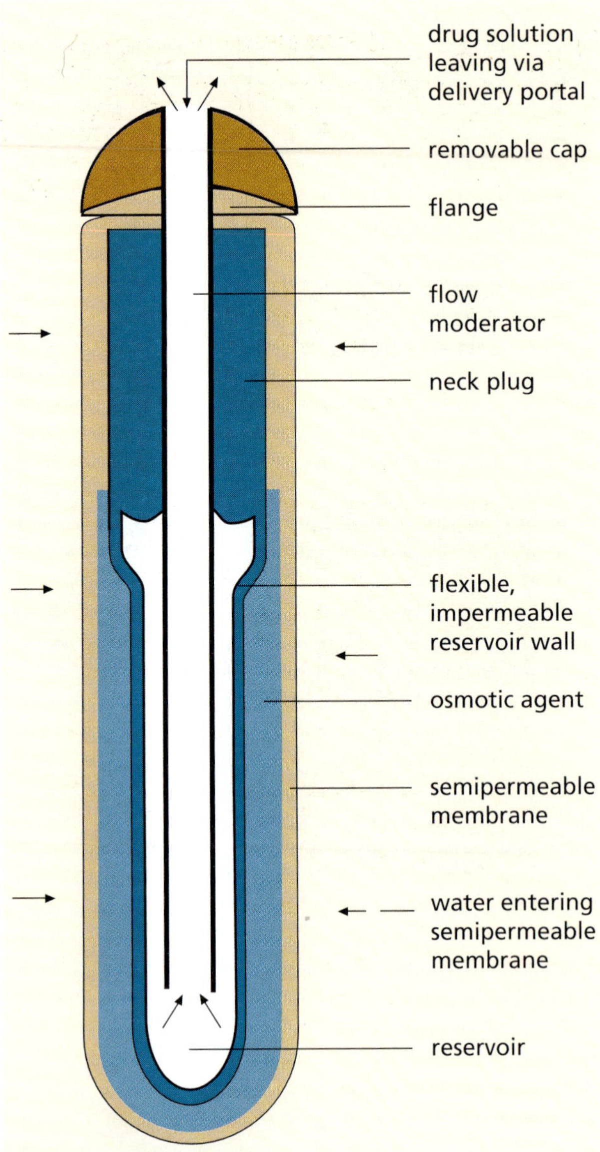

Figure 4.18. Cross section of functioning Alza Alzet osmotic minipump. Through Banerjee *et al.*, 1991.

Open loop systems: biodegradable microspheres

Polylactic acid – polyglycolic acid (PLGA) based delivery systems have been used extensively for the delivery of therapeutic peptides, in particular LHRH agonists such as leuprolide in the therapy of prostate cancer. The first LHRH agonist controlled release formulations were implants containing leuprolide with dose ranges of one to three months. Later, microspheres loaded with leuprolide were introduced and dosing intervals were prolonged for up to six months. Critical success factors for the design of these controlled release systems are: 1) the drug has to be highly potent (only a small dosage is required over the dosing interval); 2) a sustained presence in the body is required, and 3) no adverse reactions at the injection site should occur.

In 1999 FDA approved hGH containing PLGA microspheres for pediatric growth hormone deficiency (cf. Chapter 11). These microspheres are to be administered once or twice per month.

PLGA is a biodegradable polymer that degrades at the site of injection (s.c.) into lactic and glycolic acid. Degradation may take between a few weeks to over a year and depends, among other things, on the ratio between the lactic acid and glycolic acid moieties, the geometry of the spheres, and the degree of crystallinity of the polymer (crystalline versus amorphous phase). Large structures with a high lactic acid content that form a crystalline state degrade slowly.

hGH microspheres are prepared by spraying a zinc-hGH complex, suspended in a solution of PLGA in methylene chloride, into liquid nitrogen on top of a frozen ethanol layer. Microspheres with diameters around 50 µm are collected. Figure 4.19 shows single dose mean hGH concentrations in pediatric growth hormone deficiency patients. A burst release phase (releasing over 50% of the dose in the first two days) is followed by a period in which the release slowly declined (Nutropin Depot™ insert information).

New strategies for controlled release of therapeutic proteins are presently being developed. For example, Figures 4.20 and 4.21 describe a dextran-based microsphere technology for s.c. or i.m. administration that misses the strong burst effect, as observed with the PLGA technology, and

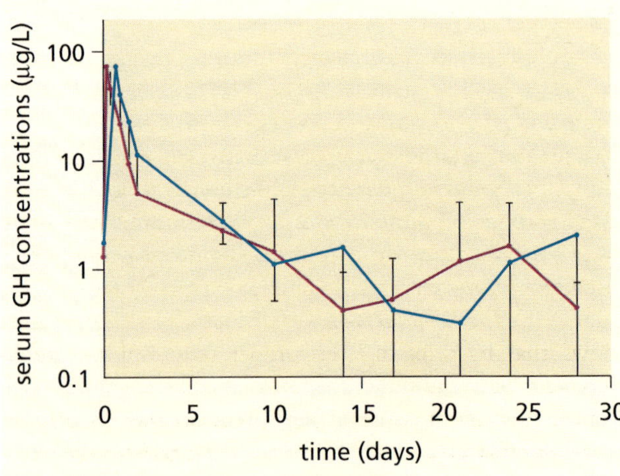

Figure 4.19. Serum hGH concentrations in pediatric patients after injection of hGH containing microspheres. In Nutropin Depot™ micronized hGH particles are embedded in biodegradable PLGA microspheres.
●—●: 0.75 mg/kg subcutaneous injection (n = 12)
●—●: 1.5 mg/kg subcutaneous injection (n = 8)

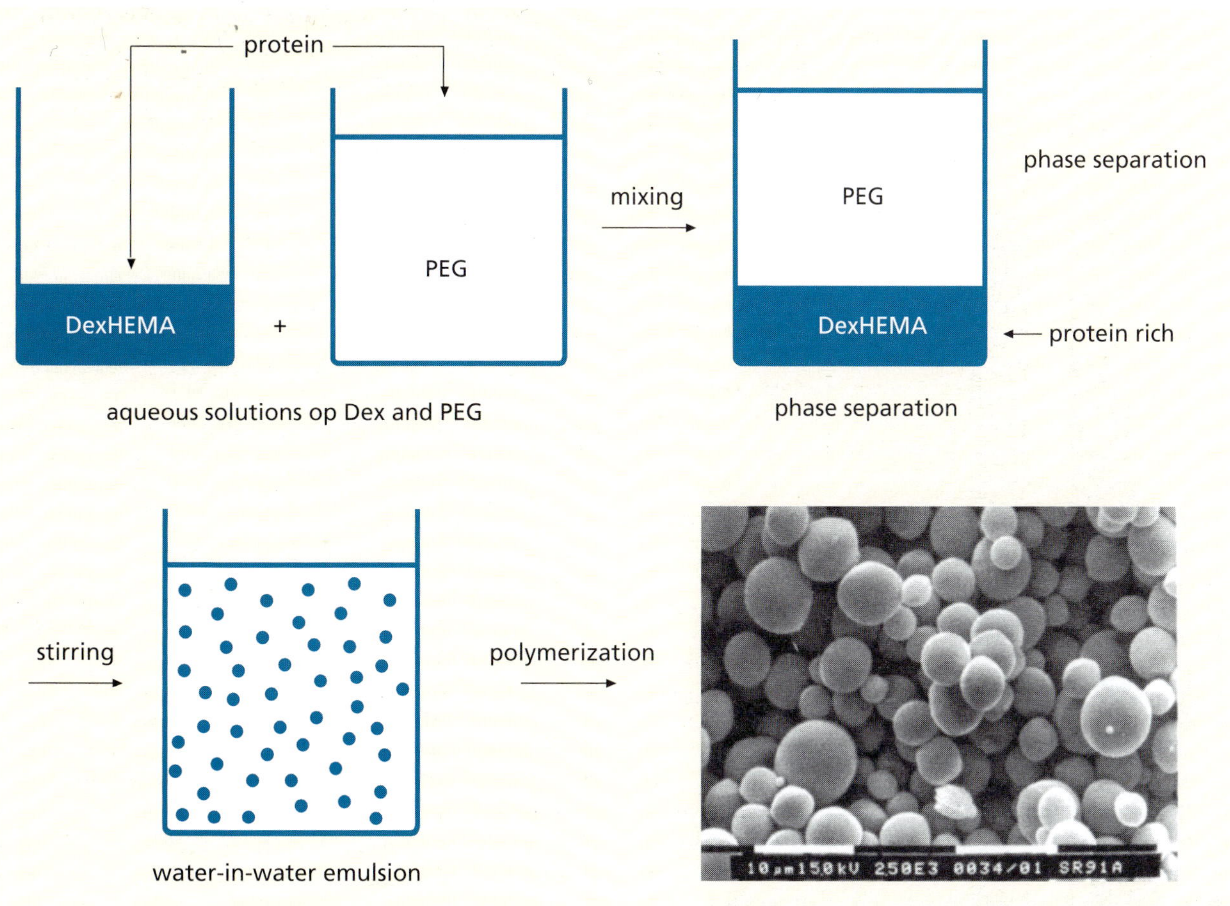

Figure 4.20. Schematic representation of the microsphere preparation process for the controlled release of therapeutic proteins from dextran (DexHEMA = modified dextran = dextran hydroxyethylmethacrylate) microspheres. No organic solvents are involved and encapsulation efficiencies (percentage of therapeutic protein ending up in the microspheres) is routinely > 90%. Polymerization: cross-linking of dextran chains through the HEMA units. (Stenekes, 2000).

has an almost 100% protein encapsulation efficiency (Figure 4.20). Here, no organic solvents are used in the preparation protocol. Thus, a direct interaction of the dissolved protein with an organic phase (as seen in many polymeric microsphere preparation schemes) is avoided. This avoidance minimizes the denaturation of the protein. Figure 4.21 shows that by selecting the proper cross-linking conditions one has a degree of control over the release kinetics. Release kinetics are mainly dependent on the degradation of the dextran matrix and the size of the protein molecule (Stenekes, 2000).

Closed loop systems: biosensor-pump combinations

If input rate control is desired to stabilize a certain body function, then this function should be monitored. This data should be converted into a drug-input rate via an algorithm and connected pump settings. These systems are called closed loop systems, as compared to the open loop systems discussed above. If there is a known relationship between the plasma level and the pharmacological effect these systems contain (Figure 4.22):

(1) a biosensor, measuring the plasma level of the protein,
(2) an algorithm, to calculate the required input rate for the delivery system, and
(3) a pump system, able to administer the drug at the required rate over prolonged periods of time.

The concept of a closed loop delivery of proteins still has to overcome many conceptual and practical problems. A simple relationship between plasma level and therapeutic

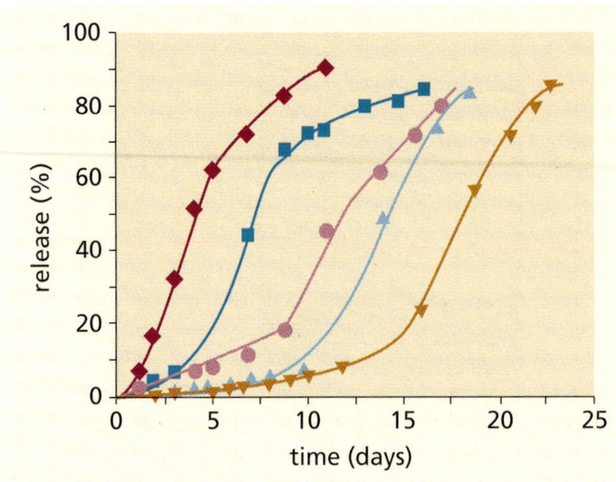

Figure 4.21. Cumulative release of IgG from degrading dexHEMA microspheres in time in vitro at pH 7, 37 °C. Water content of the dextran microspheres upon swelling: about 60%, DS 3 (◆) and water content of about 50%, DS 3 (■), DS 6 (●), DS 8 (▲) and DS 11 (▼). The values are the mean of 2 independent measurements that deviated typically less than 5% from each other. DS = degree of cross-linking (Stenekes, 2000).

effect does not always exist (see Chapter 5). There are many exceptions known to this rule, for instance, 'hit and run' drugs can have long lasting pharmacological effects after only a short exposure time. Also, drug effect-blood level relationships may be time-dependent, as in the case of the down regulation of relevant receptors on prolonged stimulation. Finally, if circadian rhythms exist, these will be responsible for variable PK/PD relationships as well.

If the PK/PD concerns expressed above do not apply, as with insulin, technical problems form the second hurdle in the development of closed loop systems. It has not yet been possible to design biosensors that work reliably *in vivo* over prolonged periods of time. Biosensor stability, robustness and absence of histological reactions still pose problems.

Protein Delivery by Self-regulating Systems

Apart from the design of biosensor-pump combinations, two other developments should be mentioned when discussing closed loop approaches: self-regulating systems and encapsulated secretory cells. At the present, time both concepts are still under development (Heller, 1993).

In self-regulating systems drug release is controlled by stimuli in the body. The majority of the research is focused on insulin release as a function of local glucose concentrations in order to stabilize blood glucose levels in diabetics. Two approaches for controlled drug release are being followed: (1) competitive desorption, and (2) enzyme-substrate reactions. The competitive desorption approach is schematically depicted in Figure 4.23.

It is based on the competition between glycosylated-insulin and glucose for concanavalin (Con A) binding sites. Con A is a plant lectin with a high affinity for certain sugars. Con A, attached to sepharose beads and loaded with glycosylated-insulin (a bio-active form of insulin), is

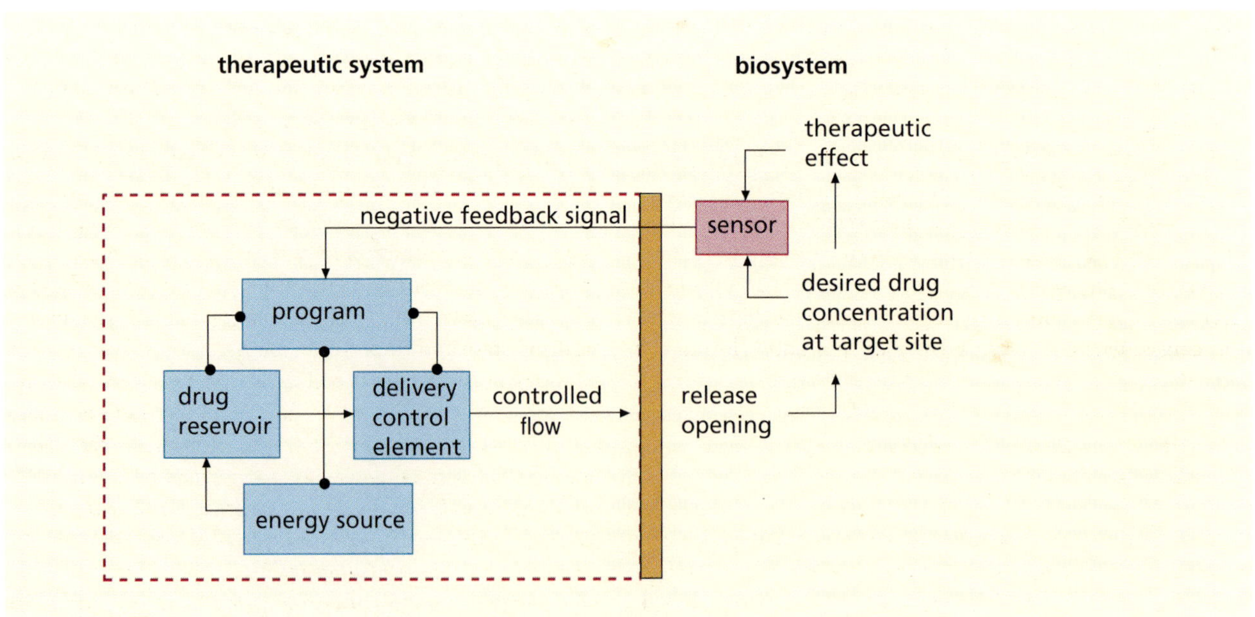

Figure 4.22. Therapeutic system with closed control loop. From Heilman, 1984.

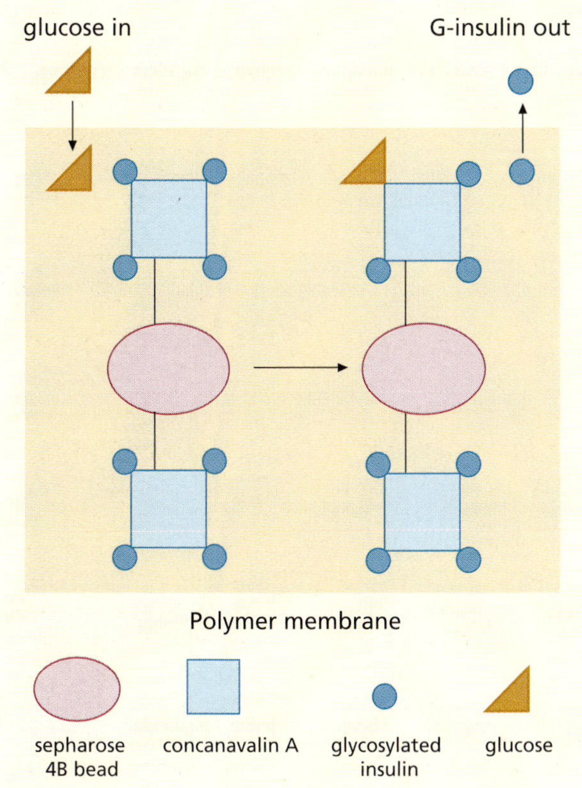

Figure 4.23. Schematic design of the Con A immobilized bead/G (glycosylated)-insulin/membrane self-regulating insulin delivery system. From Kim *et al.*, 1990.

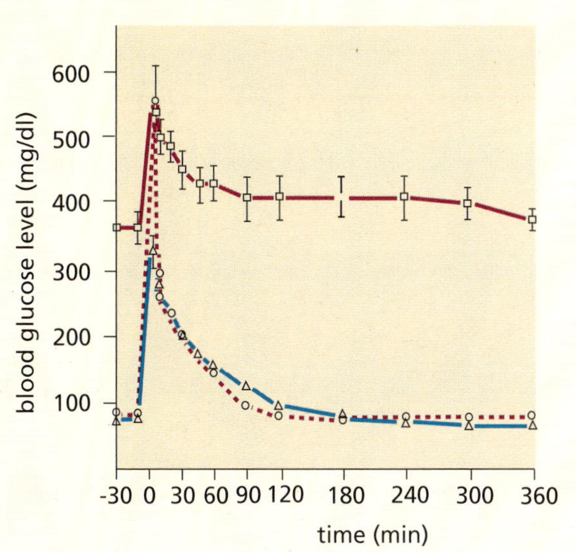

Figure 4.24. Peripheral blood glucose profiles of dogs administered bolus dextrose (500 mg/kg) during an intravenous glucose tolerance test. Normal dogs (o) had an intact pancreas, diabetic dogs (□) had undergone total pancreatectomy, and implant dogs (Δ) had been intraperitoneally implanted with a cellulose pouch containing a Con A-G-insulin complex. Blood glucose at t = –30 minutes shows the overnight fasting level 30 minutes prior to bolus injection of dextrose. Through Heller, 1993.

implanted in a pouch with a semipermeable membrane: permeable for insulin and glucose, but impermeable for the sepharose beads carrying the toxic Con A. An example of the performance of a Con A-glycosylated-insulin complex in pancreatectomized dogs is given in Figure 4.24.

Enzyme-substrate reactions for regulating insulin release from an implanted reservoir are all based on pH drops occurring when glucose is converted to gluconic acid in the presence of the enzyme glucose oxidase. This pH drop then induces changes in the structure of acid-sensitive delivery devices such as acid sensitive polymers, which start releasing insulin, lowering the glucose concentration, and consequently increasing the local pH and "closing the reservoir."

Protein Delivery by Microencapsulated Secretory Cells

The idea to use implanted, secretory cells to administer therapeutic proteins was launched long ago. A major objective has been the implantation of Langerhans cells in diabetics to restore their insulin production through bio-feedback. These implanted secretory cells should be protected from the body environment, since rejection processes would immediately start if imperfectly matched cell material were used. Besides, it is desirable to keep the cells from migrating in all different directions. When genetically modified cells are used, safety issues would be even stricter. Therefore, (micro)encapsulation of the secretory cells has been proposed (Figure 4.25)

Thin (wall thickness in µm range), robust, biocompatible and permselective polymeric membranes have been designed for these (micro)capsules (Tresco, 1994; Uludag *et al.*, 1993). The membrane should ensure the transport of nutrients (in general low M_w) from the outside medium to the encapsulated cells to keep them in a physiological, 'healthy' state and to prohibit the induction of undesirable immunological responses (rejection process). Antibodies (M_w >150 kDa) and cells belonging to the immune system (e.g. lymphocytes) should not be able to reach the encapsulated cells. The polymer membrane should have a cut off between 50 and 150 kDa, the exact number still being a matter for debate. In the case of insulin, the membrane is permeable for this relatively small sized hormone (5.4 kDa). The membrane is also permeable for glucose ('indicator' molecule), which is essential for proper bio-feedback processes. Successful studies in diabetic animals were performed.

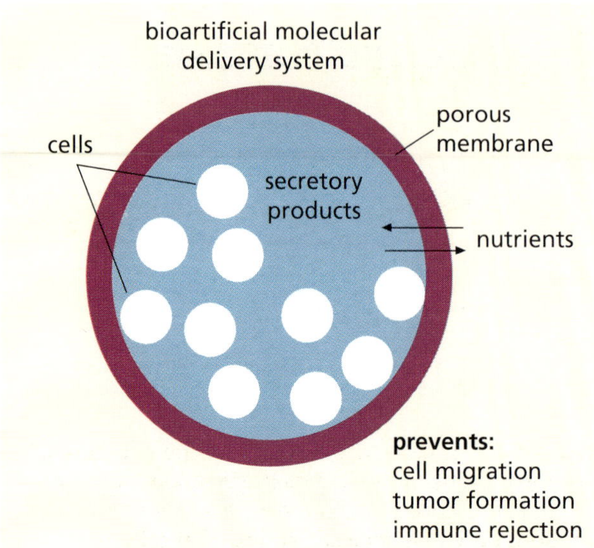

Figure 4.25. Schematic illustration of a 'bioartificial molecular delivery system'. Secretory cells are surrounded by a semi-permeable membrane prior to implantation in host tissue. Nutrients and secretory products passively diffuse through pores in the encapsulating membrane powered by concentration gradients. The use of a membrane that excludes the humoral and the cellular components of the host immune system allows immunologically incompatible cells to survive implantation without the need to administer immunosuppressive agents. Extracellular matrix material may be included depending upon the requirements of the encapsulated cells.
From Tresco, 1994.

Promising clinical data has been reported with human secretory islet cells encapsulated in alginate based microspheres (Shoon-Shiong *et al.*, 1994).

Site Specific Delivery (Targeting) of Protein Drugs

Why are we still not able to beat life-threatening diseases such as cancer with our current arsenal of drugs? Causes of failure can be summarized as follows (Crommelin *et al.*, 1992):

1) The active compound never reaches the target site, because it is rapidly eliminated intact from the body through the kidneys, or it is inactivated through metabolic action, (e.g. in the liver).
2) Only a small fraction of the drug reaches the target site. By far the largest fraction of the drug is distributed over non-target organs, where they exert side-effects; in other words, accumulation of the drug at the target site is the exception and not the rule.
3) Many drug molecules (in particular high M_w and hydrophilic molecules, i.e. many proteins) do not enter cells easily. This poses a problem, if intracellular delivery is required for their therapeutic activity.

Attempts are made to increase the therapeutic index of drugs through drug targeting:

(1) by specific delivery of the active compound at its site of action, and
(2) to keep it there until it has been inactivated and detoxified.

Targeted drug delivery should both maximize the therapeutic effect and avoid toxic effects elsewhere. The basics of the concept of drug targeting were defined already in the early days of this century by Paul Ehrlich. But only in the last decade has substantial progress been made to implement this site specific delivery concept. Recent progress can be ascribed to: (1) the rapidly growing number of technological options (e.g. safe carriers) for drug delivery; (2) many new insights gained into the pathophysiology of diseases at the cellular and molecular level, including the presence of cell specific receptors and homing devices to target to them (e.g. monoclonal antibodies); and, finally, (3) new revelations in the nature of the anatomical and physiological barriers that hinder easy access to target sites. Site specific delivery systems presently in different stages of development consist, in general, of three functionally separate units (Table 4.11).

Nature has provided us with antibodies, which exemplify a class of natural drug targeting devices. In an antibody molecule one can recognize a homing device part (antigen binding site) and 'active' parts. These active parts in the molecule are responsible for participating in the complement cascade. They also induce interactions with monocytes when antigen is bound. The rest of the molecule can be considered as carrier (cf. Figure 5.6).

Most of the drug (protein) targeting work is done with delivery systems that are designed for parenteral and, more specifically, intravenous delivery. Only a limited number of papers have dealt with the pharmacokinetics of the drug

*** an active moiety**	for: therapeutic effect
**** a carrier**	for: (metabolic) protection, changing the disposition of the drug
***** a homing device**	for: specificity, selection of the assigned target site

Table 4.11. Components for targeted drug delivery (carrier-based).

1. Drugs with high total clearance are good candidates for targeted delivery.

2. Response sites with a relatively small blood flow require carrier-mediated transport.

3. Increases in the rate of elimination of free drug from either central or response compartments tend to increase the need for targeted drug delivery; this also implies a higher input rate of the drug-carrier conjugate to maintain the therapeutic effect.

4. For maximizing the targeting effect, the release of drug from the carrier should be restricted to the response compartment.

Table 4.12. Pharmacokinetic considerations related to protein targeting.

targeting process (Hunt *et al.*, 1986). From these kinetic models a number of conclusions could be drawn for situations where targeted delivery is, in principle, advantageous (Table 4.12).

The potential and limitations of carrier-based, targeted drug delivery systems for proteins are briefly discussed. The focus is on concepts where monoclonal antibodies are being used. They can be used as the antibody itself (also in Chapter 13), in modified form when antibodies are conjugated with an active moiety, or attached to drug laden colloidal carriers such as liposomes.

Two terms are regularly used in the context of targeting: passive and active targeting. With passive targeting the 'natural' disposition pattern of the carrier system is utilized for site specific delivery. For instance, particulate carriers circulating in the blood (see below) are often rapidly taken up by macrophages in contact with the blood circulation and accumulate in the liver (Kupffer cells) and the spleen. Active targeting is the concept where attempts are made to change the natural disposition of the carrier by some sort of homing device or homing principle to select one particular tissue or cell type.

Anatomical, Physiological and Pathological Considerations Relevant for Protein Targeting

Carrier mediated transport in the body depends on the physico-chemical properties of the carrier: its charge, molecular weight/size, surface hydrophobicity and the presence of ligands for interaction with surface receptors (Crommelin and Storm, 1990). If a drug enters the circulation and the target site is outside the blood circulation, the drug has to pass through the endothelial barrier. Figure 4.26 gives a schematic picture of the capillary wall structures (under physiological conditions) present at different locations in the body.

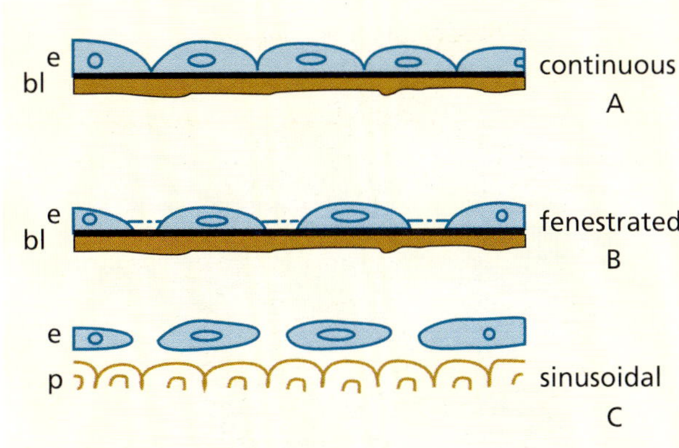

Figure 4.26. Schematic illustration of the structure of different classes of blood capillaries. A. Continuous capillary. The endothelium is continuous with tight junctions between adjacent endothelial cells. The subendothelial basement membrane is also continuous. B. Fenestrated capillary. The endothelium exhibits a series of fenestrae which are sealed by a membranous diafragm. The subendothelial basement membrane is continuous. C. Discontinuous (sinusoidal) capillary. The overlying endothelium contains numerous gaps of varying size enabling materials in the circulation to gain access to the underlying parenchymal cells. The subendothelial basement is either absent (liver) or present as a fragmented interrupted structure (spleen, bone marrow). The fenestrae in the liver are about 0.1–0.2 μm; the pores in/between the endothelial cells and those in the basement membrane outside liver, spleen and bone marrow are much smaller. From Poste, 1985.

Figure 4.26 shows a diagram of intact endothelium under normal conditions. Under pathological conditions, such as those encountered in tumors and inflammation sites, endothelium can differ considerably in appearance and endothelial permeability may be widely different from that in 'healthy' tissue. Particles with sizes up to around 0.1 μm can enter tumor tissue demonstrated with long circulating, colloidal carrier systems (long circulating liposomes). On the other hand, necrotic tissue can also hamper access to tumor tissue (Jain, 1987). In conclusion, the body is highly compartmentalized; it should not be considered as one big pool without internal barriers for transport.

Soluble Carrier Systems for Targeted Delivery of Proteins

(MONOCLONAL) ANTIBODIES (MAB) AS TARGETED THERAPEUTIC AGENTS: HUMAN AND HUMANIZED ANTIBODIES (CF. CHAPTER 13)

Antibodies are 'natural targeting devices'. Their homing ability is combined with functional activity (Crommelin *et al.*, 1992; Crommelin and Storm, 1990). MAb can affect the target cell function upon attachment. Complement can be bound via the Fc receptor and can subsequently cause lysis of the target cell. Alternatively, certain Fc receptor-bearing killer cells can induce 'antibody dependent, cell mediated cytotoxicity' (ADCC), or contact with macrophages can be established. Moreover, metabolic deficiencies can be induced in the target cells through a blockade of certain essential cell surface receptors by MAb. Structural aspects and therapeutic potential of MAb is dealt with in detail in Chapter 13.

A problem that occurs when using murine antibodies for therapy is the production of human anti-mouse (HAMA) antibodies after administration. HAMA induction may prohibit further use of these therapeutic MAb by neutralizing the antigen-binding site; anaphylactic reactions are relatively rare. Concurrent administration of immunosuppressive agents is a strategy for minimizing side-effects.

There are several other ways to cope with this immunogenicity problem. These options are dealt with in more detail in Chapter 13. Here, a brief summary of the options relevant for protein targeting will suffice. First of all, the use of $F(ab')_2$ or F(ab') fragments (Figure 4.27) avoids raising an immune response against the Fc part, but the development of humanized or human MAb minimizes the induction of HAMA even further. For the humanization of MAb several options can be considered. One can build chimeric (partly human, partly murine) molecules consisting of a human Fc part and a murine Fab part with the antigen binding sites or, alternatively, only the six complementarity determining regions (CDR) of the murine antibody can be grafted in a human antibody structure. CDR grafting minimizes the exposure to murine material.

Completely human MAb can be produced by transfecting human antibody genes into mouse cells, which subsequently produce the human MAb. Alternatively, transgenic mice can be used (cf. Chapter 6 and 13). These approaches reduce the immunogenicity compared to the existing generation of murine MAb. Even with all of these human or humanized MAb, however, anti-idiotypic immune responses against the binding site structure of the MAb can not be excluded (cf. Chapter 12).

Bispecific antibodies (cf. 13)

To enhance the therapeutic potential of antibodies, bispecific antibodies have been designed. Bispecific antibodies are manufactured from two separate antibodies to create a molecule with two different binding sites (Fanger and Guyre, 1991). Bispecific MAb bring target cells or tissue (one antigen-binding site) in contact with other structures (second antigen binding site). This second antigen binding site can bind to effector cells via cytotoxicity triggering molecules on T cells, NK (natural killer) cells, or macrophages, and thus trigger cytotoxicity.

Bispecific antibodies have been used experimentally in the clinic, for instance, to direct intraperitoneally injected autologous T-lymphocytes stimulated with recombinant interleukin-2, to intraperitoneally located ovarian carcinoma cells. This MAb combines an antigen-binding site

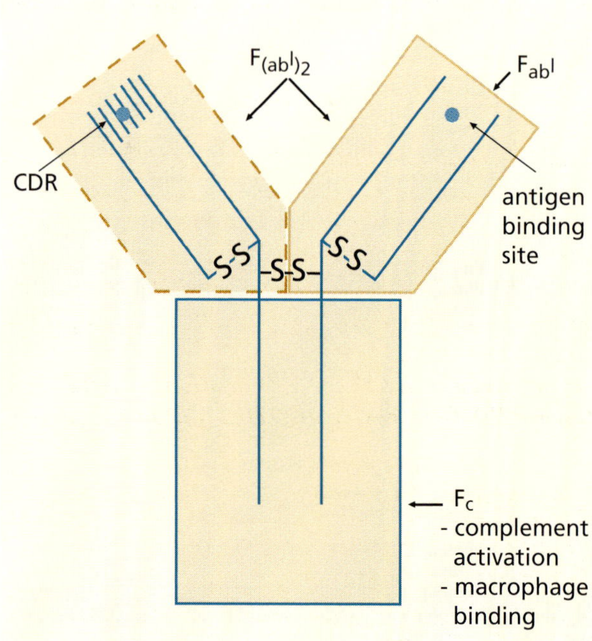

Figure 4.27. Highly simplified IgG1 structure; CDR = complementarity determining region (cf. Figure 13.2).

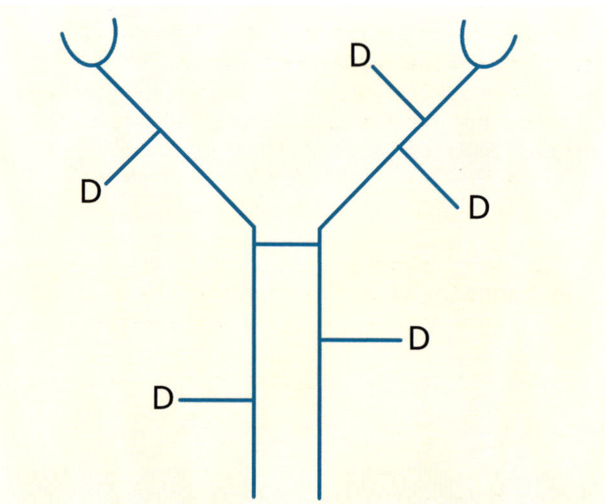

Figure 4.28. A schematic view of an immunoconjugate (D = drug molecules covalently attached to antibody (fragments)), cf. Figure 13.10.

for a carcinoma-surface antigen with an antigen-binding site with T cell affinity. The MAb are *in vitro* incubated with the stimulated T-lymphocytes prior to intraperitoneal injection (De Leij *et al.*, 1990; Crommelin and Storm, 1990).

Immunoconjugates: combinations between an antibody and an active compound

In many cases antibodies alone or bispecific antibodies have been shown to lack sufficient therapeutic activity. To enhance their activity, both conjugates of MAb and drugs have been designed. These efforts mainly focus on the treatment of cancer and no products have yet reached the market (Crommelin and Storm, 1990). To test the concept of immunoconjugates, a wide range of drugs have been covalently bound to antibodies and have been evaluated in animal tumor models. As only a limited number of antibody molecules can bind to the target cells, only conjugation of highly potent drugs will lead to sufficient therapeutic activity (cf. Figure 4.29). Table 4.13 lists a number of potential problems encountered with immunoconjugates (Crommelin *et al.*, 1992).

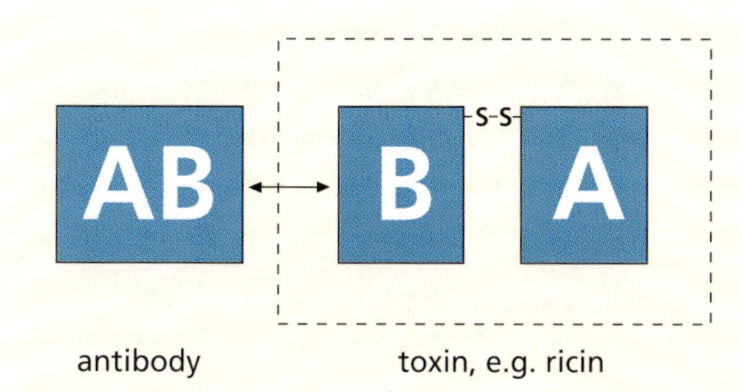

Figure 4.29. Immunotoxins are composed of antibody molecules connected to a toxin, e.g. ricin. Both the integral ricin molecule has been used as well as the A-chain alone. AB = antibody; A and B stand for the A and B chain of the ricin toxin, respectively (not in the list of abbreviations).

1. Covalent binding of the protein to the antibody can change the cytotoxic potential of the drug and decrease the affinity of the MAB for the antigen
2. The stability of the conjugate in vivo can be insufficient; fragmentation will lead to loss of targeting potential
3. The immunogenicity of the MAB and toxicity of the protein involved can change dramatically

Table 4.13. Potential problems encountered with immunoconjugates (Crommelin *et al.*, 1992).

Cytostatics with a high intrinsic cytotoxicity are needed (see above). Because the kinetic behavior of active compounds is strongly affected by the conjugating antibody, active compounds that were never used before as drugs – due to their high toxicity – in addition to existing cytostatics, should now be re-considered.

Immunoconjugated toxins are now tested as chemotherapeutic agents to treat cancer (immunotoxins). Examples of the toxin family are ricin, abrin and diphtheria toxin (Figure 4.29). These proteins are extremely toxic; they block enzymatically intracellular protein synthesis at the ribosomal level. Ricin (M_w 66 kDa) consists of an A and a B chain that are linked through a cystin bridge. The A chain is responsible for blocking protein synthesis at the ribosomes. The B chain is important for the cellular uptake of the molecule (endocytosis) and the intracellular trafficking.

In animal studies with immuno-conjugated ricin only a small fraction of these immunotoxins accumulates in tumor tissue (1%). A major fraction still ends up in the liver, the main target organ for 'natural' ricin. Moreover, in clinical phase I studies (to assess the safety of the conjugates) the first generation of immunoconjugates turned out to be immunogenic. Now attempts are being made to adapt the ricin molecule (by genetic engineering) so that liver targeting is minimized. This adapting can be done by blocking (removing or masking) on the ricin molecule ligands for galactose receptors on hepatocytes. Besides, murine MAb can be replaced by human or humanized MAb (see above) (Ramakrishnan, 1990).

Potential Pitfalls in Tumor Targeting

Upon intravenous injection only a small fraction of the homing device-carrier-drug complex is sequestered at the target site. Apart from the compartmentalization of the body (see above: anatomical and physiological hurdles) and, consequently, the carrier-dependent barriers that result, several other factors account for this lack of target site accumulation (Table 4.14).

How successful are MAb in discriminating target cells (tumor cells) from non-target cells? Do all tumor cells

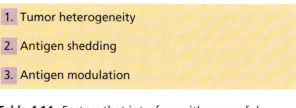

1. Tumor heterogeneity
2. Antigen shedding
3. Antigen modulation

Table 4.14. Factors that interfere with successful targeting of proteins to tumor cells.

expose the tumor-associated antigen? These questions are still difficult to answer (Hellström *et al.*, 1987). Tumor cell-surface specific molecules used for homing purposes are often differentiation antigens on the tumor cell wall. These structures are not unique since they occur in a lower density level on non-target cells, as well. Therefore, the target site specificity of MAb raised against these structures is more quantitative than qualitative in nature.

Another category of tumor associated antigens are the clone specific antigens. They are unique for the clone forming the tumor. However, the practical problem when focusing on clone specific antibodies for drug targeting is that each patient probably needs a tailor-made MAb.

The surface 'make up' of tumor cells in a tumor or a metastasis is not constant; neither in time nor between cells in the same tumor. There are many subpopulations of cells and they express different surface molecules. This heterogeneity means that not all cells in the tumor will interact with one, single targeted conjugate. Antigen shedding and antigen modulation are two other ways tumor cells can avoid recognition. Shedding of antigens means that antigens are released from the surface. They can then interact with circulating conjugates outside the target area, form an antigen-antibody complex and neutralize the homing potential of the conjugates before the target area has been reached. Finally, antigen modulation can occur upon the binding of MAb to the cell surface antigen. Upon endocytosis of the (originally exposed) surface antigen-immunoconjugate complex, modulation is the phenomenon where some of these antigens are no longer exposed on the surface; there is no replenishment of endocytosed surface antigens.

Four strategies can be implemented to solve problems related to tumor cell heterogeneity, shedding and modulation. (1) Cocktails of different MAb attached to the toxin can be used. (2) Another approach is to give up striving for complete target cell specificity and to induce so-called 'bystander' effects. In this case, the targeted system is designed in such a way that the active part is released from the conjugate after reaching a target cell, but before the antigen-conjugate complex has been taken up (is endocytosed) by the target cell. (3) Not all surface antigens show shedding or modulation. If these phenomena occur, other antigen/MAb combinations should be selected that do not demonstrate these effects. (4) At the present, injection of free MAb prior to injection of the immunoconjugate is under investigation to neutralize 'free' circulating antigen; then, the subsequently injected conjugate should not encounter shedded, free antigen.

In conclusion, targeted (modified) MAb and MAb-conjugates are now studied to assess their value in fighting life-threatening diseases such as cancer. During the last decade, the technology has evolved quickly; many different new options have become available. A lack of detailed pathophysiological and cell biological knowledge about the behavior of tumors, for instance, slows down progress. It is even possible that the whole concept of MAb-(conjugates) will turn to out to be of only limited therapeutic value, because of problems such as tumor cell heterogeneity, poor access to tumors and immunogenicity concerns.

Colloidal Particulate Carrier Systems for Targeted Delivery of Proteins

A wide range of carrier systems in the colloidal size range (diameters up to a few micrometers) has been proposed for protein targeting. Examples are: liposomes, biodegradable polycyanoacrylate nanoparticles, albumin microspheres, polylactic acid microspheres, and low density lipoproteins (LDL). Upon entering the bloodstream after i.v. injection, it is difficult for many of these particulate systems to pass through epithelial and endothelial membranes in healthy tissue, as the size cut off for permeation through these multilayered barriers is around 20 nm (excluding the liver, see above Figure 4.26). Parameters that control the fate of particulate carriers *in vivo* are listed in Table 4.15.

As a rule, cells of the mononuclear phagocyte system (MPS), such as macrophages, recognize stable, colloidal particulate systems (< 5 μm) as 'foreign body like structures' and phagocytose them. Thus, the liver and spleen, organs rich in blood circulation exposed macrophages, take up the majority of these particulates (Tomlinson, 1987; Crommelin and Storm, 1990). Larger (> 5 μm) intravenously injected particles tend to form emboli in lung capillaries on their first encounter with this organ.

Liposomes have gained considerable attention among the colloidal particulate systems proposed for the site-specific drug delivery of proteins. Liposomes are vesicular structures based on (phospho)lipid bilayers surrounding an aqueous core. The main component of the bilayer usually is phosphatidylcholine (Figure 4.30).

By selecting their bilayer constituents and one of the many preparation procedures described, liposomes can be made in sizes varying between 30 μm (e.g. by extrusion or ultrasonication) and 10 μm. The charges of liposomes can also be varied by the incorporation of a positively or

1. size
2. charge
3. surface hydrophilicity
4. presence of homing devices on their surface
5. exchange of constitutive parts with blood components

Table 4.15. Parameters controling the fate of particulate carriers *in vivo*.

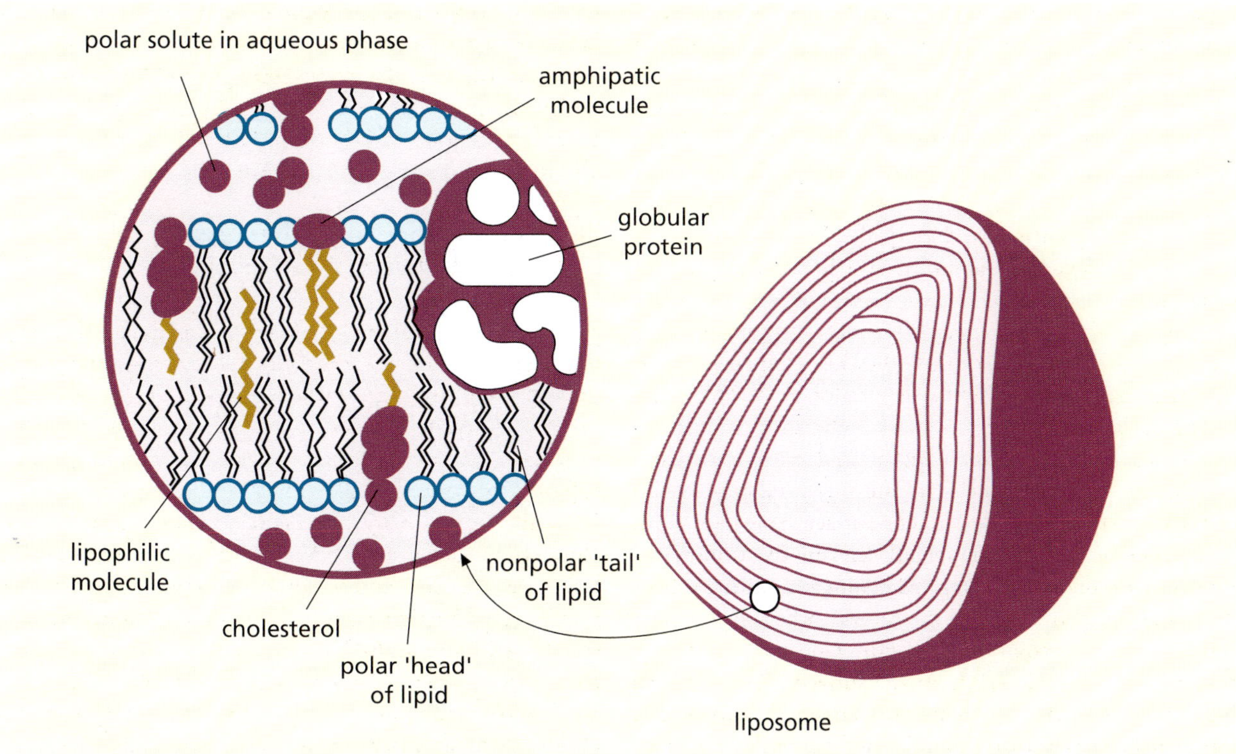

Figure 4.30. An artist's view of what a multilamellar liposome looks like. The lamellae are bilayers of (phospho)lipid molecules with their hydrophobic tails oriented inwards and their polar heads directed to, and in contact with, the aqueous medium. The bilayer may accomodate lipophilic drugs inside. Hydrophilic drugs will be found in the aqueous core and in between the bilayers. Depending on their hydrophilic/hydrophobic balance and tertiary structure proteins and peptides will be found in the aqueous phase, at the bilayer-water interface, or inside the lipid bilayer. Adapted from Fendler, 1980.

negatively charged lipid (cf. Chapter 7), Additionally, bilayer rigidity can be controlled by selecting special phospholipids or by adding lipids such as cholesterol. Liposomes can carry their proteins in the lipid core of the bilayer through partitioning, attached to the bilayer, or physically entrapped in the aqueous phase. To make liposomes target site specific, except for passive targeting to liver (Kupffer cells) and spleen macrophages, homing devices are covalently coupled to the outside bilayer leaflet (Toonen and Crommelin, 1983). In Table 4.16 three relative advantages of liposomes over other particulate systems are given.

After injection, 'standard' liposomes stay in the blood circulation only for a short time. They are taken up by macrophages in liver and spleen, or they degrade by the exchange of bilayer constituents with blood constituents. Liposome residence time in the blood circulation can be extended to many hours and even days if polyoxyethylene (PEG) chains are grafted on the surface and stable bilayer structures are used (Figure 4.31 and cf. Figure 4.17). These long circulating liposomes are able to escape macrophage uptake for prolonged periods of time and are sequestered

Liposomes stand out among other particulate carrier systems, because of:
1. their relatively low toxicity, existing safety record and experience with marketed, intravenously administered liposome products (e.g., amphothericin B, doxorubicin, daunorubicin) (Storm *et al.*, 1993)
2. the presence of a relatively large aqueous core, which is essential to stabilize the structural features of many proteins
3. the possibility to manipulate release characteristics of liposome associated proteins and to control disposition in vivo by changing preparation techniques and bilayer constituents (Crommelin and Schreier, 1994).

Table 4.16.

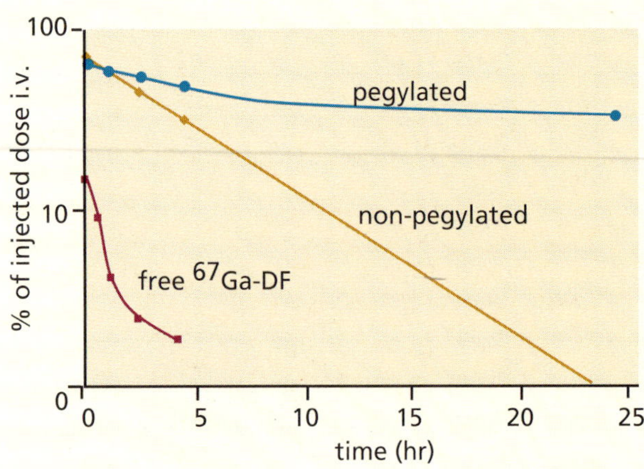

Figure 4.31. Comparison of the blood levels of free label, ^{67}Ga-DF, gallium-desferal with ^{67}Ga-DF laden pegylated (PEG) and non-pegylated liposomes upon i.v. administration in rats. From Woodle, *et al.*, 1990.

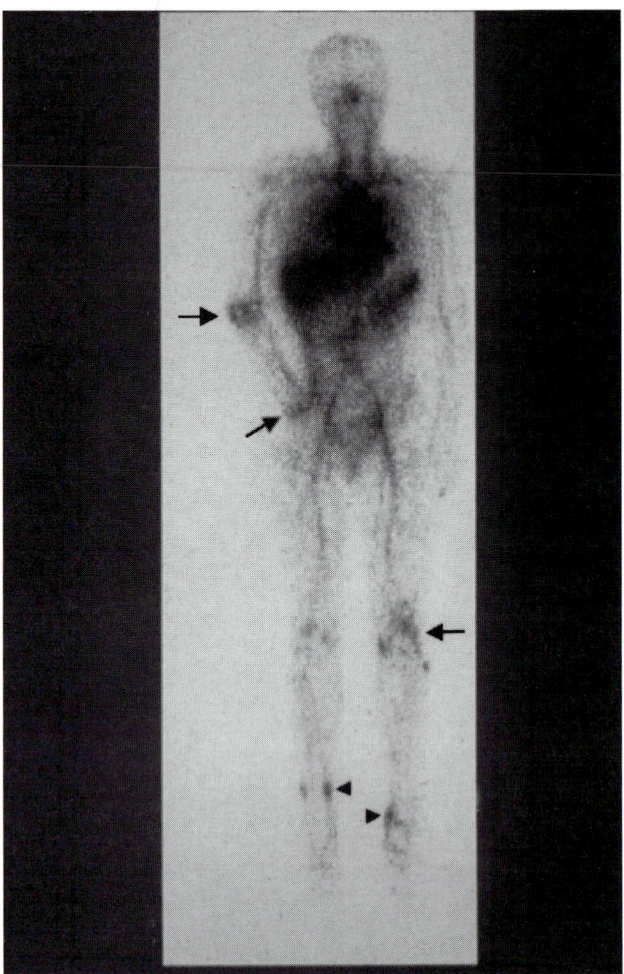

Figure 4.32. ^{99m}Tc-PEG-liposomes scintigraphy of a female patient. Anterior whole body image, 24 h post-injection, shows physiological uptake in the cardiac blood, greater veins, liver, spleen. Liposome uptake at pathological sites can be noted along synovial lining of the left elbow, left wrist, and right knee (arrows and the medial site of both ankles (arrow heads) (Storm and Crommelin, 1998).

in organs other than the liver and spleen alone, e.g. tumors and inflamed tissues. In Figure 4.32 an example is shown of the use of ^{111}Tc-labelled liposomes in the detection of inflammation sites in a patient.

The accumulation of protein-laden liposomes in macrophages (passive targeting) offers interesting therapeutic opportunities. Liposome encapsulated lymphokines and 'microbial' products, such as interferon-gamma or muramyltripeptide-phosphatidylethanolamine (MTP-PE), respectively, can activate macrophages and enable them to kill micrometastases. These products can also help to stimulate immune reactions. Moreover, reaching macrophages may help us to more effectively fight macrophage located microbial, viral or bacterial diseases (Emmen and Storm, 1987; Crommelin and Schreier, 1994).

Several attempts have been made to sequester immunoliposomes (i.e. antibody-liposome combinations) at predetermined sites in the body. Here, the aim is active targeting to the desired target site instead of passive targeting to macrophages. The concept is schematically presented in Figure 4.33.

When designing immunoliposomes, antibodies or antibody-fragments are covalently bound to the surface of liposomes through lipid anchor molecules (Toonen and Crommelin, 1983). Non-PEGylated immunoliposomes have poor access to target sites outside the blood circulation after intravenous injection. The reason is the high resistance against liposome penetration through the endothelial lining at target sites and their relatively short circulation time (cf. Figure 4.26). Therefore, target sites should be sought in the blood circulation (i.e. red blood cells, thrombi, lymphocytes, or endothelial cells exposing, under stress,

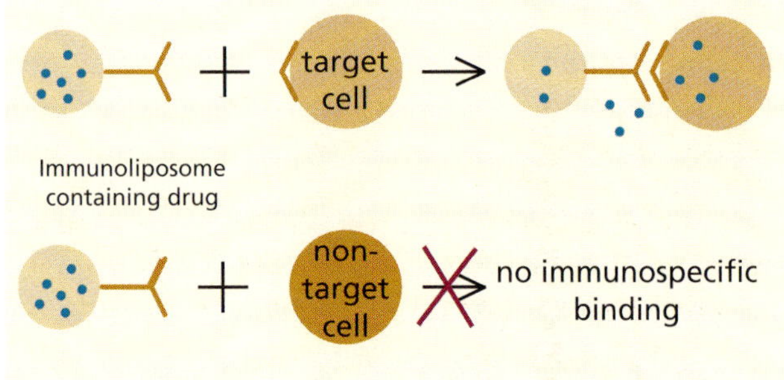

Figure 4.33. Schematic representation of the concept of drug targeting with immunoliposomes. From Nässander, *et al.*, 1990.

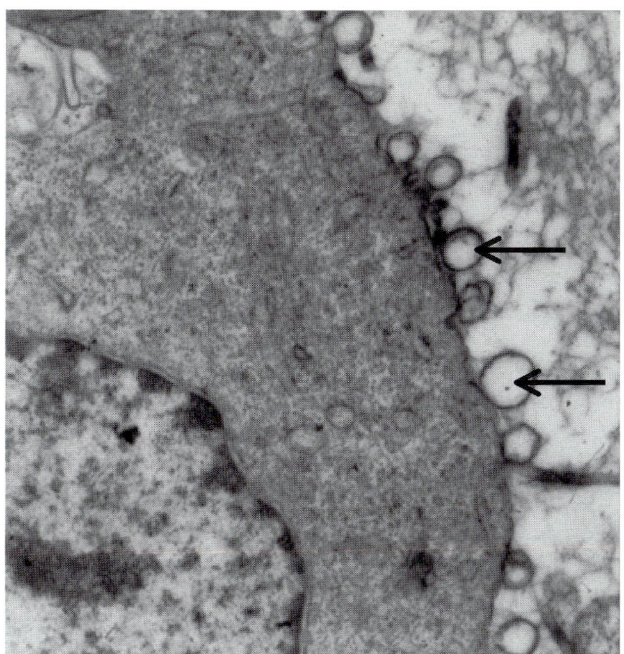

Figure 4.34. Electromicrograph showing immunoliposomes (vesicular structures) attached to human ovarian carcinoma cells (see text below).

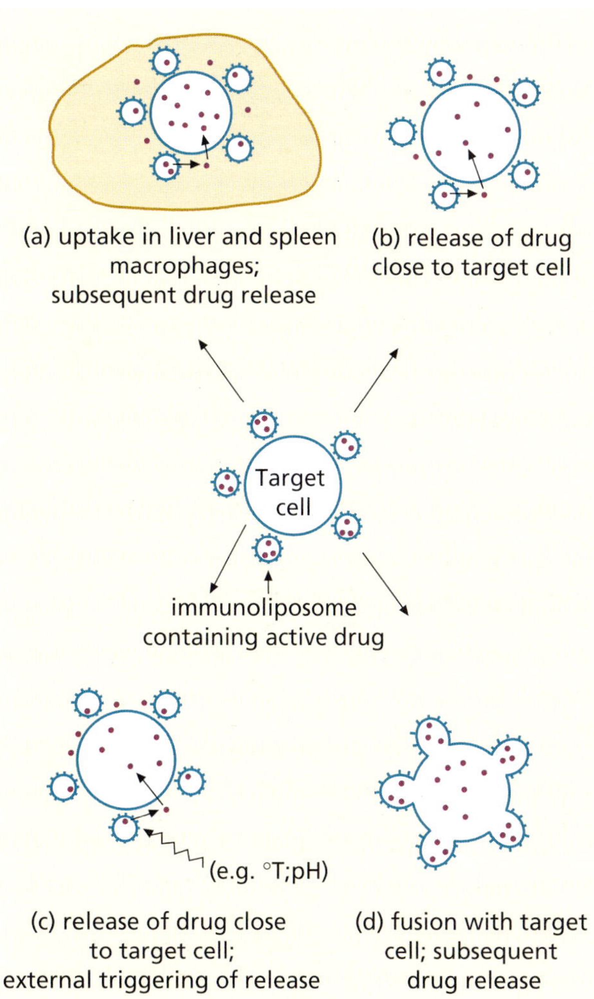

Figure 4.35. Several pathways of drug internalization after immunospecific binding of the immunoliposomes to the appropriate target cell. From Peeters *et al.*, 1987.

certain adhesion molecules, e.g. ICAM-1, intercellular cell adhesion molecule) (Vingerhoeds *et al.*, 1994; Crommelin *et al.*, 1995).

Other interesting target sites are those located in cavities, where one can locally administer the drug-carrier combination. The bladder and the peritoneal cavity are such cavities. These cavities can be the sites where the diseased tissue is concentrated. For instance, with ovarian carcinomas the tumors are confined to the peritoneal cavity for most of their lifetime. After intraperitoneal injection of immunoliposomes directed against human ovarian carcinomas in athymic, nude mice, a specific interaction between immunoliposomes and the human ovarian carcinoma was observed (Nässander and colleagues) (Figure 4.34). A new generation of liposomes is under development that combines PEG-coating (long circulation characteristic) and antibody coating (targeting).

Attaching an immunoliposome to target cells usually does not induce a therapeutic effect *per se*. After the establishment of an immunoliposome-cell interaction the protein drug has to exert its action on the cell. To do that, the protein has to be released in its active form. There are several pathways proposed to reach this goal (Figure 4.35) (Peeters *et al.*, 1987).

When the immunoliposome-cell complex encounters a macrophage, the cells and the adhering liposome are probably phagocytosed and enter the macrophage (option a). Subsequently, the liposome associated protein drug can be released. As this release will most likely happen in the 'hostile' lysosomal environment, little intact protein will become available. In the situation depicted in Figure 4.35 (option b) the drug is released from the adhering immunoliposomes in the close proximity of the target cell. In principle, release rate control is achieved by selecting the proper liposomal bilayers with delayed or sustained drug release characteristics. A third approach is depicted as option c: drug release is induced from liposomal bilayers by external stimuli (local pH change or temperature change). Finally, one can envision that immunoliposomes can be built with intrinsic fusogenic potential, which is only activated upon attachment of the carrier to the target cell. This exciting option d, Figure 4.35, resembles the behavior of certain viruses. However, this complicated technology is still in an early stage of development.

Perspectives for Targeted Protein Delivery

Protein targeting strategies have been developing at a rapid pace. A new generation of homing devices (target cell specific monoclonal antibodies) and a better insight into the anatomy and physiology of the human body under pathological conditions have been critical factors in achieving this success. A much better picture has emerged not only about the potentials, but also alout the limitations of the different targeting approaches.

Very little attention has been paid to the typically pharmaceutical aspects of advanced drug delivery systems, such as immunotoxins and immunoliposomes. These systems are now produced on a lab scale and their therapeutic potential is currently under investigation. If therapeutic benefits have been clearly proven in preclinical and early clinical trials, then scaling up, shelf life and quality assurance issues (e.g. reproducibility of technology, purity of the ingredients) will still require considerable attention. ■

References

- **Arakawa, T., Kita, Y. and Carpenter, J.F.** (1991). Protein-solvent interactions in pharmaceutical formulation. *Pharmaceutical Research,* **8**, 285–291.
- **Banerjee, P.S., Hosny, E.A. and Robinson, J.R.** (1991). Parenteral delivery of peptide and protein drugs. In V.H.L. Lee (Ed.), *Peptide and protein drug delivery* (pp. 487–543). N.Y.: Marcel Dekker, Inc.
- **Björk, E. and Edman, P.** (1988). Characterization of degradable starch microspheres as a nasal delivery system for drugs. *Int. J. Pharm.*, **62**, 187–192.
- **Brange, J. and Langkjaer, L.** (1993). Insulin structure and stability. In Y.J. Wang & R. Pearlman (Eds.), *Stability and characterization of protein and peptide drugs. Case histories* (pp. 315–350). N.Y.: Plenum Press, Inc.
- **Chien, Y.W.** (1991). Transdermal route of peptide and protein drug delivery. In V.H.L. Lee (Ed.), *Peptide and protein drug delivery* (pp. 667–689). N.Y.: Marcel Dekker, Inc.
- **Crommelin, D.J.A., Bergers, J. and Zuidema, J.** (1992). Antibody-based drug targeting approaches: perspectives and challenges. In C.G. Wermuth, N. Koga, H. König, & B.W. Metcalf (Eds.), *Medicinal chemistry for the 21st century* (pp. 351–365). Oxford: Blackwell Scientific Publications.
- **Crommelin, D.J.A., Scherphof, G. and Storm, G.** (1995). Active targeting with particulate carrier systems in the blood compartment. *Advanced Drug Delivery Reviews,* **17**, 49–60.
- **Crommelin, D.J.A. and Schreier, H.** (1994). Liposomes. In J. Kreuter (Ed.), *Colloidal drug delivery systems* (pp. 73–190). New York: Marcel Dekker, Inc.
- **Crommelin, D.J.A. and Storm, G.** (1990). Drug Targeting. In P.G. Sammes & J.D. Taylor (Eds.), *Comprehensive Medicinal Chemistry* (pp. 661–701). Oxford: Pergamon Press.
- **Cullander, C. and Guy, R.H.** (1992). Transdermal delivery of peptides and proteins. *Advanced Drug Delivery Reviews,* **8**, 291–329.
- **De Leij, L., De Jonge, M.W.A., Ter Haar, J., Spakman, H., De Vries, E., Willmese, P., Mulder, N.H., Berendsen, H., Elias, M., Smit Sibinga, C., De Lau, W., Tax, W. and The, T.H.** (1990). Bispecific monoclonal antibody (BIAB) retargeted cellular therapy for local treatment of cancer patients. In D.J.A. Crommelin & H. Schellekens (Eds.), *From Clone to Clinic* (pp. 159–165). Dordrecht: Kluwer Academic.
- **Edman, P. and Björk, E.** (1992). Nasal delivery of peptide drugs. *Advanced Drug Delivery Reviews,* **8**, 165–177.
- **Eldridge, J.H., Hammond, C.J., Meulbroek, J.A., Staas, J.K., Giley, R.M. and Tice, T.R.** (1990). Controlled vaccine release in the gut-associated lymphoid tissues. I. Orally administered biodegradable microspheres target the Peyer's patches. *J. Controlled Release,* **11**, 205–214.
- **Emmen, F. and Storm, G.** (1987). Liposomes in the treatment of infectious diseases. *Pharm. Weekblad Sci. Ed.*, **9**, 162–171.
- **Fanger, M.W. and Guyre, P.M.** (1991). Bispecific antibodies for targeted cellular cytotoxicity. *TIBTECH,* **9**, 375–380.
- **Fendler, J.H.** (1980). Optimizing drug entrapment in liposomes. Chemical and biophysical considerations. In G. Gregoriadis & A.C. Allison (Eds.), *Liposomes in biological systems* (p. 87). Chichester: Wiley, J. & Sons, Ltd.
- **Franks, F., Hatley, R.H.M. and Mathias, S.F.** (1991). Materials science and the production of shelf-stable biologicals. *Pharmaceutical Technol. Int.*, **3**.
- **Groves, M.** (1988). *Parenteral Technology Manual.* Buffalo Grove, Il: Interpharm Press, Inc.
- **Halls, N.A.** (1994). *Acheiving sterility in medical and pharmaceutical products.* N.Y.: Marcel Dekker, Inc.
- **Heilmann, K.** (1984). *Therapeutic systems. Rate controlled delivery: concept and development.* Stuttgart: G. Thieme Verlag.
- **Heller, J.** (1993). Polymers for controlled parenteral delivery of peptides and proteins. *Advanced Drug Delivery Reviews,* **10**, 163–204.
- **Hellström, K.E., Hellström, I. and Goodman, G.E.** (1987). Antibodies for drug delivery. In J.R. Robinson & V.H.L. Lee (Eds.), *Controlled drug delivery* (pp. 623–653). N.Y.: Marcel Dekker, Inc.
- **Ho, N.F.H., Barsuhn, C.L., Burton, P.S. and Merkle, H.P.** (1992). Mechanistic insights to buccal delivery of proteinaceous substances. *Advanced Drug Delivery Reviews,* **8**, 197–235.
- **Holmgren, J., Clemens, J., Sack, D., Sanchez, J. and Svennerholm, A.M.** (1989). Development of oral vaccines with special reference to cholera. In D.D. Breimer, D.J.A. Crommelin,

& K.K. Midha (Eds.), *Topics in Pharmaceutical Sciences 1989* (pp. 297–311). The Hague: International Pharmaceutical Federation (F.I.P.).

- **Hunt, C.A., MacGregor, R.D. and Siegel, R.A.** (1986). Engineering targeted in vivo drug delivery. I. The physiological and physicochemical principles governing opportunities and limitations. *Pharm. Research*, **3**, 333–344.
- **Jain, R.K.** (1987). Transport of molecules in the tumor interstitium: a review. *Cancer Research*, **47**, 3039–3051.
- **Jani, P.U., Florence, A.T. and McCarthy, D.E.** (1992). Further histological evidence of the gastrointestinal absorption of polystyrene nanospheres in the rat. *Int. J. Pharm.*, **84**, 245–252.
- **Kim, S.W., Pai, C.M., Makino, K., Seminoff, L.A., Holmberg, D.L., Gleeson, J.M., Wilson, D.A. and Mack, E.J.** (1990). Self-regulated glycosylated insulin delivery. *J. Controlled Release*, **11**, 193–201.
- **Klegerman, M.E. and Groves, M.J.** (1992). *Pharmaceutical biotechnology: Fundamentals and essentials.* Buffalo Grove, IL: Interpharm Press, Inc.
- **Kumar, S., Char, H., Patel, S., Piemontese, D., Malick, A.W., Iqbal, K., Neugroschel, E. and Behl, C.R.** (1992). In vivo transdermal iontophoretic delivery of growth hormone releasing factor GRF (1–44) in hairless guinea pigs. *J. Controlled Release*, **18**, 213–220.
- **Lee, V.H.L., Dodda-Kashi, S., Grass, G.M. and Rubas, W.** (1991). Oral route of peptide and protein drug delivery. In V.H.L. Lee (Ed.), *Peptide and protein drug delivery* (pp. 691–738). N.Y.: Marcel Dekker.
- **Lee, H.J., Riley, G., Johnson, O., Cleland, J.F., Kim, N., Charnis, M., Bailey, L., Duenas, E., Shahzamani, A., Marian, M., Jones, A.J.S. and Putney, S.D.** (1997). In vivo characterization of sustained-release formulations of human growth hormone. *J. Pharmacology and Experimental Therapeutics* **281**, 1431–1439.
- **Maberly, G.F., Wait, G.A., Kilpatrick, J.A., Loten, E.G., Gain, K.R., Stewart, R.D.H. and Eastman, C.J.** (1982). Evidence for insulin degradation by muscle and fat tissue in an insulin resistant diabetic patient. *Diabetologica* (23), 333–336.
- **Nässander, U.K., Storm, G., Peeters, P.A.M. and Crommelin, D.J.A.** (1990). Liposomes. In M. Chasin & R. Langer (Eds.), *Biodegradable Polymers as Drug Delivery Systems* (pp. 261–33). New York: Marcel Dekker.
- Neutropin Depot™ insert information.
- **O'Hagan, D.T.** (1990). Intestinal translocation of particulates – implications for drug and antigen delivery, *Advanced Drug Delivery Reviews*, **5**, 265–285.
- **Nguyen, T.H. and Ward, C.** (1993). Stability characterization and formulation development of alteplase, a recombinant tissue plasminogen activator. In Y.J. Wang & R. Pearlman (Eds.), *Stability and characterization of protein and peptide drugs. Case histories* (pp. 91–134). N.Y.: Plenum Press.
- **Patton, J.S. and Platz, R.M.** (1992). Pulmonary delivery of peptides and proteins for systemic action. *Advanced Drug Delivery Reviews*, **8**, 179–196.
- **Patton, J.S., Trinchero, P. and Platz, R.M.** (1994). Bioavailability of pulmonary delivered peptides and proteins: alpha-interferon, calcitonins and parathyroid hormones. *J. Controlled Release*, **28**, 79–85.
- **Patton, J.S., Bukar, J. and Nagarajan, S.** (1999). Inhaled insulin. *Advanced Drug Delivery Reviews*, **35**, 235–247.
- **Pearlman, R. and Bewley, T.A.** (1993). Stability and characterization of human growth hormone. In Y.J. Wang & R. Pearlman (Eds.), *Stability and characterization of protein and peptide drugs. Case histories* (pp. 1–58). N.Y.: Plenum Press.
- **Peeters, P.A.M., Storm, G. and Crommelin, D.J.A.** (1987). Immunoliposomes in vivo: state of the art. *Advanced Drug Delivery Reviews*, **1**, 249–266.
- **Pikal, M.J.** (1990a). Freeze-drying of proteins. Part I: Process Design. *BioPharm*, **3**(8), 18–27.
- **Pikal, M.J.** (1990b). Freeze-drying of proteins. Part II: Formulation selection. *BioPharm*, **3**, 26–30.
- **Poste, G.** (1985). Drug targeting in cancer therapy. In G. Gregoriadis, G. Poste, J. Senior, & A. Trouet (Eds.), *Receptor-mediated targeting of drugs* (pp. 427–474). New York: Plenum Press.
- **Pristoupil, T.I.** (1985). Haemoglobin lyophilized with sucrose: effect of residual moisture on storage. *Haematologia*, **18**, 45–52.
- **Ramakrishnan, S.** (1990). Current status of antibody-toxin conjugates for tumor therapy. In P. Tyle & B.P. Ram (Eds.), *Targeted therapeutic systems* (pp. 189–213). N.Y.: Marcel Dekker, Inc.
- **Roitt, I.M., Brostoff, J. and Male, D.K.** (1993). *Immunology*, third edition, Mosby, St. Louis, MO
- **Sage, B.H., Bock, C.R., Denuzzio, J.D. and Hoke, R.A.** (1995). Technological and developmental issues of iontophoretic transport of peptide and protein drugs. In V.H.L. Lee, M. Hashida, & Y. Mizushima (Eds.), *Trends and future perspectives in peptide and protein drug delivery* (pp. 111–134). Chur: Harwood Academic Publishers GmbH.
- **Soon-Shiong, P., Heintz, R.E., Merideth, N., Yao, Q.X., Yoa, Z., Zheng, T., Murphy, M., Moloney, M.K., Schmehl, M., Harris, M., Mendez, R., Mendez, R. and Sandford, P.A.** (1994). Insulin independence in a type 1 diabetic patient after encapsulated islet transplantation. *Lancet*, **343**, 950–951.
- **Stenekes, R.**, Nanoporous dextran microspheres for drug delivery. Thesis, Utrecht University, 2000.
- **Storm, G., Oussoren, C., Peeters, P.A.M. and Barenholz, Y.B.** (1993). Tolerability of liposomes in vivo. In G. Gregoriadis (Ed.), *Liposome Technology* (pp. 345–383.). Boca Raton: CRC Press, Inc.
- **Storm, G., Nässander, U., Vingerhoeds, M.H., Steerenberg, P.A. and Crommelin, D.J.A.** (1994). Antibody-targeted liposomes to deliver doxorubicin to ovarian cancer cells. *J. Liposome Research*, **4**, 641–666.
- **Storm, G. and Crommelin, D.J.A.** (1998). Liposomes: quo vadis? *Pharmaceutical Science & Technology Today*, **1**, 19–31.

- **Supersaxo, A., Hein, W.R. and Steffen, H.** (1990). Effect of molecular weight on the lymphatic absorption of water-soluble compounds following subcutaneous administration. *Pharm. Research*, **7**, 167–169.
- **Thurow, H. and Geisen, K.** (1984). Stabilization of dissolved proteins against denaturation at hydrophobic interfaces. *Diabetologica*, **27**, 212–218.
- **Tomlinson, E.** (1987). Theory and practice of site-specific drug delivery. *Advanced Drug Del. Reviews*, **1**, 87–198.
- **Toonen, P. and Crommelin, D.J.A.** (1983). Immunogobulins as targeting agents for liposome encapsulated drugs. *Pharm. Weekblad Sci. Ed.*, **16**, 269–280.
- **Tresco, P.A.** (1994). Encapsulated cells for sustained neurotransmitter delivery to the central nervous system. *J. Controlled Release*, **28**, 253–258.
- **Uludag, H., Kharlip, L. and Sefton, M.V.** (1993). Protein delivery by microencapsulated cells. *Adv. Drug Delivery Reviews*, **10**, 115–130.
- **Vemuri, S., Yu, C.T. and Roosdorp, N.** (1993a). Formulation and stability of recombinant alpha-antitrypsin. In Y.J. Wang & R. Pearlman (Eds.), *Stability and characterization of protein and peptide drugs. Case histories* (pp. 263–286). N.Y.: Plenum Press.
- **Vemuri, S., Yu, C.T. and Roosdorp, N.** (1993b). Formulation and stability of recombinant alpha1-antitrypsin. In Y.J. Wang & R. Pearlman (Eds.), *Stability and characterization of protein and peptide drugs* (pp. 263–286). N.Y.: Plenum Press.
- **Vingerhoeds, M.H., Storm, G. and Crommelin, D.J.A.** (1994). Immunoliposomes in vivo. *Immunomethods*, **4**, 259–272.
- **Woodle, M., Newman, M., Collins, L., Redemann, C. and Martin, F.** (1990). Improved long-circulating (Stealth®) liposomes using synthetic lipids. *Proc. Int. Symp. Control. Rel. Bioactive Mater.*, **17**, 77–78.
- **USP XXIV/NF 19** (2000). United States Pharmacopeial Convention, Inc. Rockville, MD.
- **Zhou, X.H. and Li Wan Po, A.** (1991a). Peptide and protein drugs: I. Therapeutic applications, absorption and parenteral administration. *Int. J. Pharm.*, **75**, 97–115.
- **Zhou, X.H. and Li Wan Po, A.** (1991b). Peptide and protein drugs: II. Non-parenteral routes of delivery. *Int. J. Pharm.*, **75**, 117–130.

Self-Assessment Questions

Question 1: *How does one sterilize biotech products for parenteral administration?*

Question 2: *A pharmaceutical protein, which is poorly water soluble around its i.e.p., has to be formulated as an injection. What conditions would one select to produce a water soluble, injectable solution?*

Question 3: *Why are most of the biotech proteins used in the clinic formulated in freeze-dried form? Why is, as a rule, the presence of lyoprotectants required? Why is it important to know the glass transition temperature or eutectic temperature of the system?*

Question 4: *Why is it not necessarily wise to work at the lowest possible chamber pressures?*

Question 5: *Why are (with the exception of oral vaccines) no oral delivery systems for proteins available?*

Question 6: *What alternative route of administration to the parenteral route would be the first to be looked into if a systemic therapeutic effect is pursued and if one does not wish to exploit absorption enhancing technologies?*

Question 7: *If one considers use of the iontophoretic transport route for protein delivery, what are the variables to be considered?*

Question 8: *What are the differences between the endocrine, paracrine and autocrine methods of cell communication? Why is information on the way cells communicate important in the drug formulation process?*

Question 9: *A company decides to explore the possibility for developing a feedback system for a therapeutic protein. What information should be available for estimating the chances of success?*

Question 10: *Why is the selection of the dimensions of a colloidal particulate carrier system for targeted delivery of a protein of the utmost importance?*

Question 11: *Design a targeted, colloidal carrier system and a protocol for its use to circumvent the three hurdles for achieving successful treatment of solid tumors (mentioned in Table 4.14).*

Question 12: *What are the options for inducing therapeutic actions upon the attachment of immunoliposomes to (tumor) target cells.*

Answers

Answer 1: Through aseptic manufacturing protocols; filtration through 0.2 or 0.22 μm pore filters plays an important role in reducing the degree of contamination of the protein solutions.

Answer 2: One has to go through the items listed in Table 4.1. As the aqueous solubility is probably pH dependent, information on the preferred pH ranges should be collected. If necessary, solubility enhancers (e.g. lysine, arginine and/or surfactants) and stabilizers against adsorption/aggregation should be added. As a last resort, one might consider carriers such as liposomes.

Answer 3: Chemical and physical instability of proteins in aqueous media is usually the reason to dry the protein solution. Freeze-drying is then the preferred technology, as other drying techniques do not give rapidly reconstitutable dry forms for the formulation, and/or because elevated temperatures necessary for drying jeopardize the integrity of the protein.
The glass transition/eutectic temperature should not been exceeded as otherwise collapse of the cake can be observed. Collapse reduces the drying process rate and collapsed material does not rapidly dissolve upon adding water for reconstitution.

Answer 4: Because gas conduction (one of the three heat transfer routes) depends on pressure and is reduced when the pressure is.

Answer 5: Because of the hostile environment in the GI tract regarding protein stability and the poor absorption characteristics of proteins (high molecular weight/often hydrophilic).

Answer 6: The pulmonary route.

Answer 7: Physical characteristics of the protein and medium, such a molecular weight, i.e.p., ionic strength, pH. And, in addition, electrical current options (pulsed, permanent, wave shape) and desired dose level/pattern (pulsed/constant/variable).

Answer 8: See Table 4.8. This information is important because in particular with paracrine and autocrine acting proteins targeted delivery should be considered to minimize unwanted side effects.

Answer 9:
- The desired pharmacokinetic profile (e.g. information on the PK/PD relationship/circadian rhythm)
- Chemical and physical stability of the protein on long term storage at body/ambient temperature
- Availability of a bio-sensor system (stability in vivo, precision/accuracy)
- Availability of a reliable pump system (see Table 4.10).

Answer 10: The body is highly compartmentalized and access to target sites inside and outside the blood circulation is highly dependent on the size of the carrier system involved.

Answer 11: The selection should be based on the induction of bystander effects, 'cocktails' of homing devices (e.g. monoclonal antibodies), selection of non-modulating receptors and non-shedding receptors. Neutralization of free, shed tumor antigens with free, non-conjugated monoclonal antibodies by the injection of these free antibodies before the administration of ligand-carrier-drug combinations would be an approach for avoiding the neutralization of the carrier-homing device combination.

Answer 12: Figure 4.35 gives an overview of these options.

5 Pharmacokinetics and Pharmacodynamics of Peptide and Protein Drugs

Rene Braeckman

Introduction

Pharmacokinetics is the study of the rate processes that are responsible for the time course of the level of an exogenous compound in the body. The processes involved are absorption (A), distribution (D), metabolism (M), and excretion (E) (Figure 5.1). The pharmacokinetics of peptides, peptoids (peptide-like compounds), proteins and other biotechnology products are important factors in their pharmacodynamics, i.e. the time course of their pharmacological effect. Therefore, knowledge of the pharmacokinetics and pharmacodynamics of a pharmaceutical drug in humans and laboratory animals is required when selecting dose levels and dose regimens. Similarly, the toxicokinetics (pharmacokinetics in toxicology studies, including higher doses than used clinically) and toxicodynamics (time course of undesired effects) are important for the design of toxicology studies (dose levels and dose regimens), as well as in determining safety margins and extrapolating toxicological data to humans.

In this chapter, the pharmacokinetics (PK) of protein therapeutics will be described, followed by an introduction to the complex relationship with the pharmacodynamic (PD) effect, and how plasma protein binding can influence PK and PD. Furthermore, interspecies extrapolation of PK

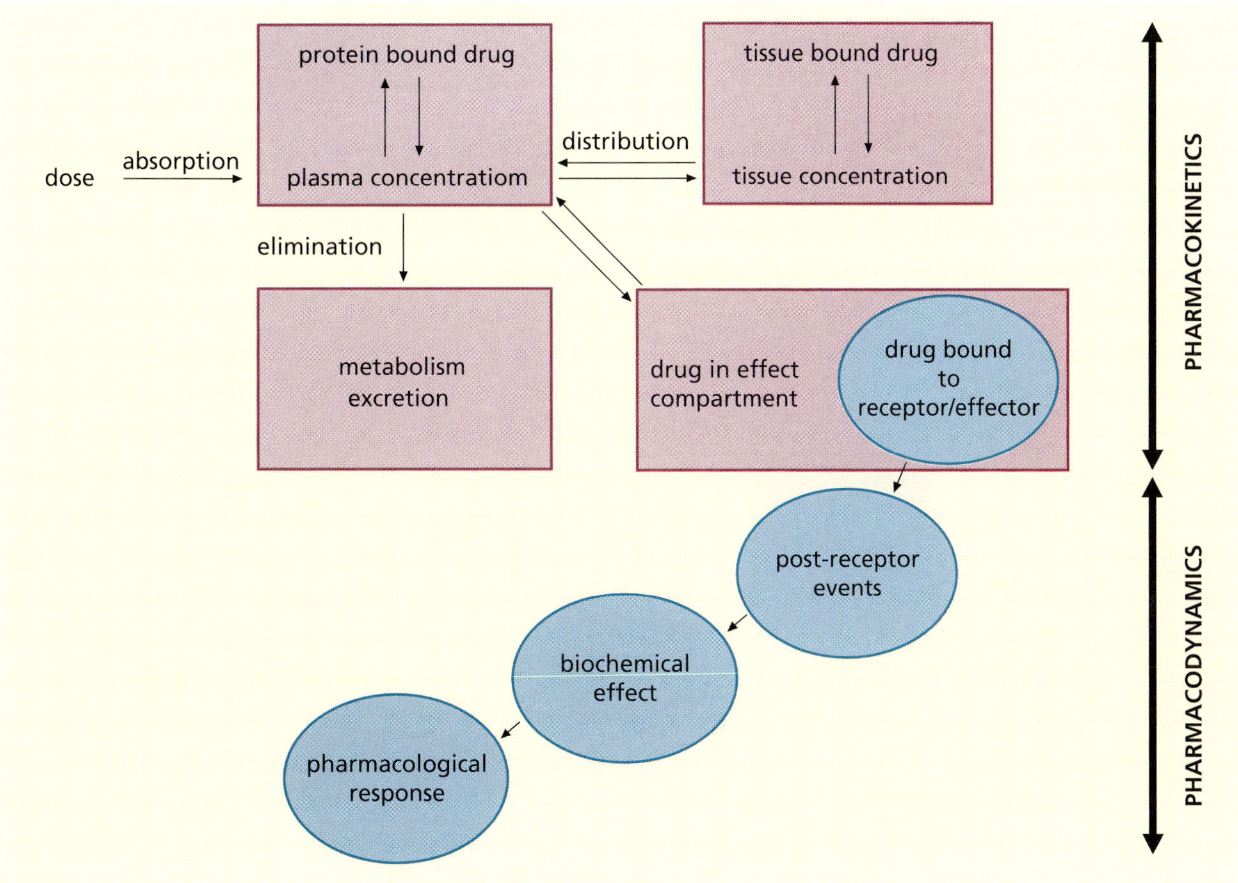

Figure 5.1. Physiological scheme of pharmacokinetic and pharmacodynamic processes.

and the influence of molecular structure on the PK characteristics of proteins will be discussed. Finally, the immunogenicity of protein therapeutics will be described, including a discussion on how antibody formation can influence PK and PD.

Elimination of Protein Therapeutics

It is commonly accepted that peptide and protein drugs are metabolized through identical catabolic pathways as endogenous and dietary proteins. Generally, proteins are broken down into amino acid fragments that can be reutilized in the synthesis of endogenous proteins. Although history has shown that proteins can be powerful and potentially toxic compounds, their end products of metabolism are not considered to be a safety issue. This is in contrast with small organic synthetic drug molecules from which potentially toxic metabolites can be formed. The study of the metabolism of protein drugs is also very complicated because of the great number of fragments that can be produced. The mechanisms for elimination of peptides and proteins are outlined in Table 5.1.

Proteolysis

Most if not all proteins are catabolized by proteolysis. Proteolytic enzymes are not only widespread throughout the body, they are also ubiquitous in nature, and therefore the potential number of catabolism sites on any protein is very large (Bocci, 1987; Bocci, 1990; Lee, 1988). It has been shown for interferon-γ (INF-γ) that truncated forms are present in the circulation after dosing of rhesus monkeys with rIFN-γ. The rate and extent of production of these metabolites may be dependent on the route of administration. This, and the cross-reactivity of these degraded forms in the ELISA may be responsible for the observation of a bioavailability of more than 100% after subcutaneous administration of rIFN-γ (Ferraiolo and Mohler, 1992). Proteolytic activity in tissue may be responsible for the loss of protein after subcutaneous administration.

Renal Excretion and Metabolism

Metabolism studies of peptide and protein drugs were performed to identify the organs responsible for metabolism (and/or excretion), and their relative contribution to the total elimination clearance. The importance of the kidney as an organ of elimination was assessed for rIL-2 (Gibbons *et al.*, 1995), M-CSF (Bauer *et al.*, 1994) and rIFN-γ (Mordenti *et al.*, 1992) in nephrectomized animals. The relative contributions of renal and hepatic clearances to the total plasma clearance of several other proteins are shown in Figure 5.2.

The different renal processes that are important for the elimination of proteins are depicted in Figure 5.3. The kidney appears to be the most dominant organ for the catabolism of small proteins (Maack *et al.*, 1979). Based on the observation that only trace amounts of albumin pass

M_W	Site of elimination	Dominating clearance mechanism	Determinant factor
< 500	blood liver	extracellular hydrolysis passive lipoid diffusion	
500 - 1,000	liver	carrier-mediated uptake passive lipoid diffusion	structure lipophilicity
1,000 - 50,000	kidney	glomerular filtration	M_W
50,000 - 200,000	kidney liver	receptor-mediated endocytosis receptor-mediated endocytosis	sugar, charge
200,000 - 400,000		opsonization	α_2-macroglobulin, IgG
> 400,000		phagocytosis	particle aggregation

Table 5.1. Clearance mechanisms for peptides and proteins as a function of molecular weight (Mw). Other determining factors are size, charge, lipophilicity, functional groups, sugar recognition, vulnerability for proteases, aggregation to particles, formation of complexes with opsonization factors, etc. The indicated mechanisms overlap, and fluid-phase endocytosis can in principle occur across the entire Mw range (after Meijer and Ziegler, 1993).

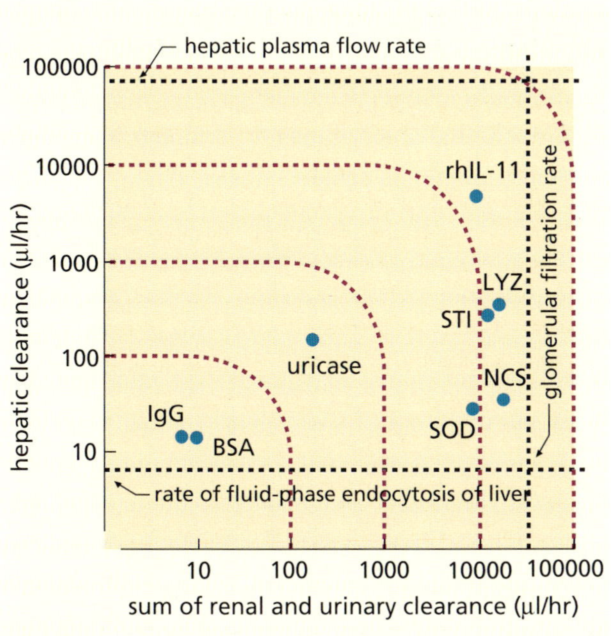

Figure 5.2. Hepatic and renal clearances of proteins in mice. LYZ: lysozyme, STI: soy bean trypsin inhibitor, NCS: neocarzinostatin, IgG: immunoglobulin G, BSA: bovine serum albumin, rhIL-11: recombinant human interleukin-11. From Takagi et al. (Takagi et al., 1995).

the glomerulus, it is believed that macromolecules have to be smaller than 69 kDa to undergo glomerular filtration (Takakura *et al.*, 1990). Glomerular filtration and excretion is most efficient, however, for proteins smaller than 30 kDa (Kompella and Lee, 1991). Peptides and small proteins (<5 kDa) are filtered very efficiently, and their glomerular filtration clearance approaches the glomerular filtration rate (GFR, ~120 mL/min in humans). For molecular weights exceeding 30 kDa, the filtration rate falls off sharply. Rather than strictly size of the molecules, it is the effective molecular radius that determines the degree of sieving by the glomerulus (Figure 5.4) (Rabkin and Dahl, 1993).

The glomerular barrier is also charge selective: the clearance of anionic molecules is impaired relative to that of neutral molecules, and the clearance of cationic macromolecules is enhanced. The influence of charge on glomerular filtration is especially important for molecules with a radius greater than 2 nm (Maack *et al.*, 1985). The charge-selectivity of glomerular filtration is related to the negative charge of the glomerular filter due to the abundance of glycosaminoglycans. Anionic proteins, such as TNF-α, INF-β, and INF-γ, are therefore repelled (Bocci, 1990).

After glomerular filtration, some peptides (melanostatin, for example) can be excreted unchanged in the urine. In contrast, complex polypeptides and proteins are actively re-absorbed by the proximal tubules by luminal endocytosis

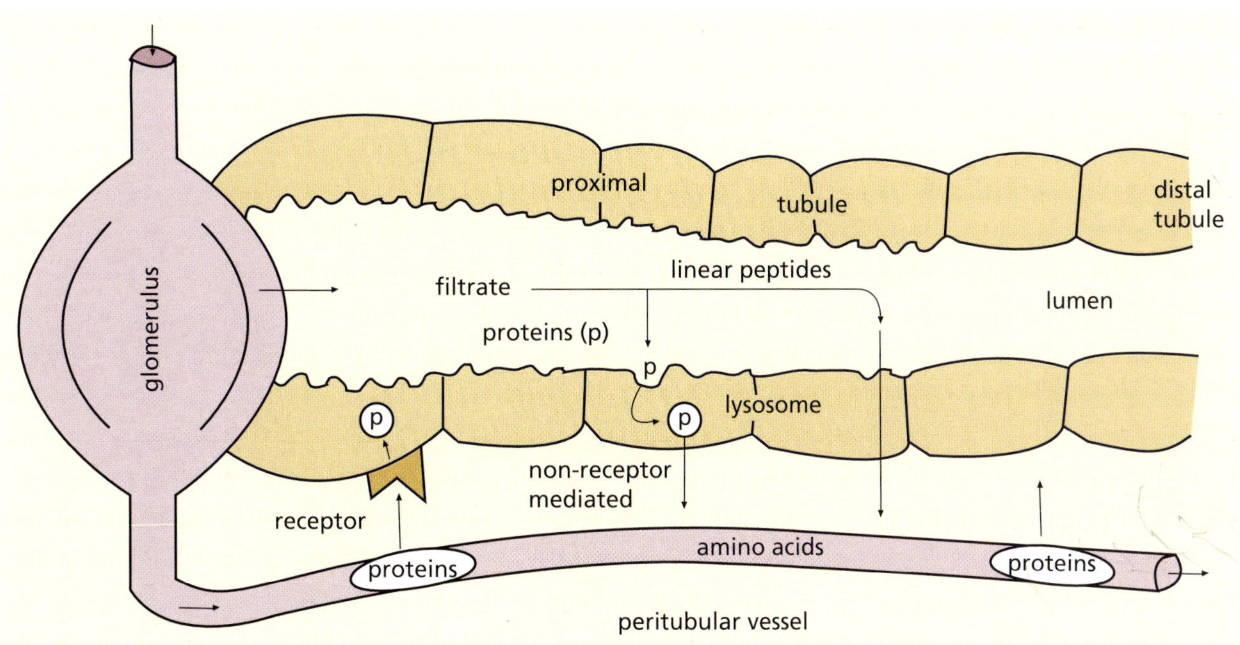

Figure 5.3. Pathways of renal elimination of proteins, including glomerular filtration, catabolism at the luminal membrane, tubular absorption followed by intracellular degradation, and postglomerular peritubular uptake followed by intracellular degradation. From Rabkin and Dahl, 1993.

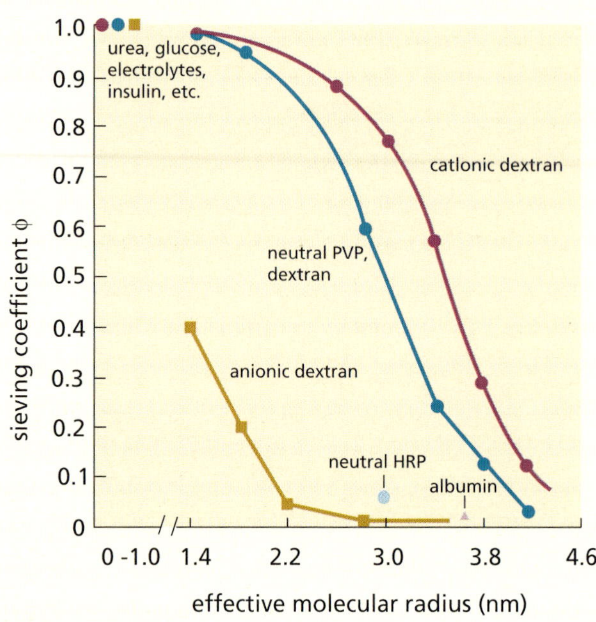

Figure 5.4. Glomerular sieving curves of several macromolecules. The different sieving coefficients reflect the influence of size, charge, and rigidity of molecules. From Arendshorst and Navar (Arendshorst and Navar, 1988).

and then hydrolyzed within the intracellular lysosomes to peptide fragments and amino acids (Maack *et al.*, 1985; Wall and Maack, 1985). The amino acids are returned to the systemic circulation. Consequently, only small amounts of intact protein are detected in the urine. The kidney appears to be the most dominant organ for the catabolism of small proteins (Maack *et al.*, 1979). Examples of proteins undergoing tubular reabsorption are calcitonin, glucagons, insulin, growth hormone, oxytocin, vasopressin, and lysozyme (Kompella and Lee, 1991). Cathepsin D, a major renal protease, is responsible for the hydrolysis of IL-2 in the kidney (Ohnishi *et al.*, 1989). Important determinants for tubular reabsorption of proteins are their physicochemical characteristics, such as net charge and number of free amino groups (Maack *et al.*, 1979). Cationic proteins are more susceptible to reabsorption than anionic proteins (Maack, 1975). Renal tubular cells also contain an active transporter for di- and tripeptides (Ganapathy and Leibach, 1986).

Small linear peptides (<10 amino acids), such as angiotensin I and II, bradykinin, and LHRH, are subjected to luminal membrane hydrolysis. They are hydrolyzed by enzymes in the luminal surface of the brush border membrane of the proximal tubules, and the small peptide fragments and amino acids are subsequently reabsorbed, further degraded intracellularly, and/or transported through the cells into the systemic circulation (Carone and Peterson, 1980).

Peritubular extraction of proteins from the postglomerular capillaries and intracellular catabolism is another renal mechanism of elimination (Rabkin and Kitaji, 1983). This route of elimination was demonstrated for IL-2 (Gibbons *et al.*, 1995), insulin (Hellfritzsch *et al.*, 1988; Rabkin *et al.*, 1984), calcitonin, parathyroid hormone, vasopressin and angiotensin II (Maack *et al.*, 1979). It is believed that the peritubular pathway exists mainly for the delivery of certain hormones to their site of action, i.e. to the receptors on the contraluminal site of the tubular cells.

Hepatic Metabolism

Besides proteolytic enzymes and renal catabolism, the liver has also been shown to contribute significantly to the metabolism of protein therapeutics. The rate of hepatic catabolism, which determines, in part, the elimination half-life, is largely dependent on the presence of specific amino acid sequences in the protein (Meijer and Ziegler, 1993). Before intracellular hepatic catabolism, proteins and peptides need to be transported from the blood stream to the liver cells. An overview of the different mechanisms of hepatic uptake of proteins is listed in Table 5.2.

Molecules of relatively small size and with highly hydrophobic characteristics permeate the hepatocyte membrane by simple non-ionic passive diffusion. Peptides of this nature include the cyclosporins (cyclic peptides) (Ziegler *et al.*, 1988). Other cyclic and linear peptides of small size (<1.4 kDa) and hydrophobic nature (containing aromatic amino acids), such as renin and cholecystokinin-8 (CCK-8; 8 amino acids), are cleared by the hepatocytes by a carrier-mediated transport (Ziegler *et al.*, 1988). After internalization into the cytosol, these peptides are usually metabolized by microsomal enzymes (cytochrome P-450IIIA for cyclosporin A) or cytosolic peptidases (CCK-8). Substances that enter the liver via carrier-mediated transport are typically excreted into the bile by the multispecific bile-acid transporter. These hepatic clearance pathways are identical to those known for most small organic hydrophobic drug molecules.

For larger peptides and proteins, there is a multitude of energy-dependent carrier-mediated transport processes available for cellular uptake. One of the possibilities is receptor-mediated endocytosis (RME), such as for insulin and EGF (Burwen and Jones, 1990; Kim *et al.*, 1988; Sugiyama and Hanano, 1989). In RME, circulating proteins are recognized by specific hepatic receptor proteins (Kompella and Lee, 1991). The receptors are usually integral membrane glycoproteins with an exposed binding domain on the extracellular side of the cell membrane. After the binding of the circulating protein to the receptor, the complex is already present or moves in coated pit regions, and the

Cell Type	Uptake mechanism	Proteins/Peptides Transported
Hepatocytes	anionic passive diffusion carrier-mediated transport	cyclic and linear hydrophobic peptides (<1.4 kDa) (cyclosporins, CCK-8)
	RME: Gal/GalNAc receptor (Asialoglycoprotein receptor)	N-acetylgalactosamine-terminated glycoproteins Galactose-terminated glycoproteins (e.g.: desialylated EPO)
	RME: Low Density Lipoprotein Receptor (LDLR)	LDL, apoE- and apoB-containing lipoproteins
	RME: LDLR-Related Protein (LRP receptor)	α_2-macroglobulin, apo-E-enriched lipoproteins, lipoprotein lipase (LpL), lactoferrin, t-PA, u-PA, complexes of t-PA and u-PA with plasminogen activator inhibitor type 1 (PAI-1), TFPI, thrombospondin (TSP), TGF-β and IL-1β bound to α_2-macroglobulin
	RME: Other receptors	IgA, glycoproteins, lipoproteins, immunoglobulins intestinal and pancreatic peptides, metallo- and hemoproteins, transferrin, insulin, glucagon, GH, EGF
	nonselective pinocytosis (non-receptor-mediated)	albumin, antigen-anti-body complexes, some pancreatic proteins, some glycoproteins
Kupffer cells	endocytosis	particulates with galactose groups
Kupffer and Endothelial Cells	RME	IgG N-acetylgalactosamine-terminated glycoproteins
	RME: Mannose receptor	Mannose-terminated glycoproteins (e.g.: t-PA, renin)
	RME: Fucose receptor	fucose-terminated glycoproteins
Endothelial Cells	RME: Scavenger receptor	negatively charged proteins
	RME: other receptors	VEGF, FGF (?)
Fat-storing Cells	RME: Mannose-6-phosphate receptor	Mannose-6-phosphate-terminated proteins (e.g.: IGF-II)

Table 5.2. Hepatic uptake mechanisms for proteins and protein complexes. From: Braeckman (Braeckman, 2000), compiled from several sources (see references in the text), including reviews by Kompella and Lee (Kompella and Lee, 1991), by Marks, Gores and Larusso (Marks *et al.*, 1995), and by Cumming (Cumming, 1991). RME = Receptor-Mediated Endocytosis.

membrane invaginates and pinches off to form an endocytotic coated vehicle that contains the receptor and ligand (internalization). The vesicle coat consists of proteins (clathrin, adaptin, and others), which are then removed by an uncoating adenosine triphosphatase (ATPase). The vesicle parts, the receptor, and the ligand dissociate and are targeted to various intracellular locations. Some receptors, such as the LDL, asialoglycoprotein and transferrin receptors, are known to undergo recycling. Since sometimes several hundred cycles are part of a single receptor's lifetime, the associated RME is of high capacity. Other receptors, such as the interferon receptor, undergo degradation. This degradation leads to a decrease in the concentration of receptors on the cell surface (receptor down-regulation). Others (insulin and EGF receptors, for example) undergo both recycling and degradation (Kompella and Lee, 1991).

For glycoproteins, if a critical number of exposed sugar groups (mannose, galactose, fucose, N-acetylglucosamine, N-acetylgalactosamine, or glucose) is exceeded, RME through sugar-recognizing receptors, is an efficient hepatic uptake mechanism (Meijer and Ziegler, 1993). Important carbohydrate receptors in the liver are the asialoglycoprotein receptor in hepatocytes and the mannose receptor in Kupffer and liver endothelial cells (Ashwell and Harford, 1982; Ashwell and Morell, 1974; Fallon and Schwartz, 1989). The high-mannose glycans in the first kringle domain of rt-PA have been implicated in its clearance, for example (Cumming, 1991).

Low density lipoprotein receptor-related protein (LRP) is a member of the low-density lipoprotein (LDL) receptor family responsible for endocytosis of several important lipoproteins, proteases, and protease-inhibitor complexes in the liver and other tissues (Strickland *et al.*, 1995). Examples of proteins and protein complexes for which hepatic uptake is mediated by LRP are listed in Table 5.2. The list includes many endogenous proteins, including some that are marketed or being developed as drugs, such as t-PA, u-PA, and tissue factor pathway inhibitor (TFPI). There are observations indicating that these proteins bound to the cell-surface proteoglycans are presented to LRP for endocytosis, thus facilitating the LRP-mediated clearance. It seems likely that proteoglycans serve to concentrate LRP ligands on the cell surface, thereby enhancing their interaction with LRP. Interestingly, none of the LRP ligands compete against each other for the LRP receptor, which is very large (~650 kDa) and contains multiple distinct binding sites (Nielsen *et al.*, 1995).

Uptake of proteins by liver cells is followed by transport to an intracellular compartment for metabolism. Proteins internalized into vesicles via an endocytotic mechanism such as RME undergo intracellular transport towards the lysosomal compartment near the center of the cell. There, the endocytotic vehicles fuse with or mature into lysosomes, which are specialized acidic vesicles that contain a wide variety of hydrolases capable of degrading all biological macromolecules. Proteolysis is started by endopeptidases (mainly cathepsin D) that act on the middle part of the proteins. Oligopeptides – as the result of the first step – are further degraded by exopeptidases. The resulting amino acids and dipeptides reenter the metabolic pool of the cell (Meijer and Ziegler, 1993). The hepatic metabolism of glycoproteins may occur more slowly than the naked protein because protecting oligosaccharide chains need to be removed first. Metabolized proteins and peptides in lysosomes from hepatocytes, hepatic sinusoidal cells and Kupffer cells may be released into the blood. Degraded proteins in hepatocyte lysosomes can also be delivered to the bile canaliculus and excreted by exocytosis.

A second intracellular pathway for proteins is the direct shuttle or transcytotic pathway (Kompella and Lee, 1991). The endocytotic vesicle formed at the cell surface traverses the cell to the peribiliary space, where it fuses with the bile canalicular membrane, releasing its contents by exocytosis into bile. This pathway, described for polymeric immunoglobulin A, bypasses the lysosomal compartment completely.

The receptor-mediated uptake of protein drugs by hepatocytes, followed by intracellular metabolism, sometimes causes dose-dependent plasma disposition curves due to the saturation of the active uptake mechanism at higher doses. As an example, EGF administered at low doses (50 μg/kg and lower) to rats showed an elimination clearance proportional to hepatic blood flow, since the systemic supply of drug to the liver is the rate limiting process for elimination. At high doses (>200 μg/kg), the hepatic clearance is saturated, and extrahepatic clearance by other tissues is the dominant factor in the total plasma clearance. At intermediate doses of EGF, both hepatic blood flow and EGF receptors responsible for the active uptake affect the total plasma clearance (Murakami *et al.*, 1994).

For some proteins, receptor-mediated uptake by the hepatocytes is so extensive that hepatic blood clearance approaches its maximum value, liver blood flow. As examples, recombinant tissue-type and urokinase-type plasminogen activator (rt-PA and ru-PA, respectively) have been shown to behave as high clearance drugs, and both reductions and increases in liver blood flow affect their clearance in the same direction (van Griensven *et al.*, 1995; van Griensven *et al.*, 1996). This affection may be important for patients with myocardial infarction who may have variations in liver perfusion caused by diminished cardiac function or concomitant vasoactive drug treatment. Also, liver blood flow decreases during exercise, and increases after food intake.

Receptor-Mediated Elimination by Other Cells

For small synthetic drugs, the fraction of the dose bound to receptors at each moment after administration is usually negligible, and receptor binding is reversible, mostly without internalization of the receptor-drug complex. For protein drugs, however, a substantial part of the dose may be bound to the receptor, and receptor-mediated uptake by specialized cells, followed by intracellular catabolism, may play an important part in the total elimination of the drug from the body. A derivative of granulocyte colony-stimulating factor (G-CSF), nartograstim, and most likely G-CSF itself, is taken up by bone marrow through a saturable receptor-mediated process (Kuwabara *et al.*, 1995). It has been demonstrated for macrophage colony-stimulating factor (M-CSF) that besides the linear renal elimination pathway, there is a saturable non-linear elimination pathway that follows Michaelis-Menten kinetics (Bartocci *et al.*, 1987; Bauer *et al.*, 1994). The importance of the non-linear elimination pathway was demonstrated by a steeper dip in the plasma concentration profile at lower M-CSF concentrations (Figure 5.5). At higher levels, linear renal

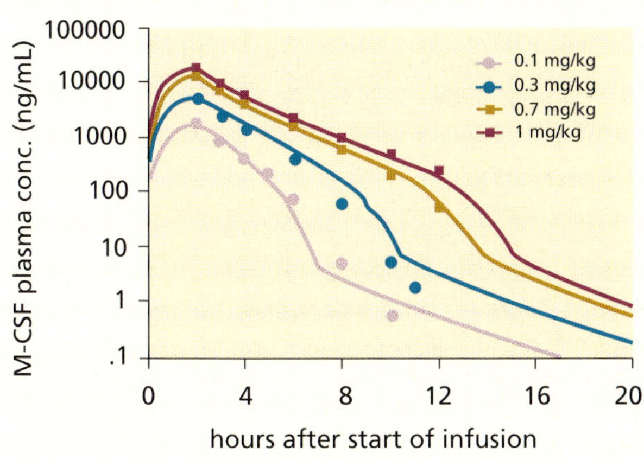

Figure 5.5. Observed and predicted plasma concentration-time profiles of M-CSF after 2-hour intravenous infusions of 0.1–1 mg/kg in cynomolgus monkeys. A two-compartmental pharmacokinetic model with a linear clearance pathway and a parallel Michaelis-Menten elimination pathway was used.

elimination was dominant, and the non-linear pathway was saturated. The non-linear pathway could be blocked by coadministration of carrageenan, a macrophage inhibitor, indicating that receptor-mediated uptake by macrophages was likely responsible for the non-linear elimination (Bauer *et al.*, 1994). This result is especially relevant since M-CSF stimulates the proliferation of macrophages. It is also possible that the receptor-mediated uptake and the effect of M-CSF are closely linked. Indeed, it was observed that after chronic administration of M-CSF, the non-linear elimination was probably induced by autoinduction, since M-CSF increases circulating levels of macrophages. Although autoinduction and, consequently, the accelerated metabolism of most drugs is related to a loss of their pharmacological effect, for M-CSF, it may be an indication of sustained pharmacodynamic activity. Similar kinetics were observed for other hematopoietic stimulating factors, such as G-CSF (Tanaka and Kaneko, 1991) and granulocyte macrophage colony-stimulating factor (GM-CSF) (Petros *et al.*, 1992). Michaelis-Menten (saturable) elimination was also described for t-PA (Tanswell *et al.*, 1990), and recently for a recombinant amino-terminal fragment of bactericidal/permeability-increasing protein ($rBPI_{23}$) (Bauer *et al.*, 1997).

Distribution of Protein Therapeutics

Once a molecule reaches the blood stream, it encounters the following processes for intracellular biodistribution: distribution through the vascular space, transport across the microvascular wall, transport through the interstitial space, and transport across cell membranes. The biodistribution of macromolecules is determined by the physicochemical properties of the molecule, and by the structural and physicochemical characteristics of the capillaries responsible for transendothelial passage of the molecule from the systemic circulation to the interstitial fluid. In addition, the presence of receptors determines the biodistribution to certain tissues, including extracellular association and/or intracellular uptake. Capillary endothelia are of three types, listed in increasing order of permeability: continuous (non-fenestrated), fenestrated, and discontinuous (sinusoidal) (Kompella and Lee, 1991; Taylor and Granger, 1984). The most likely dominant mode of transport of macromolecules in non-fenestrated capillaries is through interendothelial junctions. Through these junctions, there are two modes of transport (Jain and Baxter, 1993): The convective transport, often the most important for macromolecules, is dependent on a pressure difference between the vascular and interstitial spaces. The diffusive transport is driven by a concentration gradient.

Capillaries selectively sieve macromolecules based on their effective molecular size, shape, and charge. Because of the large size of proteins, their apparent volume of distribution is usually relatively small. The initial volume of distribution after intravenous injection is approximately equal to or slightly higher than the total plasma volume. The total volume of distribution is generally twice or less than twice the initial volume of distribution. Although this is sometimes interpreted as a low tissue penetration, it is difficult to generalize. Indeed, adequate concentrations may be reached in a single target organ because of receptor-mediated uptake, but the contribution to the total volume of distribution may be rather small.

Besides size, it appears that the charge-selective nature of continuous capillaries and cell membranes may also be important for the biodistribution of proteins. Information for this is available from studies with different types of Cu,Zn-superoxide dismutase (Cu,Zn-SOD), which are similar in molecular weight (33 kDa), but have different net surface charges, and are isolated from different species (Omar *et al.*, 1992). Tissue equilibration of the positively charged sheep Cu,Zn-SOD was much faster than for the negatively charged bovine Cu,Zn-SOD. In addition, the positively charged Mn-SOD equilibrated much faster than the negatively charged human Cu,Zn-SOD, although Mn-SOD is much bigger (88 kDa). A trend towards increasing anti-inflammatory activity, for which interstitial concentrations are important, was observed with increasing isoelectric point. It was suggested that the electrostatic attraction between positively charged proteins and negatively charged cell membranes might increase the rate and extent of tissue biodistribution. Most cell surfaces are negatively charged because of the abundance of glycosaminoglycans in the extracellular matrix.

Tissue binding is also important for the biodistribution of the heparin-binding proteins, including the fibroblast growth factor family (such as FGF-1 and FGF-2) (Medalion *et al.*, 1997), vascular endothelial growth factor (VEGF) (Shen *et al.*, 1997), platelet-derived growth factor (PDGF), tissue factor pathway inhibitor (TFPI) (Narita *et al.*, 1995), amphiregulin, and epidermal growth factor (EGF). Proteins of this group contain a highly positively charged tail, which electrostatically binds to low-affinity binding sites consisting of heparin sulfate proteoglycans (acidic glycosaminoglycans) (Templeton, 1992; Yanagishita and Hascall, 1992). These binding sites are abundant on the vascular endothelium and liver, and are responsible for the majority of cell surface binding of these proteins. The rapid and extensive binding to the vascular endothelium of protein drugs in this class is most likely the explanation for their rapid distribution phase after iv injection, and their relatively large volume of distribution. Binding of growth factors to proteoglycans has been proposed to provide a mechanism for growth factor recruitment at the cell surface, presentation to specific receptors, regulation of their action on target cells at short range, and establishment of a growth factor gradient within a tissue.

A major *in vivo* pool of some of the heparin-binding proteins is probably associated with the vascular endothelium, and is released into the circulation quickly after an injection of heparin. Since heparin is structurally similar to the cell-surface glycosaminoglycans, the proteins bind to circulating heparin, depleting the intravascular pool. This was demonstrated, for example, for TFPI (Hansen *et al.*, 1996; Sandset *et al.*, 1988) and basic FGF (FGF-2) (Medalion *et al.*, 1997).

Biodistribution studies with the measurement of the protein drug in tissues are necessary to establish tissue distribution. These studies are usually performed with radiolabeled compounds. Biodistribution studies are imperative for small organic synthetic drugs, since long residence times of the radioactive label in certain tissues may be an indication of tissue accumulation of potentially toxic metabolites. Because of the possible re-utilization of amino acids from protein drugs in endogenous proteins, such a safety issue does not exist. Therefore, biodistribution studies for protein drugs are usually performed to assess drug targeting to specific tissues, or to detect the major organs of elimination (usually kidneys and liver).

If the protein contains a suitable amino acid such as tyrosine or lysine, an external label such as ^{125}I can be chemically coupled to the protein (Ferraiolo and Mohler, 1992). Although this coupling is easily accomplished and a highly specific activity can be obtained, the protein is chemically altered. Therefore, it may be better to label proteins and other biotechnology compounds by introducing radioactive isotopes during their synthesis by which an internal atom becomes the radioactive marker (internal labeling). For recombinant proteins, internal labeling can be accomplished by growing the production cell line in the presence of amino acids labeled with ^{3}H, ^{14}C, ^{35}S, etc. This method is not routinely used because of the prohibition of radioactive contamination of fermentation equipment. Moreover, internally labeled proteins may be less desirable than iodinated proteins because of the potential re-utilization of the radiolabeled amino acid fragments in the synthesis of endogenous proteins and cell structures. Irrespective of the labeling method, but more so for external labeling, the labeled product should have demonstrated physicochemical and biological properties identical to the unlabeled molecule (Bennett and McMartin, 1979).

In addition, as for all types of radiolabeled studies, it needs to be established whether the measured radioactivity represents intact labeled protein, or radiolabeled metabolites, or the liberated label. Trichloro-acetic acid-precipitable radioactivity is often used to distinguish intact protein from free label or low-molecular-weight metabolites, which appear in the supernatant after centrifugation. Proteins with re-utilized labeled amino acids and large protein metabolites can only be distinguished from the original protein by techniques such as PAGE, HPLC, specific immunoassays, or bioassays (cf. Chapter 2). This discussion also implies that the results of biodistribution studies with autoradiography can be very misleading. Autoradiography is a technique where tissue samples are brought into contact with X-ray sensitive films to visualize radioactively labeled molecules or fragments of molecules. Although autoradiography is becoming more quantitative, one never knows what is being measured qualitatively (original molecules or its degradation products) without specific assays. It is therefore sometimes better to perform biodistribution studies by the collection of the tissues and the specific measurement of the protein drug in the tissue homogenate.

A method was developed to calculate early-phase tissue uptake clearances based on plasma and tissue drug measurements during the first five minutes after intravenous administration (Kim *et al.*, 1988). The short time interval has the advantage that metabolism and the tissue efflux clearance can presumably be ignored. As an example, with this method, dose-independent (non-saturable) uptake clearance values were observed for a recombinant derivative of hG-CSF, nartograstim, for kidney and liver (Kuwabara *et al.*, 1995). In contrast, a dose-dependent reduction in the uptake clearance by bone marrow with increasing doses of nartograstim was observed. These findings suggested that receptor mediated endocytosis of the G-CSF receptor in bone marrow may participate in the non-linear properties of nartograstim. Since G-CSF is one of the growth factors that stimulates the proliferation and differentiation of neutropoietic progenitor cells to granulocytes in bone marrow, the distribution aspects of nartograstim into bone marrow are especially relevant for the pharmacodynamics.

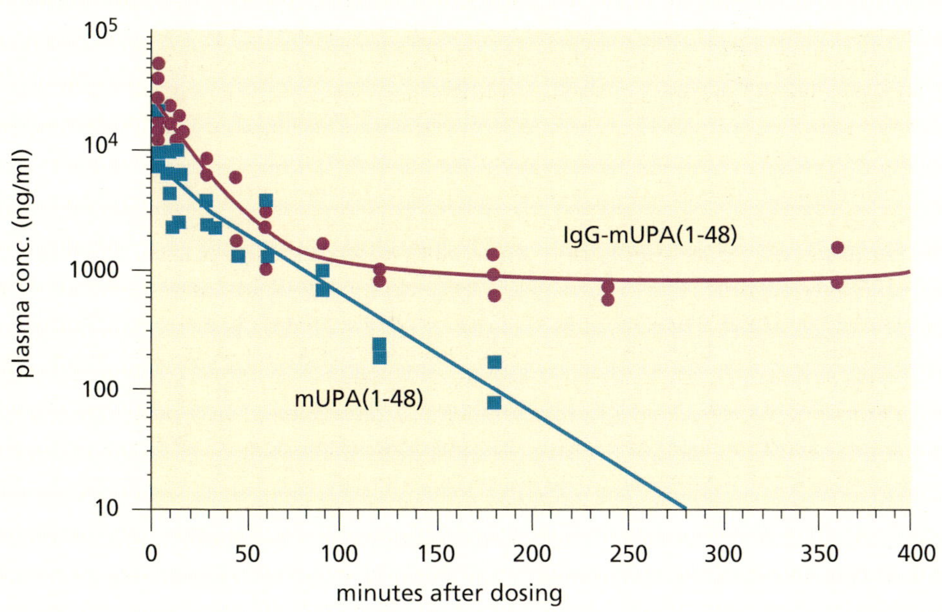

Figure 5.6. Fusion of the murine urokinase EGF-like peptide of 48 amino acids with human IgG (IgG-mUPA(1-48)) resulted in a much longer half-life than the original peptide (mUPA(1-48)). The data were modeled according to a linear compartmental model.

In addition, since G-CSF and nartograstim are catabolized in the bone marrow cells after receptor-mediated uptake, the biodistribution into bone marrow is also a pathway for the elimination of these molecules. Unlike for classical small synthetic drugs, it is not uncommon for biotechnology-derived drugs that biodistribution, pharmacodynamics, and elimination are closely connected.

Besides receptor-mediated uptake into target organs and tissues, other proteins, or macromolecules in general, distribute into tissues in more non-specific ways. It was demonstrated in at least one study with tumor-bearing mice that high total systemic exposure of target-non-specific macromolecules was the most important factor that determines the extent of tissue uptake (Takakura *et al.*, 1990). Consequently, molecules with physicochemical characteristics that minimize hepatic and renal elimination clearances showed the highest tumoral exposure. Compounds with relatively low molecular weights (approximately 10 kDa) or positive charges were rapidly eliminated and showed lower tumor radioactivity accumulation; large (>70 kDa) and negatively charged compounds (carboxymethyl dextran, BSA, mouse IgG) showed prolonged retention in the circulation, and high tumoral levels. A typical example is the murine urokinase (muPA) EGF-like domain peptide of 48 amino acids, muPA(1–48). This peptide is a urokinase receptor antagonist under consideration as an anticancer drug, since urokinase has been implicated in invasive biological processes, such as tumor metastasis, trophoblast implantation, and angiogenesis. Scientists at Chiron have fused muPA(1–48) to the human IgG constant region. The fused molecule (IgG-muPA(1–48)) retained its activity of inhibition of the murine UPA receptor, but had a much longer *in vivo* elimination half-life (79 versus 0.5 hours; Figure 5.6). The half-life increase was due to both a decrease in elimination clearance (4.3 versus 95 mL/hr/kg) and an increase in the peripheral volume of distribution (434 versus 43 mL/kg). Although the fused molecule was substantially larger, tissue distribution increased, possibly because of substantial tissue binding. This is in contrast with some polyethylene glycol-modified (PEGylated) molecules such as PEG IL-2 (polyethylene glycol-modified interleukin-2) for which the size increase resulted in a smaller distribution volume compared to the original molecule (see below).

As discussed earlier (Figure 4.12), biodistribution into the lymphatics after subcutaneous (sc) injection deserves special attention since it is a rather unique transport pathway for macromolecules. Following sc administration, the drug can be transported to the systemic circulation by absorption into the blood capillaries or by the lymphatics. Since the permeability of macromolecules through the capillary wall is low, they were found to enter blood indirectly through the lymphatic system (Supersaxo *et al.*, 1988; Supersaxo *et al.*, 1990). Compounds with a molecular weight larger than 16 kDa are absorbed mainly (>50%) by the lymphatics, while compounds smaller than 1 kDa are hardly absorbed by the lymphatics at all. Lymph recovery after sc dosing was apparently linearly related to molecular weight up to 19 kDa (Figure 4.12) (Supersaxo *et al.*, 1990). Negatively charged proteins had increased lymph absorption, as compared to positively charged proteins with similar molecular weight (Xie and Hale, 1996). After lymphatic absorption, compounds circulate within the lymph and are gradually returned to the blood. As a result, lymph concentrations for these proteins may be higher than blood concentrations. Targeting of the lymphatics may be beneficial for proteins that act on the immune system, such as for IL-2. It was shown that sc administration of IL-2 in a pig model resulted in higher lymph levels compared to blood, and at higher doses, absorption was exclusively through lymph (Chen *et al.*, 2000). The IL-2 receptor-positive T-lymphocytes, that are thought to be primarily associated with efficacy, reside largely in the lymphoid organs. On the other hand, natural killer cells and neutrophils in blood produce cytokines, reactive oxygen intermediates, and proteases, all of which have been shown to be necessary to produce Il-2 toxicities. Therefore, adverse *in vivo* activity of Il-2 may be related to blood levels, while beneficial activity may be associated to lymph concentrations (Chen *et al.*, 2000).

Biodistribution into target organs, usually receptor-mediated, is important for the pharmacodynamics of protein drugs. For some proteins, saturable receptor-mediated tissue uptake in target organs is responsible for non-linear kinetics (Kato *et al.*, 1997). For example, the uptake clearance of rhEPO by bone marrow and spleen exhibited clear saturation in rats. Also, a single high dose of rhEPO caused a reduction of uptake clearance by bone marrow and spleen, while repeated injections caused an increase of the tissue uptake clearance, especially by the spleen, in a dose-dependent manner (Kato *et al.*, 1997). Hematopoietic parameters such as hematocrit and hemoglobin concentration changed accordingly, suggesting that changes in the uptake clearance were caused by down- or upregulation of EPO receptors.

Pharmacodynamics of Protein Therapeutics

Although the time course of the compound at the receptor or effector site represents the desired knowledge for predicting or explaining the pharmacodynamics (PD), accurate drug level data at that site are difficult to obtain. In most cases, pharmacokinetic (PK) data are limited to plasma concentration data. Pharmacokinetic models are widely used to describe and predict the time course of the drug in plasma and tissues. These models include compartmental models and physiological models.

During the last decade, the application of PD models for *in vivo* effect data has increased tremendously (Girard *et al.*, 1990). In addition, the PD models have been linked to PK models, and this approach has made integrated PK/PD analysis possible. PK/PD modeling has been reviewed extensively for small drug molecules (Colburn and Blue, 1992; Derendorf and Hochhaus, 1995; Holford, 1990; Kroboth *et al.*, 1991; Schwinghammer and Kroboth, 1988; Steimer *et al.*, 1993), but relatively few publications are available for proteins, or biotechnological therapeutics in general (Colburn, 1991). PD models are based on the law of mass action of drug-receptor interaction, classically called the occupancy theory (Kenakin, 1993). These models that express the effect as a function of drug concentration have been known for a long time from the classical *in vitro* pharmacological experiments wherein receptors in organ baths or tissue strips were exposed to a drug concentration. A similar situation occurs *in vivo* when the effect concentration is the concentration in plasma, an effect compartment or biophase (Holford and Sheiner, 1981).

Direct Effects

Sometimes, the effect concentration in the PD model equations can be set equal to the plasma concentration when there is a direct relationship between the plasma drug concentration and the pharmacological effect. These are the direct effect PK/PD models. Figure 5.7 shows one example

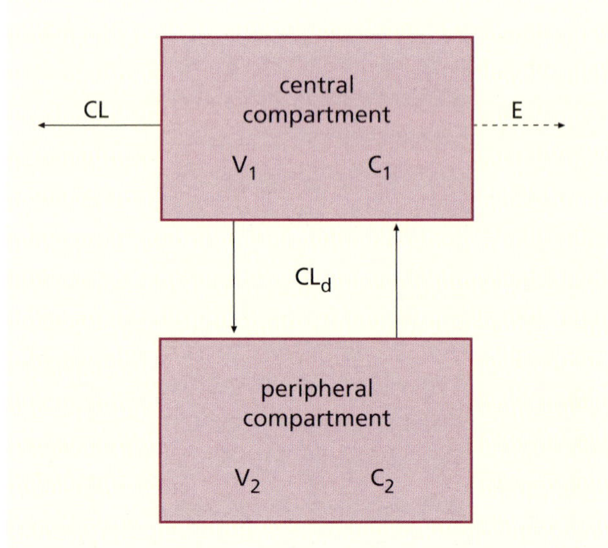

Figure 5.7. Example of a direct effect PK/PD model. The PK model is a typical two-compartmental model with a linear elimination clearance from the central compartment (CL) and a distributional clearance (CL_d). C_1 and C_2 are the concentrations in the central and peripheral compartments, and V_1 and V_2 are their respective apparent volumes of distribution. The effect (E) is a function of C_1.

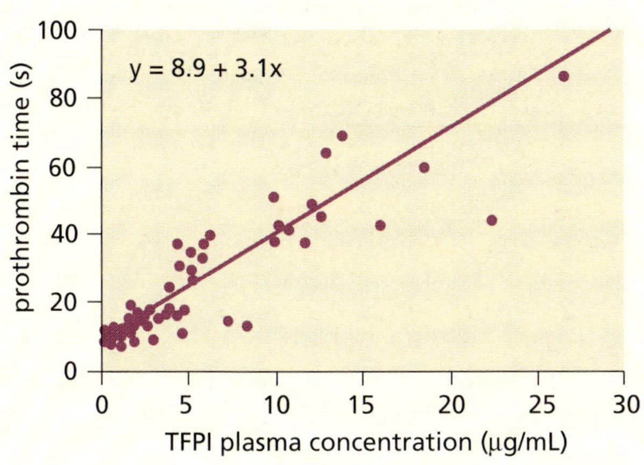

Figure 5.8. Direct relationship of the increase in prothrombin time (PT) and the plasma concentrations of TFPI after continuous iv infusion of TFPI in cynomolgus monkeys.

of a PK/PD model wherein the effect is directly related to the concentration in the central compartment (the plasma concentration). Any appropriate compartmental model or other PK model that predicts the plasma concentration-time curve can be used. In the direct effect PK/PD models, the effect-time profile follows the plasma-concentration profile, and the maximum effect occurs at the time of the peak plasma concentration.

A typical example is the thrombolytic effect of tissue factor pathway inhibitor (TFPI). The increase of the prothrombin time (PT) during continuous infusion of *E. Coli* derived recombinant human TFPI in a two-week toxicology study in cynomolgus monkeys was directly related to the TFPI plasma concentrations (Figure 5.8) (Childs *et al.*, 1996). The PD model equation is

$$E = E_0 + S\ C$$

where E is the effect (PT); E_0 is the baseline effect (predose PT), C is the TFPI plasma concentration, and S is the slope of the effect-concentration curve. The slope represents the sensitivity of the effect or the potency, i.e. change in PT (in seconds) per unit change of concentration (µg/mL). An integrated PK/PD analysis according to a two-compartmental PK model and a direct effect PD model explained the observed data.

Indirect Effects

For most effects after administration of peptides and proteins, however, no such direct relationship can be observed. In a lot of cases, the maximum effect is reached at times later than the maximum plasma concentration, and sometimes, a considerable effect can still be measured at times where the plasma drug levels have fallen below the limit of detection. The temporal differences between drug exposure and onset/duration of effect has created the idea that for peptides and proteins, there is no relationship between plasma drug levels and effect. The opposite is true: if the effect is drug related, there must be a relationship between plasma drug concentrations and the time course of effect intensity. A plot of the concentration-effect relationship from non-steady state conditions, i.e. when the plasma concentrations rise and fall, such as following an iv infusion or an extravascular dose, is a helpful diagnostic of the temporal features of drug effect. In such plots, effect delays manifest themselves as (counterclockwise) *hysteresis*. Delays caused between the appearance of the drug in plasma and the appearance of the pharmacodynamic response, by processes such as distribution into the biophase or cascade-type post-receptor events (Figure 5.1), may cause hysteresis. The relationship can be described by more complicated combined PK/PD models. Two basic approaches are available. The first one is the family of PK/PD link models, the second approach uses the indirect effect PK/PD models.

PK/PD Link Models

The temporal delay of the effect appearance and duration in the PK/PD link models is explained by a distributional delay (Holford and Sheiner, 1981). In this case, drug concentrations in a slowly equilibrating tissue compartment with plasma are directly related to the effect intensity. Since the peak level of drug in the biophase is reached later than the time of the peak plasma concentration, the peak effect also occurs later than the plasma peak level. Although theoretically the biophase drug concentration may equal the drug concentration in a peripheral compartment, it rarely happens that a peripheral pharmacokinetic compartment acts as the biophase or effect compartment. More often the biophase is a small part of a pharmacokinetic compartment that from a pharmacokinetic point of view cannot be distinguished from other tissues within that compartment. Compartmental modeling with plasma concentration-time data is just not sensitive enough to isolate the biophase as a separate compartment without the availability of measured drug concentration data in the biophase.

The solution to this problem has been to postulate a hypothetical effect compartment linked to the central compartment (or to a peripheral compartment in some cases) (Figure 5.9). The drug distributes into the effect compartment (this is the link) but since the amount of drug in the effect compartment is rather small, no actual mass transfer is implemented in the pharmacokinetic part of the PK/PD model. The drug concentration in the effect compartment is then plugged into the pharmacodynamic part of the PK/PD model. Although this PK/PD model is constructed

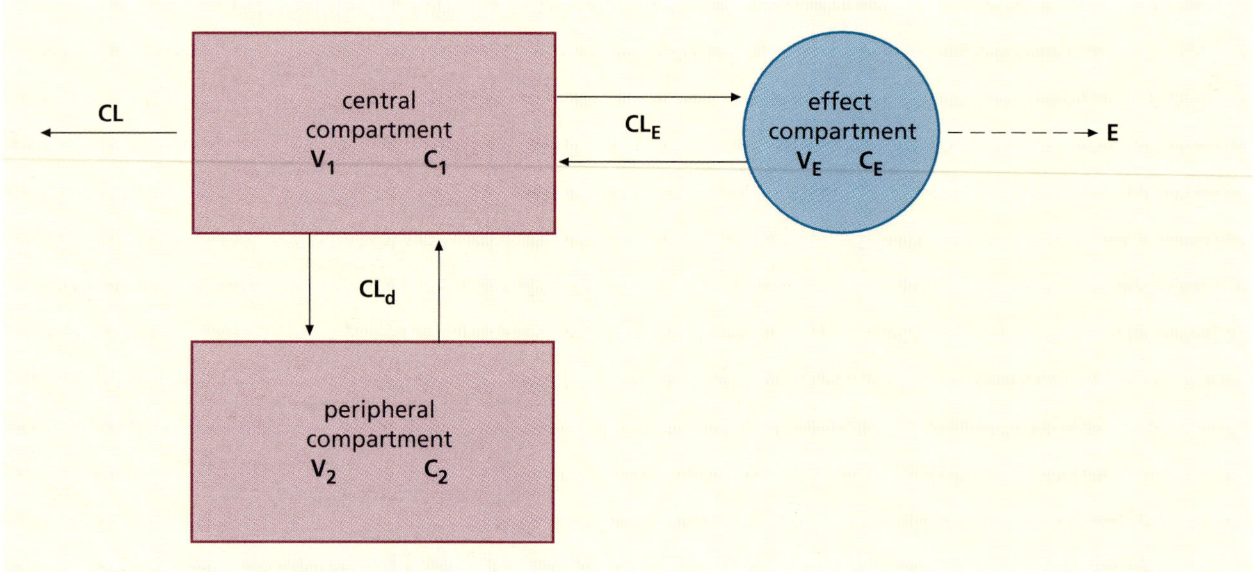

Figure 5.9. Example of a typical PK/PD link model. A hypothetical effect compartment is linked to the central compartment of a two-compartmental pharmacokinetic model. The concentration in the effect compartment (C_e) drives the intensity of the pharmacodynamic effect (E). CL_e is the linear clearance for distribution of drug to the effect compartment and elimination from the effect compartment. V_e is the apparent volume of distribution in the effect compartment. All PK parameters are identical to those used in Figure 5.7.

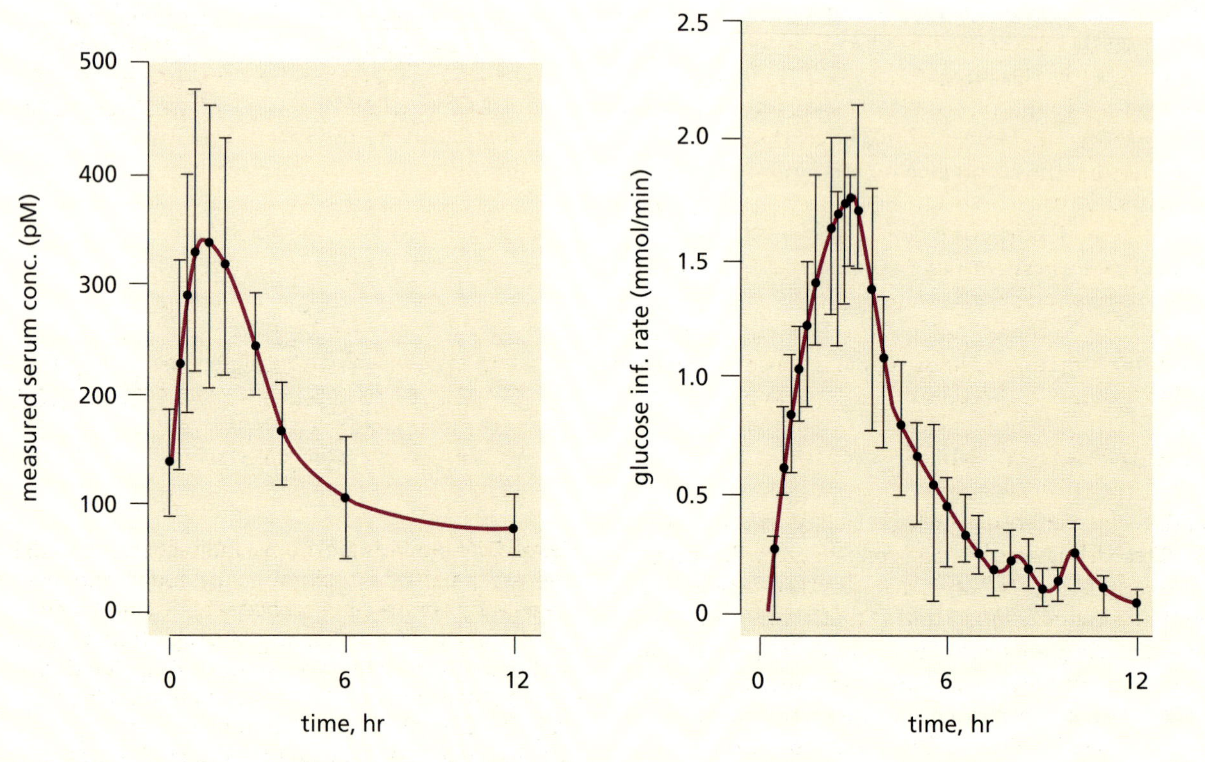

Figure 5.10. Mean measured serum insulin concentrations after a single 10-U subcutaneous dose of regular insulin in 10 volunteers (left panel); corresponding glucose infusion rates needed to maintain euglycemia (right panel). From Woodworth et al. (Woodworth et al.,1994).

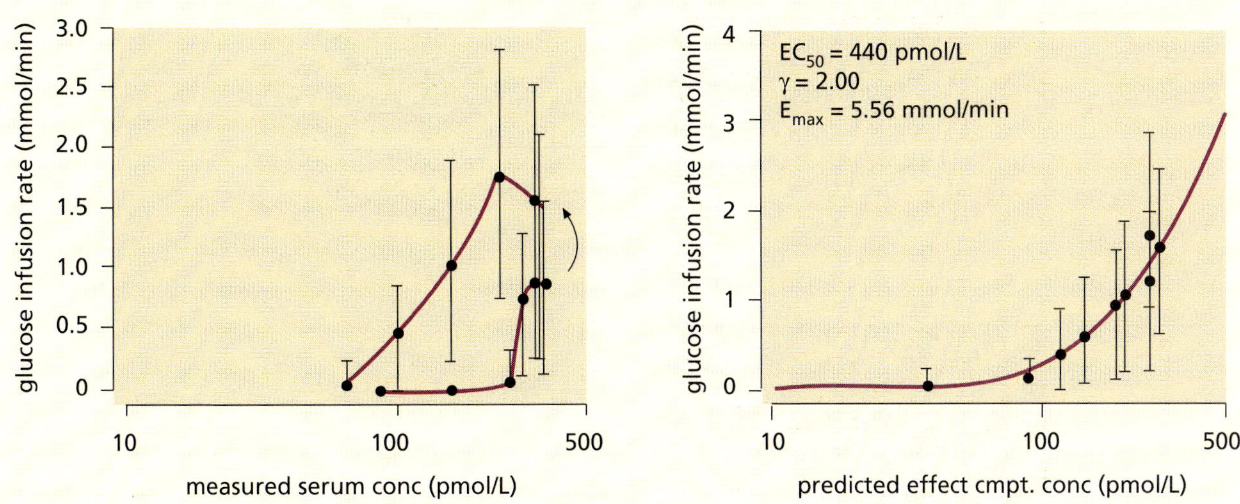

Figure 5.11. Relationship between the glucose infusion rate to maintain euglycemia versus serum insulin concentrations after a single subcutaneous dose of 10 U regular insulin in 10 volunteers (left panel). The time-dependent hysteresis, which is an indication of the indirect nature of the effect, is indicated by the arrow. The right panel shows the sigmoidal relationship between the effect and the predicted effect compartment concentration, demonstrating the collapse of the hysteresis loop. From Woodworth et al. (Woodworth et al.,1994).

with tissue distribution as the reason for the delay of the effect, the distribution clearance to the effect compartment can be interpreted differently, including other reasons of delay, such as transduction processes and secondary post receptor events. The hypoglycemic effect of insulin has been modeled by this type of PK/PD model (Hooper, 1991; Woodworth *et al.*, 1994). Figure 5.10 shows the mean serum concentration profile of insulin after a single sc injection of 10 U in 10 volunteers, and the corresponding effect measured as the glucose infusion rate to maintain an euglycemic state. Figure 5.11 shows the hysteresis in the effect-concentration relationship, and how a typical sigmoidal effect-concentration curve is obtained with the hypothetical effect concentration from a one-compartmental PK/PD link model (Woodworth *et al.*, 1994).

Indirect Effect Models

Another and better approach to include effect delays in PK/PD modeling based on post receptor events has been the indirect effect models (Dayneka *et al.*, 1993; Jusko and Ko, 1994; Nagashima *et al.*, 1968; O'Reilly and Levy, 1970). In this modeling approach, the observed effect is an indirect effect, i.e. is not the primary effect, but rather a consequence of rate-limiting transduction and other post receptor events. In the simplest indirect effect model, the effect is maintained by a balance of two processes (Figure 5.12), which together form the biosignal flux. The first process is the production of the effect, determined by a zero-order production rate. The second process is the decrease or disappearance of

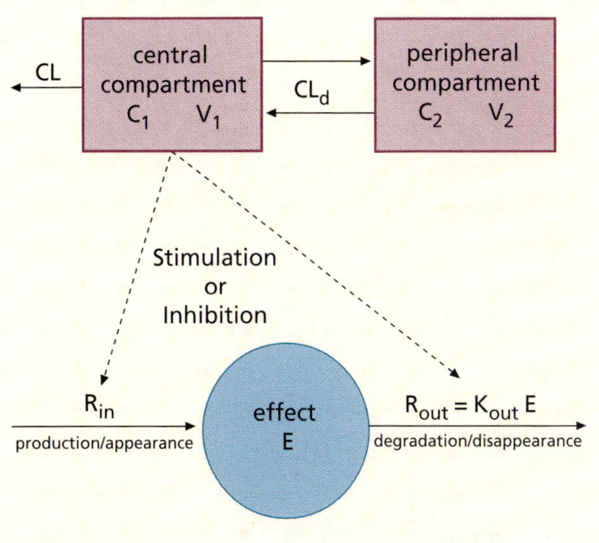

Figure 5.12. Pharmacodynamic indirect effect model wherein the effect is maintained by equilibrium between a zero-order appearance rate, R_{in}, and a first-order disappearance rate, R_{out}. A drug effect is caused by stimulation or inhibition of R_{in} or R_{out}. The degree of stimulation or inhibition is dependent on the plasma drug concentration. The PD parameters are R_{in}, K_{out} (the first order rate constant for effect disappearance), EC_{50} (the concentration that produces 50% of maximum inhibition or stimulation), and Emax (the maximum inhibition or stimulation). The pharmacokinetic model is identical to the one presented in Figure 5.7.

the effect by a first-order dissipation rate. In a normal (predose; no drug present) situation, both processes are in equilibrium and homeostasis of the effect is maintained (baseline effect). Drug effect is caused by the stimulation or inhibition of either the production or disappearance rate. The degree of stimulation or inhibition is determined by the plasma concentration.

This model was used to describe the effect of filgrastim (r-methionine-hG-CSF) on neutrophilic granulopoiesis after the sc dosing of human volunteers for ten days (Roskos *et al.*, 1998). The transient decrease of blood neutrophils in the first hour after dosing is due to rapid distribution of neutrophils into the marginal blood pool (disappearance process in Figure 5.12). The increase in neutrophil count is modeled as a filgrastim concentration-dependent flux into the circulating neutrophil pool (appearance process in Figure 5.12). The PK part of the model also includes a receptor-mediated increase of filgrastim clearance. This combined PK/PD model accurately describes the accession of absolute neutrophil count (ANC) to steady-state levels (Figure 5.13).

A double indirect effect model was applied for the effects of IL-2 treatment in HIV patients (Piscitelli *et al.*, 1996). The PK model for IL-2 included two compartments with a time-varying serum clearance, which was related to concentrations of the soluble IL-2 receptor (sIL2R). Increasing circulating sIL2R levels were used as a surrogate marker for the upregulation of the cell-based IL-2 receptor, which probably causes an increase of the receptor-mediated clearance of IL-2 after chronic dosing. Indirect PK/PD models with IL-2 stimulation of the formation rates were used for sIL2R, as well as for the serum levels of tissue necrosis factor-α (TNFα), which were increased by IL-2.

Complex PK/PD Models

Many protein therapeutics have multiple and/or biphasic responses that are indirect in nature. In some cases, more complicated PK/PD models based on the basic models described above are necessary. An example is a model that was developed to explain the effects of subcutaneous PEG IL-2 (polyethylene glycol-modified interleukin-2) in rats. An early moderate decrease of the number of blood lymphocytes was followed by a pronounced increase of the blood lymphocyte count. The model (Figure 5.14) describes

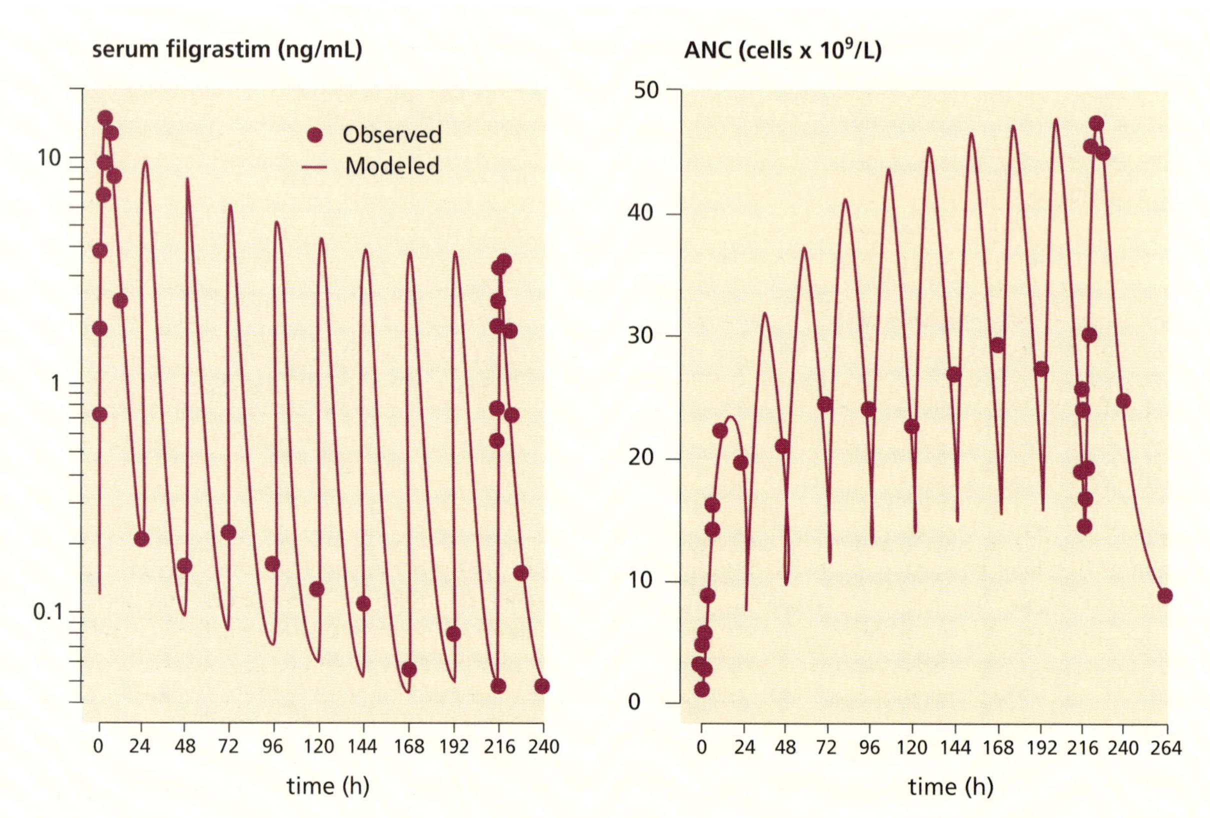

Figure 5.13. Simultaneous PK/PD modeling of serum filgrastim levels and mean absolute neutrophil counts (ANC) response in normal volunteers receiving sc filgrastim 300 μg/day) for 10 days (Roskos et al., 1998).

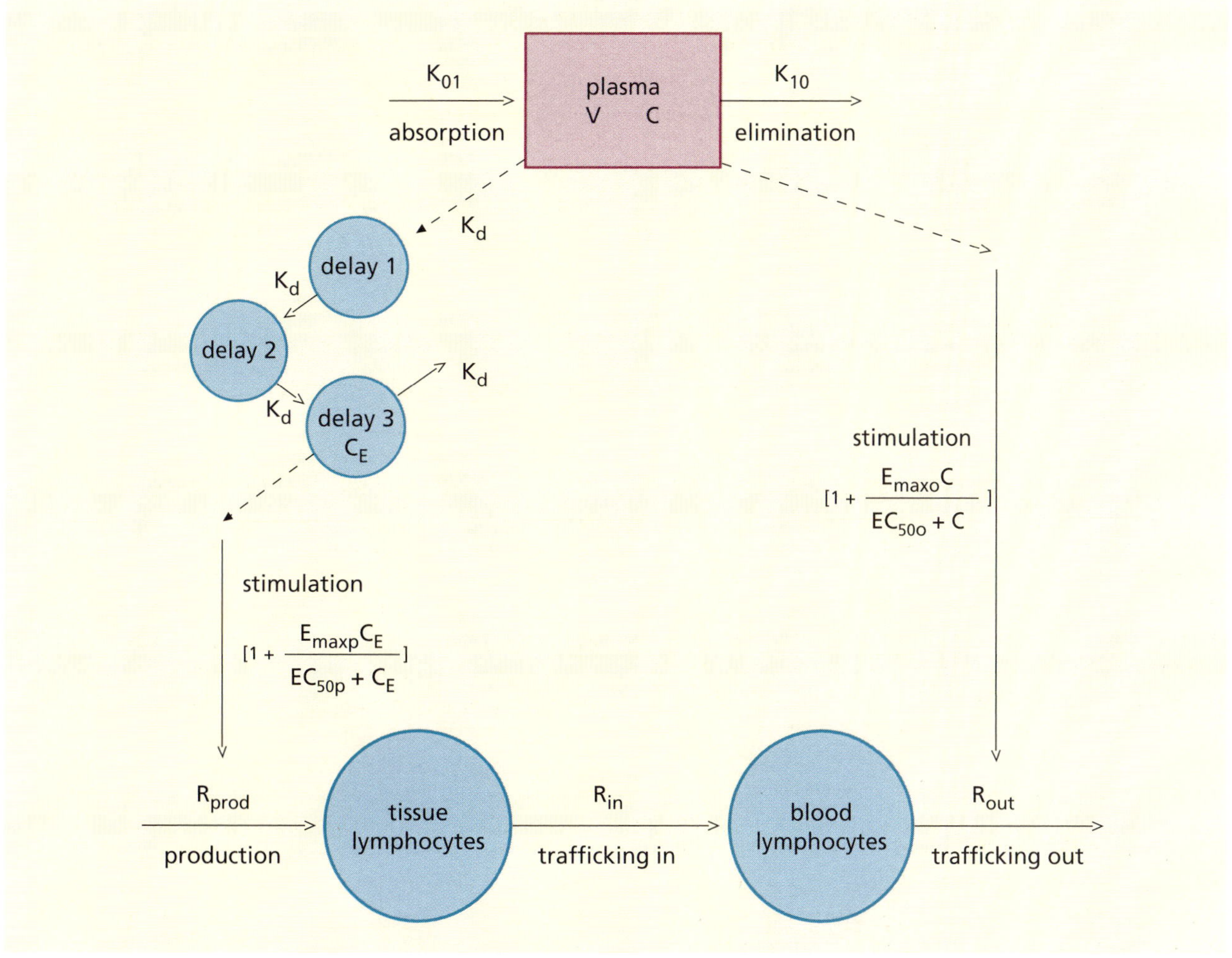

Figure 5.14. PK/PD model for changes in blood lymphocytes after sc administration of PEG IL-2 in rats. The PK model is a one-compartmental model with first-order absorption (rate constant K_{01}) and elimination (rate constant K_{10}). PEG IL-2 stimulates the trafficking out of blood and/or catabolism of lymphocytes (first-order rate R_{out}) according to an E_{max} model (parameters E_{maxo} and EC_{50o}), which is a function of the PEG IL-2 plasma concentration (C). The delayed increase of blood lymphocytes is modeled in two consecutive ways: 1. Three delay compartments with first-order input and output rates (rate constant K_d) resembling distribution and transduction delays; 2. Stimulation of lymphocyte production in tissues according to an E_{max} model (parameters E_{maxp} and EC_{50p}), which is a function of the effect concentration C_E. Tissue lymphocytes traffic into the blood pool (first-order rate R_{in}).

the production of lymphocytes in tissues, after which they traffic into the blood pool, followed by trafficking out of blood and subsequent degradation. The indirect, but relatively early decrease of the number of blood lymphocytes after PEG IL-2 administration is caused by a stimulation of the lymphocyte traffic out of blood. The indirect, delayed increase of the blood lymphocytes is modeled by a stimulation of the production rate of lymphocytes. The delay effect relative to the maximum plasma levels of PEG IL-2 is caused by distributional and post receptor events through three delay compartments. An additional delay is caused by the fact that the lymphocytes need to travel from their site of production to blood before an increase can be measured. Figure 5.15 does not only demonstrate the goodness-of-fit of the modeling, but also shows that the blood lymphocyte increase on Day 3 post dosing occurs after most of the PEG IL-2 is eliminated. PK/PD models like this one link the effect to drug exposure in a quantitative way, which allows extrapolations to other dose levels and routes of administration. It is obvious that a better understanding of the receptor-mediated and post receptor transduction mechanisms of protein drugs may contribute to the creation of representative and useful PK/PD models.

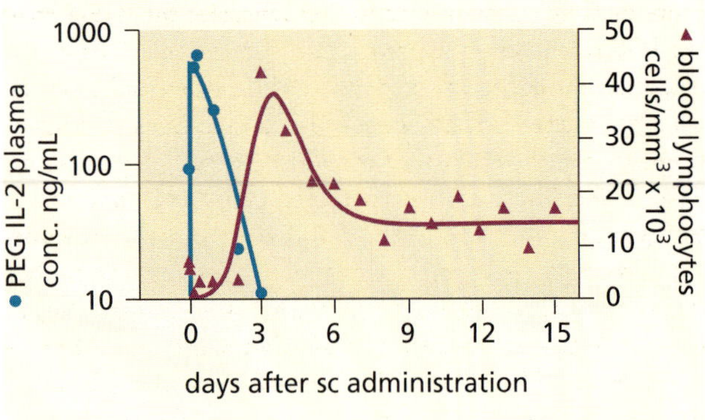

Figure 5.15. PEG IL-2 pharmacokinetics and pharmacodynamics (changes in blood lymphocyte count) after subcutaneous administration of 10 MIU/kg in rats, modeled according to the PK/PD model depicted in Figure 5.14.

The stimulation of erythropoiesis by recombinant human erythropoietin (EPO) therapy in patients with uremic anemia was analyzed with a different PD model (Uehlinger *et al.*, 1992). The model assumes a linear stimulatory effect of EPO on the production rate of red blood cells (RBC) as measured by hematocrit. In the first stage (Figure 5.16), EPO increases the hematocrit because red cells are produced at an increased rate and none of the newly produced red cells die yet. However, after reaching one life span, the red cells start dying at the increased rate at which they were produced and a new steady state is reached. Although the effect of EPO is almost immediate after dosing initiation, it takes time to develop fully. This is an alternate mechanism responsible for hysteresis in concentration-effect curves.

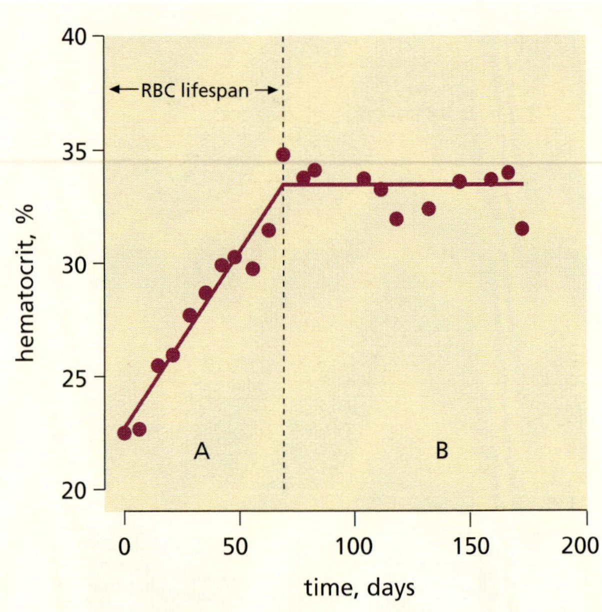

Figure 5.16. Hematocrit (Hct) in an uremic patient on a constant EPO dose of 3 × 4000 U/week. Stage A: Hct increases because EPO stimulates erythrocyte production and none of the newly formed red cells are old enough to die; Stage B: EPO maintains increased red cell production, but red cells die at a faster rate since newly formed cells from Stage A exceed their average life span. Consequently a new steady state is reached. From Uehlinger et al. (Uehlinger et al., 1992).

Dose-Response and Concentration-Response Curves

PK/PD modeling is especially useful in Phase II studies wherein the relationship between dose (and/or concentration) and response for new drug candidates needs to be established. The outcome from these studies does not only convince the sponsors and the regulatory agencies of an existing drug effect, but also assists in the selection of the optimal dose for Phase III trials. For many biotechnology-derived drugs, the Phase II trial was non-existent or too small (one dose level for example) to design a successful or optimal Phase III trial. To complicate this matter even more, it is believed that biotechnology drugs (and potentially all types of drugs) sometimes show bell-shaped dose-response curves, i.e. there is a dose that gives a maximum response, and any increase beyond this dose level results in a further decrease of the response. As an example, lower doses of rINF-γ in multiple myeloma patients seemed to induce a greater increase in natural killer activity than higher doses (Einhorn *et al.*, 1982). Bell-shaped dose-response curves were also observed for superoxide dismutase (SOD) in four different animal models of myocardial infusion, *in vivo* and *in vitro*, using different SOD preparations (Figure 5.17) (Omar *et al.*, 1992).

Protein Binding of Protein Therapeutics

The binding of drugs to circulating plasma proteins can influence both the distribution and elimination of drugs, and consequently their pharmacodynamics. Since it is generally accepted for small drug molecules, including small proteins, that only the unbound drug molecules can pass through membranes, distribution and elimination clearances of total drug are usually smaller than those of free drug. Accordingly, the activity of the drug is more closely related to the unbound drug concentration than to the total plasma concentration. For other protein drugs however, plasma binding proteins may act as facilitators of cellular uptake processes, especially for drugs that pass membranes by active processes. When a binding protein facilitates the interaction of the protein therapeutic with receptors or other cellular sites of action, the amount of bound drug influences the pharmacodynamics directly.

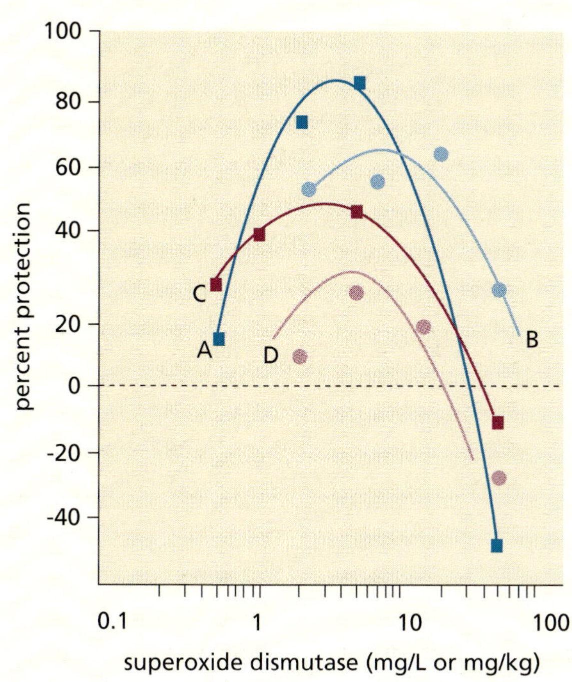

Figure 5.17. Bell-shaped dose-response curves for superoxide dismutase (SOD) in four animal models of myocardial reperfusion injury: A. Ischemic rabbit hearts treated with hrMn-SOD, monitoring recovery of developed tension; B. hypoxic rat hearts treated with yeast Cu,Zn-SOD, monitoring creatine kinase release; C. hypoxic rabbit hearts treated with hrCu,Zn-SOD, monitoring lactate dehydrogenase release; D. rabbit hearts with ligated coronary arteries in vivo treated with hrCu,Zn-SOD, monitoring infarct size (Omar et al., 1992).

Numerous examples of binding proteins are reported for proteins: IGF-I and IGF-II, t-PA, growth hormone, DNase (Mohler *et al.*, 1993), nerve growth factor, etc. (Mohler *et al.*, 1992). Some proteins have their own naturally occurring binding proteins that specifically bind the protein. As an example, six specific binding proteins are identified for IGF-I, denoted as IGFBP-1 to IGFBP-6 (Baxter, 1993; Clemmons, 1993). The IGFBPs are high affinity, soluble carrier proteins that transport IGF-I (and IGF-II) in the circulation (Clemmons, 1993). In humans, IGFBP-3 appears to be the most important binding protein for IGF-I since it is the most abundant in serum and tissues. At least 95% of the total human serum concentration of IGF-I is bound to IGFBP-3 (Baxter and Martin, 1989). IGFBP-3 seems to act as a reservoir for IGF-I and, as such, protects the organism against acute insulin-like hypoglycemic effects. Indeed, the hypoglycemic effect is related to the free IGF-I plasma concentration. In this case, the binding protein limits the accessibility of IGF-I to receptors since all binding proteins have substantially higher affinities for IGF-I than the IGF receptors (Clemmons *et al.*, 1992). In contrast, the delayed, indirect effects of IGF-I, such as its anabolic effects, may be related to the bound IGF-I levels. This relation is supported by evidence that the IGFBPs may play an active role in the interaction with target cells, and may act as facilitators for the delivery of IGF-I to certain receptors (Clemmons, 1993). One example is the demonstration that the affinity of the binding protein for IGF-I (IGFBP-6) at the cell surface is lower than in solution, which would make it easier for IGF-I to leave its association with the binding protein and to engage in binding with a cell-based receptor. As such, the IGFBPs may act as inhibitors for certain IGF-I effects, and as stimulators for other IGF-I effects.

It has been demonstrated that the elimination half-life of bound IGF-I is significantly prolonged relative to that of free IGF-I (Cohen and Nissley, 1976; Mohler *et al.*, 1992; Zapf *et al.*, 1986). This prolonged half-life suggests that only unbound IGF-I is available for elimination by routes such as glomerular filtration and peritubular extraction. The binding proteins for IGF-I are also responsible for the complicated pharmacokinetic behavior of IGF-I. The IGFBPs can be saturated at high IGF-I plasma concentrations, typically reached after endogenous therapeutic administration of IGF-I. At high doses, the binding proteins saturate and leave a larger proportion of free protein available for elimination. Additionally, the non-linear pharmacokinetics of IGF-I are complicated by the fact that the concentrations and relative ratios of the IGFBPs change with time during chronic dosing. The binding proteins are also very different between species, which makes interspecies scaling of the IGF-I pharmacokinetics impossible.

Another example is growth hormone (GH), for which a specific high-affinity binding protein homologous with the extra cellular domain of the growth hormone receptor is present in human plasma (Herington *et al.*, 1986; Leung, 1987). At least two GH-binding proteins (GHBP) have been identified in plasma with respectively high and low binding affinities for GH (Mohler *et al.*, 1992). GHBP binds about 40–50% of circulating GH at low GH concentrations of about 5 ng/mL (Baumann *et al.*, 1988). At higher circulating GH levels, the binding proteins become saturated (Figure 5.18). The clearance of bound GH is about ten-fold slower than that of free GH (Baumann *et al.*, 1988). Consequently, the binding proteins prolong the elimination half-life of GH and, as a result, enhance or prolong its activity. On the other hand, the plasma binding of GH prevents access of free GH to its receptors, and this could decrease its activity (Mohler *et al.*, 1992).

Other protein therapeutics seem to bind to circulating proteins in a more non-specific way. As an example, a recombinant derivative of hG-CSF, nartogastrim, showed 92% binding in rat plasma, presumably to albumin (Kuwabara *et al.*, 1995).

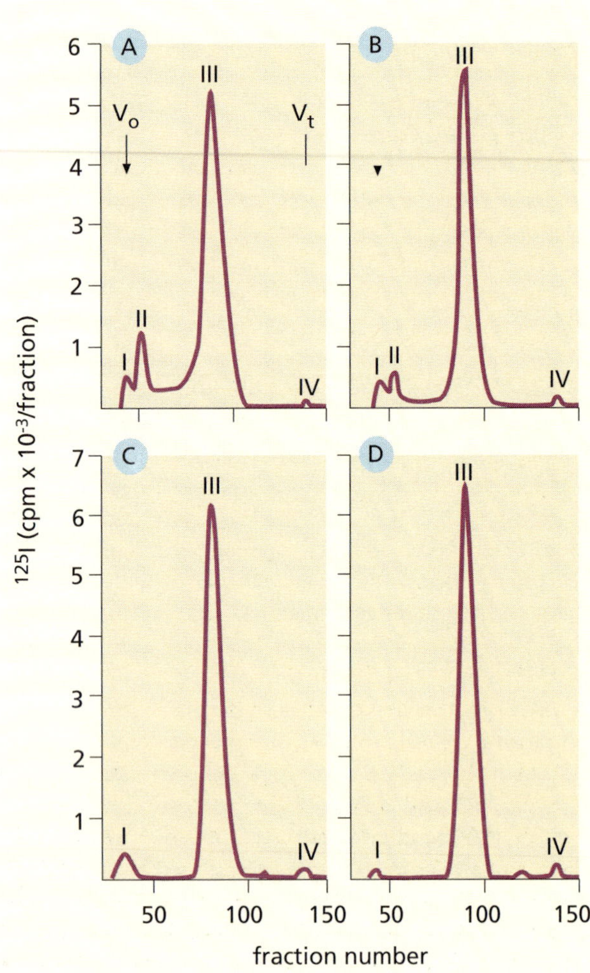

Figure 5.18. Gel filtration profiles of ^{125}I-hGH in plasma on Sephadex G-100. V_0 and V_t are the void and total volumes, respectively. A. Blank plasma with endogenous level of hGH only; B.126 ng/mL hGH added; C. 10 µg/mL hGH added; D. Tracer only (no plasma). Peak III corresponds to monomeric hGH; peak II and the plateau region between peaks II and III refer to the plasmabound hGH; peak IV is free iodide. Higher hGH concentrations saturate the binding proteins as peak II becomes smaller relative to peak III (C versus B versus A). From Clemmons (Clemmons, 1993).

Interspecies Scaling

Techniques for the prediction of pharmacokinetic parameters in one species from data derived from other species have been applied for many years (Boxenbaum, 1986; Dedrick, 1973). Such scaling techniques use various allometric equations based on body weight using the following allometric equation:

$$P = a.W^b$$

where P is the pharmacokinetic parameter being scaled, W is the body weight, a is the allometric coefficient, and b is the allometric exponent. Although a and b are specific constants for any compound and for each pharmacokinetic parameter, the exponent b seems to average around 1 for volume terms, such as the volume of distribution and 0.75 for rates such as elimination and distribution clearances. Since the elimination half-life of any drug is proportional to the volume of distribution and inversely proportional to the elimination clearance, b is about 0.25 for elimination half-lives. Allometric scaling of pharmacokinetic parameters has been difficult for small synthetic drug molecules, especially for those drugs with a high hepatic clearance and quantitative and/or qualitative interspecies differences in metabolism. In contrast, the biochemical and physiological processes that are responsible for the pharmacokinetic fate of biologics such as peptides and proteins are better conserved across mammalian species. As such, allometric scaling for those compounds has been more reliable and accurate (Mordenti *et al.*, 1991). It is our experience that the systemic exposure in humans of proteins that follow linear pharmacokinetics can be predicted within a factor of two from pharmacokinetic data from three to four animal species. As a typical example, we could scale the pharmacokinetic parameters for IL-2 and PEG IL-2, as demonstrated in Figure 5.19, for the elimination clearance. Notice that the regression lines for both compounds are parallel, which is expected if PEGylation decreases the clearance to the same degree in all species.

A helpful although potentially less accurate prediction can be made based on pharmacokinetic data from one species to another, based on the average allometric exponents for volumes and clearances. Interspecies scaling is helpful in the prediction of doses for pharmacological animal models of disease, toxicology studies, and the first human studies. Indeed, if the efficacious concentration of a protein drug is known from *in vitro* studies, one might predict the dose needed to reach these levels in an animal efficacy or toxicology model when pharmacokinetic data are known from another species. Similarly, if an estimation of the maximum tolerated exposure can be made, allometric scaling may be helpful to determine the highest dose in toxicology studies. The dose that results in efficacious concentrations may be taken as the lowest dose in the toxicology studies. Additionally, the efficacious dose in humans can be estimated from the animal pharmacokinetic data. A starting dose in the first human study (usually a dose-escalation study) can be chosen as this estimated efficacious dose, divided by a factor of two or more, based on conservative safety considerations.

It needs to be emphasized that allometric scaling techniques are useful tools for predicting a dose that will assist in the planning of dose-ranging studies, but are not a replacement for such studies. The advantage of including such

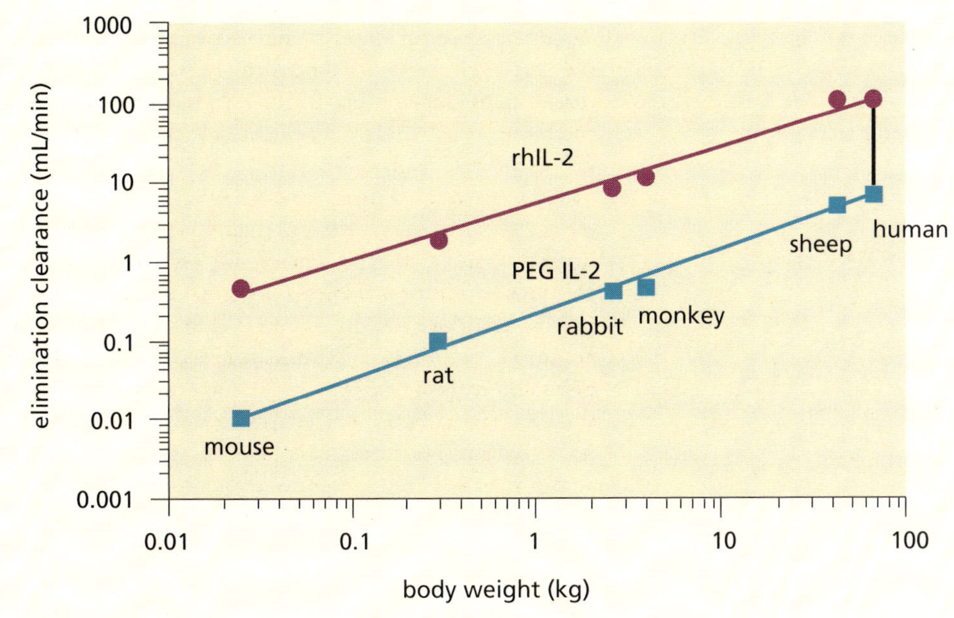

Figure 5.19. Allometric interspecies scaling of the elimination clearance of IL-2 and PEG IL-2.

dose prediction in the protocol design of dose-ranging studies is that a smaller number of doses need to be tested before finding the final dose level. Interspecies dose predictions simply narrow the range of doses in the initial pharmacological efficacy studies, the animal toxicology studies, and the human safety and efficacy studies.

Heterogeneity of Protein Therapeutics

The identity, purity and potency of small synthetic drugs can be demonstrated analytically, and consequently, they are usually completely defined in terms of their chemical structure. Peptides, proteins, and other biotechnologically derived compounds are usually more complex compounds, and it is generally not possible to define them as discrete chemical entities with unique compositions. As described in Chapter 2, the physicochemical and biochemical characteristics of proteins are not only dependent on the amino acid sequence (primary structure), but also on the shape and folding (secondary and tertiary structures), and the relationship between the protein molecules themselves, such as the formation of aggregates (quaternary structure). Biotechnologically-derived and endogenous proteins may be heterogeneous at each structural level. For natural IFN-γ, for example, six naturally occurring C-terminal sequences have been identified (Pan *et al.*, 1987; Rinderknecht and Burton, 1985; Rinderknecht *et al.*, 1984).

In addition, post-translational modifications of proteins, such as the degree of glycosylation of amino acid residues, may be different. The secreted and membrane-associated proteins of almost all eukariotic cells are glycosylated (Kukuruzinska and Lennon, 1998; Reuter and Gabius, 1999), and different glycoproteins also have different carbohydrate contents, from ~3% for serum IgG to >40% for erythropoietin (EPO). EPO has three N-linked and one O-linked sugar chains. The degree of glycosylation differs according to the cell line used for production. For example, GM-CSF and M-CSF are non-glycosylated in bacterial cell lines such as *E. Coli*, moderately glycosylated in yeast, and heavily glycosylated in mammalian cell lines (see Chapter 3). Receptor binding studies with GM-CSF have shown that the receptor affinity decreases with an increase of the level of glycosylation (Stoudemire, 1992).

Another classical example is recombinant human tissue-plasminogen activator (t-PA). Although the active enzyme was first derived from *E. coli* cultures, this cell line lacks several desirable biological activities, such as glycosylation ability and the ability to form the correct three-dimensional t-PA structure. Finally, recombinant t-PA was cloned into a Chinese hamster ovary (CHO) cell line. These mammalian cells carried out the glycosylation, disulfide bond formation, and proper folding similar to human cells (Ogez *et al.*, 1991).

Besides the importance of correct glycosylation for activity, differences in glycosylation may also have an influence on the pharmacokinetics. A typical example is that the removal of terminal sialic acid residues from the sugar chains of EPO (asialo-EPO) causes complete loss of *in vivo* biological activity, but increases *in vitro* activity. The loss of *in vivo* activity of asialo-EPO was explained by a rapid removal from the systemic circulation, which resulted from hepatic uptake mediated by galactose-recognizing receptors (cf. Chapter 17).

Chemical Modifications of Protein Therapeutics

Besides the mostly unwanted heterogeneity of protein drugs introduced by the manufacturing process, other chemical modifications of protein and peptide drugs are intentional for obtaining molecules with specified characteristics. Variant proteins can be engineered that differ from natural proteins by exchange, deletion, or insertion of single amino acids, or longer sequences up to entire domains. Small changes in the chemical structure of proteins may cause differences in pharmacokinetics and pharmacodynamics. In addition, mutations may affect glycosylation patterns and conformational changes, which in turn may affect clearance and receptor interactions. A single amino acid mutation in t-PA or the removal of carbohydrate on a single amino acid in t-PA resulted in plasma concentration profiles that were very different from natural t-PA (Figure 5.20) (Tanswell, 1992).

Modification of peptide and protein drugs with the aim of changing the pharmacological activity may at the same time affect the pharmacokinetic behavior of the molecules. In other instances, the increase of duration of response may be exclusively attributed to a change in the pharmacokinetics, such as an increase in residence time. Such modifications include amino acid substitution, deletions and additions, cyclization, drug conjugation, glycosylation or deglycosylation, etc.

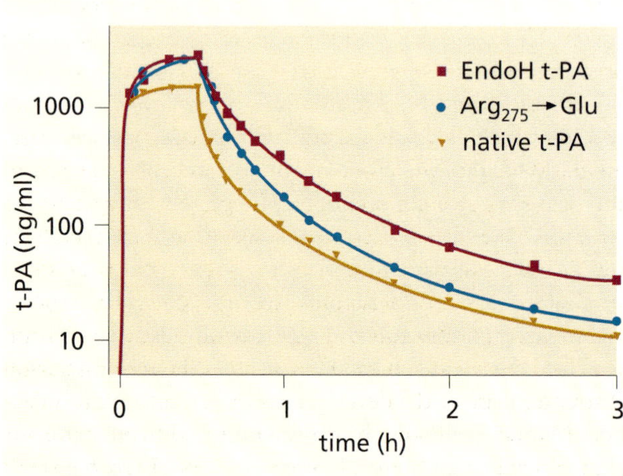

Figure 5.20. t-PA plasma concentrations after 30-min IV infusions of 0.6 mg/kg t-PA in groups of 4 rabbits. The figure shows the marked effect on clearance of a single amino acid mutation (Arg_{275}->Glu) or of removal of a carbohydrate with a high mannose content at Asn_{114} by the enzyme endoglycosidase H (EndoH t-PA), as compared to native t-PA. From Tanswell (Tanswell, 1992).

The elimination half-life of many peptide and protein drugs is rather short. Consequently, frequent dosing or continuous infusion is necessary to maintain efficacious plasma levels of the drug. Several approaches have been applied to decrease the elimination clearance of biotechnological drugs. One approach is chemical modification such as PEGylation, i.e. the attachment of monomethoxy polyethylene glycol polymer (PEG) to the protein. An example is PEG IL-2, which usually consists of a mixture of rhIL-2 molecules (M_W 15 kDa) with one to five or more PEG polymers attached to each molecule on the ε-amino portions of the lysine residues. The production process determines the average number of PEG residues attached, but any process results in a mixture. With each PEG addition, the molecular weight increases with about 7 kDa, but because of the attraction of water molecules, the hydrodynamic size increases even more (95–250 kDa). Increasing the degree of PEGylation decreases the elimination clearance and the volume of distribution (Figure 5.21). Since the elimination clearance usually decreases relatively more than the decrease in volume of distribution, the elimination half-life of PEG IL-2 is longer than for IL-2. Based on the relationship between elimination clearance and effective molecular weight, it is possible to calculate the optimal degree of PEGylation for obtaining the desired systemic exposure (Bauer *et al.*, 1992; Knauf *et al.*, 1988).

The effect of prosthetic sugar groups on elimination and targeting is illustrated by the comparison of the pharmacokinetics of native glucose-oxidase (GO), deglycosylated GO (dGO), and galactosylated GO (gGO) in mice (Demignot and Domurado, 1987). A saturable mechanism was responsible both for GO and dGO uptake by mononuclear phagocytes, although there was a substantial difference in elimination half-life (ten minutes for GO; 100 minutes for dGO). In contrast, gGO had a half-life of four minutes and was taken up preferably by hepatocytes, presumably through hepatic galactose receptors. This is an example where receptor-mediated endocytosis through sugar-recognizing receptors is an efficient hepatic uptake mechanism for glycoproteins. However, when terminal sialic acid residues on the carbohydrate moieties of glycoproteins shield the receptor-binding sugars, hepatic receptor-mediated endocytosis is lower than the desialylated analogues (Meijer and Ziegler, 1993). This has been demonstrated for rEPO and rGM-CSF (Cumming, 1991). The protection by sialic residues appears to be a natural mechanism essential for the normal survival of enzymes, acute-phase proteins

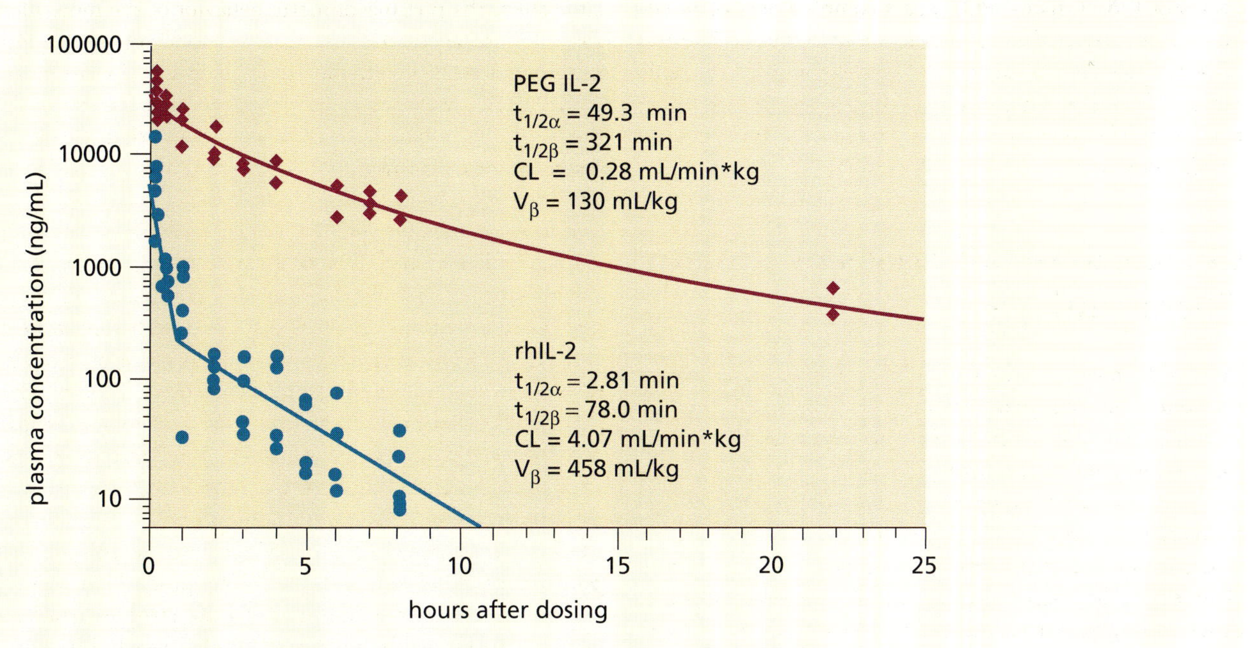

Figure 5.21. Pharmacokinetics of recombinant human interleukin-2 (rhIL-2) and its PEGylation form (PEG IL-2) in rats after IV bolus administration of 0.25 mg/kg. The data were described by a linear two-compartmental pharmacokinetic model.

(such as α_1-acid glycoprotein), and most plasma proteins of the immune system (cf. Chapter 17).

Immunogenicity

Immunogenicity is the ability to induce the formation of antibodies or immune lymphocytes. Immunogenicity is an important property distinguishing most biologic products from most small drug molecules. An immunogenic response to heterologous (non-host) proteins is expected, as antibody formation is also often observed after chronic dosing of human proteins in animal studies. However, recombinant human proteins may also stimulate the production of circulating antibodies in chronic human therapy and clinical studies. In this case, immunogenic responses are sometimes associated with the formation of protein aggregates, altered protein forms or fragments – such as acetylated protein – or proteins with broken disulfide bridges (for interferons, for example). In other cases, impurities from cell substrates or media components are either directly immunogenic or act as adjuvants to stimulate antibody formation against the protein.

Immunogenic responses can cause a wide variety of unwanted effects, with different degrees of severity. Safety issues include the potential for injection site reactions, systemic hypersensitivity reactions, and anaphylactic shock in some cases. As an example, bovine Cu,Zn-superoxide dismutase (Cu,Zn-SOD) (Orgotein) as a treatment for various arthritic diseases was withdrawn from the market in several European countries because of hypersensitivity. Asparaginase from bacterial origin (*E. coli*), indicated in the therapy of acute lymphocytic leukemia, causes a very high level of allergic reactions (3–73% incidence) (Zoon *et al.*, 1999). The manufacturer of asparaginase has a scheme for skin testing and desensitization should skin tests be positive prior to therapy. Another one of the few non-human proteins on the market is the thrombolytic streptokinase, produced in group C β-hemolytic streptococci. Levels of anti-streptokinase antibodies can be present in patients as a result of a recent streptococcus infection and, therefore, allergic reactions have been noticed (1–4% incidence), some anaphylactic and anaphylactoid responses (Zoon *et al.*, 1999). The manufacturer cautions against re-administration within a period of five days to 12 months of either administration of streptokinase or the development of a streptococcus infection. Human antibodies have been observed to recombinant human proteins for human interferons (IFN), human growth hormone (hGH), human insulin, and human factor VIII. However, hypersensitivity reactions are rather rare. In general, for human recombinant proteins, immunogenicity has not been the primary limitation for their clinical use; poor PK and PD are frequently the major obstacles for efficacy.

Immunogenicity can be a problem in the study (and use) of protein drugs since the presence of antibodies can complicate the interpretation of preclinical and clinical studies by inactivating (neutralizing) the biological activity of the protein drug. Additionally, protein-antibody complex formation may affect the distribution, metabolism, and elimination of the protein drug. Neutralizing antibodies may inactivate the biological activity of the protein by blocking its active site or by a change of the tertiary structure by steric effects. Antibodies are most likely to be induced when the protein is foreign to the host. Examples of such situations are when mouse-derived monoclonal antibodies are administered to humans, or when human recombinant proteins are tested for safety in animals. Extravascular injections (e.g. sc, im) are also more likely to stimulate antibody production than intravenous administrations, presumably because of the higher degree of protein precipitation and aggregation at the injection site. This was demonstrated for IL-2 (Krigel *et al.*, 1988) and INF-β (Konrad *et al.*, 1987; Larocca *et al.*, 1989).

Antibodies may directly neutralize the activity of the protein. This neutralization has been observed for interferons in the presence of neutralizing IgG, for example. If neutralization occurs, it indicates that at least some fraction of the antibody population binds at or near the active site, which blocks activity (Working, 1992). Irrespective of the neutralizing capabilities of the antibodies formed, they may also indirectly affect the efficacy of a protein drug by changing its pharmacokinetic profile (Figure 5.22) Elimination clearances of protein drugs may be either increased or decreased by antibody formation and binding. An increase of the clearance is observed if the protein-antibody complex is eliminated more rapidly than the unbound protein (Rosenblum *et al.*, 1985). This increase may occur when high levels of the protein-antibody complex stimulate its clearance by the mononuclear phagocyte system (Sell, 1987). In other situations, the serum concentration of a protein can be increased if binding to an antibody slows down its rate of clearance because the protein-antibody complex is eliminated more slowly than the unbound protein (Working, 1992). In this case, the complex may act as a depot for the protein and, if the antibody is not neutralizing, a longer duration of the pharmacological action may occur. For example, the clearance of rIFN-α2a in cancer patients was increased because of an antibody response. In contrast, human leukocyte INF-β in rats was decreased 15-fold when circulating antibodies were present. A decrease of clearance in the presence of antibody titers was also detected for t-PA in dogs (Working, 1992).

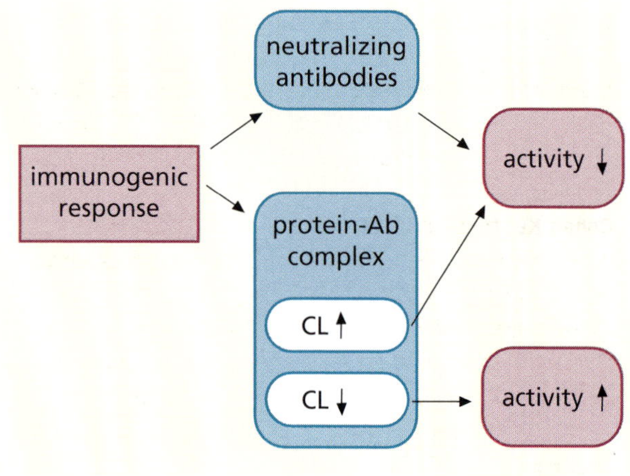

Figure 5.22. Effect of antibody formation on pharmacokinetics and pharmacodynamics of protein drugs.

Both an increased and decreased clearance is possible for the same protein, dependent on the dose level administered. At low doses, protein-antibody complexes delay clearance because their elimination is slower than the unbound protein. In contrast, at high doses, higher levels of protein-antibody complex result in the formation of aggregates, which are cleared more rapidly than the unbound protein.

The most worrisome situation occurs when neutralizing antibodies are formed during chronic therapy with a protein drug, and when the antibodies cross-react with the endogenous protein or with another endogenous factor (Zoon *et al.*, 1999). This cross-reaction is especially a safety concern if the endogenous protein has a unique type of activity and there is no redundant mechanism to compensate for the activity loss of the neutralized factor. As an example, humans dosed with thrombopoietin (TPO) developed long-term thrombocytopenia, which is believed to be caused by the neutralizing activity of antibodies against endogenous TPO (Zoon *et al.*, 1999). Apparently, TPO is the only factor really important for the formation of platelets. Some patients appeared to have pre-existing antibodies to TPO. Pre-existing antibodies were also detected for interferons in cancer and HIV patients.

Besides the route of administration and product characteristics, other immunogenic determinants are dose and regimen, disease, and concomitant medications. Typically, larger proteins are more immunogenic than smaller ones. The effect of dose size on the antibody response is unpredictable, although the cumulative dose may be more important than the daily dose. With interferons, for example, a higher cumulative dose resulted in less neutralizing antibodies. Time, more than dosing frequency, is important, since any antibody response needs weeks to months to develop fully. In humans, IgM levels appear after five to seven days, while IgG serum concentrations peak three to four weeks after dosing initiation. Patients with infectious diseases, presumably because of a stimulated immune system, showed higher antibody levels than cancer patients, who are typically immunosuppressed. Similarly, autoimmune disease state is a factor that might stimulate immunogenicity responses, while a lower response is possible in patients with kidney and liver disease. Immunosuppressants such as cyclosporin as concomitant medication may diminish the immunogenic response.

Due to the different possible effects of an immunogenicity response on the PK/PD of protein drugs the study of an antibody response is very important in the drug development process. However, the presence of an immunogenic response in animal studies is rarely a prediction of a similar occurrence in humans. More importantly, the value of certain preclinical toxicology studies may be questioned when large titers of neutralizing antibodies are measured, because a lack of toxicity findings may be caused by the neutralization of the toxicodynamic effect. For the situation in humans, the measurement of antibody, and neutralizing antibody titers, in chronic clinical studies is important. ■

References

- **Arendshorst WJ, Navar LG.** (1988). Renal circulation and glomerular hemodynamics. In *Diseases of the kidney*, edited by RW Schrier and CW Gottschalk. Little, Brown, Boston, pp. 65–117
- **Ashwell G, Harford J.** (1982). Carbohydrate-specific receptors of the liver. *Annual Review of Biochemistry*, 51, 531–554
- **Ashwell G, Morell AG.** (1974). The role of surface carbohydrates in the hepatic recognition and transport of circulating glycoproteins. *Advances in Enzymology*, 41, 99–128
- **Bartocci A, Mastrogiannis DS, Migliorati G, Stockert RJ, Wolkoff AW, Stanley ER.** (1987). Macrophages specifically regulate the concentration of their own growth factor in the circulation. *Proc Natl Acad Sci USA*, 84, 6179–6183
- **Bauer RJ, Der K, Ottah-Ihejeto N, Barrientos J, Kung AHC.** (1997). The role of liver and kidney on the pharmacokinetics of a recombinant amino terminal fragment of bactericidal/permeability-increasing protein in rats. *Pharmaceutical Research*, 14, 224–229
- **Bauer RJ, Gibbons JA, Bell DP, Luo Z-P, Young JD.** (1994). Nonlinear pharmacokinetics of recombinant human macrophage colony-stimulating factor (M-CSF) in rats. *J Pharmacol Exper Ther*, 268, 152–158
- **Bauer RJ, Winkelhake JL, Young JD, Zimmerman RZ.** (1992). Protein drug delivery by programmed pump infusion: Interleukin-2. In *Therapeutic proteins. Pharmacokinetics and pharmacodynamics*, edited by AHC Kung, RA Baughman, JW Larrick. W.H. Freeman and Company, New York, pp. 239–253
- **Baumann G, Amburn K, Shaw MA.** (1988). The circulating growth hormone (GH)-binding protein complex: A major constituent of plasma GH in man. *Endocrinology*, 122, 976–984
- **Baumann G, Shaw MA, Buchanan TA.** (1988). In vivo kinetics of a covalent growth hormone-binding protein complex. *Metabolism*, 38, 330–333
- **Baxter RC.** (1993). Circulating binding proteins for the insulinlike growth factors. *Trends Endocrinol Metab*, 4, 91–96
- **Baxter RC, Martin JL.** (1989). Structure of the Mr 140,000 growth hormone-dependent insulin-like growth factor binding protein complex: determination by reconstitution and affinity labeling. *Proc Natl Acad Sci USA*, 86, 6898–6902
- **Bennett HPJ, McMartin C.** (1979). Peptide hormones and their analogues: distribution, clearance from the circulation, and inactivation *in vivo*. *Pharmacol Reviews*, 30, 247–292
- **Bocci V.** (1987). Metabolism of anticancer agents. *Pharmacol Ther*, 34, 1–49
- **Bocci V.** (1990). Catabolism of therapeutic proteins and peptides with implications for drug delivery. *Adv Drug Del Rev*, 4, 149–169
- **Boxenbaum H.** (1986). Time Concepts in Physics, Biology and Pharmacokinetics. *Journal of Pharmaceutical Sciences*, 75, 1053–1062
- **Braeckman R.** (2000). Pharmacokinetics and Pharmacodynamics of Protein Therapeutics. In *Peptide and Protein Drug Analysis*, edited by RE Reid. Marcel Dekker, New York, pp. 633–669
- **Burwen SJ, Jones AL.** (1990). Hepatocellular processing of endocytosed proteins. *J Electron Microsc Tech*, 14, 140–151
- **Carone FA, Peterson DR.** (1980). Hydrolysis and transport of small peptides by the proximal tubule. *Am J Physiol*, 238, F151–F158
- **Chen SA, Sawchuk RJ, Brundage RC, Horvath C, Mendenhall HV, Gunther RA, Braeckman RA.** (2000). Plasma and lymph pharmacokinetics of recombinanat human interleukin-2 and polyethylene-modified interleukin-2 in pigs. *JPET*, 293, 248–259
- **Childs A, Grevel J, Baron DA, Reynolds DL, McCabe RD, Burton EG, Johnson DE, Braeckman RA.** (1996). Population PK/PD of tissue factor pathway inhibitor (TFPI) in cynomolgus monkeys during a 12-day toxicology study. *Fund Appl Toxicol*, 30, 104
- **Clemmons DR.** (1993). IGF binding proteins and their functions. *Molecular Reproduction and Development*, 35, 368–375
- **Clemmons DR, Dehoff MH, Busby WH, Bayne ML, Cascieri MA.** (1992). Competition for binding to IGFBP-2, 3, 4 and 5 by the insulin-like growth factors and IGF analogs. *Endocrinology*, 132, 890–895
- **Cohen KL, Nissley SP.** (1976). The serum half-life of somatomedin activity: Evidence for growth hormone dependence. *Acta Endocrinol*, 83, 243–258
- **Colburn WA.** (1991). Peptide, peptoid, and protein pharmacokinetics/pharmacodynamics. In *Peptides, peptoids, and proteins. Pharmacokinetics and pharmacodynamics*, edited by PD Garzone, WA Colburn, M Mokotoff. Harvey Whitney Books, Cincinnati, pp. 93–115
- **Colburn WA, Blue JW.** (1992). Using pharmacokinetics and pharmacodynamics to direct pharmaceutical research and development. *Applied Clinical Trials*, 1, 42–46

- **Cumming DA.** (1991). Glycosylation of recombinant protein therapeutics: control and functional implications. *Glycobiology,* 1, 115–130
- **Dayneka NL, Garg V, Jusko WJ.** (1993). Comparison of Four Basic Models of Indirect Pharmacodynamic Responses. *Journal of Pharmacokinetics and Biopharmaceutics,* 21, 457–478
- **Dedrick RL.** (1973). Animal Scale-Up. *Journal of Pharmacokinetics and Biopharmaceutics,* 1, 435–461
- **Demignot S, Domurado D.** (1987). Effect of prosthetic sugar groups on the pharmacokinetics of glucose-oxidase. *Drug design and delivery,* 1, 333–348
- **Derendorf H, Hochhaus G,** Eds. (1995). *Handbook of Pharmacokinetic/Pharmacodynamic Correlation.* Handbooks of Pharmacology and Toxicology. London, CRC Press.
- **Einhorn S, Ahre A, Blomgren H, Johansson B, Mellstedt H, Strander H.** (1982). Interferon and natural killer activity in multiple myeloma. Lack of correlation between interferon-induced enhancement of natural killer activity and clinical response to human interferon-a. *Int J Cancer,* 30, 167–172
- **Fallon RJ, Schwartz AL.** (1989). Receptor-mediated delivery of drugs to hepatocytes. *Advanced Drug Delivery Reviews,* 4, 49–63
- **Ferraiolo BL, Mohler MA.** (1992). Goals and analytical methodologies for protein disposition studies. In *Protein pharmacokinetics and metabolism,* edited by BL Ferraiolo, MA Mohler, CA Gloff. Plenum Press, New York, pp.
- **Ganapathy V, Leibach FH.** (1986). Carrier-mediated reabsorption of small peptides in renal proximal tubule. *Am J Physiol,* 25, F945–F953
- **Gibbons JA, Luo Z-P, Hannon ER, Braeckman RA, Young JD.** (1995). Quatitation of the renal clearance of interleukin-2 using nephractomized and ureter-ligated rats. *J Pharmacol Exp Ther,* 272, 119–125
- **Girard P, Nony P, Boissel JP.** (1990). The place of simultaneous pharmacokinetic pharmacodynamic modeling in new drug development: trends and perspectives. *Fundamental and Clinical Pharmacology,* 4, 103s–115s
- **Hansen J-B, Sandset PM, Raanaas Huseby K, Huseby N-E, Nordoy A.** (1996). Depletion of intravascular pools of Tissue Factor Pathway Inhibitor (TFPI) during repeated or continuous intravenous infusion of heparin in man. *Thrombosis and Haemostasis,* 76, 703–709
- **Hellfritzsch M, Nielsen S, Christensen EI, Nielsen JT.** (1988). Basolateral tubular handling of insulin in the kidney. *Contrib Nephrol,* 68, 86–91
- **Herington AC, Ymer S, Stevenson J.** (1986). Identification and characterization of specific binding proteins for growth hormone in normal human sera. *J Clin Invest,* 77, 1817–1823
- **Holford NHG.** (1990). Concepts and usefulness of pharmacokinetic-pharmacodynamic modelling. *Fundamental and Clinical Pharmacology,* 4, 93s–101s
- **Holford NHG, Sheiner LB.** (1981). Pharmacokinetic and Pharmacodynamic Modeling in Vivo. *Critical Reviews in Bioengineering,* 5, 273–322
- **Holford NHG, Sheiner LB.** (1981). Understanding the Dose-Effect Relationship: Clinical Application of Pharmacokinetic-Pharmacodynamic Models. *Clinical Pharmacokinetics,* 6, 429–453
- **Hooper S.** (1991). Pharmacokinetics and Pharmacodynamics of Intravenous Regular Human Insulin. In *Pharmacokinetics and Pharmacodynamics. Peptides, Peptoids, and Proteins,* edited by PD Garzone, WA Colburn, M Mokotoff. Harvey Whitney Books, Cincinnati, OH, pp. 128–137
- **Jain RK, Baxter LT.** (1993). Extravasation and interstitial transport in tumors. In *Biological Barriers to Protein Delivery,* edited by KL Audus and TJ Raub. Plenum Press, New York, pp. 441–465
- **Jusko WJ, Ko HC.** (1994). Pharmacodynamics and Drug Action. Physiologic Indirect Response Models Characterize Diverse Types of Pharmacodynamic Effects. *Clinical Pharmacology and Therapeutics,* 56, 406–419
- **Kato M, Kamiyama H, Okazaki A, Kumaki K, Kato Y, Sugiyama Y.** (1997). Mechanism for the nonlinear pharmacokinetics of erythropoietin in rats. *Journal of Pharmacology and Experimental Therapeutics,* 283, 520–527
- **Kenakin T.** (1993). Drug-Receptor Theory. In *Pharmacologic Analysis of Drug-Receptor Interaction,* edited by T Kenakin. Raven Press, New York, pp. 1–38
- **Kim DC, Sugiyama Y, Satoh H, Fuwa T, Iga T, Hanano M.** (1988). Kinetic analysis of *in vivo* receptor-dependent binding of human epidermal growth factor by rat tissues. *J Pharm Sci,* 77, 200–207
- **Knauf MJ, Bell DP, Hirtzer P, Luo Z-P, Young JD, Katre NV.** (1988). Relationship of effective molecular size to systemic clearance in rats of recombinant interleukin-2 chemically modified with water-soluble polymers. *J Biological Chem,* 263, 15064–15070
- **Kompella UB, Lee VHL.** (1991). Pharmacokinetics of peptide and protein drugs. In *Peptide and protein drug delivery,* edited by VHL Lee. Marcel Dekker, New York, pp. 391–484
- **Konrad M, Childs A, Merigan T, Bordon E.** (1987). Assessment of the antigenic response in humans to a recombinant mutant interferon beta. *J Clin Immunol,* 7, 365–375
- **Krigel RL, Padavic-Shaller KA, Rudolph AR, Litwin S, Konrad M, Bradley EC, Comis RL.** (1988). A Phase I study of recombinant interleukin-2 plus recombinant b-interferon. *Cancer Res,* 48
- **Kroboth PD, Schmith VD, Smith RB.** (1991). Pharmacodynamic Modelling – Application to New Drug Development. *Clinical Pharmacokinetics,* 20, 91–98
- **Kukuruzinska MA, Lennon K.** (1998). Protein N-glycosylation: Molecular genetics and functional significance. *Crit Rev Oral Biol Med,* 9, 415–448
- **Kuwabara T, Uchimura T, Takai K, Kobayashi H, Kaboyashi S, Sugiyama Y.** (1995). Saturable uptake of a recombinant human granulocyte colony-stimulating factor derivative, nartograstim, by the bone marrow and spleen of rats *in vivo. J Pharmacol Exper Ther,* 273, 1114–1122

- **Larocca AP, Leung SC, Marcus SG, Colby CB, Borden EC.** (1989). Evaluation of neutralizing antibodies in patients treated with recombinant interferon-b_{ser}. *J Interferon Res*, 9(Suppl. 1), S51–S60
- **Lee VHL.** (1988). Enzymatic barriers to peptide and protein absorption. *CRC Crit Rev Ther Drug Carrier Syst*, 5, 69–97
- **Leung DW.** (1987). Growth hormone receptor and serum binding: Purification, clonong and expression. *Nature*, 330, 537–543
- **Maack T.** (1975). Renal handling of low molecular weight proteins. *Am J Med*, 58, 57–64
- **Maack T, Johnson V, Kau ST, Figueiredo J, Sigulem D.** (1979). Renal filtration, transport, and metabolism of low-molecular weight protein: a review. *Kidney Int*, 16, 251–270
- **Maack T, Park CH, Camergo MJF.** (1985). Renal filtration, transport, and metabolism of proteins. In *The kidney: Physiology and pathophysiology*, edited by DW Seldin and G Giebisch. Raven Press, New York, pp. 1173–1803
- **Marks DL, Gores GJ, LaRusso NF.** (1995). Hepatic processing of peptides. In *Peptide-based drug design. Controlling transport and metabolism*, edited by MD Taylor and GL Amidon. Amrican Chemical Society, Washington, DC, pp. 221–248
- **Medalion B, Merin G, Aingorn H, Miao H-Q, Nagler A, Elami A, Ishai-Michaeli R, Vlodavski I.** (1997). Endogenous basic fibroblast factor displaced by heparin from the luminal surface of human blood vessels is preferentially sequestered by injured regions of the vessel wall. *Circulation*, 95, 1853–1863
- **Meijer DKF, Ziegler K.** (1993). Mechanisms for the hepatic clearance of oligopeptides and proteins. In *Biological barriers to protein delivery*, edited by KL Audus and TJ Raub. Plenum Press, New York, pp. 339–408
- **Mohler M, Cook J, Lewis D, Moore J, Sinicropi D, Championsmith A, Ferraiolo B, Mordenti J.** (1993). Altered pharmacokinetics of recombinant human deoxyribonuclease in rats due to the presence of a binding protein. *Drug Metabol Dispos*, 21, 71–75
- **Mohler MA, Cook JE, Baumann G.** (1992). Binding proteins of protein therapeutics. In *Protein pharmacokinetics and metabolism*, edited by BL Ferraiolo, MA Mohler, CA Gloff. Plenum Press, New York, pp. 35–71
- **Mordenti J, Chen SA, Moore JA, Ferraiolo BL, Green JD.** (1991). Interspecies Scaling of Clearance and Volume of Distribution Data for Five Therapeutic Proteins. *Pharmaceutical Research*, 8, 1351–1359
- **Mordenti J, Chen SC, Ferraiolo BL.** (1992). Pharmacokinetics of interferon-gamma. In *Therapeutic proteins. Pharmacokinetics and pharmacodynamics*, edited by AHC Kung, RA Baughman, JW Larrick. W.H. Freeman and Company, New York, pp. 187–199
- **Murakami T, Misaki M, Masuda S, Higashi Y, Fuwa T, Yata N.** (1994). Dose-dependent plasma clearance of human epidermal growth factor in rats. *J Pharm Sci*, 83, 1400–1403
- **Nagashima R, O'Reilly RA, Levy G.** (1968). Kinetics of pharmacologic effects in man: The anticoagulant action of warfarin. *Clinical Pharmacology and Therapeutics*, 10, 22–35
- **Narita M, Bu G, Olins GM, Higuchi DA, Herz J, Broze GJJ, Schwartz AL.** (1995). Two receptor systems are involved in the plasma clearance of tissue factor pathway inhibitor *in vivo*. *Journal of Biological Chemistry*, 270, 24800–24804
- **Nielsen MS, Nykjaer A, Warshawsky I, Schwartz AL, Gliemann J.** (1995). Analysis of ligand binding to the a_2-macroglobulin receptor/low density lipoprotein receptor-related protein. *Journal of Biological Chemistry*, 270, 23713–223719
- **Ogez JR, van Reis R, Paoni N, Builder SE.** (1991). Recombinant human tissue-plasminogen activator: biochemistry, pharmacology, and process development. In *Peptides, peptoids, and proteins*, edited by PD Garzone, WA Colburn, M Mokotoff. Harvey Whitney Books, Cincinnati, pp. 170–188
- **Ohnishi H, J.T.Y. C, Lin KK, Lee H, Chu TM.** (1989). Role of the kidney in metabolic change of interleukin-2. *Tumor Biol*, 10, 202–214
- **Omar BA, Flores SC, McCord JM.** (1992). Superoxide dismutase. In *Therapeutic Proteins. Pharmacokinetics and Pharmacodynamics*, edited by AHC Kung, RA Baughman, JW Larrick. W.H. Freeman and Company, New York, pp. 295–315
- **O'Reilly RA, Levy G.** (1970). Kinetics of the anticoagulant effect of bishydroxycoumarin in man. *Clinical Pharmacology and Therapeutics*, 11, 378–384
- **Pan Y-CE, Stern AS, Familletti PC, Khan FR, Chizzonite R.** (1987). Stuctural characterization of human interferon gamma. *Eur J Biochem*, 166, 145–149
- **Petros WP, Rabinowitz J, Stuart AR, Gilbert CJ, Kanakura Y, Griffin JD, Peters WP.** (1992). Disposition of recombinant human granulocite-macrophage colony-stimulating factor in patients receiving high-dose chemotherapy and autologous bone marrow support. *Blood*, 80, 1135–1140
- **Piscitelli SC, Forrest A, Vogel S, Metcalf J, Baseler M, Stevens R, Kovacs JA**. (1996). A novel PK/PD model for infused interleukin-2 (IL-2), in HIV-infected patients. Ninety-Seventh Annual Meeting of the American Society for Clinical Pharmacology and Therapeutics, Lake Buena Vista, Florida
- **Rabkin R, Dahl DC.** (1993). Renal uptake and disposal of proteins and peptides. In *Biological barriers to protein delivery*, edited by KL Audus and TJ Raub. Plenum Press, New York, pp. 299–338
- **Rabkin R, Kitaji J.** (1983). Renal metabolism of peptide hormones. *Mineral Electrolyte Metab*, 9, 212–226
- **Rabkin R, Ryan MP, Duckworth WC.** (1984). The renal metabolism of insulin. *Diabetologica*, 27, 351–357
- **Reuter G, Gabius H-J.** (1999). Eukariotic glycosylation: whim of nature or multipurpose tool? *Cell Mol Life Sci*, 55, 386–422
- **Rinderknecht E, Burton LE.** (1985). Biochemical characterization of natural and recombinant IFN-gamma. In *The biology of the interferon system 1984*, edited by H Kirchner and H Schellenkens. Elsevier, Amsterdam, pp. 397–402
- **Rinderknecht E, O'Connor BH, Rodriguez H.** (1984). Natural human interferon-gamma: complete amino acid sequence and dtermination of sites of glycosylation. *J Biol Chem*, 259, 6790–6797

- **Rosenblum MG, Unger BW, Gutterman JU, Hersh EM, David GS, Fincke JM.** (1985). Modification of human leucocyte interferon pharmacology with monoclonal antibody. *Cancer Res*, 45, 2421–2424
- **Roskos LK, Cheung EN, Vincent M, Foote M, Morstyn G.** (1998). Pharmacology of Filgrastim (r-metHuG-CSF). In *Filgrastim (r-metHuG-CSF) in Clinical Practice*, edited by G Morstyn, TM Dexter, M Foote. Marcel Dekker, New York, pp. 51–71
- **Sandset PM, Abildgaard U, Larsen ML.** (1988). Heparin induces release of extrinsic coagulation pathway inhibitor (EPI). *Thrombosis Research*, 50, 803–813
- **Schwinghammer TL, Kroboth PD.** (1988). Basic Concepts in Pharmacodynamic Modeling. *Journal of Clinical Pharmacology*, 28, 388–394
- **Sell S**. (1987). *Immunology, immunopathology and immunity.* Amsterdam, Elsevier.
- **Shen BQ, DeGuzman GG, Zioncheck TZ**. (1997). Characterization of vascular endothelial growth factor binding to rat liver sinusoidal cells *in vitro*. Western Regional Meeting of the American Association of Pharmaceutical Scientists, South San Francisco
- **Steimer J-L, Ebelin M-E, Van Bree J.** (1993). Pharmacokinetic and Pharmacodynamic data and models in clinical trials. *European Journal of Drug Metabolism and Pharmacokinetics*, 18, 61–76
- **Stoudemire JB.** (1992). Pharmacokinetics and metabolism of hematopoietic proteins. In *Protein pharmacokinetics and metabolism*, edited by BL Ferraiolo, MA Mohler, CA Gloff. Plenum Press, New York, pp. 189–222
- **Strickland DK, Kounnas MZ, Argraves WS.** (1995). LDL receptor-related protein: a multiligand receptor for lipoprotein and proteinase catabolism. *Faseb J*, 9, 890–8
- **Sugiyama Y, Hanano M.** (1989). Receptor-mediated transport of peptide hormones and its importance in the overall hormone disposition in the body. *Pharm Res*, 6, 192–202
- **Supersaxo A, Hein W, Gallati H, Steffen H.** (1988). Recombinant human interferon alpha-2a: delivery to lymphoid tissue by selected modes of application. *Pharm Res*, 5, 472–476
- **Supersaxo A, Hein WR, Steffen H.** (1990). Effect of molecular weight on the lymphatic absorption of water-soluble compounds following subcutaneous administration. *Pharm Res*, 7, 167–169
- **Takagi A, Masuda H, Takakura Y, Hashida M.** (1995). Disposition characteristics of recombinant human interleukin-11 after a bolus intravenous administration in mice. *J Pharmacol Exper Ther*, 275, 537–543
- **Takakura Y, Fujita T, Hashida M, Sesaki H.** (1990). Disposition characteristics of macromolecules in tumor-bearing mice. *Pharm Res*, 7, 339–346
- **Tanaka H, Kaneko T.** (1991). Pharmacokinetics of recombinant human granulocyte colony-stimulating factor in the rat. *Drug Metabol Dispos*, 19, 200–204
- **Tanswell P.** (1992). Tissue-type plasminogen activator. In *Therapeutic proteins. Pharmacokinetics and pharmacodynamics*, edited by AHC Kung, RA Baughman, JW Larrick. W.H. Freeman and Company, New York, pp. 255–281
- **Tanswell P, Heinzel G, Greischel A, Krause J.** (1990). Nonlinear pharmacokinetics of tissue-type plasminogen activator in three animal species and isolated perfused rat liver. *Journal of Pharmacology and Experimental Therapeutics*, 255, 318–324
- **Taylor AE, Granger GN.** (1984). In *Handbook of physiology*, edited by EM Renkin and CC Michel. American Physiological Society, Bethesda, MD, pp. 467–520
- **Templeton DM.** (1992). Proteoglycans in cell regulation. *Critical Reviews in Clinical Laboratory Science*, 29, 141–184
- **Uehlinger DE, Gotch FA, Sheiner LB.** (1992). A pharmacodynamic model of erythropoietin therapy for uremic anemia. *Clinical Pharmacology and Therapeutics*, 51, 76–89
- **van Griensven JMT, Burggraaf KJ, Gerloff J, Gunzler WA, Beier H, Kroon R, Huisman LGM, Schoemaker RC, Kluft K, Cohen AF.** (1995). Effects of changing liver blood flow by exercise and food on kinetics and dynamics of saruplase. *Clin Pharmacol Ther*, 57, 381–389
- **van Griensven JMT, Huisman LGM, Stuurman T, Dooijewaard G, Kroon R, Schoemaker RC, Kluft K, Cohen AF.** (1996). Effect of increased liver blood flow on the kinetics and dynamics of recombinant tissue-type plasminogen activator. *Clin Pharmacol Ther*, 60, 504–511
- **Wall DA, Maack T.** (1985). Endocytic uptake, transport, and catabolism of proteins by epithelial cells. *Am J Physiol*, 248, C12–C20
- **Woodworth JR, Howey DC, Bowsher RR.** (1994). Establishment of time-action profiles for regular and NPH insulin using pharmacodynamic modeling. *Diabetes Care*, 17, 64–69
- **Working PK.** (1992). Potential effects of antibody induction by protein drugs. In *Protein pharmacokinetics and metabolism*, edited by BL Ferraiolo, MA Mohler, CA Gloff. Plenum Press, New York, pp. 73–92
- **Xie D, Hale VG.** (1996). Factors affecting the lymphatic absorption of macromolecules following extravascular administration. *Pharm Res*, 13, S-396
- **Yanagishita M, Hascall VC.** (1992). Cell surface heparan sulfate proteoglycans. *Journal of Biological Chemistry*, 267
- **Zapf J, Hauri C, Waldvogel M, Froesch ER.** (1986). Acute metabolic effects and hslf-lives of intravenous insulin-like growth factor I and II in normal and hypophysectomized rats. *J Clin Invest*, 77, 1768–1775
- **Ziegler K, Polzin G, Frimmer M.** (1988). Hepatocellular uptake of cyclosporin A by simple diffusion. *Biochim Biophys Acta*, 938, 44–50
- **Zoon K, Stein K, Bekisz J, Schwieterman A.** (1999). Immune Reactions Against Therapeutic and Diagnostic Biological Products. Meeting of the Biological Response Modifiers Advisory Committee, Bethesda, MD

Self-Assessment Questions

Question 1: *What are the major elimination pathways for protein drugs after administration?*

Question 2: *Which pathway of absorption is rather unique for proteins after sc injection?*

Question 3: *Explain counterclockwise hysteresis in plasma concentration-effect plots.*

Question 4: *What is the role of plasma binding proteins for natural proteins?*

Question 5: *How do the sugar groups on glycoproteins influence hepatic elimination of these glycoproteins?*

Question 6: *In which direction might elimination clearance of protein drug change when antibodies are produced after chronic dosing with protein drugs? Why?*

Answers

Answer 1: Proteolysis, glomerular filtration followed by tubular reabsorption and catabolism, renal peritubular absorption followed by catabolism, receptor-mediated endocytosis followed by metabolism in the liver and possibly other cells.

Answer 2: Biodistribution from the injection site into the lymphatics.

Answer 3: Counterclockwise hysteresis is an indication of the indirect nature of the effects seen for many protein drugs. It can be explained by delays between the appearance of drug in plasma and the appearance of the pharmacodynamic response, by processes such as distribution into the biophase or cascade-type post-receptor events.

Answer 4: Plasma proteins may act as circulating reservoirs for the proteins that are their ligands. Consequently, the protein ligands may be protected from elimination and distribution. In some cases, protein binding may protect the organism from undesirable, acute effects; in other cases, receptor binding may be facilitated by the binding protein.

Answer 5: In some cases, the sugar groups are recognized by hepatic receptors (galactose by the galactose receptor, for example), facilitating receptor-mediated uptake and metabolism. In other cases, sugar chains and terminal sugar groups (terminal sialic acid residues, for example) may shield the protein from binding to receptors and hepatic uptake.

Answer 6: Clearance may increase of decrease by binding to antibodies. A decrease of clearance occurs when the antibody-protein complex is eliminated slower than free drug. An increase of clearance occurs when the protein-antibody complex is eliminated more rapidly than the unbound protein, such as when reticuloendothelial uptake is stimulated by the complex.

6 Genomics, Proteomics and Additional Biotechnology-Related Techniques

Robert D. Sindelar

Introduction

Until recently, the techniques made available by advances in molecular biology and biotechnology that have provided currently approved therapeutic agents generally fell into two broad areas: recombinant DNA (rDNA) technology and hybridoma techniques (to produce monoclonal antibodies). A wealth of additional and innovative biotechnologies, however, have been, and will continue to be, developed in order to explore the human genome, better understand the relationship between genetics and biological function, unravel the causes of disease, and enhance pharmaceutical research. These revolutionary technologies and additional biotechnology-related techniques are improving the very competitive process of drug discovery and development of new medicinal agents and diagnostics. Some of the technologies and techniques described in this chapter are both well-established and commonly used applications of biotechnology producing potential therapeutic products now in clinical trials. Still more applications are evolving as you read this text. Their full impact on the future of molecular medicine has yet to be imagined.

No meaningful discussion of pharmaceutical biotechnology and 21st century healthcare can occur without mention of genomics and proteomics. Research in genomics and proteomics is heralded as the next important supply source of innovative future drug design targets. With the Human Genome Project rapidly approaching closure, researchers are turning increasingly to the task of converting the DNA sequence data into information that will potentially improve, and perhaps even revolutionize, drug discovery (see Figure 6.1) and pharmaceutical care. Pharmaceutical scientists are poised to take advantage of this scientific breakthrough by incorporating state-of-the-art genomics and proteomics techniques along with the associated technologies utilized in bioinformatics and pharmacogenomics into a new drug discovery and development paradigm.

Techniques such as genetically engineered animals (including transgenic animals and knockout mice), protein engineering, peptide chemistry and peptidomimetics, nucleic acid technologies (including antisense technology, aptamer technology, and ribozyme catalysis), catalytic antibodies, the rapidly emerging field of glycobiology, and tissue engineering are directly influencing the pharmaceutical sciences and are well positioned to impact significantly modern pharmaceutical care. These additional techniques in biotechnology and molecular biology are being rapidly exploited to bring new drugs to market.

It is not the intention of this author to detail each and every biotechnology technique exhaustively, since numerous specialized resources already meet that need. Rather,

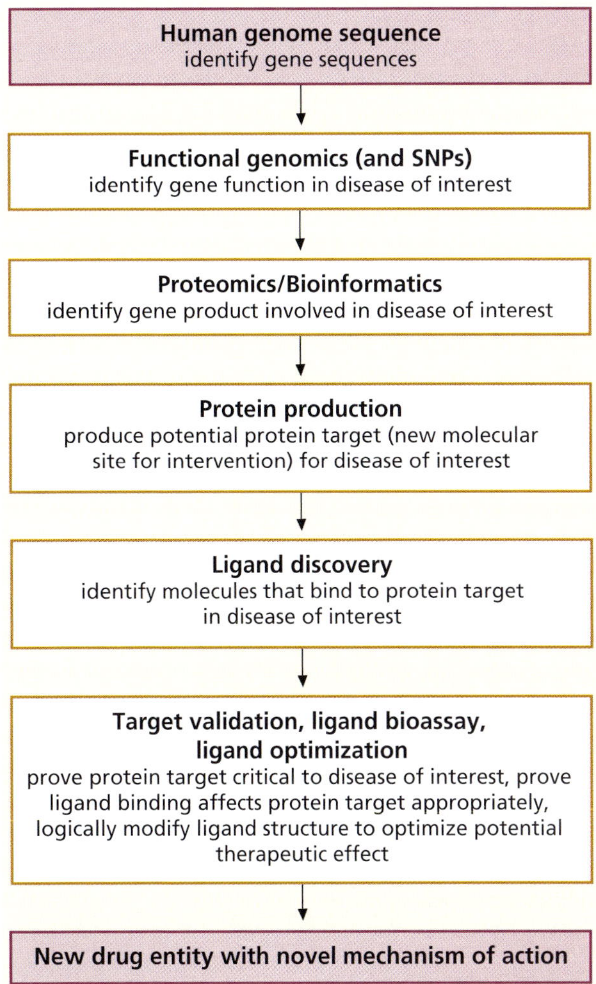

Figure 6.1. The genomics strategy for new drug discovery and individualized optimized medicine.

this chapter will illustrate and enumerate various biotechnologies that should be of key interest to pharmacy students, practising pharmacists, and pharmaceutical scientists because of their effect on many aspects of pharmacy.

Genomics, Proteomics and Pharmacogenetics/Genomics

Since the discovery of DNA's overall structure in 1953, the world's scientific community has continued to gain a better understanding of the genetic information encoded by DNA and the genetic information carried by a cell or organism. In the 1980s and 1990s, biotechnology techniques produced novel therapeutics and a wealth of information about the mechanisms of various diseases such as cancer. Yet the etiology of many other diseases, including obesity and heart disease, remained unknown at the genetic and the molecular level, presenting no obvious target to attack with a small molecule drug or biotechnology-produced therapeutic agent. The answers were hidden in what was unknown about the human genome. Despite the increasing knowledge of DNA structure and function in the 1990s, the genome, the entire collection of genes and all other functional and non-functional DNA sequences in the nucleus of an organism, had yet to be sequenced. DNA may well be the largest, naturally occurring molecule known. Successfully meeting the challenge of sequencing the entire human genome is one of history's great milestones and heralds enormous potential. While the genetic code for transcription and translation has been known for years, sequencing the human genome provides a blueprint for all human proteins and the sequences of all regulatory elements that govern the developmental interpretation of the genome. The potential significance includes identifying genetic determinants of common and rare diseases, providing a methodology for their diagnosis, suggesting interesting new molecular sites for intervention (see Figure 6.1), and the development of new biotechnologies to bring about their eradication. Unlocking the secrets of the human genome may lead to a paradigm shift in clinical practice toward true targeted molecular medicine and patient-specific therapy.

Structural Genomics and the Human Genome Project

Genomics is the comparative study of the complete genome sequence and its function from different organisms (Wiley, 1998; Brown, 1999). Initially, genetic analysis focused on structural genomics, basically the characterization of the structure of the genome. Structural genomics intersects the techniques of DNA sequencing, cloning, PCR, protein expression, crystallography, and data analysis. Proposed in the late 1980s, the publicly funded Human Genome Project (HGP) or Human Genome Initiative (HGI) was officially sanctioned in October 1990 to map the structure and to sequence human DNA (Collins and Galas, 1993; Cantor and Smith, 1999). As described in Table 6.1, HGP structural genomics was envisioned to proceed through increasing

Human genome project goals	Base pair resolution
Detailed genetic linkage map Comments: Poorest resolution; depicts relative chromosomal locations of DNA markers, genes, or other markers and the spacing between them on each chromosome.	2 Mb *)
Complete physical map Comments: Instead of relative distances between markers, maps actual physical distance in base pairs between markers; lower resolution = actual observance of chromosomal banding under microscope; higher resolution is "restriction map" generated in presence of restriction enzymes.	0.1 Mb
Complete DNA sequence Comments: The ultimate goal; determine the base sequence of the genes and markers found in mapping techniques along with the other segments of the entire genome; techniques commonly used include DNA amplification methods such as cloning, PCR and other techniques described in Chapter 1 along with novel sequencing and bioinformatics techniques.	1 bp **)

Table 6.1. The increasing levels of genetic resolution obtained from structural genomic studies of the HGP. *) Mb = megabase = 1 million base pairs, **) bp = base pair

levels of genetic resolution: detailed human genetic linkage maps [approximately 2 megabase pairs (Mb = million base pairs) resolution], complete physical maps (0.1 Mb resolution), and ultimately complete DNA sequencing of the approximately 3.5 billion base pairs (23 pairs of chromosomes) in a human cell nucleus [1 base pair (bp) resolution] (Griffiths *et al.*, 2000). Projected for completion in 2003, the goal of the project was to learn not only what was contained in the genetic code, but also how to "mine" the genomic information to cure or help prevent the estimated 4000 genetic diseases afflicting humankind. In May 1999, 700 million base pairs of the human genome were deposited in public archives. After merely fifteen months of additional studies, the figure had increased to greater than 4 billion base pairs (Pennisi, 2000). Two years earlier than projected, a milestone in genomic science was reached on June 26, 2000, when researchers at the privately funded Celera Genomics and the Genome International Sequencing Consortium (the international collaboration associated with the HGP) jointly announced that they had completed sequencing 97 to 99% of the human genome. The journal *Science* rates the mapping of the human genome as its "breakthrough of the year" in its December 22, 2000 issue. The two groups published their results in 2001 (Vinter *et al.*, 2001; The Genome International Sequencing Consortium, 2001).

The genome sequencing strategies of the HGP and Celera Genomics differed (Brown, 2000). HGP utilized a "nested shotgun" approach. The human DNA sequence was "chopped" into segments of ever decreasing size and the segments put into rough order. Each segment was further "blasted" into small fragments. Each small fragment was sequenced and the sequenced fragments assembled according to their known relative order. The Celera researchers employed a "whole shotgun" approach where they "blasted" the whole genome into small fragments. Each fragment was sequenced and assembled in order by identifying where they overlapped. Each approach required unprecedented computer resources (the field of bioinformatics is described later in this chapter). Regardless of genome sequencing strategies, the collective results are impressive. More than 27 million high quality sequence reads provided a 5-fold coverage of the entire human genome. Genomic studies have identified over 1 million single nucleotide polymorphisms (SNPs), binary elements of genetic variability (SNPs are described later in this chapter). While original estimates of the number of human genes in the genome varied consistently between 80,000–120,000, the genome researchers unveiled a number far short of biologist's predictions; 32,000 (Vinter *et al.*, 2001; The Genome International Sequencing Consortium, 2001). Within months, others suggested that the human genome possesses between 65,000 and 75,000 genes (Wright *et al.*, 2001). Further research is needed to establish the actual number of human genes.

Functional and Comparative Genomics

Sequencing the entire genome may now be a reality, but the chore of sorting through human and pathogen diversity factors and correlating them with genomic data to provide real pharmaceutical benefits has barely begun. Pharmaceutical company drug pipelines are loaded with promising therapeutic agent leads, due in large part to the application of biotechnology to the discovery process. Early supporters of the human genome project characterized it as a potential medical panacea that would rapidly add to the pipeline. However, translating genomics discoveries from the bench top to the patient's bedside requires a clear understanding of the direct relationship between genes and their function. The DNA sequence information itself rarely provides definitive information about the function and regulation of that particular gene. Yet there is little doubt that completing the human genome sequence will dramatically alter prevention, treatment, and even our definition of disease (Temple *et al.*, 2001). One approach to solve this disconnect is the study of functional genomics (Hunt and Livesey, 2000). Functional genomics is a new approach to genetic analysis that focuses on genome-wide patterns of gene expression, the mechanisms by which gene expression is coordinated, and the interrelationships of gene expression when a cellular environmental change occurs. After genome sequencing, this approach is the next step in the knowledge chain to identify functional gene products that are potential biotech drug leads and new drug discovery targets (see Figure 6.1).

To relate functional genomics to therapeutic clinical outcomes, the human genome sequence must reveal the thousands of genetic variations among individuals that will become associated with diseases in the patient's lifetime. Sequencing alone is not the end, simply the end of the beginning of the genomic medicine era. Determining gene functionality in any organism opens the door for linking a disease to specific genes or proteins, which become targets for new drugs or methods to detect organisms (i.e. new diagnostic agents).

The face of biology has changed forever with the sequencing of the genomes of numerous organisms. Biotechnologies applied to the sequencing of the human genome are also being utilized to sequence the genomes of comparatively simple organisms as well as other mammals. Often, the proteins encoded by the genomes of lesser organisms and the regulation of those genes closely resemble the proteins and gene regulation in humans. Since model organisms are much easier to maintain in a laboratory setting, researchers are actively pursuing "comparative" genomics studies (Clark, 1999). To date, genome sequencing is completed for *Drosophila melanogaster* (fruit fly; 180 Mb), *Saccharomyces cerevisiae* (baker's yeast; 12.1 Mb), and *Caenorhabditis elegans* (nemotode; 97 Mb). The Mouse

Genome Sequencing Network and other laboratories are actively working on the mouse genome. Unlocking genomic data for each of these organisms provides valuable insight into the molecular basis of inherited human disease (Karow, 2000). *S. cerevisiae* is a good model for studying cancer and is a common organism used in rDNA methodology. For example, it has become well known that women who inherit a gene mutation of the *BRCA1* gene have a high risk, perhaps as high as 85%, of developing breast cancer before the age of 50 (source: www.ncbi.nlm.nih.gov). The first diagnostic product generated from genomic data was the *BRCA1* test for breast cancer predisposition. The gene product of *BRCA1* is a well-characterized protein implicated in both breast and ovarian cancer. Evidence has accumulated suggesting that the Rad9 protein of *S. cerevisiae* is distantly, but significantly, related to the *BRCA1* protein. The fruit fly possesses a gene similar to *p53*, the human tumor suppressor gene. Much of our early knowledge of apoptosis, the normal biological process of programmed cell death, has been learned by studying *C. elegans*. Greater than 90% of the proteins identified thus far from a common laboratory animal, the mouse, have structural similarities to known human proteins.

Not all comparative genomic studies are looking for similarities to the human genome. For example, some may provide the basis for creating new and novel potential antibiotic targets for drug design (Guild, 1999). Comparative genomics is being used to provide a compilation of genes that code for proteins that are essential to the growth or viability of a pathogenic organism, yet differ from any human protein. Assuring selective toxicity to the organism, not the human patient, this genomic mining of new targets for drug design may aid the quest for new antibiotics in a clinical environment of increasing incidence of antibiotic resistance.

Proteomics

Functional genomics research will provide an unprecedented information resource for the study of biochemical pathways at the molecular level. Certainly a large number of the 32,000 genes identified in sequencing the human genome will be shown to be functionally important in various disease states. This will result in the identification of a vast array of proteins implicated as playing pivotal roles in disease processes. Some have anticipated 10,000 therapeutic targets resulting from the genome sequence information (Edwards *et al.*, 2000). These key identified proteins will serve as potential new sites for therapeutic intervention (see Figure 6.1). A new research area called proteomics seeks to define the function and correlate that with expression profiles of all proteins encoded within a genome (Blackstock and Weit, 1999; Borman, 2000; Edwards *et al.*, 2000; Persidis, 1998a). Less than a decade old, the concept of proteomics requires determination of the structural, biochemical and physiological repertoire of all proteins. Proteomics may be a greater scientific challenge than genomics due to the intricacy of protein expression and the complexity of 3-D protein structure as it relates to biological activity (Saeks, 2001). Protein expression, isolation, purification, identification, and characterization are among the key procedures utilized in proteomics research. To perform these procedures, technology platforms such as 2-D gel electrophoresis, mass spectrometry, chip-based microarrays (discussed later in this chapter), X-ray crystallography (discussed later in this chapter), protein nmr (also discussed later in this chapter), and phage displays are employed. Pharmaceutical scientists anticipate that many of the proteins identified by proteomic research will be entirely novel, possessing unknown functions. This scenario offers not only a unique opportunity to identify previously unknown molecular targets, but also to develop new ultrasensitive diagnostics to address unmet clinical needs.

Today's methodology does not allow us to identify valid drug targets and new diagnostic methodologies simply by examining gene sequence information. However, "in silico proteomics", the computer-based prediction of 3-D protein structure, intermolecular interactions, and functionality is currently a very active area of research (Roberts and Swinton, 2001).

Often, multiple genes and their protein products are involved in a single disease process. Since few proteins act alone, studying protein interactions will be paramount to a full understanding of functionality. Also, many abnormalities in cell function may result from over-expression of a gene and/or protein, under-expression of a gene and/or protein, a gene mutation causing a malformed protein, and post-translation modification changes that alter a protein's function. Therefore, the real value of human genome sequence data will only be realized after every protein coded by the 32,000 genes has a function assigned to it.

Bioinformatics

Structural genomics, functional genomics, and proteomics studies have generated an enormous volume of data to store. The entire encoded human DNA sequence alone requires computer storage of approximately 10^9 bits of information: the equivalent of a thousand 500-page books! The HGP and other genome sequencing research organizations continue to produce some of the largest databases in the world. GenBank (managed by the National Center for Biotechnology Information, NCBI, of the National Institutes of Health), the European Molecular Biology Laboratory (EMBL), and the DNA Data Bank of Japan (DDBJ) are three of the centers worldwide that collaborate on collecting DNA sequences. GenBank alone stores more than 12 million sequences. Once stored, analyzing the wealth of genomic and proteomic data, (i.e. comparing and relating information from various sources) to identify useful characteristics or trends, such as selecting a group of drug targets from all proteins in the human body, presents a Herculean task.

Scientists have applied advances in information technology, innovative software algorithms and massive parallel computing to the on-going research in genetics, genomics, proteomics, and related areas to give birth to the new field of bioinformatics (Emmett, 2000; Felton, 2001; Watkins, 2001). Bioinformatics is the application of computer technologies to the biological sciences with the object of discovering knowledge. With bioinformatics, a researcher can now better exploit the tremendous flood of genomic and proteomic data, more cost-effectively data mining for a drug discovery "needle" in that massive data "haystack". In this case, data mining refers to the bioinformatics approach to "sifting" through volumes of raw data, identifying and extracting relevant information, and developing useful relationships among them. Modern drug discovery will utilize bioinformatics techniques to gather information from multiple sources (such as the HGP, functional genomic studies, proteomics, phenotyping, patient medical records, and bioassay results), integrate the data, apply life science developed algorithms, and generate useful target identification and drug lead identification data. Another goal of bioinformatics is to be able to study the molecules and processes discovered by genomics and proteomics research in silico: that is, to be able to predict chemical and physical structure and properties by computer.

The massive scientific effort embodied in the Human Genome Project and the development of bioinformatics technologies have catalyzed fundamental changes in the practice of modern biology (Aderem and Hood, 2001). Biology has become an information science defining all the elements in a complex biological system and placing them in a database for comparative interpretation. As seen in Figure 6.2, the hierarchy of information collection goes well beyond the biodata contained in the genetic code that is transcribed and translated.

DNA Microarrays and Oligonucleotide Microarrays

The biochips known as DNA microarrays and oligonucleotide microarrays are a surface collection of hundreds to thousands of immobilized DNA sequences or oligonucleotides created with specialized equipment that can be simultaneously examined to conduct expression analysis (Khan *et al.*, 1999; Lipschutz *et al.*, 1999; Ramsey, 1998; Southern, 2001). Biochips may contain representatives of a particular set of gene sequences (i.e. sequences coding for all human cytochrome P450 isozymes) or may contain sequences representing all genes of an organism.

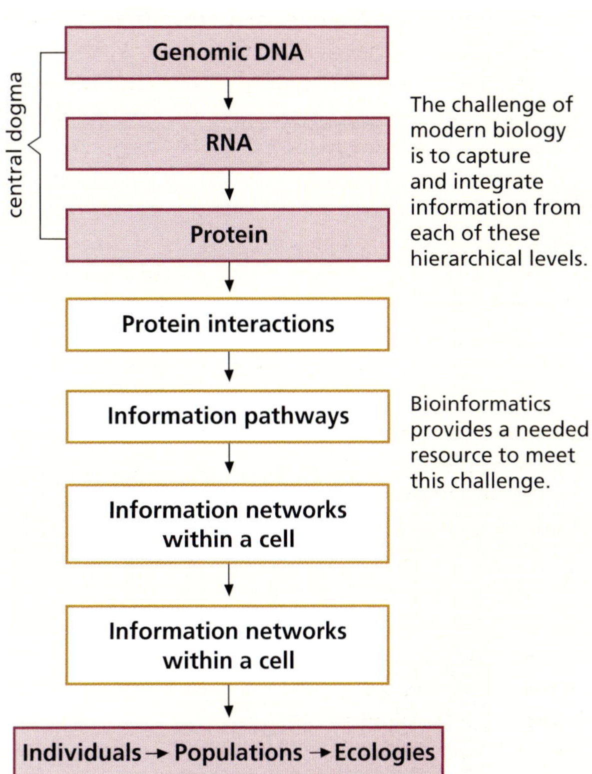

Figure 6.2. The information challenge of systems biology in the genomics era (see Aderem and Hood, 2001).

Commonly, arrays are prepared on non-porous supports, such as glass microscope slides. DNA microarrays generally contain high-density microspotted cDNA sequences approximately 1 Kb in length representing thousands of genes. The field was advanced significantly when technology was developed to synthesize closely spaced oligonucleotides on glass wafers using semiconductory industry photolithographic masking techniques (see Figure 6.3). Oligonucleotide microarrays (often called oligonucleotide arrays or DNA chips) contain closely spaced synthetic gene-specific oligonucleotides representing thousands of gene sequences. Microarrays can provide expression analysis for mRNAs. Screening of DNA variation is also possible. Thus, biochips can provide polymorphism detection and genotyping as well as hybridization-based expression monitoring.

Microarray analysis has gained increasing significance as a direct result of the genome sequencing studies. Array technology is a logical tool for studying functional genomics since the results obtained may link function to expression. Microarray technology's potential to study key areas of molecular medicine is unlimited at this stage of development. For example, gene expression levels of thousands of mRNA species may be studied simultaneously in normal versus cancer cells, each incubated with potential anticancer drug candidates.

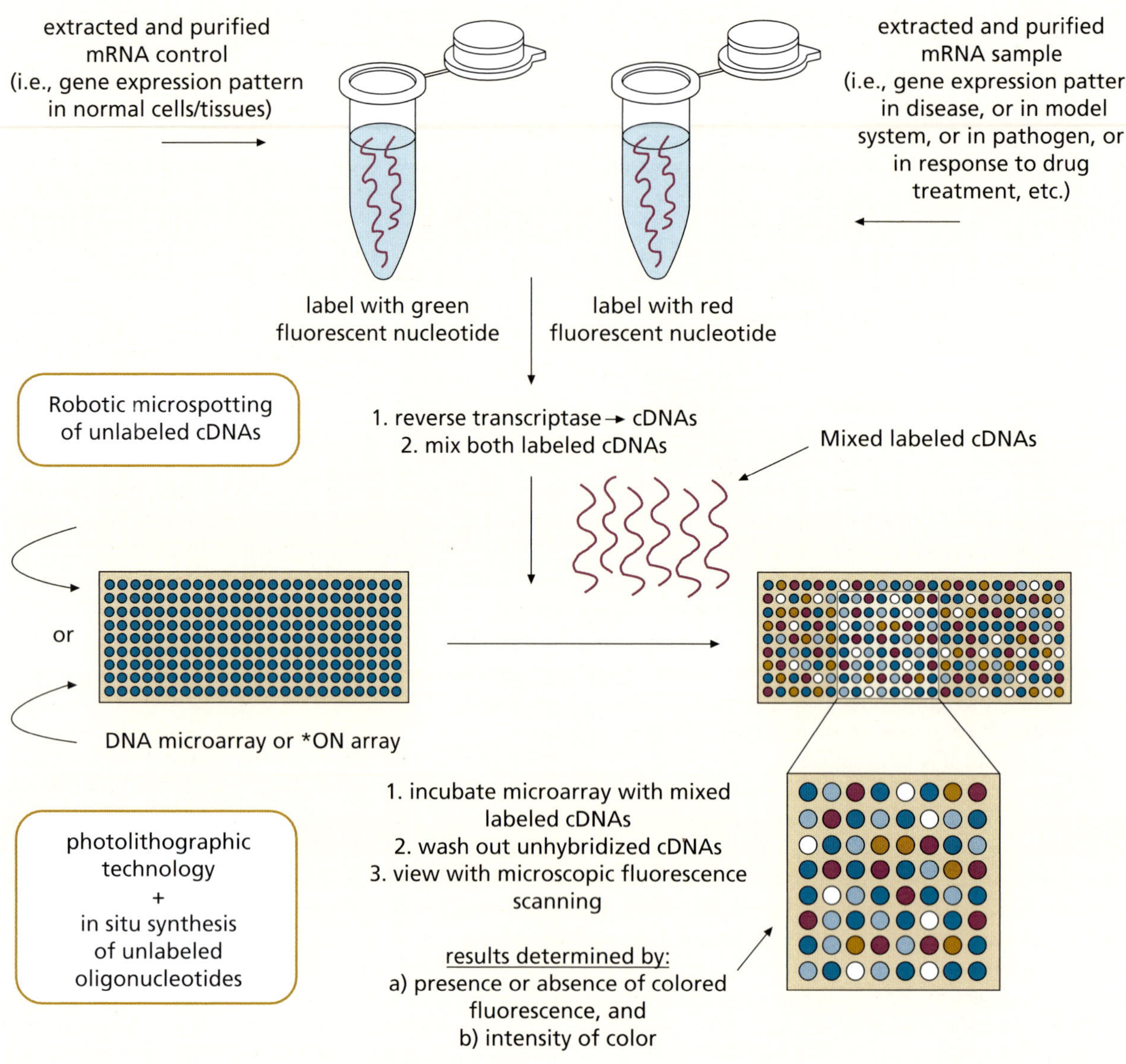

Figure 6.3. Principle of operation of a representative DNA microarray or oligonucleotide (*ON) microarray.

Single Nucleotide Polymorphisms (SNPs)

While comparing the base sequences in the DNA of two individuals reveals them to be approximately 99.9 per cent identical, base differences, or polymorphisms, are scattered throughout the genome. The best-characterized human polymorphisms are single nucleotide polymorphisms (SNPs) occurring approximately once every 1000 bases in the 3.5 billion base pair human genome (Cargill *et al.*, 1999; Silber, 2001). Commonly referred to as "snips", these subtle sequence variations account for most of the genetic differences observed among humans. Thus, they can be utilized to determine inheritance of genes in successive generations.

Research suggests that, in general, humans tolerate SNPs as a probable survival mechanism. This tolerance may result because most SNPs occur in non-coding regions of the genome. Identifying SNPs occurring in gene coding regions (cSNPs) and/or regulatory sequences may hold the key for elucidating complex, polygenic diseases such as cancer, heart disease, and diabetes, and understanding the differences in response to drug therapy observed in individual patients (Grant and Phillips, 2001; also see SNP Consortium website, http://snp.cshl.org/). Some cSNPs do not result in amino acid substitutions in their gene's protein product(s) due to the degeneracy of the genetic code. These cSNPs are referred to as synonymous cSNPs.

Other cSNPs, known as non-synonymous, can produce conservative amino acid changes, such as similarity in sidechain charge or size, or more significant amino acid substitutions.

SNPs, when associated with epidemiological and pathological data, can be used to track susceptibilities to common diseases such as cancer, heart disease, and diabetes (Pfost *et al.*, 2000; Gura, 2001). Biomedical researchers have recognized that discovering SNPs linked to diseases will lead potentially to the identification of new drug targets and diagnostic tests. The projected impact of SNPs on our understanding of human disease led to the formation of the SNP Consortium in 1999, an international research collaboration involving pharmaceutical companies, academic laboratories, and private support.

Pharmacogenetics and Pharmacogenomics

Tremendous advances in biotechnology are causing a dramatic shift in the way new pharmaceuticals are discovered, developed, and monitored during patient use. Pharmacists will utilize the knowledge gained from genomics and proteomics to tailor drug therapy to meet the needs of their individual patients employing the fields of pharmacogenetics and pharmacogenomics (Ball and Borman, 1997; Persidis, 1998b; Evans and Relling, 1999; Lau and Sakul, 2000; Pettipher and Holford, 2000).

Pharmacogenetics is the study of how an individual's genetic differences influence drug action, usage, and dosing. A detailed knowledge of a patient's pharmacogenetics in relation to a particular drug therapy may lead to enhanced efficacy and greater safety. Table 6.2 provides some examples of therapeutic drug classes for which patient response to drugs is considered poor or no response is observed in as many as 70% of patients administered. Pharmacogenetics analysis may identify the responsive patient population prior to administration.

The field of pharmacogenetics is almost 50 years old, but is undergoing renewed, exponential growth at this time. Of particular interest in the field of pharmacogenetics is our understanding of the genetic influences on drug pharmacokinetic profiles such as genetic variations among patients affecting liver enzymes such as the cytochrome P450 group (Nelson, 2000). It is well recognized that specific drug metabolizer phenotypes may cause adverse drug reactions. For instance, some patients lack an enzymatically active form, have a diminished level, or possess a modified version of CYP2D6 (a cytochrome P450 allele) and will metabolize certain classes of pharmaceutical agents differently to other patients expressing the native active enzyme. All pharmacogenetic polymorphisms examined to date differ in frequency among racial and ethnic groups. For example, CYP2D6 enzyme deficiencies may occur in $\leq$ 2% Asian patients, $\leq$ 5% black patients and $\leq$11% white patients (Freeman, 2001). A diagnostic test to detect CYP2D6 deficiency could be used to identify patients that should not be administered drugs metabolized predominantly by CYP2D6. Also, pharmacogenetics represents one of many genetic responses to environmental impacts affecting human biochemistry and drug action (Kalow, 1997).

A classic application of pharmacogenetics is our present understanding of the potentially fatal hematopoietic toxicity that occurs in some patients administered standard doses of the antileukemic agents azathioprine, mercaptopurine and thioguanine (Lennard, 1998). These drugs are metabolized by the enzyme thiopurine methyltransferase (TPMT) to the inactive S-methylated products. Gene mutations (polymorphisms) may occur in as many as 11% of patients resulting in decreased TPMT-mediated metabolism of the thiopurine drugs. A diagnostic test for TPMT is now available. Identified patients with poor TPMT metabolism may need their drug dose lowered 10–15 fold.

While sometimes used interchangeably (especially in pharmacy practice literature), pharmacogenetics and

Therapeutic drug class	Disease state	% poor or no response
butyrophenones, dibenzodiazepines, benzisoxazoles	schizophrenia	25–75%
histamine H2 antagonists, proton pump inhibitors	duodenal ulcer	20–70%
HMGCoA reductase inhibitors	hyperlipidemia	30–75%
sulfonylureas, glitazones	type II diabetes	50–75%
thiazides, ACE inhibitors, beta-blockers	hypertension	10–70%

Table 6.2. Examples of poor or no response to pharmacotherapy in as many as 70% of patients (Data from Silber, 2001).

pharmacogenomics are subtly different (Kalow, 2001). Pharmacogenomics introduces the additional element of our present technical ability to pinpoint patient-specific DNA variation using genomics techniques. While overlapping fields of study, pharmacogenomics is a much newer term that correlates an individual patient's DNA variation (SNP level of variation knowledge rather than gene level of variation knowledge) with his or her response to pharmacotherapy.

Individualized optimized molecular medicine utilizing pharmacogenomic knowledge would not only spot disease before it occurs in a patient, increase drug efficacy upon pharmacotherapy, and reduce drug toxicity, it would also facilitate the drug development process (see Figure 6.1) including improving clinical development outcomes, reducing overall cost of drug development, leading to development of new diagnostic tests that impact on therapeutic decisions, etc. Individualized optimized pharmacotherapy would first require a detailed genetic analysis of a patient, assembling a comprehensive list of SNPs. Pharmacogenomic tests would be administered to pre-identify responsive patients before dosing with a specific agent. The impact of the patient's SNPs on the use of new or existing drugs would thus be predicted, and individualized drug therapy would be identified that assures maximal efficacy and minimal toxicity. This will become especially important in cases where the cost of testing is either less than the cost of the drug, or the cost of correcting adverse drug reactions caused by the drug. Pharmaceutical care would begin by identifying a patient's susceptibility to a disease, then administering the right drug to the right patient at the right time. For example, the monoclonal antibody trastuzumab (Herceptin) is a breast cancer therapy specifically directed to the HER2 gene product (25–30% of human breast cancers over-express the human epidermal growth factor receptor, HER2 protein). Exhibiting reduced side-effects as compared to standard chemotherapy due to this protein target specificity, trastuzumab is not prescribed to treat a breast cancer patient unless the patient has first tested positive for HER2 over-expression. While currently an immunohistochemical assay, not a sophisticated DNA microarray assay, the example shows the power of such future tests.

Genetically Engineered Animals

For thousands of years, man has selectively bred animals and plants either to enhance or to create desirable traits in numerous species. The explosive development of recombinant DNA technology and other molecular biology techniques have made it possible to engineer species possessing particular unique and distinguishing genetic characteristics. The genetic material of an animal can be manipulated so that extra genes may be inserted (transgenes), replaced (i.e. human gene homologs coding for related human proteins), or deleted (knockout). Theoretically, these approaches enable the introduction of virtually any gene into any organism. A greater understanding of specific gene regulation and expression will contribute to important new discoveries made in relevant animal models. Such genetically altered species have found utility in a myriad of research and potential commercial applications including the generation of models of human disease, protein drug production, creation of organs and tissues for xenotransplantation, and a host of agricultural uses (Brooks, 1998).

Engineered animal models are proving invaluable to pharmaceutical research since small animal models of disease are often poor mimics of that disease in human patients. Genetic engineering can predispose an animal to a particular disease under scrutiny and the insertion of human genes into the animal can initiate the development of a more clinically relevant disease condition. Also, it is possible to screen potential drug candidates *in vivo* against a human receptor target inserted into an animal model. The number of examples of transgenic animal models of human disease useful in drug discovery and development efforts is growing rapidly (Swanson *et al.*, 1994). Such models have potential to increase the efficiency and decrease the cost of drug discovery and development by reducing the time it takes to move a medicinal agent from discovery into clinical trials. Table 6.3 provides a list of some selected examples of genetically engineered animal models of human disease.

Transgenic Animals

Transgenic animals contain either foreign DNA (a transgene) that has been incorporated into their genome or endogenous genomic DNA that has had its molecular structure manipulated (Isola and Gordon, 1991; Lodish *et al.*, 2000). While there are some similarities between transgenic technology and gene therapy (see Chapter 7), it is important to distinguish clearly between them. Technically speaking, the introduction of foreign DNA sequences into a living cell is called gene transfer. Thus, one method to create a transgenic animal involves gene transfer (transgene incorporated into the genome). Gene therapy is also a gene transfer procedure and, in a sense, produces a transgenic human. In transgenic animals, however, the foreign gene is transferred indiscriminately into all cells, including germ line cells. The process of gene therapy differs generally from transgenesis since it involves a transfer of the desired gene in such a way that involves only specific somatic and hematopoietic cells, and not germ cells. Thus unlike in gene therapy, the genetic changes in transgenic organisms are conserved in any offspring according to the general rules of Mendelian inheritance (see Chapter 7).

The production of transgenic animals is not a new technology. They have been produced since the 1970s. However, modern biotechnology has greatly improved the

Genetic Engineering	Gene a)	Disease model
knockout	*BRCA1, BRCA2*	breast cancer
knockout	apolipoprotein E	atherosclerosis
knockout	glucocerebrosidase	Gaucher's disease
knockout	HPRT	Lesch-Nyhan syndrome
knockout	hexokinase A	Tay-Sachs disease
knockout	human CFTR	cystic fibrosis
knockout	p53	cancer suppressor gene deletion
knockout	P-glycoprotein	multidrug resistance (MDR)
knockout	α-globin and β-globin	sickle cell anemia
knockout	urate oxidase	gout
knockout	retinoblastoma-1	familial retinoblastoma
transgene	c-*neu* oncogene	cancer
transgene	c-*myc* oncogene	cancer
transgene	growth hormone	dwarfism
transgene	H-*ras* oncogene	cancer
transgene	histocompatibility antigens	autoimmunity
transgene	HIV *tat*	Kaposi sarcoma
transgene	human APP	Alzheimer's disease
transgene	human β-globin	thalassemia
transgene	human CD4 expression	HIV infection
transgene	human β-globin mutant	sickle cell anemia
transgene	human CETP	atherosclerosis
transgene	LDL receptor	hypercholesterolemia

Table 6.3. Some selected examples of genetically engineered animal disease models.
a) Key abbreviations: BRCA1, BRCA2 = suspected breast cancer genes; CETP = cholesterol (cholesteryl) ester transfer protein; CFTR = cyctic fibrosis transport regulator; HIV = human immunodeficiency virus; HPRT = hypoxanthine phosphoribosyl transferase; LDL = low-density lipoprotein.

methods of inducing the genetic transformation. While the mouse has been the most studied animal species, transgenic technology has been applied to cattle, fish, goats, poultry, rabbits, rats, sheep, swine, and various lower animal forms. Transgenic animals have already made valuable research contributions to studies involving regulation of gene expression, the function of the immune system, genetic diseases, viral diseases, cardiovascular disease, and the genes responsible for the development of cancer. Each of these applications is used in the drug discovery and development process.

Production of transgenic animals by DNA microinjection and random gene addition

The production of transgenic animals has most commonly involved the microinjection (also called gene transfer) of 100–200 copies of exogenous transgene DNA into the larger, more visible male pronucleus (as compared to the female pronucleus) of a recipient fertilized embryo (see Figure 6.4). The transgene contains both the DNA encoding the desired target amino acid sequence along with regulatory sequences that will mediate the expression of the added gene. The microinjected eggs are then implanted into the reproductive tract of a female and allowed to develop into embryos. The foreign DNA generally becomes randomly inserted at a single site on just one of the host chromosomes (i.e. the founder transgenic animal is heterozygous). Thus each transgenic founder animal (positive transgene incorporated animals) is a unique species. Interbreeding of founder transgenic animals where the transgene has been incorporated into germ cells may result in the birth of a homozygous progeny provided the transgene incorporation did not induce a mutation of an essential endogenous gene. All cells of the transgenic animal will contain the transgene if DNA insertion occurs prior to the first cell division. However, usually only 20%–25% of the offspring contain detectable levels of the transgene. Selection of neonatal animals possessing an incorporated transgene can readily be accomplished either by the direct identification of specific DNA or mRNA sequences or by the observation of gross phenotypic characteristics.

Production of transgenic animals by retroviral infection

The production of the first genetically altered laboratory mouse embryos was by insertion of a transgene via a modified retroviral vector. The non-replicating viral vector binds to the embryonic host cells, allowing subsequent transfer and insertion of the transgene into the host genome. Many of the experimental human gene therapy trials employ the same viral vectors (see Chapter 7 for further details on the use and types of viral vectors). Advantages of this method of transgene production are the ease with which genes can be introduced into embryos at various stages of development, and the characteristic that only a single copy of the transgene is usually integrated into the genome. Disadvantages include possible genetic recombination of the viral vector with other viruses present, the size limitation of the introduced DNA (up to 7kb of DNA, less than the size of some genes), and the difficulty in preparing certain viral vectors.

Production of transgenic animals by homologous recombination in embryonic stem cells following microinjection of DNA

Transgenic animals can also be produced by the *in vitro* genetic alteration of pluripotent embryonic stem cells (ES cells) (see Figure 6.5) (Sedivy and Joyner, 1992). ES cell technology is more efficient at creating transgenics than microinjection protocols. ES cells, a cultured cell line derived from the inner cell mass (blastocyst) of a blastocyte (early preimplantation embryo), are capable of having their genomic DNA modified while retaining their ability to contribute to both somatic and germ cell lineages. The desired gene is incorporated into ES cells by one of several methods such as microinjection. This is followed by introduction of the genetically modified ES cells into the blastocyst of an early preimplantation embryo, selection and culturing of targeted ES cells which are transferred subsequently to the reproductive tract of the surrogate host animal. The resulting progeny is screened for evidence that the desired genetic modification is present and selected appropriately. In mice, the process results in approximately 30% of the progeny containing tissue genetically derived from the incorporated ES cells. Interbreeding of selected founder animals can produce species homozygous for the mutation.

While transforming embryonic stem cells is more efficient than the microinjection technique described first, the desired gene must still be inserted into the cultured stem cell's genome to ultimately produce the transgenic animal. The gene insertion could occur in a random or in a targeted process. Non-homologous recombination, a random process, readily occurs if the desired DNA is introduced into the ES cell genome by a gene recombination process that does not require any sequence homology between genomic DNA and the foreign DNA. While most ES cells fail to insert the foreign DNA, some do. Those that do are selected and injected into the inner cell mass of the animal blastocyst and thus eventually lead to a transgenic species. In still far fewer ES cells, homologous recombination occurs by chance. Segments of DNA base sequence in the vector find homologous sequences in the host genome and the region between these homologous sequences replaces the matching region in the host DNA. A significant advance in the production of transgenic animals in ES cells is the advent of targeted homologous recombination techniques. Homologous recombination, while much more rare to this point in transgenic research than non-homologous recombination, can be favored when the researcher carefully designs (engineers) the transferred DNA to have specific

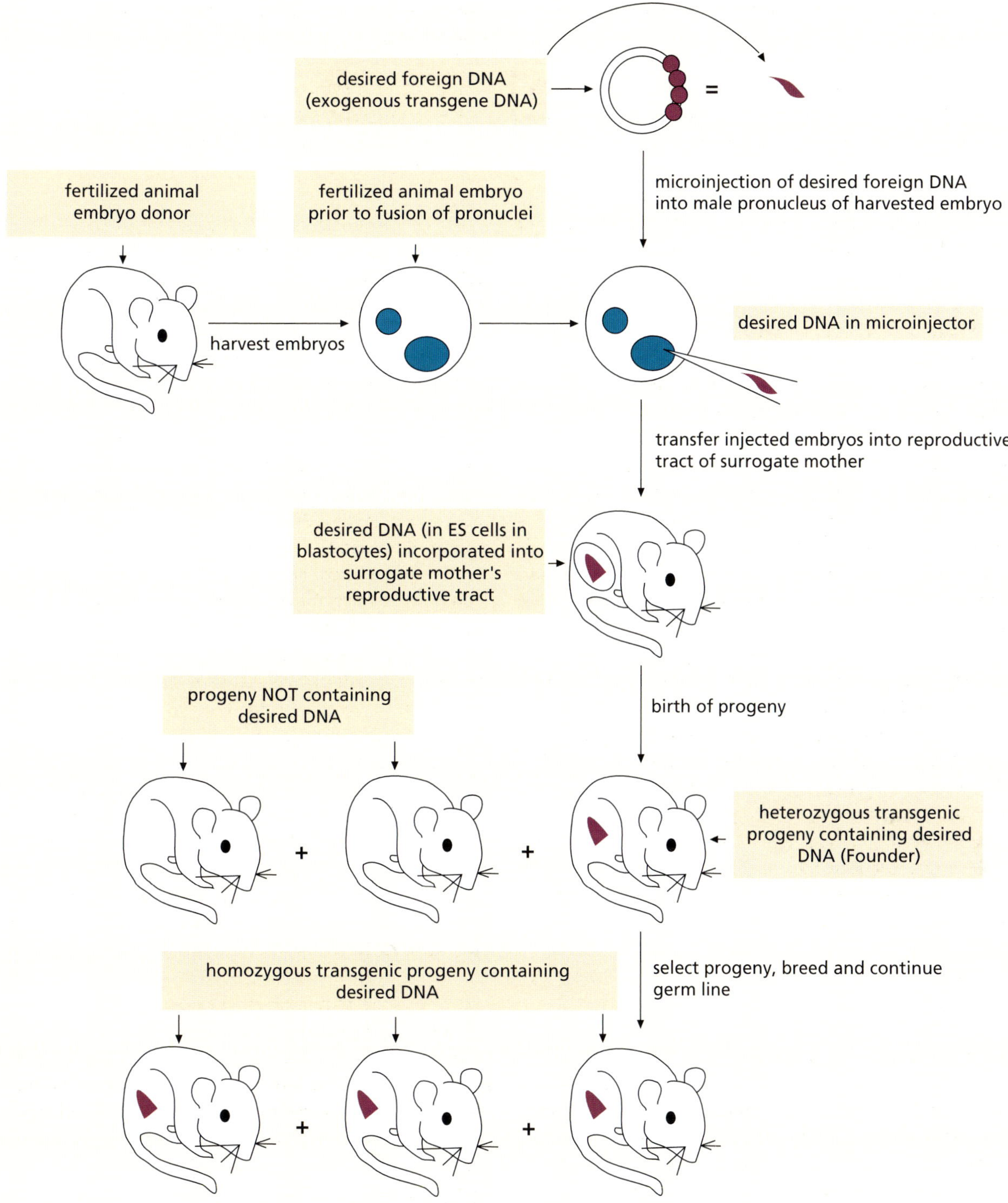

Figure 6.4. Schematic representation of the production of transgenic animals by DNA microinjection.

sequence homology to the endogenous DNA at the desired integration site and also carefully selects the transfer vector conditions. This targeted homologous recombination at a precise chromosomal position provides an approach to very subtle genetic modification of an animal or can be used to produce knockout mice (to be discussed later).

A modification of the procedure involves the use of hematopoietic bone marrow stem cells rather than pluripotent

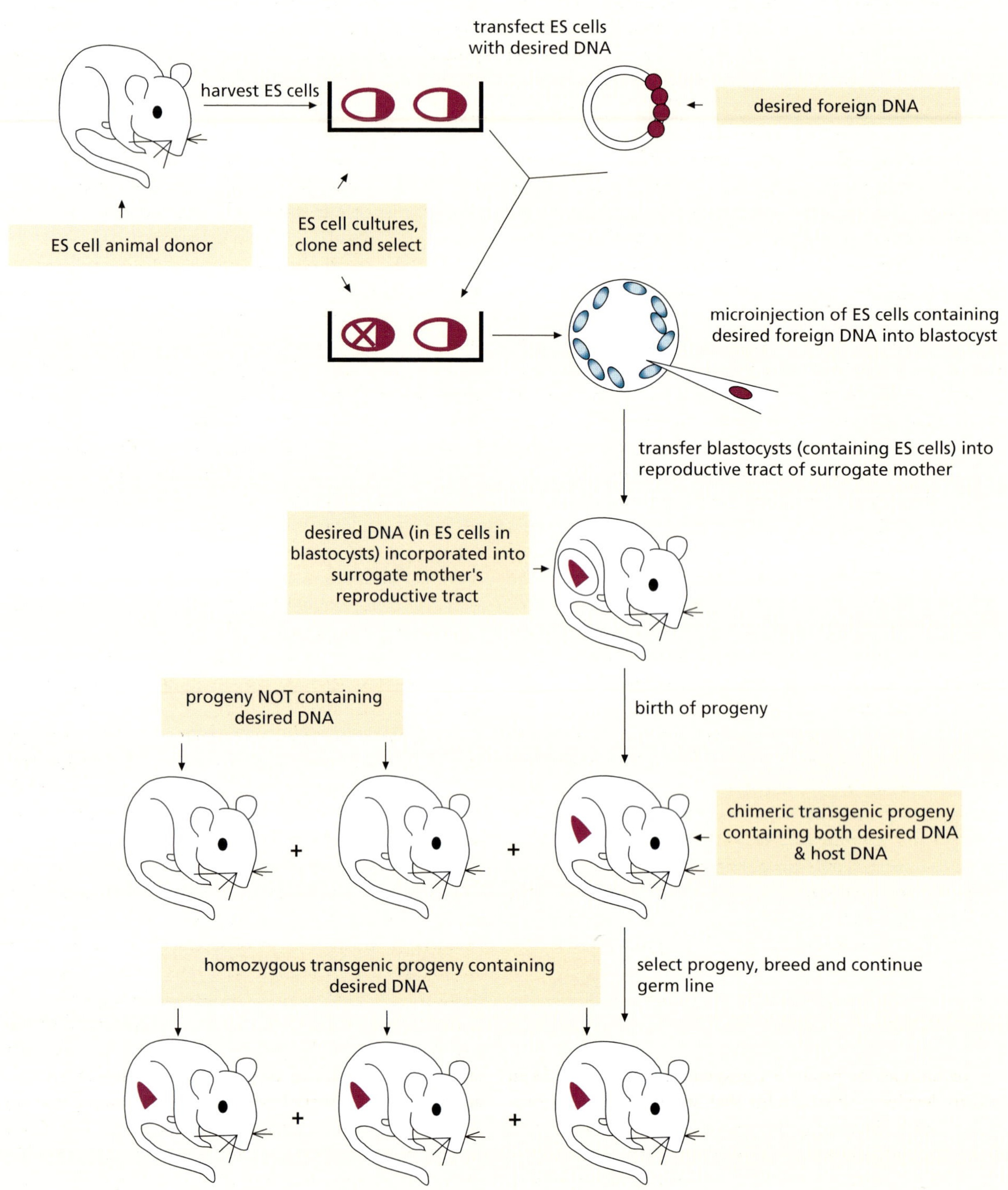

Figure 6.5. Schematic representation of the production of transgenic animals by pluripotent embryonic stem cell methodology.

embryonic stem cells. The use of ES cells results in changes to the whole germ line, while hematopoietic stem cells modified appropriately are expected to repopulate a specific somatic cell line or lines (more similar to gene therapy).

The science of cloning and the resulting ethical debate surrounding it is well beyond the scope of this chapter. Yet it is important to place the concept of animal cloning within the pharmaceutically important context of transgenic animal production. The technique of microinjection (and its variations) has formed the basis for commercial transgenic animal production. While successful, the microinjection process is limited to the creation of only a small number of transgenic animals in a given birth. The slow process of conventional breeding of the resulting transgenic progeny must follow to produce a larger number of transgenic animals with the same transgene as the original organism. To generate a herd (or a flock, etc.), an alternative approach would be advantageous. The technique of nuclear transfer, the replacement of the nuclear genomic DNA of an oocyte (immature egg) or a single-cell fertilized embryo with that from a donor cell is such an alternative breeding methodology. Animal "cloning" can result from this nuclear transfer technology. Judged Science's most important breakthrough of 1997 (Sailor, 1997), creating the sheep Dolly, the first cloned mammal, from a single cell of a 6-year old ewe was a feat many had thought impossible. Dolly was born after nuclear transfer of the genome from an adult mammary gland cell. Since this announcement, commercial and exploratory development of nuclear transfer technology has progressed rapidly. It is important to note that the cloned sheep Dolly is NOT a transgenic animal. While Dolly is a clone of an adult ewe, she does not possess a transgene. However, cloning could be used to breed clones of transgenic animals, or to directly produce transgenic animals (if prior to nuclear transfer, a transgene was inserted into the genome of the cloning donor). For example, human factor IX (a blood factor protein) transgenic sheep were generated by nuclear transfer from transfected fetal fibroblasts (Schniecke *et al.*, 1997). Several of the resulting progeny were shown to be transgenic (i.e. possessing the human factor IX gene) and one was named Polly. Thus, animal cloning can be utilized not only for breeding, but also for the production of potential human therapeutic proteins and other useful pharmaceutical products. A number of cloned animals with various transgenes have now been produced.

PROTEIN PRODUCTION IN TRANSGENIC ANIMALS

The techniques to produce transgenic animals have been used to develop animal strains that secrete important proteins in milk. During such large animal "gene farming", the transgenic animals serve as bioreactors to synthesize recoverable quantities of therapeutically useful proteins. Among the advantages of expressing protein in animal milk is that the protein is generally produced in sizable quantities and can be harvested manually or mechanically by simply milking the animal. Protein purification from the milk requires the usual separation techniques as described in Chapter 3. In general, recombinant genes coding for the desired protein product are fused to the regulatory sequences of the animal's milk-producing genes. The animals are not endangered by the insertion of the recombinant gene. The logical fusion of the protein product gene to the milk-producing gene targets the transcription and translation of the protein product exclusively in mammary tissues normally involved in milk production and does not permit gene activation in other, non-milk producing tissues in the animal. Transgenic strains are established and perpetuated by breeding the animals since the progeny of the original transgenic animal (founder animal) usually also produce the desired recombinant protein.

Yields of protein pharmaceuticals produced transgenically are expected to be 10–100 times greater than those achieved in recombinant cell culture (Thayer, 1996). Protein yields from transgenic animals are generally good [conservative estimates of 1 gram/Liter (g/L) with a 30% purification efficiency] with milk yield from various species per annum estimated at: cow = 10,000 L; sheep = 500 L; goat = 400 L; and pig = 250 L (Rudolph, 1995). PPL Therapeutics has estimated that the cost to produce human therapeutic proteins in large animal bioreactors could be as much as 75% less expensive than cell culture. In addition, should the desired target protein require post-translational modification, the large mammals used in milk production of pharmaceuticals would be a bioreactor capable of adding those groups (unlike a recombinant bacterial culture).

Some examples of human long peptides and proteins under development in the milk of transgenic animals (see Table 6.4) include growth hormone, interleukin-2, calcitonin, insulin-like growth factor, alpha 1 antitrypsin, the anti-clotting protein antithrombin III, clotting Factor VIII, clotting Factor IX, tissue plasminogen activator (tPA), lactoferrin and various human monoclonal antibodies (such as those from the Xenomouse) (Garner and Colman, 1998; Rudolph, 1999). The first clinical trial of a recombinant product isolated from the milk of transgenic animals was initiated by Genzyme Transgenics in the Fall, 1996. Apart from the production of pharmaceuticals, research is underway to produce various nutraceuticals (specialty nutritional products) in genetically engineered animal systems.

An innovative use of transgenics for the production of useful proteins is the generation of clinically transplantable transgenic animal organs. Several research groups in academia and industry have pioneered the transgenic engineering of animals (especially pigs) expressing both human complement inhibitory proteins as well as key human blood group proteins (antigens) (Fodor *et al.*, 1994; Tsuji *et al.*, 1994). Transgenic pigs for xenotransplatation have now been produced by cloning (see discussion in Lewis, 2000). Cells, tissues and organs from these double transgenic animals appear to be very resistant to the humoral immune system mediated reactions of both primates and humans. These findings begin to pave the way for potential xenograft transplantation of animal components into humans with a lessened chance of acute rejection.

Species	Protein product	Potential indication(s)
cow	collagen	burns, bone fracture
cow	human fertility hormones	infertility
cow	human serum albumin	surgery, burns, shock, trauma
cow	lactoferrin	bacterial GI infection
goat	α-1-anti-protease inhibitor	inherited deficiency
goat	α-1-antitrypsin	anti-inflammatory
goat	anti-thrombin III	associated complications from genetic or acquired deficiency
goat	growth hormone	pituitary dwarfism
goat	human fertility hormones	infertility
goat	human serum albumin	surgery, burns, shock, trauma
goat	LAtPA[2)]	venous status ulcers
goat	monoclonal antibodies	colon cancer
goat	t-PA[2)]	myocardial infarct, pulmonary embolism
pig	Factor IX	hemophilia
pig	Factor VIII	hemophilia
pig	fibrinogen	burns, surgery
pig	human hemoglobin	blood replacement for transfusion
pig	protein C	deficiency, adjunct to tPA
rabbit	insulin-like growth factor	wound healing
rabbit	interleukin-2	renal cell carcinoma
rabbit	protein C	deficiency, adjunct to tPA
sheep	α-1-antitrypsin	antiinflammatory
sheep	Factor VIII	hemophilia
sheep	Factor IX	hemophilia
sheep	fibrinogen	burns, surgery
sheep	protein C	deficiency, adjunct to tPA

Table 6.4. Some examples of human proteins under development in the milk of transgenic animals.
[1)] Data from Rudolph, 1995; Garner and Colman, 1998; and Rudolph, 1999.
[2)] Abbreviations: t-PA = tissue plasminogen activator, LAtPA = long acting tissue plasminogen activator.

Knockout Mice

While a mouse carrying an introduced transgene is called a transgenic mouse, transgenic technologies can also produce a knockout animal (mice are the most studied animal species). A knockout mouse, also called a gene knockout mouse or a gene-targeted knockout mouse, is an animal in which an endogenous gene (genomic wild-type allele) has been specifically inactivated by replacing it with a null allele (Lodish *et al.*, 2000). A null allele is a nonfunctional allele of a gene generated by either deletion of the entire gene or mutation of the gene resulting in the synthesis of an inactive protein. Recent advances in intranuclear gene targeting and embryonic stem cell technologies as described above are expanding the capabilities to produce knockout mice routinely for studying certain human genetic diseases or elucidating the function of a specific gene product.

The procedure for producing knockout mice basically involves a four-step process. A null allele (i.e. knockout allele) is incorporated into one allele of murine ES cells. Incorporation is generally quite low; approximately one cell in a million has the required gene replacement. However, the process is designed to impart neomycin and ganciclovir resistance only to those ES cells in which homologous gene integration has resulted. This facilitates the selection and propagation of the correctly engineered ES cells. The resulting ES cells are then injected into early mouse embryos creating chimeric mice (heterozygous for the knockout allele) containing tissues derived from both host cells and ES cells. The chimeric mice are mated to confirm that the null allele is incorporated into the germ line. The confirmed heterozygous chimeric mice are bred to homogeneity producing progeny that are homozygous knockout mice.

For example, knockout mice have been engineered that have extremely elevated cholesterol levels while being maintained on normal chow diets due to their inability to produce apolipoprotein E (apo E) (Zhang *et al.*, 1992; Breslow, 1994). Apo E is the major lipoprotein component of very low-density lipoprotein (VLDL) responsible for liver clearance of VLDL. These engineered mice are being examined as animal models of atherosclerosis useful in cardiovascular drug discovery and development. Table 6.3 provides a list of some additional selected examples of knockout mouse disease models.

The knockout mouse is becoming the basic tool for researchers to determine gene function *in vivo* in numerous biological systems. For example, knockout mouse technology has helped transform our understanding of the immune response (Mak *et al.*, 2001). The study of single and multiple gene knockout animals have provided new perspectives on T-cell development, co-stimulation and activation. In addition, high-throughput DNA sequencing efforts, positional cloning programs, and novel embryonic stem cell-based gene discovery research areas all exploit the knockout mouse as their laboratory.

Genetic Ablation

Genetic ablation, also called cell ablation and genetic amputation, is another genetic engineering technique used to suppress selectively the growth of a specified cell line or cell type in an animal rather than suppress the activity of an individual gene (O'Kane and Moffat, 1992; Saito *et al.*, 2001). The transgene inserted into the animal is under the control of a gene promoter that is known to be active only in a certain cell population. This promoter would regulate the expression of a cytotoxic protein (such as the A-chain of diphtheria toxin) that would therefore destroy only the targeted cell line or type. Also, specific cell ablation is a useful method for analyzing the *in vivo* function of cells (Saito *et al.*, 2001). For example, genetic ablation suppresses choroidal melanocytes during a study of malignancies of the eye originating in the retinal pigment of transgenic mice (Mintz and Klein-Szanto, 1992).

Protein Engineering

Many early biotechnology-produced protein drug candidates failed in clinical trials due to their short biological half-life, low affinity for their receptor, or immunogenicity (McCafferty and Glover, 2000). Recombinant DNA technology has made it possible to engineer specifically altered or new and novel protein molecules possessing tailored chemical and biological characteristics. Termed protein engineering, the deliberate design and construction of unique proteins with enhanced or novel molecular properties is a result of specifying the exact amino acid sequence (protein primary structure) of that protein (Narang, 1990, Richardson and Richardson, 1990, Cleland and Craik, 1996). When applied to enzymes, the process is often called enzyme engineering.

As described in Chapter 2, the primary structure affects the protein's conformation. The conformation of each and every amino acid component present in the protein influences the protein's complex three-dimensional structure. The conformational preference of the protein chain residues determines the protein's secondary structure including α-helices and β-sheets or reverse turns. The local secondary structures are folded into three-dimensional tertiary structures made up of domains. The domains are not only structural units, but are also functional units often containing intact ligand binding (in a receptor) or enzyme catalytic sites. Thus, protein engineering provides an approach to modify a native protein's structure specifically or to create a unique, new protein with a particular structure. Protein engineering has numerous powerful theoretical and practical implications for examining and modifying protein structure and function, probing enzyme mechanisms, investigating protein folding and conformation, enhancing protein stability, introducing detectable groups into proteins as an analytical tool, producing improved second generation tailored biopharmaceuticals, and in the case of enzymes, improving catalytic function (Fothergill-Gilmore, 1993; Nixon *et al.*, 1998).

Engineered proteins have been prepared by many different approaches. Direct chemical synthetic routes for small proteins with modified amino acid sequences have been devised using either solution chemistry or solid supports (chemistry occurring while reactants are attached to resin beads) techniques. Peptide synthesizers have been designed to automate the process. Dugas provides a useful overview of the chemistry of protein engineering (including site-directed mutagenesis) (Dugas 1999). The synthesis of gene fragments coding for the mutation(s) is another approach to produce engineered proteins (Johnson and Reitz, 1998). Completely synthetic genes of as many as 100 nucleotides coding for the desired mutation can be inserted into a gene of a prokaryotic (such as Phage M13) or eukaryotic expression vector. The resulting mutant gene (hybrid gene) is then cloned and expressed producing the engineered protein. The genetic route to engineered proteins is limited to the repertoire of the 20 natural amino acids. The purely chemical route allows for the introduction of alternative structures (e.g. non-natural amino acids) in the peptide chain (see section "Peptide Chemistry and Peptidomimetics").

Site-Directed Mutagenesis

Site-directed mutagenesis (also called site-specific mutagenesis) is a protein engineering technique allowing specific amino acid residue (site-directed) alteration (mutation) to create new protein entities (Johnson and Reitz, 1998). Mutagenesis at a single amino acid position in an engineered protein is called a point mutation. Therefore, site-directed mutagenesis techniques can aid in the examination at the molecular level of the relationship between 3-D structure and function of interesting proteins.

Figure 6.6 suggests an excellent example of possible theoretical mutations of the active site of a model serine

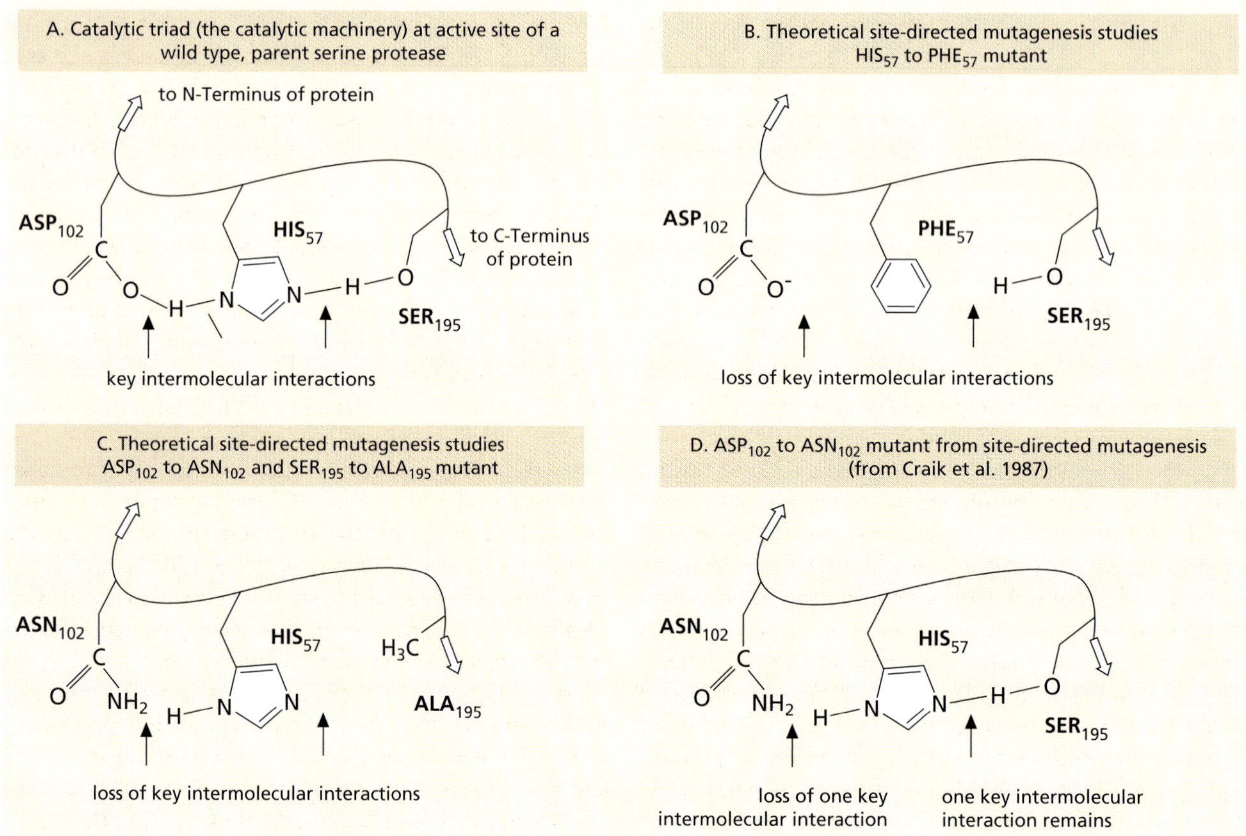

Figure 6.6. Some possible site-directed mutations of the amino acids composing the catalytic triad of a serine protease: influence on key hydrogen bonding.

protease enzyme that could be engineered to probe the mechanism of action of the enzyme. Structures B and C of Figure 6.6 represent a theoretical mutation to illustrate the technique. Craik and co-workers have actually tested the role of the aspartic acid residue in the serine protease catalytic triad Asp, His, and Ser. They replaced Asp ^{102} (carboxylate anion side chain) of trypsin with Asn (neutral amide side chain) by site-directed mutagenesis and observed a pH dependent change in the catalytic activity compared to the wild-type parent serine protease (see Figure 6.6, structure D) (Craik *et al.*, 1987). Site-directed mutagenesis studies also provide invaluable insight into the nature of intermolecular interactions of ligands with their receptors. For example, studies of the effect of the site-directed mutagenesis of various key amino acid residues on the binding of neurotransmitters to G-protein coupled receptors has helped define more accurate models for alpha-adrenergic, D2-dopaminergic, 5HT2a-serotonergic and both M1 and M3 muscarinic receptors (Bikker, *et al.*, 1998).

Enzyme Engineering

Enzyme engineering is the application of protein engineering techniques to enzymatic molecules. Enzyme engineering can optimize catalytic reactions, improve an enzyme's function under abnormal conditions, and enhance or change the catalytic reaction of unnatural substrates (Nixon, *et al.*, 1998).

An exciting application of protein engineering is the preparation of enzymes that have improved catalytic activity and stability in organic solvents, rather than requiring an aqueous environment. In that case, site-directed mutagenesis replaces hydrophilic, charged amino acids and hydrogen bonding residues at the surface of the enzyme with amino acids that stabilize the conformational stability of the protein at the organic solvent-protein surface interface.

The generation of enzyme hybrids, enzymes composed of elements of more than one enzyme, is an exciting area of current study using enzyme engineering techniques. Some examples include the hybridization of the enzyme trypsin to hydrolyze either trypsin and chymotrypsin substrates, and the modification of the substrate specificity of lactate dehydrogenase (pyruvate) to include also oxaloacetate (Nixon, *et al.*, 1998). While enzyme engineering is a powerful technique, it is difficult to engineer, via site-directed mutagenesis, a new catalytic function into an existing enzyme because of the precise spatial arrangement required for the catalytic functional groups at the active site. Fusion molecules (see below), however, are examples of protein-engineered products that may possess more than one activity or property. By fusing the secondary-structural elements or whole domains of enzymes, one could theoretically construct hybrid enzymes (or other proteins) capable of catalysing reactions not observed in nature.

Fusion Proteins

Using ligation chemistry to fuse the gene-coding region for one protein with that of another protein, researchers have created chimeric proteins that combine the properties and activities of the two individual parents. The molecule created is called a fusion protein. Fusion proteins contain portions, or the entire amino acid sequences, of both parent proteins. Fusion proteins have found use in improving the gene expression of a target protein, creating molecules with additive biological activities, and assessing the structure-activity relationships of regions in a protein important to its function.

Creating a fusion protein as an intermediate may facilitate gene expression of therapeutically useful proteins (or any protein). Human recombinant proinsulin is expressed highly by cloning a fusion gene consisting of the codes for both proinsulin and the enzyme galactosidase. After recovering the fusion protein from *E. coli* culture, cleavage of the methionine peptide bond linking the two proteins with the chemical cyanogen bromide yields the free proinsulin.

Ligation chemistry can create DNA coding for fusion molecules with additive properties in comparison to the individual parent proteins. Numerous fusion proteins have been created that contain a toxin fused to another protein. Cutaneous T-cell lymphoma (CTCL) is a general term for a group of low-grade non-Hodgkin's lymphomas affecting approximately 1000 new patients/year. For many patients, CTCL is a persistent, disfiguring and debilitating disease that requires multiple treatments over time. Malignant CTCL cells express one or more of the components of the IL-2 receptor. Thus, the IL-2 receptor may be a homing device to attract a "killer." The IL-2 fusion protein DAB_{389} IL-2 (also called IL-2 fusion toxin) is a recombinant protein consisting of amino acid residues 2–133 of human IL-2 (the IL-2 residues replace the amino acids of the receptor-binding domain of the native diphtheria toxin) "fused" to the first 389 amino acid residues of diphtheria toxin (catalytic and lipophilic domains) (VanderSpek *et al.*, 1993). Denileukin diftitox (Ontak) is such a FDA-approved rDNA-derived cytotoxic IL-2 "fusion" protein. The drug targets IL-2 receptors (the IL-2 portion), and brings the diphtheria toxin directly to the cell to kill the CTCL targets. Studies have observed 30% of patients treated with Denileukin diftitox experience at least 50% reduction of tumor burden sustained for at least 6 weeks.

Many additional variations of diphtheria toxin-containing fusion proteins have been engineered including DAB_{389} CD4 (containing amino acids 1–178 contained in the V1 and V2 domains of human CD4; studied for the treatment of chronically HIV-infected cells), DAB_{389} IL-4 (linked to interleukin 4; treatment of myeloma and Kaposi's sarcoma), DAB_{389} IL-6 (linked to interleukin 6; therapy of autoimmune diseases and cancer), DAB_{389} EGF (containing the amino acid sequence of epidermal growth factor; prevention of restenosis), and DAB_{389} hGM-CSF (fused peptide sequence of human GM-CSF; potential as an antileukemic agent).

Antibody Engineering

A pharmaceutically important application of protein engineering is the production of chimeras to examine the structure-activity relationships of a protein. An example is the engineering of humanized monoclonal antibodies (MAbs). These altered MAbs are prepared by expressing a chimeric antibody gene containing the code for both human and murine portions of the resulting antibody protein. The differences between species in the structure-activity relationships and the structure-function relationships of these chimeric antibodies can be examined by studying properties such as antigen specificity, affinity, and avidity (see Chapter 13) (Pluckthun, 1992).

The application of protein engineering to the synthesis of new antibodies is called antibody engineering (Adair, 1992; Borrebaeck, 1992; Chamow and Ashkenazi, 1999). The production of humanized antibodies is one example of the application of antibody engineering.

Immunoadhesins are antibody engineered fusion proteins containing the immunoglobulin Fc effector domain and a molecule that will adhere specifically to other target molecules. Examples include the replacement of the variable region of an antibody with either the helper T-cell CD4 surface protein or tumor necrosis factor receptor (see Figure 6.7). These immunoadhesins would retain the antibody's Fc effector region (see Chapter 13), but would display specificity for HIV or tumor necrosis factor, respectively. Tumor necrosis factor-alpha is a proinflammatory cytokine released during various immune challenges. A soluble TNF-alpha receptor could bind to circulating TNF and remove the proinflammatory protein. The biopharmaceutical Etanercept (Enbrel) was approved for the reduction of signs and symptoms in rheumatoid arthritis patients refractory to disease-modifying antirheumatic drugs. It is a fusion protein combining a rDNA, soluble p75 TNF receptor (this portion acts as natural antagonist to TNF) fused with a human IgG Fc region. Thus, the drug binds excess circulating TNF preventing it from binding to its membrane receptor.

Alternatively, a fused protein can be produced that consists of an antibody with an intact variable region to recognize and bind a specific target (i.e. an antifibrin antibody) along with an enzyme (i.e. tissue plasminogen activator, tPA) resulting in a more specific and potent agent (i.e. a fibrin specific thrombolytic agent). In other words, the antibody first attaches the enzyme (tPA) specifically to fibrin clots. tPA will activate circulating plasminogen by converting it from plasminogen into plasmin. This plasmin locally attacks fibrin clots and dissolves them. The concept is called antibody-directed enzyme prodrug therapy, ADEPT.

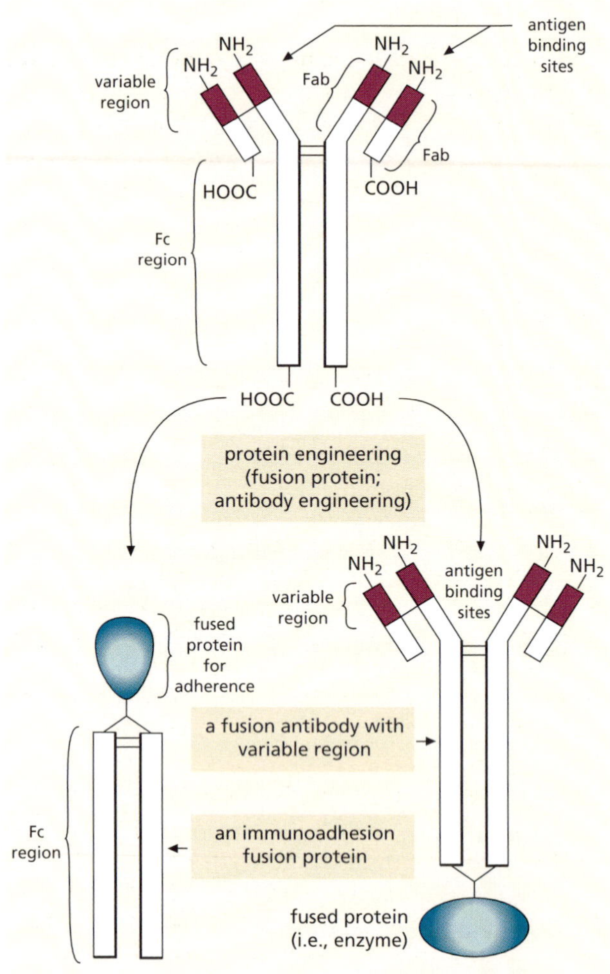

Figure 6.7. Protein engineering (antibody engineering) to produce fusion antibodies.

3D Structures of Engineered Proteins

A variety of techniques can produce structural information about the engineered protein. Among the techniques available, only protein X-ray crystallography and nuclear magnetic resonance (NMR) spectroscopy have the routine ability to determine directly the experimental three-dimensional arrangement of atoms comprising the protein at atomic resolution. A computer can be used for protein modeling, when insufficient quantities of the engineered protein are available, or if X-ray crystallography and NMR are not amenable. While a detailed discussion of each of these techniques is well beyond the scope of this chapter, a very brief introduction of each is valuable to introduce the concepts. The references cited will provide the reader with useful resources to further explore these techniques in detail.

PROTEIN X-RAY CRYSTALLOGRAPHY

Protein X-ray crystallography is a tremendously powerful technique (Ducruis and Giege, 1992; McRee, 1993; McPherson, 1995). Following formation of appropriate crystals of the protein, an X-ray diffraction pattern is obtained for the crystal. An electron density map is derived from the diffraction data, which subsequently provides the atom positions in the protein. While the X-ray structure obtained is a structure averaged over all of the mutant protein molecules found in the crystal (various subtle conformational differences among chemically identical molecules of the engineered protein), the technique provides a view of the spatial arrangement of the protein's atoms. Molecular interactions (i.e. ligand-protein binding) and the mechanism of catalytic reactions can be studied at the molecular level.

Protein X-ray crystallography is severely limited by the availability of appropriate crystals for analysis. Other limitations include the inability to get most hydrogen positional information and the fact that the X-ray structure represents a crystal structure, which is not necessarily equal to a solution structure. An exciting recent advance that may overcome the serious handicap of the necessity for growing quality protein crystals to solve a 3D structure is the use of high resolution single molecule diffraction images (Miao, *et al.*, 2001). This new methodology utilizes a powerful X-ray free electron laser (X-FEL) and an algorithm that can solve protein structures from the X-FEL-produced diffraction patterns from single biomolecules rather than multiple molecules held in a specific crystal lattice. Should the need to obtain quality protein crystals be eliminated, there would be an explosive increase in the number of high-resolution 3D protein structures available for use in rational, structure-based drug design.

NUCLEAR MAGNETIC RESONANCE (NMR) SPECTROSCOPY

The concurrent development of nuclear magnetic resonance (NMR) techniques and molecular biology has led to an increased study of the three-dimensional structure and dynamics of proteins in solution (Archer *et al.*, 1996; Craik, 1996; Markley and Opella, 1997; Clore and Gronenborn, 1998). Like X-ray crystallography, NMR spectroscopy generates information directly about the proximity of atoms and about the lifetimes of the through-space interactions of those atoms. Significant advantages of the protein NMR approach over X-ray crystallography include its ability to study proteins in solution, to obtain structural information about dynamic (flexible) portions of the molecule and to look specifically at hydrogen atoms. X-ray crystallography, unlike NMR, provides spatial information about all non-hydrogen atoms.

PROTEIN MODELING

Protein modeling (in the broader sense, molecular modeling) is a collection of computer techniques, including computer graphics, computational chemistry, statistical methods and database management, applied to the description, analysis, and prediction of protein structures and protein properties (Veerapandian, 1995; Charifson, 1997; Murcko *et al.*, 1999). Protein folding (including prediction of 3-D structures), dynamics simulations, protein function and protein-molecule (ligand, DNA, protein, etc.) interactions are some of the problems that are being studied currently by protein modeling. Protein modelers often study products from protein engineering. The 3-D protein structures used in modeling are frequently derived from X-ray crystallography and NMR analyses. When structures are not available from these structural techniques, either *de novo* methods or homology modeling approaches must be used (Greer *et al.*, 1994; Charifson, 1997). *De novo* methods involve the prediction of secondary protein structure from an analysis of the amino acid sequence. Homology modeling uses the known structures of homologous or similar proteins as 3-D templates on which one constructs the framework of the protein being studied. Validation of the computer model resulting from either of these methods with experimental observations is necessary. The limited success rate for homology modeling approaches to accurately predict a protein's three-dimensional structure (ascertained by comparing a protein's homology modeling predicted structure with its experimentally determined X-ray crystallographic structure) has limited their broader use until more recent enhancements to the homology algorithms (Peitsch, 1997).

Peptide Chemistry and Peptidomimetics

Peptide chemistry and biology have become very popular fields of study since the discovery that a large number of hormones, neurotransmitters and other endogenous chemical mediators are peptides (some examples are listed in Table 6.5). Peptide receptors are attractive targets in drug discovery and design efforts. Thus, both peptides and proteins have the potential to be developed into useful therapeutic agents. Peptides, like the larger proteins, may be produced by various genetic methods (as described for proteins in Chapter 1, 3 and earlier in this chapter). As smaller molecules, however, chemical synthesis is quite viable. Both classical solution methods and newer solid phase approaches based on the technique originally developed by Merrifield (the chemistry occurs while the growing peptide chain is anchored onto a polymeric bead) have been applied to the synthesis of thousands of peptides of diverse structure (Gutte, 1995; Seneci, 2000). Peptides of 50 amino acids or

Peptide	# Amino Acids
angiotensin II	8
β-endorphin	31
bradykinin	9
cholecystokinin	33
corticotropin	39
dynorphin B	17
endothelin-1	21
gastrin	17
glucagon	29
insulin	51 (two chains)
leu-enkephalin	5
met-enkephalin	5
neuropeptide Y	36
neurotensin	13
oxytocin	9
somatostatin	14
somatostatin	14
substance P	11
thyrotropin-releasing factor	3
tuftsin	4

Table 6.5. Some endogenous peptide hormones, neurotransmitters and chemical mediators.

greater are synthesized by automated solid phase peptide synthesizers.

Despite their achievable synthesis, peptides suffer from a number of characteristics that make them less suitable as drugs than the classical small organic molecule agents. In most cases, peptide pharmaceuticals are characterized by low oral bioavailability, poor passage through the blood-brain barrier (for CNS targeted peptides), metabolic instability catalyzed by endogenous peptidases (hydrolysis of the amide bond), and rapid urinary and biliary excretion (Luthman and Hacksell, 1996). Also, the inherent flexibility of peptide molecules allows them to adopt multiple, low energy conformations or shapes. This property permits a peptide drug to interact with several different similar peptide receptors. Side effects and low affinity can result from this lack of selectivity at target receptor sites. Numerous peptide modifications have been studied to overcome the limitations that make peptides poorly suited as drugs (Goodman and Ro, 1995; Luthman and Hacksell, 1996; Nakanishi and Kahn 1996; Abell, 1999).

Peptidomimetics

The isolation and structure elucidation of two endogenous morphine-like pentapeptides, leu-enkephalin and met-enkephalin, formally introduced the study of peptidomimetics (Hughes *et al.*, 1975). Morphine, a narcotic alkaloid, and the enkephalins were conclusively demonstrated to elicit their analgesia by binding to the same opioid receptor (see Figure 6.8). Therefore, morphine acts as a narcotic analgesic because it is a nature-synthesized mimic of the endogenous pentapeptides. Peptidomimetics (sometimes called peptide mimetics and nonpeptide mimetics) are substitutes for peptides that possess not only the peptide's affinity for interactions with receptors and/or enzymes, but also efficacy. Numerous reviews on the topic are available (Luthman and Hacksell, 1996; Nakanishi and Kahn, 1996; Giannis and Rubsam, 1997; Ripka and Rich, 1998).

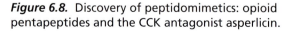

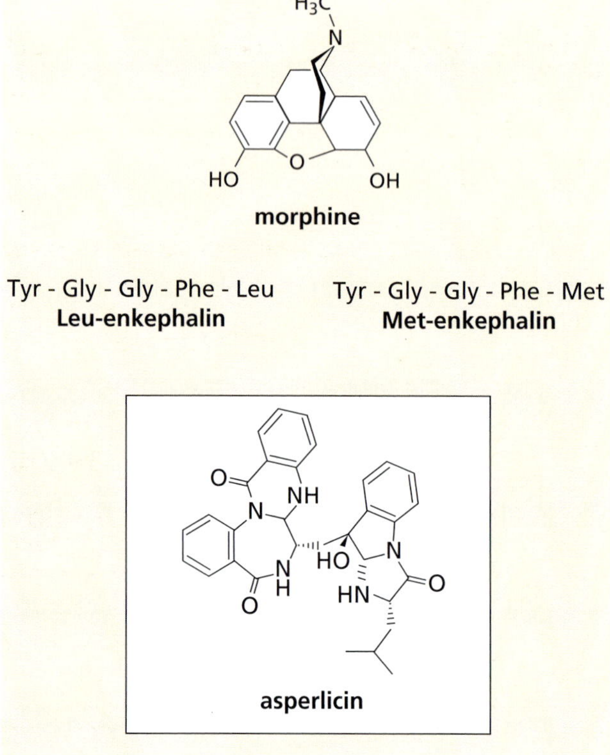

Figure 6.8. Discovery of peptidomimetics: opioid pentapeptides and the CCK antagonist asperlicin.

There are a number of approaches to the discovery of peptidomimetics that interact with specific peptide receptors (Obrecht *et al.*, 1999). An empirical approach to peptidomimetic discovery is the screening of pure compound libraries and complex mixtures (from natural product extracts, microbial fermentations or combinatorial chemistry) (Giannis and Rubsam, 1997; Gron and Hyde-DeRuyscher, 2000). A screening success was the discovery of the potent cholecystokinin (CCK) receptor antagonist asperlicin (see Figure 6.8) from a fermentation and the subsequent medicinal chemistry development of additional agents (Wiley and Rich 1993). This nonpeptide natural product containing a 1,4-benzodiazepine moiety acts as a peptidomimetic antagonist at a receptor for a neuroactive peptide ligand (CCK). Computer-aided molecular modeling is often used to design better analogs (exhibiting improved affinity and selectivity) of the lead molecule discovered via such an empirical approach.

Peptidomimetic Approaches

The peptidomimetic approach known as "pseudopeptides" is an attempt to improve the biostability of peptides (Hirschmann *et al.*, 1995). Numerous pseudopeptides (also called amide bond surrogates) have been prepared that substitute an amide bond bioisostere for the amide peptide bond. A bioisostere is a replacement of an atom or groups of atoms while retaining a broadly similar bioactivity. Examples of some bioisosteric peptide bond replacements are shown in Figure 6.9 (Luthman and Hacksell, 1996). This

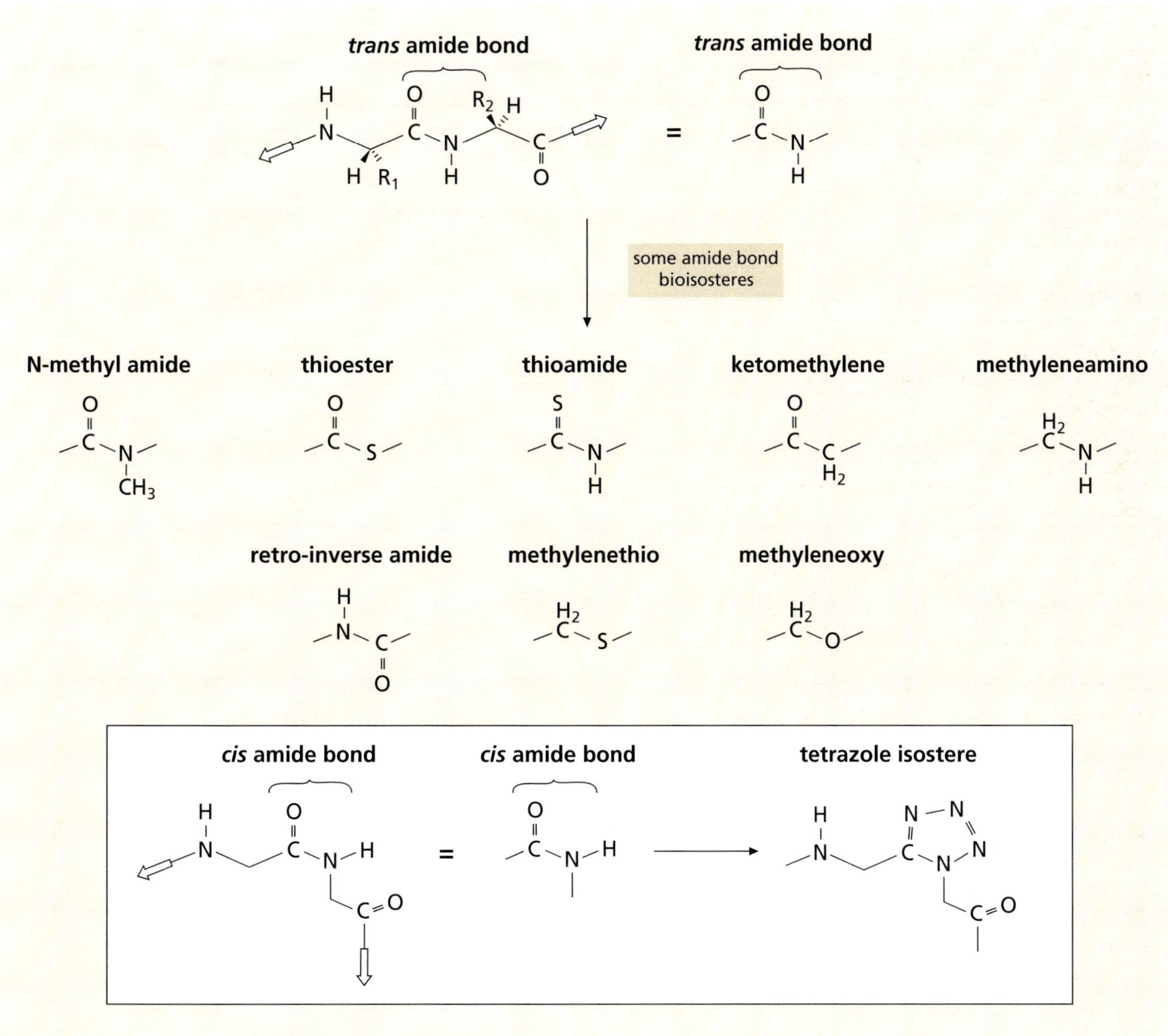

Figure 6.9. Pseudopeptides: examples of some bioisosteric peptide bond replacements (adapted from Goodman and Ro 1995 and Luthman and Hacksell 1996).

type of substitution changes the backbone of the peptide and may alter its conformation. Bioisosteric pseudopeptides do exhibit decreased endogenous peptidase-mediated hydrolysis, however, many still suffer from insufficient oral bioavailability. An interesting amide bond bioisostere is the tetrazole analog (a five-membered ring with four nitrogens, see Figure 6.9) that also serves to restrict the backbone conformation of the peptide amide bond to the *cis*-orientation (see Chapter 2).

Another peptidomimetic approach is the introduction of local conformational constraints into a peptide's backbone and/or α-carbon side chain groups (the R-group attached to the α-carbon of the amino acid residues; i.e., R = $-CH_3$ in alanine and R = $-CH_2OH$ in serine, etc.) resulting in improved receptor selectivity. Decreased conformational flexibility leads to fewer possible multiple receptor interactions. Also, local conformational constraints may decrease a peptide's biodegradation (Liskamp, 1994). Examples of various types of conformationally restricted analogs are shown in Figure 6.10. Backbone modifications include the introduction of carbon-carbon double bonds (olefinic analogs) and rings (benzene, carbohydrates, lactams, and azoles) (Hirschmann *et al.*, 1993; Graf von Roedern and Kessler, 1994; Borg *et al.*, 1995). Replacing a peptide amide bond

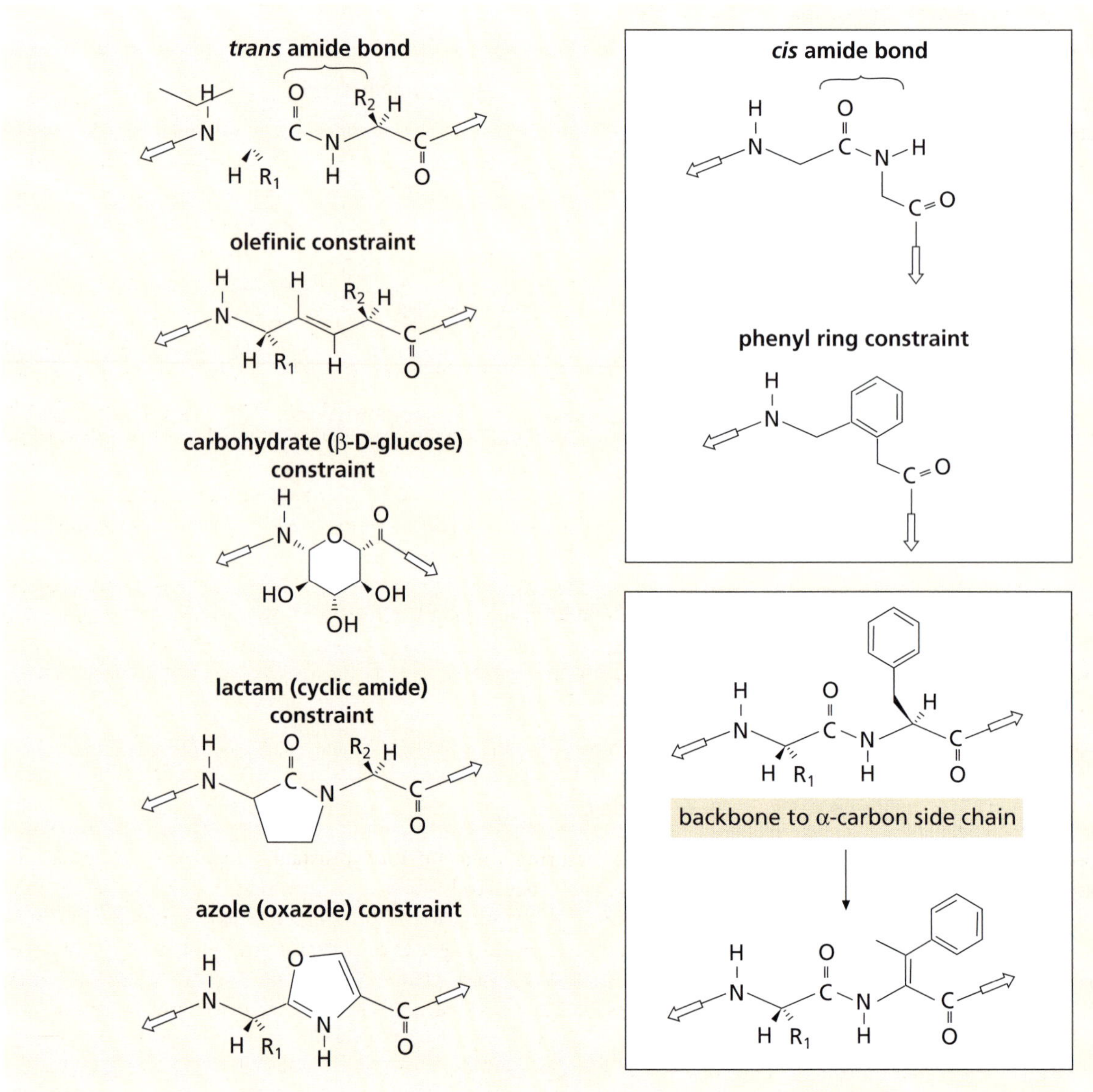

Figure 6.10. Examples of local conformational constraints of peptide backbone and α-carbon sidechain groups: olefinic analog, rings, and backbone-α-carbon sidechain link.

with an *ortho*-substituted benzene ring results in a *cis*-amide mimic, while a β-D-glucose scaffold provides a *trans*-amide mimic with less conformational flexibility. The backbone of a peptide may be covalently linked to a portion of an α-carbon side chain thus fixing the local conformational orientation of both to each other.

Nucleic Acid Technologies

Nucleic acid technologies encompass all the techniques based on oligonucleotides and their analogs including gene therapy (Ramabhadran, 1994). Nucleic acids are polymers of nucleotides. While early nucleic acid technology targeted genetic deficiency diseases with replacement gene therapy (discussed in detail in Chapter 7), antisense and triplex technologies, aptamer technology and the study of ribozymes have become dominant themes in many research and development laboratories around the world. Tremendous effort has been spent the last few years to develop oligonucleotides and oligonucleotide analogs into useful therapeutic products. The Pharmaceutical Research and Manufacturers of America recently listed seven oligonucleotide drugs being studied in Phase I-Phase III clinical trials and one FDA-approved drug, formivirsen (Vitravene) for the second-line treatment of cytomegalovirus-induced retinitis in AIDS patients (The Pharmaceutical Research and Manufacturers of America, 2000).

Oligonucleotides

Biochemistry

Oligonucleotides (or "oligos" as they are sometimes called) are short polymeric segments of deoxyribonucleic acid (DNA) or ribonucleic acid (RNA), generally 100 or fewer bases long. As described briefly in Chapter 1, the genetic information necessary for a cell to synthesize specific proteins is retained in discrete genes within the linear molecules of 2'-deoxyribonucleic acid (DNA) making up the chromosomes in the cell nucleus. The genes consist of double helical strands of DNA. The exact nucleic acid base sequence of the nuclear DNA contains the genetic code to make a specific protein.

Each base is linked through a phosphate bond at the 5'-position of a 2'-deoxyribose sugar to the 3'-end of the deoxyribose portion on the next nucleotide (Figure 6.11). The combination of a pyrimidine or purine base plus a sugar moiety is a nucleoside, while a nucleotide is a base plus a sugar moiety and a phosphate. The pyrimidines thymine (T) and cytosine (C) and the purines adenine (A) and guanine (G) are the only nucleic acid bases found in DNA. The specific hydrogen bonding interactions of complementary bases on each oligodeoxyribonucleotide strand (A only with T, G only with C) hold the two strands of DNA together to form double-helical DNA with the sugar-phosphate backbones directed toward the outside (see Chapter 1). Oligodeoxyribonucleotides are also called oligodeoxynucleotides and ODNs. In oligoribonucleotides, the pyrimidine base uracil (U) is substituted for T and hydrogen bonds with A.

The nomenclature for oligonucleotides follows a consistent pattern. For a monomer, dimer, trimer up to a decamer, the names would be mononucleotide, dinucleotide, trinucleotide, etc. Beyond that, the name of an oligonucleotide is given by its length as a number followed by "-mer". Thus a 21-base containing oligonucleotide would be a 21-mer (twenty one-mer).

Physiochemical properties of oligonucleotides

Normal oligodeoxyribonucleotides and oligoribonucleotides containing the five bases, unmodified sugars and the phosphate group are limited in their potential therapeutic applications because they are highly susceptible to rapid degradation by structurally nonspecific intracellular nucleases (Stein and Narayanan, 1996). Upon hydrolysis, the resulting smaller oligos and nucleotide pieces are not expected to retain their previous biological activity, nor specificity. Also, each of the phosphate groups of the oligonucleotide phosphate-sugar backbone (chemically, a phosphodiester linkage) possesses a negative charge preventing passive diffusion through cellular and nuclear membranes. Numerous modifications of the parent oligonucleotide structure have been undertaken to circumvent the degradation and cellular permeation limitations. Natural oligonucleotides have been shown to accumulate in cells by receptor-mediated endocytosis. This process, however, is not very efficient. Microinjection and liposome encapsulation appear to be the most effective routes of administration of normal and modified oligonucleotides.

Chemical Modifications to Enhance Drug Properties

Chemical manipulation of the oligonucleotides by substituting more nuclease resistant and lipophilic groups for the negatively charged oxygen on the phosphodiester linkages results in a series of modified oligonucleotides with improved physiochemical properties potentially more useful to enhance bioavailability and stability (Crooke, 1995a; Crooke, 1995b; Lebedev and Wickstrom, 1996; Crooke, 1998). Figure 6.12 illustrates chemical changes of a parent oligonucleotide structure resulting in phosphorothioate, alkyl phosphonate and phosphoamidate analogs, each possessing an additional asymmetric center on the phosphorus atom. These chemical changes increase lipophilicity and

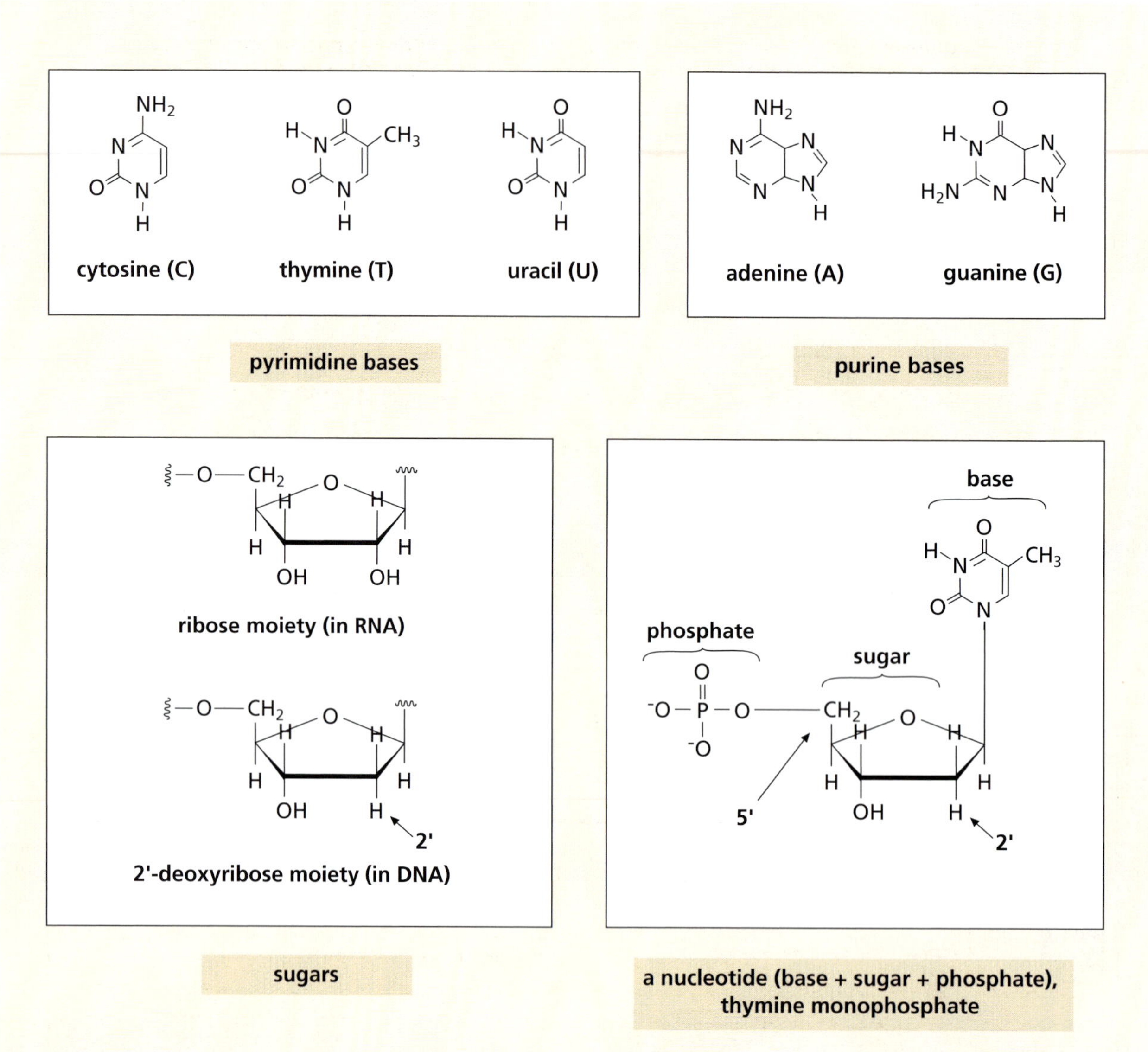

Figure 6.11. Molecular units found in nucleotides.

decrease nuclease hydrolysis. For example, the parent oligonucleotide half-life of 1 hour is increased to more than 24 hours by preparing the phosphorothioate derivative. Neutral derivatives such as the alkyl phosphonates cross the blood-brain barrier.

A peptide nucleic acid (PNA) is a more recent variation of the phosphate-sugar backbone of oligonucleotides (Nielsen 1999; Nielsen and Egholm, 1999). A PNA is a DNA/RNA mimic with a pseudopeptide backbone holding the pyrimidine and purine bases in their proper spatial arrangement. Generally, aminoethyl glycine (gly-NH-CH_2-CH_2-gly) units serve as the backbone of the polymer. These highly modified oligonucleotide analogs have improved physiochemical characteristics.

Antisense Technology and Triplex Technology

Normal cell activity: DNA makes RNA and RNA makes protein

As described in Chapter 1, during the normal process of transcription, the double-stranded DNA separates into two strands, the sense DNA strand (coding strand or plus strand) and the antisense DNA strand (template strand or minus strand). The antisense DNA strand then serves as the template for the mRNA responsible for the code for protein synthesis in the ribosome. The sense DNA strand may infrequently also code for RNA and this molecule is called

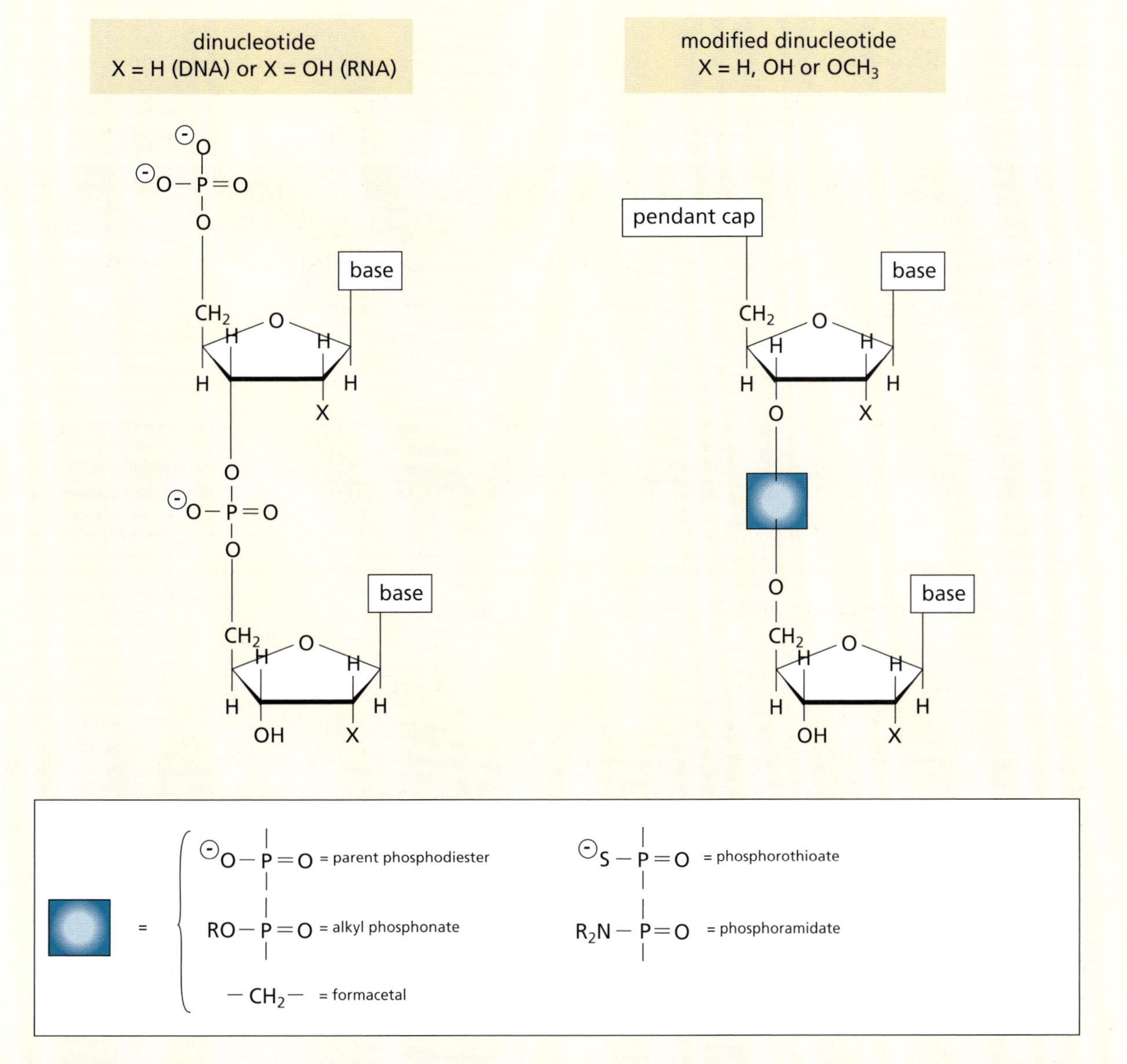

Figure 6.12. Useful chemical modifications to a dinucleotide.

antisense RNA. Antisense sequences were first described as a naturally occurring event in which an endogenous antisense RNA is formed complementary to a cellular mRNA resulting in a repressor of gene expression (Murray and Crockett, 1992).

RATIONALE FOR ANTISENSE TECHNOLOGY

The discovery that nature can regulate gene expression, and thus protein synthesis, using antisense RNA suggested that exogenous antisense oligonucleotides might also be useful in regulating gene expression. Antisense oligonucleotide interactions occur when the bases of the synthetic, specifically designed antisense oligonucleotide sequence align in a precise, sequence-specific manner with a complementary series of bases in the target mRNA (Figure 6.13) (Crooke, 1995a; Crooke, 1995b; Tidd, 1996; Kool, 1996; Crooke, 1999). The potential antisense oligonucleotide drug is chemically modified in one or more ways as described earlier.

Antisense oligonucleotide interruption of the flow of genetic information may occur at the mRNA level in the

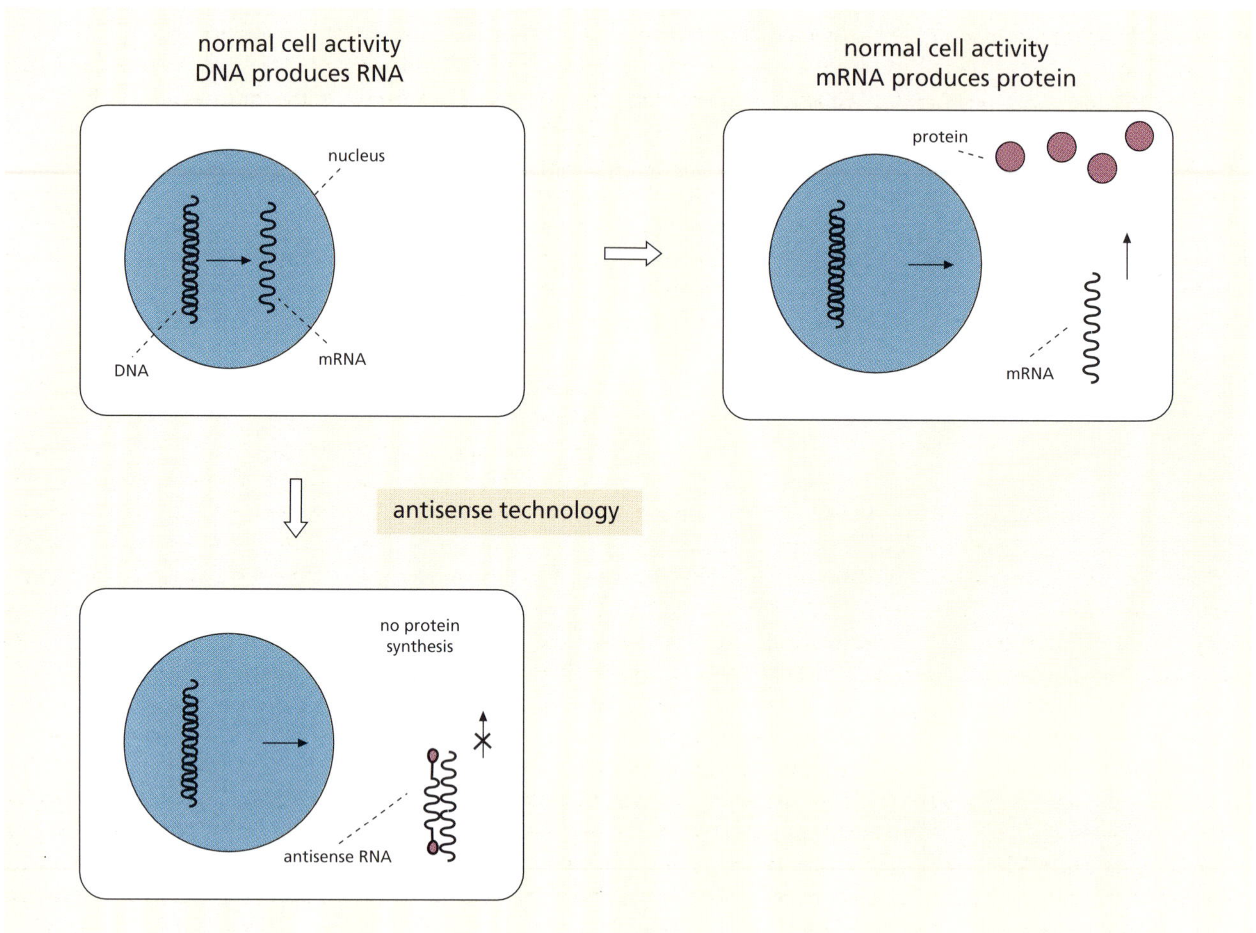

Figure 6.13. The process of antisense technology. Protein synthesis is blocked when an antisense oligonucleotide molecule binds to messenger RNA.

cytoplasm or by interacting with the mRNA precursor in the nucleus. Antisense RNA would be oligoribonucleotides that are complementary for the mRNA sequence that is targeted. Antisense DNA would be single stranded oligodeoxyribonucleotides that are, again, complementary to mRNA. There are several mechanisms by which antisense molecules ultimately disrupt gene expression and thus protein synthesis. A transient inhibition may occur by masking the ribosome binding site on mRNA preventing protein synthesis. A permanent inhibition may result from cross-linking the oligonucleotide to the target mRNA. The most important mechanism, however, appears to be through the action of an enzyme found in most cells, ribonuclease H (RNase H), which recognizes the DNA-RNA duplex (antisense DNA interacting with mRNA) or RNA-RNA duplex (antisense RNA interacting with mRNA), disrupts the base pairing, and digests the RNA-part of the double helix. Inhibition of gene expression occurs since the digested mRNA is no longer competent for translation and resultant protein synthesis.

THERAPEUTIC ANTISENSE MOLECULES

While most traditional drug molecules illicit their effect by interacting with an important enzyme or protein receptor (thus defining a receptor loosely to mean any target molecule with which a drug interacts to produce an effect rather than a strict pharmacological definition for receptor reserved for the agonist or antagonist interactions of the regulatory type), antisense technology involves the blocking of genetic messages to stop the production of disease-producing proteins at the source (Agrawal, 1996). Antisense oligonucleotide genetic-code blocking drugs might control disease by inhibiting deleterious or malfunctioning genes, differing from gene therapy which inserts needed genetic information (see Chapter 7).

Fomivirsen (Vitravene), the first antisense biotech drug to be approved and marketed, is a 21-mer phosphorothiolate oligodeoxynucleotide. This nucleic acid agent is indicated for the treatment of human cytomegalovirus (CMV) induced retinitis in AIDS patients. CMV infection is especially problematic in immunocompromised individuals. Fomivirsen inhibits CMV, a herpes virus, by both a base sequence specific antisense mechanism and a sequence non-specific binding to viral coat proteins preventing CMV adsorption to host cells (Anderson *et al.*, 1996). As stated earlier, seven oligonucleotide drugs are being studied in Phase I-Phase III clinical trials (The Pharmaceutical Research and Manufacturers of America, 2000). Some additional potential therapeutic targets under examination in the current clinical trials are cancer including chronic myelogenous leukemia (CML) in accelerated phase or blast crisis, HIV infection and AIDS, and inflammatory diseases.

Triplex technology

The general term "antigene nucleic acids" has been applied to any oligonucleotides that bind to single-stranded or double stranded DNA. An antigene nucleic acid approach related to antisense technology is triple helix (triplex) technology in which short oligodeoxyribonucleotides of 15–27 nucleotides in length can bind sequence-specifically to complementary segments of duplex DNA (Dervan, 1989; Helene *et al.*, 1992). The resulting triple helices inhibit DNA replication, thus blocking genetic information flow at the information processing level. While antisense RNA drugs would have to inhibit thousands of copies of the synthesized target mRNA present in a cell, triplex inhibition of transcription requires the inactivation of only one or possibly two copies of the genomic DNA found in each cell. Even though triple helices have been known for over 30 years, modern oligonucleotide chemistry has provided the opportunity to synthesize selectively the required specific sequences in sufficient yield.

Aptamer Technology

Aptamers are single-stranded or double-stranded sequences of oligonucleotides that bind to proteins (rather than nucleic acids) or other small molecules (Ellington and Szostak, 1990). From the Latin *aptus* meaning to fit, aptamers are being studied as potential therapeutic agents capable of binding to proteins such as transcription factors and thus blocking gene expression and protein synthesis. Laboratory studies have identified specific oligonucleotide sequences that bind to the NF-□B transcription factor in B- and T-cells, the adenosine deaminase enhancer in T-cells and human thrombin (Stull and Szoka, 1995). Currently, to this author's knowledge, there are no aptamer drugs in clinical trials.

Ribozymes

Ribozymes are catalytic RNAs that cleave covalent bonds, generally degrading a target RNA (for reviews applicable to pharmaceutical research and applications see: Krueger, 1995; Stull and Szoka, 1995; Marr, 1996). Until the Nobel Prize-winning discovery in the mid-1980s of these self-cleaving and splicing RNAs, proteins were thought to be the only types of molecules capable of functioning as biocatalysts. There are a number of naturally occurring, structurally complex ribozymes that have been isolated, including group I intron, group II intron, RNAse P and VS RNA. Pharmaceutical research has centered on three structurally smaller ribozymes for adaptation; the hammerhead, hairpin and HDV ribozymes.

Modern oligonucleotide chemistry or various genetic techniques have provided the opportunity to engineer selectively the required specific ribozyme sequences in sufficient yield (Bramlage *et al.*, 1998). While still a developing technology, ribozymes have the potential to be powerful therapeutic agents. They should be able to both intercept mRNA coding for harmful proteins in a sequence-specific fashion and destroy them via the ribozyme's enzymatic activity, thus leaving the patient's normal mRNA untouched. Cancer-causing oncogene transcripts (such as in the *ras* oncogene) and the RNA retrovirus HIV-1 are particularly attractive therapeutic targets. Drugs in development for the treatment of HIV are presently in early clinical trials. A catalytic ribozyme drug would contain a nucleotide sequence that targets a highly conserved nucleotide region in the RNA of the target cell, thus providing specificity. While they have not been discovered in nature, researchers have used combinatorial chemistry techniques to produce single stranded DNA with enzymatic function (Rawls, 1997).

Catalytic Antibodies (Abzymes)

A prime example of research at the interface of chemistry and immunology is the development of catalytic antibodies (Lerner *et al.*, 1991). Catalytic antibodies or "abzymes" have been considered as a new class of designer enzymes catalyzing reactions for which no natural enzyme exists. Catalytic antibody technology is another example of antibody engineering. Numerous recent reviews and key papers are available to provide an excellent overview of this field and serve as the sources for the discussion that follows (Benkovic, 1992; Schultz and Lerner, 1993; Sudhir, 2000; Blackburn, 2000).

Catalytic antibodies may have potential as pharmaceuticals that would enzymatically cleave specific surface proteins or sugars on viruses, or tumor cells thereby disrupting the invaders. Anti-inflammatory abzymes could be generated that break down pro-inflammatory proteins such as certain cytokines. Diagnostic applications may exist where catalytic antibodies are used as biosensors and the resulting enzymatic reaction product(s) are analyzed and quantified.

Catalytic antibodies are expected to have better pharmacokinetic and distribution properties than many structurally larger enzymes or enzyme-antibody conjugates.

Antibody Catalysis – Historical Comments

Benkovic provides an excellent review of the historical development of catalytic antibodies (Benkovic, 1992). Nearly 50 years ago, Nobel Laureate Linus Pauling suggested that an enzymatic reaction accelerates if the catalytic site is more structurally complementary to the high-energy transition state of the reaction than to its substrate or product ground states. The transition state is a transitory structural entity created from the substrate and present at the energy barrier for the reaction. The better the complementarity between the enzyme and the transition state, the lower the activation energy for the transformation. Thus, the reaction rate should be facilitated.

Each chemically distinct antibody molecule is able to bind to particular molecular configurations on the invading microorganism (antigen) that stimulated their biosynthesis. A variable region on the antibody provides for the generation of an infinite diversity of antigen recognition. Essentially, an antibody can be considered to contain "programmable" chemical binding sites. While an antibody is a soluble protein capable of ligand-specific binding, the ligand is bound in its low energy ground state. Therefore, normal antibodies lack catalytic activity. The development of hybridoma technology (see Chapter 13) and also protein engineering (earlier in this chapter) provides the ability to produce homogeneous, monoclonal antibodies and modified antibodies in the quantities necessary to reproducibly purify potential abzymes and characterize their properties. The result was the independent production of antibodies with catalytic activity by the Lerner and the Schultz groups in 1986.

Chemistry of Catalytic Antibodies

Since antibodies bind selectively to the antigens that stimulated their synthesis, the key to the production of a catalytic antibody is using a carefully designed, stable transition state analog as the antigen. Hybridoma techniques are used to fuse the polyclonal catalytic antibody-producing murine spleen cells (from a hapten-carrier immunized mouse) with murine myeloma cells. Following screening, selection and cloning, monoclonal catalytic antibodies are synthesized. Newer methods of production include the use of phage libraries (see Chapter 13). The antibody so produced would have high affinity for the transition state mimic and thus also the transition state of the studied reaction. The newly generated catalytic antibody should accelerate the transformation of substrate to product. Because antibodies against nearly any molecule (stable transition state analog) can be generated, catalytic antibody technology provides a powerful tool to improve rates of chemical reactions and cause reactions that might possibly not occur otherwise.

Chemists, using carefully designed transition state mimics and X-ray crystallographic techniques, have developed general strategies to induce catalytic activity into antibody binding sites by introducing reactive nucleophilic, electrophilic, acidic, or basic groups precisely in complementary key locations optimal for binding the transition state and catalyzing the reaction with the substrate. The literature reports a wide range of reactions catalyzed by abzymes. Many early experiments focused on antibodies produced to catalyze ester and amide hydrolysis reactions (esterase-like and amidase-like activities). For example, accelerations in ester hydrolysis reaction rates of 6×10^6 have been observed for some reactions. The stable transition state analog was generally a phosphorus-containing molecule that resembled the tetrahedral transition state of esters or amides when they are hydrolyzed (for an illustration, see Figure 6.14).

In addition to ester and amide hydrolyses/transacylations, reactions examined include enantioselective reactions (creating chiral products), proton transfers, Claisen rearrangements, β-eliminations, bimolecular amide bond formation, lactone ring formation, redox reactions and Diels-Alder reactions. Only the chemist's imagination and their understanding of reaction mechanisms probably limit the diversity of reactions. There are now catalytic antibody reagents commercially available from chemical supply houses for use in everyday laboratory reactions.

Tissue Engineering

Tissue engineering, the multidisciplinary field of varied strategies to regenerate natural or grow new human tissues and organs, has burgeoned over the past decade (Mooney and Mikos, 1999; Brownlee, 2001; Lipp, 2001; Petit-Zeman, 2001; Stock and Vacanti, 2001). Recently, a popular news magazine predicted that tissue engineering would be the hottest employment opportunity of the 21st Century. Sometimes referred to as the more general term "regenerative medicine", tissue engineering has integrated biotechnology, clinical medicine, cell biology, developmental biology, and biomaterials engineering into an effort to overcome the challenges associated with conventional surgical approaches to tissue and organ repair or replacement. Each year, over eight million surgeries are performed in the US alone to repair or replace human tissues and organs at staggering costs and significant patient discomfort (Lipp, 2001). Only a fraction of patients admitted to the hospital

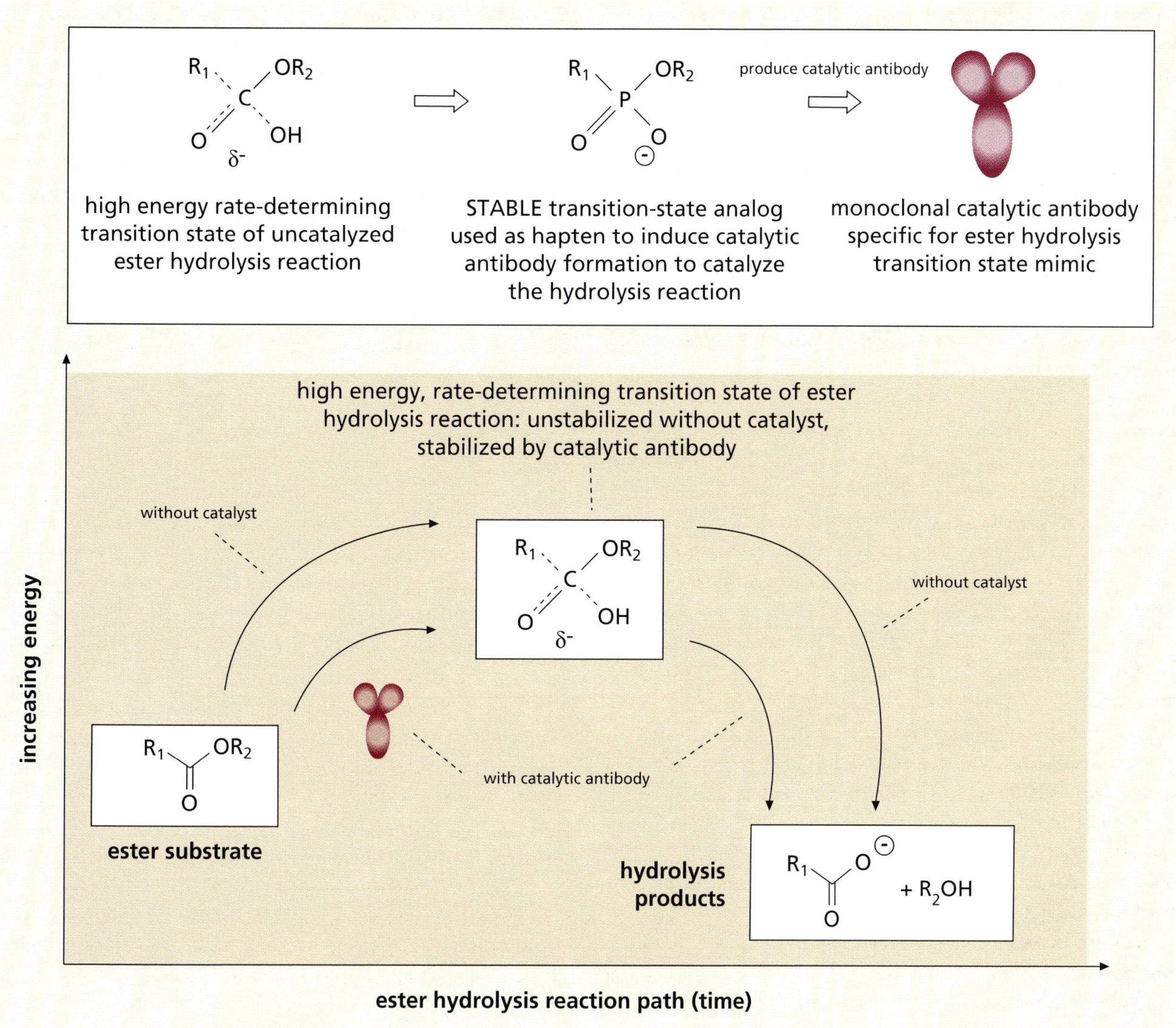

Figure 6.14. Catalytic antibodies produced to catalyze ester hydrolysis reactions. The stable transition state mimic is a phosphorus-containing molecule that resembles the tetrahedral transition state of esters when they are hydrolyzed.

in need of organs receive them due to the dearth of transplantable organs. Advances in biotechnology have created opportunities for the science of tissue engineering to address these challenges and improve health care.

Some Products of Tissue Engineering

Regenerative medicine has had success in stimulating the body's own repair mechanisms by mimicking the action of endogenous growth factors. For example, recombinant DNA technology has produced such drugs as epoetin alfa, filgrastim, and sargramostim that accomplish just that in the hematopoietic system (see Chapter 8). Research is underway to test new tissue growth factors for their ability to regenerate human tissue. Active research programs are studying the effect of growth factors on wound healing, bone repair, blood vessel generation, and nerve regeneration. Successes in genomics and proteomics should have a major impact on tissue engineering as new growth factor genes are discovered.

Several products of tissue engineering are now available for use as replacement skin and cartilage. The leading skin product is graftskin (Apligraf), approved by the FDA in 1998. It is a living skin equivalent indicated for the treatment of foot and leg ulcers. Generated in tissue culture and started from cells of human foreskin removed during infants' circumcisions, graftskin possesses a dermis, epidermis and structural matrix like normal human skin tissue. In addition to skin replacement, tissue engineering has created cartilage replacements. Autologous cultured chondrocytes (Carticel) is an approved product/procedure to repair clinically significant, symptomatic painful knee cartilage damage (medial, laterial, or trochlear) caused by acute or repetitive trauma. The patient's orthopedic surgeon sends the manufacturer a biopsy of the patient's own cartilage, which is then cultured for reinjection into the knee.

Tissue engineers are actively exploring ways to create specialized tissues and vital organs. An exciting approach is the use of a scaffold made from a biodegradable polymer matrix shaped to fit the need (for example, in the shape of a nose or an ear, etc). An important pharmaceutical area of study is the use of hydrogels for scaffold development (Lee and Mooney, 2001). The patient's own cells, donor cells or engineered cells are used to seed the scaffold. The cell-seeded scaffold is treated with requisite growth factors and placed in an appropriate growth environment so that the cells can multiply and differentiate into the appropriate different cell types. The biopolymer degrades after transplantation providing functioning tissue or organ.

Currently, there are several clinical trials underway testing novel technologies to replace damaged bone. Transgenic pigs and other animals are being engineered to provide organs for xenotransplantation to human patients that do not cause the immune system to initiate rejection mechanisms. Methodologies to introduce genes into patients to repair tissues "on-site" are being studied. Another area of active investigation is the development of technologies that can rejuvenate old tissues by manipulation of the cell's own aging mechanisms.

Pluripotent Stem Cells

Stem cell research is advancing at a rapid pace and is the subject of significant scientific, ethical, and political discussion. A timely, informative discussion of pluripotent stem cells and their potential for repair of tissues and organs is well beyond the scope of this chapter. For general information about stem cells, the reader is encouraged to research the topic in any biology textbook and a plethora of websites. Specialized stem cell topics can be studied using readily available online databases (journal and abstract) and website search engines. The US National Institutes of Health (NIH) has a valuable resource on stem cells that can be found at www.nih.gov/news/stemcell/index.htm. While published in 1999, and thus somewhat dated for such a rapidly advancing area of research, the introductory review of embryonic stem cells for regenerative medicine by Pedersen is valuable (Pedersen, 1999). A brief introduction follows solely to provide the reader with insights into the unproven potential of pluipotent stem cell research in advancing tissue engineering capabilities.

During normal human development, a single cell is produced from the joining of a sperm cell and an egg cell (please see source for this introduction at NIH *Stem Cell Primer*, www.nih.gov/news/stemcell/primer.htm). This single cell, capable of forming an entire human, initially undergoes division into two identical daughter cells. These are totipotent cells. Each totipotent cell has the capability to differentiate into the embryo, extraembryonic membranes and tissues, and all postembryonic tissues and organs. Placing one of the identical cells (or both for identical twins) in a woman's uterus has the potential to develop into a fetus. Several cycles of cell division cause the beginning of cell specialization and the formation of a blastocyst, a hollow sphere of cells. The placenta and other supporting tissues needed for fetal development in the uterus is formed from the outer layer of cells of the blastocyst while the inner cell layer can become virtually every cell type found in the human body; "virtually" every cell type. The inner cell mass is pluripotent, that is, they are capable of giving rise to many types of cells, but not all cells and not an embryo. Their potential is not total (totipotent). Further cell divisions and specializations result in cells that are committed to give rise to cells that perform specialized functions. These multipotent stem cells are extremely important to the process of cell proliferation and differentiation occurring during early human development. Types are also found in children and adults. Stem cells are cells that possess the ability to divide into daughter cells and multiply for infinite periods in culture giving rise to daughter cells with identical developmental potential and/or a cell with less potential. A totipotent stem cell can give rise to daughter totipotent stem cells and/or pluripotent stem cells. Likewise, a pluripotent stem cell can give rise to daughter pluripotent stem cells and/or multipotent stem cells, etc. For example, hematopoietic stem cells are multipotent stem cells that give rise to mutipotent hematopietic stem cells and/or white blood cells, red blood cells and platelets (see Chapter 8). Therefore, pluripotent stem cells are of real potential value to tissue engineering and regenerative medicine because of their pluripotent capabilities.

Fundamental discoveries remain to be made before this bench top research can be translated into bedside clinical medicine. Predicting what the future of stem cell research will hold is fraught with risk. However, biotechnology has experienced exponential advances in capabilities since the first edition of this text was written. If the natural requisite growth factors and appropriate differentiation/proliferation conditions can be identified and mimicked reproducibly, tissue engineering with pluripotent stem cells may give rise to repairing virtually all cells, tissues and organs including bone marrow, nerve cells, heart muscle, breast replacements, pancreatic islet cells, skin, a liver, etc. Researchers are also attempting to determine if there are conditions in which multipotent stem cells that are already more differentiated and committed to particular cell types can be converted to pluripotent capabilities.

Glycobiology

The novel scientific field of glycobiology may be defined most simply as the study of the structure, synthesis and biological role of glycans (may be referred to as oligosaccharides or polysaccharides, depending on size) and glycoconjugates in simple and complex systems (Varkin *et al.*, 1999; Fukuda and Hindsgauld, 2000; Alper, 2001). The application of glycobiology is sometimes called glycotechnology to distinguish it from biotechnology (referring to glycans rather than proteins and nucleic acids). However, many in the biotech arena consider glycobiology one of the research fields encompassed by the term biotechnology. Like proteins and nucleic acids, glycans are biopolymers. While once referred to as the last frontier of pharmaceutical discovery, recent advances in the biotechnology of discovering, cloning, and harnessing sugar cleaving and synthesizing enzymes have enabled glycobiologists to analyze and manipulate complex carbohydrates more easily (Brush, 1999).

Many of the proteins produced by animal cells contain attached sugar moieties, making them glycoproteins. Bacterial hosts for recombinant DNA could produce the animal proteins with identical or nearly identical amino acid sequences. The bacteria, however, lacked the "machinery" to attach sugar moieties to proteins (a process called glycosylation). Many of the non-glycosylated proteins differed in their biological activity as compared to the native glycoprotein. The production of animal proteins that lacked glycosylation provided an unexpected opportunity to study the functional role of sugar molecules on glycoproteins.

Basic Principles of Glycobiology

The complexity of the field can best be illustrated by reviewing some basic principles. The building blocks of glycans are simple carbohydrates (called saccharides or sugars) and their derivatives (i.e. amino sugars). Simple carbohydrates can be attached to other types of biological molecules to form glycoconjugates including glycoproteins (predominantly protein), glycolipids and proteoglycans (about 95% polysaccharide and 5% protein). While carbohydrate chemistry and biology have been active areas of research for centuries, advances in biotechnology have provided techniques and added energy to the study of glycans. Oligosaccharides found conjugated to proteins (glycoproteins) and lipids (glycolipids) display a tremendous structural diversity. The linkages of the monomeric units in proteins and in nucleic acids are generally consistent in all such molecules. Glycans, however, exhibit far greater variability in the linkage between monomeric units than that found in the other biopolymers. As an example, Figure 6.15 illustrates the common linkage sites to create polymers of glucose. Glucose can be linked at four positions: C-2, C-3, C-4 and C-6 and also can take one of two possible anomeric configurations at C-2 (α and β). The effect of multiple linkage arrangements is seen in the estimate of Kobata (Kobata, 1996). He has estimated that for a 10-mer (oligomer of length 10) the number of structurally-distinct linear oligomers for each of the biopolymers is: DNA (with 4 possible bases), 1.04×10^6; protein (with 20 possible amino acids), 1.28×10^{13}; and oligosaccharide (with eight monosaccharide types), 1.34×10^{18}.

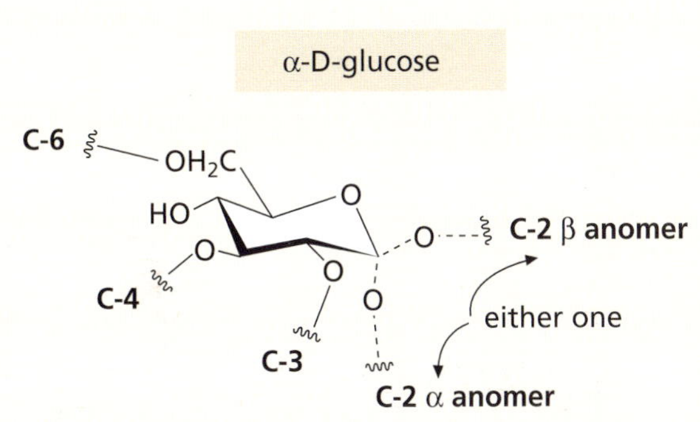

Figure 6.15. Illustration of the common linkage sites to create biopolymers of glucose. Linkages at four positions: C-2, C-3, C-4 and C-6 and also can take one of two possible anomeric configurations at C-2 (α and β).

Glycosylation and Medicine

Patterns of glycosylation affect significantly the biological activity of proteins (Paulson, 1999; McAuliffe and Hindsgaud, 2000). Many of the therapeutically used recombinant DNA-produced proteins are glycosylated including erythropoietin, glucocerebrosidase and tissue plasminogen activator. Without the appropriate carbohydrates attached, none of these proteins will function therapeutically as does the parent glycoprotein. Glycoforms (variations of the glycosylation pattern of a glycoprotein) of the same protein may differ in physicochemical and biochemical properties. For example, erythropoietin has one O-linked and three N-linked glycosylation sites. The removal of the terminal sugars at each site destroys *in vivo* activity and removing all sugars results in a more rapid clearance of the molecule and a shorter circulatory half-life (Takeuchi *et al.*, 1990). Yet, the opposite effect is observed for the deglycosylation of the hematopoietic cytokine granulocyte-macrophage colony-stimulating factor (GM-CSF) (Cebon *et al.*, 1990). In that case, removing the carbohydrate residues increases the specific activity six-fold.

Carbohydrate	Indication
fructose analog (example: Topamax)*	epilepsy
G_{D2}/KLH conjugate	melanoma (anticancer vaccine)
G_{M2}/G_{D2}/KLH conjugate	melanoma and breast cancer (anticancer vaccine)
imino sugar analog	Gaucher's Disease
low molecular weight heparins (example: Lovenox)*	cardiovascular disease
oligosaccharide conjugate	*E. coli* O157:H7 infection
sialic acid analog (example: Relenza)*	influenza
sialyl Le^x/sCR1 conjugate	reperfusion injury
sialyl-Tn antigen conjugate	metastatic breast cancer (anticancer vaccine)
swainsonine analog	cancer and viral infections

Table 6.6. Some examples of carbohydrate therapeutics approved by the FDA or in clinical trials (see Paulson *et al.*, 1999; McAuliffe and Hindsgaul, 2000; Alper, 2001)
*) FDA-approved
Abbreviations/glossary: CR1 = extracellular portion of complement receptor 1 protein; G_{M2}/G_{D2}/KLH = cancer antigens; imino sugar = nitrogen containing sugar; sialyl Le^x/ = a complex carbohydrate; sialyl-Tn = a breast cancer antigen; swainsonine = nitrogen containing sugar natural product.

The sugars of glycoproteins are known to play a role in the recognition and binding of biomolecules to other molecules in disease states such as asthma, rheumatoid arthritis, cancer, HIV-infection, the flu and other infectious diseases. A study of which oligosaccharides are involved in the recognition and binding processes associated with a disease state may lead to new molecular targets for possible therapeutic intervention (Musser *et al.*, 1995). Tools such as carbohydrate engineering, carbohydrate analysis and computer-aided molecular modeling will contribute to those efforts. Significant efforts are being employed to develop complex carbohydrate-based therapeutic agents to address many of the diseases mentioned above (see Table 6.6). Many are in preclinical development, several in early clinical trials, and a fructose analog (Topamax) has been approved and marketed recently for the control of epilepsy.

Biotechnology and Drug Discovery

Pharmaceutical scientists have taken advantage of every opportunity or technique available to aid in the long, costly drug discovery process (see Chapter 20). In essence, Chapter 6 is an overview of some of the many applications of biotechnology and related techniques useful in drug discovery or design, lead optimization, and development. In addition to recombinant DNA and hybridoma technology, the techniques described throughout Chapter 6 have changed the way drug research is conducted, refining the process that optimizes the useful pharmacological properties of an identified novel chemical lead. The promise of genomics, proteomics, pharmacogenomics/pharmacogenetics, and bioinformatics to radically change the drug discovery paradigm is eagerly anticipated (Beeley *et al.*, 2000; Ohlstein *et al.*, 2000). Figure 6.16 shows schematically the interaction of three key elements that are essential for modern drug discovery: new targets identified by genomics and related technologies; rapid, sensitive bioassays utilizing high-throughput screening methods; and new molecule creation employing a host of approaches. The key elements are underpinned at each point by bioinformatics. Several of the technologies, methods and approaches listed in Figure 6.16 have been described previously in this chapter. Others will be described below.

Screening and Synthesis

Traditionally, drug discovery programs relied heavily upon random screening followed by analog synthesis and lead

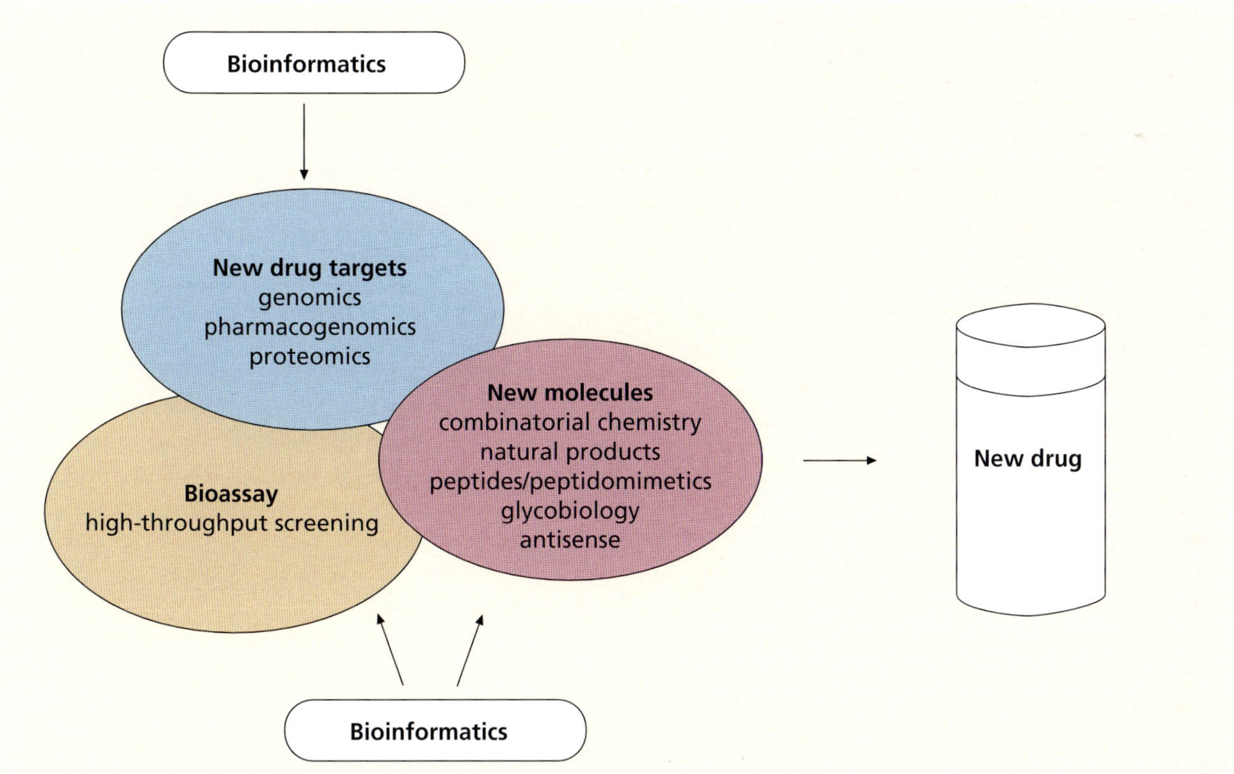

Figure 6.16. Elements of modern drug discovery: impact of biotechnology.

optimization via structure-activity relationship studies. The search for novel, efficacious, and safer medicinal agents is an increasingly costly and complex process. Therefore, any method allowing for a reduction in time and money is extremely valuable. Advances in biotechnology have contributed to a greater understanding of the cause and progression of disease and have identified new therapeutic targets forming the basis of novel drug screens. These advances have facilitated the discovery of new agents with novel mechanisms of action for diseases that were previously difficult or impossible to treat. In an effort to decrease the cost of identifying useful, quality drug leads against a pharmaceutically important target, researchers have implemented high-throughput screening and high-throughput synthesis methods.

ADVANCES IN SCREENING: HIGH-THROUGHPUT SCREENING (HTS)

Recombinant DNA technology has provided the ability to clone, express, isolate and purify receptor enzymes, membrane bound proteins, and other binding proteins in larger quantities than ever before. Instead of using receptors present in animal tissues or partially-purified enzymes for screening, *in vitro* bioassays now utilize the exact human protein target. Applications of biotechnology to *in vitro* screening include the improved preparation of: 1) cloned membrane-bound receptors expressed in cell-lines carrying few endogenous receptors; 2) immobilized preparations of receptors, antibodies and other ligand-binding proteins; and 3) soluble enzymes and extracellular cell-surface expressed protein receptors.

Previously, libraries of synthetic compounds along with natural products from microbial fermentation, plant extracts, marine organisms and invertebrates provide a diversity of molecular structures were screened randomly. Screening can be made more directed if the compounds to be investigated are selected on the basis of structural information about the receptor or natural ligand. The development of sensitive radioligand binding assays and the access to fully automated, robotic screening techniques have accelerated the screening process.

High-throughput screening (HTS) provides for the bioassay of thousands of compounds in multiple assays at the same time (Kenny *et al.*, 1998; Oldenburg, 1998). The process is automated with robots and utilizes multi-well microtiter plates. While 96-well microtiter plates are a versatile standard in HTS, the development of 1536- and 3456-well nanoplate formats and enhanced robotics brings greater miniaturization and speed to cell-based and biochemical assays. Now, companies can conduct 100,000 bioassays a day. In addition, modern drug discovery and lead optimization with DNA microarrays allows researchers to track hundreds to thousands of genes. Enzyme inhibition assays and radioligand binding assays are the most common biochemical tests employed. In most cases today, biotechnology contributes directly to the understanding, identification and/or the generation of the drug target being screened (e.g. radioligand binding displacement from a cloned protein receptor).

HIGH-THROUGHPUT SYNTHESIS: COMBINATORIAL CHEMISTRY

Traditionally, small drug molecules were synthesized by joining together structural pieces in a set sequence to prepare

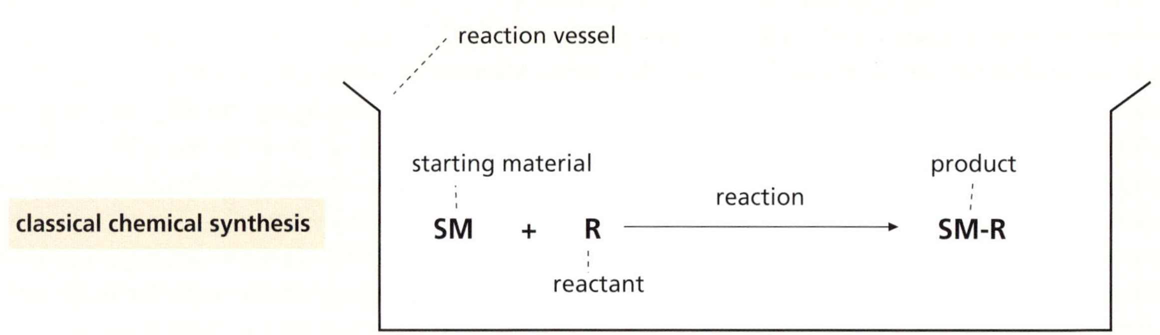

In classical chemical synthesis, a coupling reaction of one starting material (SM) with one reactant (R) would yield just one product, SM-R. One or several reactions may be run simultaneously in separate reaction vessels

combinatorial chemical synthesis: example = coupling reaction

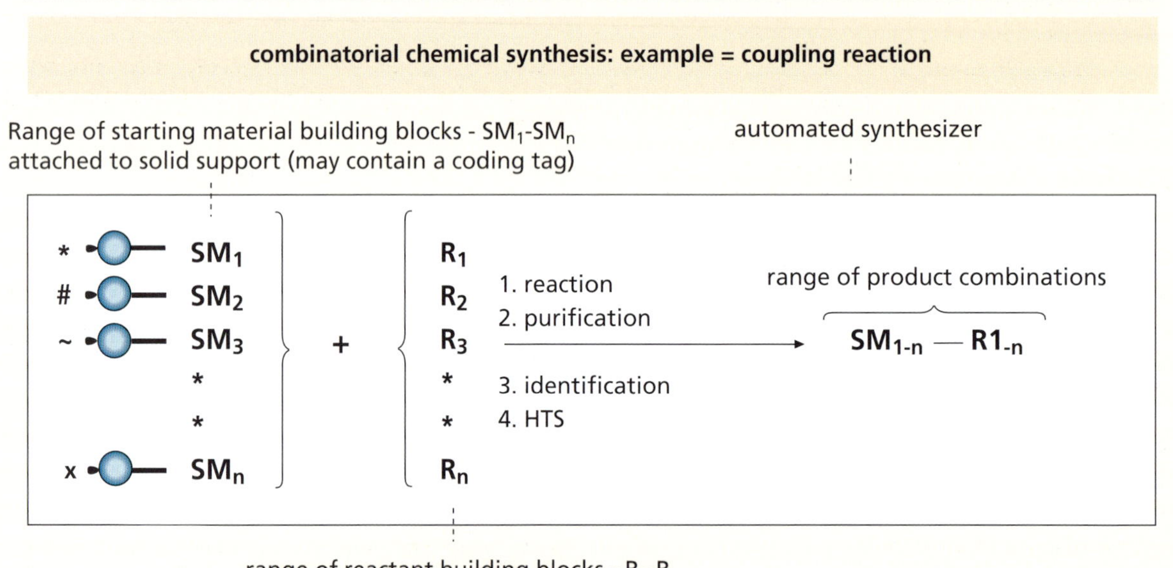

In a combinatorial chemical synthesis such as a coupling reaction, a range of starting material building blocks are reacted with a range of reactant building blocks yielding any or all possible product combinations, $SM_{1\text{-}n}$ $R_{1\text{-}n}$. The automated reactions may occur in the same reaction vessel (and coding tag used to separate/identify) or may each occur in small, separate reaction vessels (parallel synthesis)

Figure 6.17. A schematic representation of a coupling reaction: difference between classical chemical synthesis and combinatorial chemistry.

one product. One of the most powerful tools to optimize drug discovery is automated high-throughput synthesis. When conducted in a combinatorial approach, high-throughput synthesis provides for the simultaneous preparation of hundreds or thousands of related drug candidates (Czarnik and DeWitt, 1997; Gordon and Kerwin, Jr, 1998; Fenniri, 2000; Sucholeiki, 2001). The molecular libraries generated are screened in high-throughput screening assays for the desired activity, and the most active molecules are identified and isolated for further development.

There are two overall approaches to high-throughput synthesis (Bunin *et al.*, 1999). True combinatorial chemistry applies methods to substantially reduce the number of synthetic operations or steps needed to synthesize large numbers of compounds. Combichem, as it is sometimes referred to, is conducted on solid supports (resins) to facilitate the manipulations required to reduce labor. Differing from combinatorial chemistry, parallel procedures apply automation to the synthetic process, but the number of operations needed to carry out a synthesis is practically the same as the conventional approach. Thus, the potential productivity of parallel methods is not as high as combinatorial chemistries. Parallel chemistries can be conducted on solid-phase supports or in solution.

Figure 6.17 provides an illustration of a combinatorial mix-and-match process in which a simple building block (a starting material such as an amino acid, peptide, heterocycle, other small molecule, etc.) is joined to one or more other simple building blocks in every possible combination. Assigning the task to automated synthesizing equipment results in the rapid creation of large collections or libraries (as large as 10,000 compounds) of diverse molecules. Ingenious methods have been devised to direct the molecules to be synthesized, to identify the structure of the products, to purify the products via automation, and to isolate compounds. When coupled with high-throughput screening, thousands of compounds can be generated, screened, and evaluated for further development in a matter of weeks.

Building blocks include amino acids, peptides, nucleotides, carbohydrates, and a diversity of small molecule scaffolds or templates. A selection of reaction types used in combinatorial chemistry to produce compound libraries is found in Table 6.7.

Compound types
α,β-unsaturated ketones
α-hydroxy acids
acyl piperidines
azoles
β-mercaptoketones
β-turn mimetics
benzisothiazolones
benzodiazepines
biaryls
cyclopentenones
dihydropyridines
γ-butyrolactones
glycosylamines
hydantoins
isoxazoles
isoxazolines
modified oligonucleotides
peptoids
piperazinediones
porphyrins
1,3-propanediols
protease inhibitors
pyrrolidines
sulfamoylbenzamides
tetrahydrofurans
thiazole
thiazolidinones

Table 6.7 A sample of the diversity of compounds capable of being synthesized by combinatorial chemistry methods.

Conclusion

Tremendous advances have occurred in biotechnology since Watson and Crick determined the structure of DNA. Improved pharmaceuticals, novel therapeutic agents, unique diagnostic products, and new drug design tools have resulted from the escalating achievements of pharmaceutical biotechnology. While recombinant DNA technology and hybridoma techniques have received most of the press in the 1990s, a wealth of additional and innovative biotechnologies have been, and will continue to be, developed in order to enhance pharmaceutical research. Genomics, proteomics, pharmacogenomics/genetics, genetically engineered animals, protein engineering, peptide chemistry and peptidomimetics, nucleic acid technologies, catalytic antibodies, glycobiology, tissue engineering, high-throughput screening and high-speed synthesis are directly influencing the pharmaceutical sciences and are well positioned to significantly impact modern pharmaceutical care. Application of these and yet to be discovered biotechnologies will rapidly improve the competitive process of drug discovery and development of new medicinal agents and diagnostics. Pharmacists, pharmaceutical scientists and pharmacy students should be poised to take advantage of the products and techniques made available by the unprecedented scope and pace of discovery in biotechnology in the 21st Century. ■

Further Reading

- **Baxevanis AD, Ouellette BFF.** (1998). *Bioinformatics: A practical Guide to the Analysis of Genes and Proteins.* New York, New York: Wiley-Interscience
- **Crooke ST.** (2001). *Antisense Drug Technology: Principles, Strategies, and Applications.* New York, New York: Marcel Dekker, Inc.
- **Dean PM, Jolles G, Newton CG.** (1995). *New Perspectives in Drug Design.* San Diego, California: Academic Press
- **Dunn MJ.** (2000). *From Genome to Proteome: Advances in the Practice and Application of Proteomics.* Weinheim, Federal Republic of Germany: Wiley-VCH
- **Hartl DL, Jones EW.** (2001). *Genetics: Analysis of Genes and Genomes.* Sudbury, Massachusetts: Jones and Bartlett Publishers
- **Houdebine LM.** (1997). *Transgenic Animals – Generation and Use.* Amsterdam: Harwood Academic Publishers
- **Kalow W, UA Meyer and RF Tyndale.** (2001). *Pharmacogenomics.* New York, New York: Marcel Dekker, Inc.
- **Lodish H, Berk A, Zipursky SL, Matsudaira P, Baltimore D, Darnell J.** (2000). *Molecular Cell Biology* 4th Ed. New York, New York: W.H. Freeman and Company
- **Maulik S, Patel SD.** (1997). *Molecular Biotechnology – Therapeutic Applications and Strategies.* New York, New York: Wiley-Liss
- **Patrick Jr. CW, Mikos AG, McIntire LV.** (1998). *Frontiers in Tissue Engineering.* Oxford, UK: Pergamon Press
- **Pennington SR, Dunn MJ.** (2001). *Proteomics: From protein sequence to function.* New York, New York: Bios Scientific Publishers Limited
- **Schena M, Heller RA, Theriault TP, Konrad K, Lachenmeier E, Davis RW.** (1998). Microarrays: biotechnology's discovery platform for functional genomics. *Trends Biotechnol.*, 16, 301–306
- **Southern EM.** (2001). DNA Microarrays. In *DNA Arrays: Methods and Protocols*, edited by JB Rampal. Totowa, New Jersey: Humana Press, pp. 1–13
- **Swanson ME, Grass DS, Ciofalo VB.** (1994). Transgenic and Gene Targeting Technology in Drug Discovery. *Ann. Rep. Med. Chem.* 29, 265–274

References

- **Abell A.** (1999). *Advances in Amino Acid Mimetics and Peptidomimetics*, Volume 2. Stamford, Connecticut: JAI.
- **Adair JR.** (1992). Engineering antibodies for therapy. *Immunol. Rev.*, 130, 5–40.
- **Aderem A, Hood L.** (2001). Immunology in the post-genomic era. *Nature Immunol.* 2, 373–375.
- **Alper J.** (2001). Searching for Medicine's Sweet Spot. *Science*, 291, 2338–2343.
- **Anderson KP, Fox MC, Brown-Driver V.** (1996). Inhibition of human cytomegalovirus immediate-early gene expression by an oligonucleotide complementary to immediate early RNA. *Antimicrob. Agents Chemother.*, 40, 2004–2011.
- **Agrawal A.** (1996). *Antisense Therapeutics.* Totowa, New Jersey: Humana Press.
- **Ball S, Borman N.** (1997). Pharmacogenomics and drug metabolism. *Nature Biotech.*, 15, 925–926.
- **Beeley LJ, Duckworth DM, Southan C.** (2000). The impact of genomics on drug discovery. *Prog. Med. Chem.*, 37, 1–43.
- **Bikker JA, Trumpp-Kallmeyer S, Humblet C.** (1998). G-Protein Coupled Receptors: Models, Mutagenesis, and Drug Design. *J. Med. Chem.*, 41, 2911–2927.
- **Blackstock WP, Weir MP.** (1999). Proteomics: quantitative and physical mapping of cellular proteins. *TIBECH*, 17, 121–127.
- **Borg S, Estenne-Bouhton G, Luthman K, Csöregh I, Hesselink W, Hacksell U.** (1995). Synthesis of 1,2,4-oxadiazole, 1,3,4-oxadiazole, and 1,2,4-triazole-derived dipeptidomimetics. *J. Org. Chem.*, 60, 3112–3120.
- **Borman S.** (2000). Proteomics: Taking Over Where Genomics Leaves Off. *Chem. Eng. News*, 78(July 31), 31–37.
- **Borrebaeck CAK.** (1992). *Antibody Engineering: A Practical Guide.* New York, New York: WH Freeman and Company.
- **Bramlage B, Luzi E, Eckstein F.** (1998). *IIBECH*, 16, 434–438.
- **Breslow J.** (1994). Lipoprotein and heart disease: transgenic mice models helping in the search for new therapies. *Bio/ Technology*, 12, 665–370.
- **Brooks G.** (1998). Potential use of transgenic animals in health and disease. In *Biotechnology in Healthcare – An introduction to biopharmaceuticals*, edited by G Brooks. London, England: Pharmaceutical Press, pp. 131–146.
- **Brown K.** (2000). The Human Genome Business Today. *Sci. Amer.*, 283, 50–55.
- **Brown TA.** (1999). *Genomes.* New York, New York: Wiley-Liss.
- **Brownlee C.** (2001). The Mechanics of Tissue Engineering. *Mod. Drug Discov.*, 4, 35–38.
- **Bunin BA, Dener JM, Livingston DA.** (1999). Applications of Combinatorial and Parallel Synthesis to Medicinal Chemistry. *Ann. Rep. Med. Chem.* 34, 267–286.
- **Bush M.** (1999). Sugars and Splice – Glycobiology: The Next Frontier. *The Scientist*, July 19, 22–23.
- **Cantor CR, Smith CL.** (1999). *Genomics – The Science and Technology Behind the Human Genome Project.* New York, New York: John Wiley & Sons, Inc.
- **Cargill M, Altshuler A, Ireland J, Sklar P, Ardlie K, Patil N, Lane CR, Lim EP, Kalyanaraman N, Ziaugra L, Friedland**

L, Rolfe A, Warrington J, Lipshutz R, Daley GQ, Lander E. (1999). Characterization of single-nucleotide polymorphisms in coding regions of human genes. *Nature Genet.*, 22, 231–238.
- **Cebon J, Nicola N, Ward M, Gardner I, Dempsey P, Layton J, Duhrsen U, Burgess AW, Nice E, Morstyn G.** (1990). Granulocyte-macrophage colony stimulating factor from human lymphocytes. *J. Biol. Chem.*, 265, 4483–4491.
- **Chamow SM, Ashkenazi A.** (1999). *Antibody Fusion Proteins.* New York, New York: John Wiley and Sons. Inc.
- **Charifson PS.** (1997). *Practical Application of Computer-Aided Drug Design.* New York, New York: Marcel Dekker, Inc.
- **Clark MS.** (1999). Comparative genomics: the key to understanding the Human genome Project. *Bioessays*, 21, 121–130.
- **Cleland JL, Craik CS.** (1996). *Protein Engineering. Principles and Practice.* New York, New York: Wiley-Liss.
- **Clore GM, Gronenborn AM.** (1998). Determining the structures of large proteins and protein complexes by NMR. *TIBECH*, 16, 22–34.
- **Collins F, Galas D.** (1993). A new five-year plan for the U.S. Human genome. *Science*, 262, 43–46.
- **Craik CS, Roczniak S, Largman C, Rutter WJ.** (1987). The catalytic role of the active site aspartic acid in serine proteases. *Science*, 237, 909–913.
- **Craik DJ.** (1996). *NMR in Drug Design*, Boca Raton, Florida: CRC Press.
- **Crooke ST.** (1995a). Oligonucleotide Therapeutics. In *Burger's Medicinal Chemistry, Fifth Edition*, Vol. 1, edited by M.E. Wolff. New York, New York: John Wiley & Sons, Inc., pp. 863–900.
- **Crooke ST.** (1995b). The Future of Antisense Technology. *Pharmaceut. News*, 2, 8–11.
- **Crooke ST.** (1998). An overview of progress in antisense therapeutics. *Antisense Nucl. Acid Drug Dev.*, 8, 115–122.
- **Crooke ST.** (1999). Molecular mechanisms of action of antisense drugs. *Biochim. Biophys. Acta*, 1489, 31–43.
- **Czarnik AW, DeWitt SH.** (1997). *A Practical Guide to Combinatorial Chemistry.* Washington, DC: American Chemical Society.
- **Dervan PB.** (1989). Oligonucleotide Recognition of Double-helical DNA by Triple-helix Formation. In *Oligodeoxynucleotides: Antisense Inhibitors of Gene Expression*, edited by JS Cohen. Boca Raton, Florida: CRC Press, pp. 197–210.
- **Ducruis A, Giege R.** (1992). *Crystallization of Nucleic Acids and Proteins – A Practical Approach.* Oxford, England: IHL Press.
- **Dugas H.** (1999). *Bioorganic Chemistry: A Chemical Approach to Enzyme Action*, 3rd ed. New York, New York: Springer-Verlag.
- **Edwards AM, Arrowsmith CH, Pallieres B.** (2000). Proteomics: New tools for a new era. *Mod. Drug Discov.*, 3(September), 34–44.
- **Ellington AD, Szostak JW.** (1990). *In vitro* selection of RNA molecules that bind specific ligands. *Nature*, 346, 818–822.
- **Emmett A.** (2000). The State of Bioinformatics. *The Scientist*, 14(23), 1, 10, 12, 19.
- **Evans WE, Relling MV.** (1999). Pharmacogenomics: Translating functional genomics into rational therapies. *Science*, 286, 487–491.
- **Felton MJ.** (2001). Bioinformatics: The child of success. *Mod. Drug Discov.*, 4(January), 25–28.
- **Fenniri H.** (2000). *Combinatorial Chemistry: A Practical Approach.* Oxford, UK: Oxford University Press.
- **Fodor WL, William BL, Matis LA, Madri JA, Rollins SA, Knight JW, Velander W, Squinto SA.** (1994). Expression of a functional human complement inhibitor in a transgenic pig as a model for the prevention of xenogeneic hyperacute organ rejection. *Proc. Natl. Acad. Sci. USA*, 91, 11153–11157.
- **Fothergill-Gilmore LA.** (1993). Recombinant protein technology. In *Protein Biotechnology*, edited by F Franks. Totowa, New Jersey: Humana Press, pp. 467–487.
- **Freeman TR.** (2001). Pharmacogenomics: Opening New Vistas in Pharmacotherapy. *J. Am. Pharmaceut. Assoc.*, 41, 629–630.
- **Fukuda M, Hindsgaul O.** (2000). *Molecular and CellularGlycobiology.* Oxford, UK: Oxford University Press.
- **Garner I, Colman A.** (1998). Therapeutic Proteins form Livestock. In *Animal Breeding-Technology for the 21st Century*, edited by AJ Clark. Amsterdam: Harwood Academic Publishers, 215–227.
- **Giannis A, Rubsam F.** (1997). Peptidomimetics in drug design. *Adv. Drug Res.*, 29, 1–78.
- **Goodman M, Ro S.** (1995). Peptidomimetics for Drug Design. In *Burger's Medicinal Chemistry, Fifth Edition*, Vol. 1, edited by ME Wolff. New York, New York: John Wiley & Sons, Inc., pp. 803–861.
- **Gordon EM, Kerwin JF.** (1998). *Combinatorial Chemistry and Molecular Diversity in Drug Discovery.* New York, New York: Wiley-Liss, Inc.
- **Graf von Roedern E, Kessler H.** (1994). A sugar amino acid as a novel peptidomimetic. *Angew. Chem. Int. Ed. Engl.*, 33, 687–689.
- **Grant DM, Phillips MS.** (2001). Technologies for Analysis of Single-Nucleotide Polymorphisms. In *Pharmacogenomics*, edited by W Kalow, UA Meyer and RF Tyndale. New York, New York: Marcel Dekker, Inc., pp. 183–189.
- **Gron H, Hyde-DeRuyscher R.** (2000). Peptides as tools in drug discovery. *Curr. Opin. Drug Discovery Dev.*, 3, 636–645.
- **Greer J, Erickson JW, Baldwin JJ, Varney, MD.** (1994). Application of the Three-Dimensional Structures of Protein Target Molecules in Structure-Based Drug Design. *J. Med. Chem.*, 37, 1035–1054.
- **Griffiths AJF, Miller JH, Suzuki DT, Lewontin RC, Gelbart WM.** (2000). *An Introduction to Genetic Analysis*, 7th Ed. New York, New York: W.H. Freeman and Company.
- **Guild BC.** (1999). Genomics, Target Selection, Validation, and Assay Considerations in the Development of Antibacterial Screens. *Ann. Rep. Med. Chem*, 34, 227–236.
- **Gura T.** (2001). Can SNPs Deliver on Susceptibility Genes? *Science*, 293, 593–595.

- **Gutte B.** (1995). *Peptides: Synthesis, Structures, and Applications.* San Diego, California: Academic Press.
- **Helene C, Thuong NT, Harel-Bellan A.** (1992). Control of Gene Expression by Triple Helix-Forming Oligonucleotides. *Ann. N.Y. Acad. Sci.*, 660, 27–36.
- **Hirschmann R, Nicolaou KC, Pietranico S, Leahy EM, Salvino J, Arison B, Cichy MA, Spoors PG, Shakespeare WC, Sprengler PA, Hamley P, Smith III AB, Reisine T, Raynor K, Maechler L, Donaldson C, Vale W, Freidinger RM, Cascieri MR, Strader CD.** (1993). *De novo* design and synthesis of somatostatin non-peptide peptidomimetics utilizing □-D-glucose as a novel scaffolding. *J. Am. Chem. Soc.*, 115, 12550–12568.
- **Hirschmann R, Smith III AB, Sprengeler PA.** (1995). Some Interactions of macromolecules with Low Molecular Weight Ligands: Recent Advances in Peptidomimetic Research. In *New Perspectives in Drug Design*, edited by PM Dean, G Jolles, CG Newton. San Diego, California: Academic Press, pp. 1–14.
- **Hunt SP, Livesey FJ.** (2000). Functional genomics: approaches and methodologies. In *Functional Genomics*, edited by SP Hunt and FJ Livesey. Oxford, England: Oxford University Press, pp. 1–7.
- **Isola LM, Gordon JW.** (1991). Transgenic animals: a new era in developmental biology and medicine. In *Transgenic Animals*, edited by NL First and FP Haseltine. Boston, Massachusetts: Butterworth-Heinemann, pp. 3–20.
- **Johnson AC, Reitz M.** (1998). Site-Directed Mutagenesis. In *Recombinant DNA Principles and Methodologies*, edited by JJ Greene and VB Rao. New York, New York: Marcel Dekker, Inc., pp. 699–719.
- **Kalow W.** (1997). Pharmacogenetics in biological perspective. *Pharmacol. Rev.*, 49, 369–379.
- **Kalow W.** (2001). Historical Aspects of Pharmacogenetics. In *Pharmacogenomics*, edited by W Kalow, UA Meyer and RF Tyndale. New York, New York: Marcel Dekker, Inc., pp. 1–9.
- **Kenny BA, Bushfield M, Parry-Smith DJ, Fogarty S, Treherne JM.** (1998). The application of high-throughput. screening to novel lead discovery. *Prog. Drug Res.*, 51, 245–269.
- **Karow J.** (2000). The "Other" Genomes. *Sci. Am.*, 283, 53.
- **Khan J, Bittner ML, Chen Y, Meltzer PS, Trent JM.** (1999). DNA microarray technology: the anticipated impact on the study of human disease. *Biochim Biophys Acta*, 1423, M17–M28.
- **Kobata A.** (1991). Function and pathology of the sugar chains of human immunoglobulin G. *Glycobiology*, 1, 5–8.
- **Kool ET.** (1996). Topological modification of oligonucleotides for potential ınhibition of gene expression. *Perspectives Drug Discov. Design*, 4, 61–75.
- **Krueger RJ.** (1995). Ribozymes: RNA as a Therapeutic Agent. *Amer. Pharm.*, NS35, No. 1, 12–13.
- **Lau KF, Sakul H.** (2000). Pharmacogenomics. *Ann. Rep. Med. Chem.*, 36, 261–269.
- **Lebedev AV, Wickstrom E.** (1996). The chirality problem in P-substituted oligonucleotides. *Perspectives Drug Discov. Design*, 4, 17–40.
- **Lee KY, Mooney DJ.** (2001). Hydrogels for Tissue Engineering. *Chem. Rev.*, 101, 1869–1879.
- **Lennard L.** (1998). Clinical implications of thiopurine methyltransferase – optimization of drug dosage and potential drug interactions. *Ther. Drug Monit.*, 20, 527–531.
- **Lewis R.** (2000). Porcine Possibilities – Can transgenic technology reduce the risks of xenotransplants. *The Scientist*, 14, 1 and 10–11.
- **Lipp E.** (2001). Tissue Engineering and Repair Technologies. *Genet. Eng. News*, 21(16), 1, 53, 77.
- **Lipschutz RJ, Fodor SPA, Gingeras TR, Lockhart DJ.** (1999). High density synthetic oligonucleotide arrays. *Nature Genet.*, 21(suppl.), 20–24.
- **Liskamp RMJ.** (1994). Conformationally restricted amino acids and dipeptides, (non)peptidomimetics and secondary structure mimetics. *Recl. Trav. Chim. Pays-Bas*, 113, 1–19.
- **Lodish H, Berk A, Zipursky SL, Matsudaira P, Baltimore D, Darnell J.** (2000). *Molecular Cell Biology, 4th ed.* New York, New York: Scientific American Books, 281–290.
- **Luthman K, Hacksell U.** (1996). Peptides and Peptidomimetics. In *A Textbook of Drug Design and Development*, 2nd Edition, edited by P Krogsgaard-Larsen, T Liljefors, and U Madsen. Amsterdam, The Netherlands: Harwood Academic Publishers GmbH, pp. 386–406.
- **Mak TW, Penninger JM, Ohashi PS.** (2001). Knockout mice: A paradigm shift in modern immunology. *NatureRev. – Immunol.*, 1, 11–19.
- **Markley JL, Opella SJ.** (1997). *Biological NMR Spectroscopy.* Oxford, England: Oxford University Press.
- **Marr JJ.** (1996). Ribozymes as therapeutic agents. *Drug Discov. Today*, 1, 94–102.
- **McAuliffe JC, Hindsgaul JC.** (2000). Carbohydrates in medicine. In *Molecular and CellularGlycobiology edited by M* Fukuda and O Hindsgaul. *Oxford*, UK: Oxford University Press, pp 249–285.
- **McCafferty J, Glover DR.** (2000). Engineering therapeutic proteins. *Curr. Opin. Struct. Biol.*, 10, 417–420.
- **McPherson A.** (1995). The Role of X-Ray Crystallography in Structure-Based Rational drug Design. In *Chemical and Structural Approaches to Rational Drug Design*, edited by DB Weiner and WB Williams. Boca Raton, Florida: CRC Press pp. 161–213.
- **McRee DE.** (1993). *Practical Protein Crystallography.* San Diego, California: Academic Press.
- **Miao J, Hodgson KO, Sayre D.** (2001). An approach to three-dimensional structures of biomolecules by using single-molecule diffraction images. *Proc. Natl. Acad. Sci. USA*, 98, 6641–6645.
- **Mintz B, Klein-Szanto AJ.** (1992). Malignancy of eye melanomas originating in the retinal pigment epithelium of transgenic mice after genetic ablation choroidal melanocytes. *Proc. Natl. Acad. Sci. USA*, 89, 11421–11425.
- **Mooney DJ, Mikos AG.** (1999). Growing New Organs. *Sci. Amer.*, 281, 60–65.

- **Murcko MA, Caron PR, Charifson PS.** (1999). Structure-Based Drug Design. *Ann. Rep. Med. Chem.* 34, 297–306.
- **Murray JAH, Crockett N.** (1992). Antisense techniques: an overview. In *Antisense RNA and DNA,* edited by JAH Murray. New York, New York: Wiley-Liss, pp. 1–49.
- **Musser JH, Fügedi P, Anderson MB.** (1995). Carbohydrate-based Therapeutics. In *Burger's Medicinal Chemistry, Fifth Edition,* Vol. 1, edited by ME Wolff. New York, New York: John Wiley & Sons, Inc., pp. 901–947.
- **Nakanishi H, Kahn M.** (1996). Design of peptidomimetics. In *The Practice of Medicinal Chemistry,* edited by CG Wemuth. San Diego, California: Academic Press, pp. 570–590.
- **Narang SA.** (1990). *Protein Engineering, Approaches to the Manipulation of Protein Folding.* Stoneham, Massachusetts: Butterworth Publishers.
- **Nelson R.** (2000). Genome Pharmacy. *Drug Topics' Hosp. Pharmacist Rep.,* 14(10), 22–24.
- **Nielsen PE.** (1999). Peptide Nucleic Acid. A Molecule with Two Identities. *Acc. Chem. Res.,* 32, 624–630.
- **Nielsen PE, Egholm M.** (1999). *Peptide Nucleic Acids: Protocols and Applications.* Wymondham, UK: Horizon Scientific Press.
- **Nixon AE, Ostermeier M, Benkovic SJ.** (1998). Hybrid enzymes: manipulating enzyme design. *TIBECH,* 16, 258–264.
- **Obrecht D, Altorfer M, Robinson JA.** (1999). Novel Peptide Mimetic Building Blocks and Strategies for Efficient Lead Finding. *Adv. Med. Chem.,* 4, 1–68.
- **Ohlstein EH, Ruffolo Jr RR, Elliott JD.** (2000). Drug discovery in the next millennium. *Annu. Rev. Pharmacol. Toxicol.,* 40, 177–191.
- **O'Kane CJ, Moffat KG.** (1992). Selective cell ablation and genetic surgery. *Curr. Opin. Genet. Dev.,* 2, 602–606.
- **Oldenburg KR.** (1988). Current and Future Trends in High Throughput Screening for Drug Discovery. *Ann. Rep. Med. Chem.* 33, 301–311.
- **Paulson JC.** (1999). Glycobiology in Biotechnology and Medicine. In *Essentials of Glycobiology,* edited by A Varki, R Cummings, J Esko, H Freeze, G Hart, J Marth. LaJolla, California: Cold Spring Harbor Laboratory Press, pp. 625–634.
- **Pedersen RA.** (1999). Embryonic Stem Cells for Medicine. *Sci. Amer.,* 281, 68–73.
- **Peitsch MC.** (1997). Comparative Protein Modeling. In *Practical Application of Computer-Aided Drug Design,* edited by PS Charifson. New York, New York: Marcel Dekker, Inc., pp. 227–242.
- **Pennisi E.** (2000). Genomics Comes of Age. *Science,* 290, 2220–2221.
- **Persidis A.** (1998a). Proteomics. *Nature Biotech.,* 16, 393–394.
- **Persidis A.** (1998b). Pharmacogenomics and diagnostics. *Nature Biotech.,* 16, 791–792.
- **Petit-Zeman S.** (2001). Regenerative medicine. *Nature Biotech.,* 19, 201–206.
- **Pettipher R, Holford R.** (2000). Pharmacogenetics Paves the Way. *Drug Discov. Develop.,* (January/February), 53–54.
- **Pfost DR, Boyce-Jacino MT, Grant DM.** (2000). A SNPshot: pharmacogenetics and the future of drug therapy. *TIBTECH,* 18, 334–338.
- **Pharmaceutical Research and Manufacturers of America.** (2000). *Biotechnology Medicines In Development.* Washington, DC.
- **Pluckthun A.** (1992). Mono- and bivalent antibody fragments produced in *Escherichia coli*: engineering, folding and antigen binding. *Immunol. Rev.,* 130, 151–18.
- **Ramabhadran TV.** (1994). *Pharmaceutical Design and Development. A Molecular Biology Approach.* New York, New York: Springer-Verlag, pp. 246–277.
- **Ramsey G.** (1998). DNA chips: State-of-the-art. *Nature Biotech.,* 16, 40–44.
- **Rawls R.** (1997). Catalytic DNA. *Chem. Eng. News,* 75(Feb 3), 33–35.
- **Richardson JS, Richardson DC.** (1990). The *de novo* synthesis of proteins. In *Proteins: Form and* Function, edited by RA Bradshaw and M Purton Cambridge, England: Elsevier Trends Journal, pp. 173–182.
- **Ripka AS, Rich DH.** (1998). Peptidomimetic sesign. *Curr. Opin. Chem. Biol.,* 2, 441–452.
- **Roberts GW, Swinton J.** (2001). In silico proteomics: Playing by the rules. *Curr. Drug Discov.,* August, 30–33.
- **Rudolph NS.** (1995). Advances Continue in Production of Proteins in Transgenic Animal Milk. *Genet. Eng. News,* October 15, 8–9.
- **Rudolph NS.** (2000). Biopharmaceutical production in transgenic livestock. *TIBTECH,* 17, 367–374.
- **Saeks J.** (2001). Towards a proteomic future. *Curr. Drug Discov.,* August, 9–10.
- **Sailor MJ.** (1997). The Lamb That Roared. *Science,* 278, 2038–2039.
- **Saito M, Iwawaki T, Taya C, Yonekawa H, Noda M, Yoshiaki I, Mekada E, Kimata Y, Tsuru A, Kohno K.** (2001). Diphtheria toxin receptor-mediated conditional and targeted cell ablation in transgenic mice. *Nature Biotech.,* 19, 746–750.
- **Schniecke AE, Kind AJ, Ritchie WA, Mycock K, Scott AR, Ritchie M, Wilmut I, Colman A, Campbell KHS.** (1997). Human Factor IX Transgenic Sheep Produced by Transfer of Nuclei from Transfected Fetal Fibroblasts. *Science,* 278, 2130–2133.
- **Sedivy JM, Joyner AL.** (1992). *Gene Targeting.* New York, New York: W.H. Freeman & Co.
- **Seneci P.** (2000). *Solid-Phase Synthesis and Combinatorial Technologies.* New York, New York: Wiley-Interscience.
- **Silber BM.** (2001). Pharmacogenomics, Biomarkers, and the Promise of Personalized Medicine. In *Pharmacogenomics,* edited by W Kalow, UA Meyer and RF Tyndale. New York, New York: Marcel Dekker, Inc., pp. 11–31.
- **Stein CA, Narayanan R.** (1996). Antisense oligodeoxynucleotides: Internalization, compartmentalization and non-sequence specificity. *Perspectives in Drug Discovery and Design,* 4, 41–50.

- **Stock UA, Vacanti JP.** (2001). Tissue engineering: current state and prospects. *Annu. Rev. Med.*, 52, 443–451.
- **Stull RA, Szoka Jr FC.** (1995). Antigene, Ribozyme and Aptamer Nucleic Acid Drugs: Progress and Prospects. *Pharmaceut. Res.*, 12, 465–483.
- **Sucholeiki I.** (2001). *High-Throughput Synthesis: Principles and Practices.* New York, New York: Marcel Dekker, Inc.
- **Takeuchi M, Takasaki S, Shimada M, Kobata A.** (1990). Role of sugar chains in the in vitro biological activity in human erythropoietin produced in recombinant Chinese hamster ovary cells. *J. Biol. Chem.*, 265, 12127–12130.
- **Temple LKF, McLeod RS, Gallinger S, Wright JG.** (2001). Defining Disease in the Genomics Era. *Science*, 293, 807–808.
- **Thayer A.** (1996). Firms boost prospects for transgenic drugs. *Chem. Eng. News*, August 26, 23–24.
- **The Genome International Sequencing Consortium.** (2001). Initial sequencing and analysis of the human genome. *Nature*, 409, 860–921.
- **Tidd DM.** (1996). Specificity of antisense oligonucleotides. *Perspectives Drug Discov. Design*, 4, 51–60.
- **Tsuji S, Kaji K, Nagasawa S.** (1994). Decay-accelerating factor on human umbilical vein endothelial cells. *J. Immunol.*, 152, 1404–1410.
- **VanderSpek JC, Mindell JA, Finkelstein A, Murphy JR.** (1993). Structure/function analysis of the transmemberane domain of DAB_{389}-interleukin-2, an interleukin-2 receptor-targeted fusion toxin. The amphipathic helical region of the transmembrane domain is essential for the efficient delivery of the catalytic domain to the cytosol of target cells. *J. Biol. Chem.*, 268, 12077–12082.
- **Varki A, Cummings R, Esko J, Freeze H, Hart G, Marth J.** (1999). *Essentials of Glycobiology.* LaJolla, California: Cold Spring Harbor Laboratory Press.
- **Veerapandian, B.** (1995). Three Dimensional Structure-Aided Drug Design. In *Burger's Medicinal Chemistry, Fifth Edition,* edited by ME Wolff. New York, New York: John Wiley & Sons, Inc., Vol. 1, pp. 303–348.
- **Venter JC, *et al.*** (2001). The sequence of the Human Genome. *Science*, 291, 1304–1351.
- **Watkins KJ.** (2001). Bioinformatics: Making sense of information mined from the human genome is a massive undertaking for a fledgling industry. *Chem Eng News*, 79(Feb 19), 29–45.
- **Wiley RA, Rich DH.** (1993). Peptidomimetics derived from natural products. *Med. Res. Rev.*, 13, 327–384.
- **Wiley SR.** (1998). Genomics in the Real World. *Curr. Pharmaceut. Design*, 4, 417–42.
- **Wilmut I.** (1998). Cloning for Medicine. *Sci. Am.*, 280, 58–63.
- **Wright FA, *et al.*** (2001). A draft annotation and overview of the human genome. *Genome Biol.*, 2, 1–18.
- **Zhang SH, Reddick RL, Piedrahita JA, Maeda N.** (1992). Spontaneous Hypercholesterolemia and Arterial Lesions in Mice Lacking Apolipoprotein E. *Science*, 258, 468.

Self-Assessment Questions

Question 1: *What were the increasing levels of genetic resolution of the human genome planned for study as part of the HGP?*

Question 2: *What is functional genomics?*

Question 3: *What is proteomics?*

Question 4: *What are SNPs?*

Question 5: *What is the difference between pharmacogenetics and pharmacogenomics?*

Question 6: *Why are engineered animal models valuable to pharmaceutical research?*

Question 7: *What two techniques are commonly used to produce transgenic animals?*

Question 8: *What is a knockout mouse?*

Question 9: *What is site-directed mutagenesis?*

Question 10: *How does point mutation differ from a site-directed mutation?*

Question 11: *What are fusion proteins?*

Question 12: *What structural techniques can provide information about the 3-D structure of a protein?*

Question 13: *Define the term peptidomimetic.*

Question 14: *Name are some of the techniques that comprise nucleic acid technology.*

Question 15: *What chemical modifications have been made to improve the physiochemical properties of oligonucleotides?*

Question 16: *What are the mechanisms by which antisense oligonucleotides act?*

Question 17: *What are ribozymes?*

Question 18: *What are the key technologies that allowed for the development of catalytic antibodies?*

Question 19: *What is tissue engineering?*

Question 20: *What are stem cells?*

Question 21: *What is glycobiology?*

Question 22: *What is high-throughput screening?*

Question 23: *What are two approaches to high-throughput synthesis of drug leads and how do they differ?*

Answers

Answer 1: HGP structural genomics was envisioned to proceed through increasing levels of genetic resolution: detailed human genetic linkage maps [approx. 2 megabase pairs (Mb = million base pairs) resolution], complete physical maps (0.1 Mb resolution), and ultimately complete DNA sequencing of the approximately 3.5 billion base pairs (23 pairs of chromosomes) in a human cell nucleus [1 base pair (bp) resolution].

Answer 2: Functional genomics is a new approach to genetic analysis that focuses on genome-wide patterns of gene expression, the mechanisms by which gene expression is coordinated, and the interrelationships of gene expression when a cellular environmental change occurs.

Answer 3: A new research area called proteomics seeks to define the function and correlate that with expression profiles of all proteins encoded within a genome.

Answer 4: While comparing the base sequences in the DNA of two individuals reveals them to be approximately 99.9 per cent identical, base differences, or polymorphisms, are scattered throughout the genome. The best-characterized human polymorphisms are single nucleotide polymorphisms (SNPs) occurring approximately once every 1000 bases in the 3.5 billion base pair human genome.

Answer 5: Pharmacogenetics is the study of how an individual's genetic differences influence drug action, usage, and dosing. A detailed knowledge of a patient's pharmacogenetics in relation to a particular drug therapy may lead to enhanced efficacy and greater safety. While sometimes used interchangeably (especially in pharmacy practice literature), pharmacogenetics and pharmacogenomics are subtly different. Pharmacogenomics introduces the additional element of our present technical ability to pinpoint patient-specific DNA variation using genomics techniques. While overlapping fields of study, pharmacogenomics is a much newer term that correlates an individual patient's DNA variation (SNP level of variation knowledge rather than gene level of variation knowledge) with his or her response to pharmacotherapy.

Answer 6: Engineered animal models are proving invaluable since small animal models of disease are often poor mimics of that disease in human patients. Genetic engineering can predispose an animal to a particular disease under scrutiny and the insertion of human genes into the animal can initiate the development of a more clinically-relevant disease condition.

Answer 7: 1) DNA microinjection and random gene addition; and 2) homologous recombination in embryonic stem cells.

Answer 8: A knockout mouse, also called a gene knockout mouse or a gene-targeted knockout mouse, is an animal in which an endogenous gene (genomic wild-type allele) has been specifically inactivated by replacing it with a null allele.

Answer 9: Site-directed mutagenesis (also called site-specific mutagenesis) is a protein engineering technique allowing specifically (site-direct) alteration (mutation) of the primary amino acid sequence of proteins to create new chemical entities.

Answer 10: Site directed mutagenesis at a single amino acid position in an engineered protein is called a point mutation.

Answer 11: Fusion proteins contain portions or the entire amino acid sequences of both parent proteins fused together.

Answer 12: Protein X-ray crystallography and nuclear magnetic resonance (NMR) spectroscopy.

Answer 13: Peptidomimetic (sometimes called peptide mimetics and nonpeptide mimetics) are defined as structures that serve as appropriate substitutes for peptides in interactions with receptors and enzymes. The mimetic must possess not only affinity, but also efficacy or substitute function.

Answer 14: Gene therapy, antisense and triplex technologies, aptamer technology and ribozymes.

Answer 15: Chemical changes resulting in phosphorothioate, alkyl phosphonate, phosphoamidate, and formacetal analogs. Additional modifications include changes to the heterocyclic bases, derivatization of the ribose moiety and pendant cap groups.

Answer 16: There are several mechanisms. A transient inhibition by masking the ribosome binding site on mRNA. A permanent inhibition from cross-linking the oligonucleotide to the target mRNA. The most important mechanism, however, appears to be through the action of RNase H, which recognizes the DNA-RNA duplex or RNA-RNA duplex, disrupts the base pairing, and digests the RNA-part of the double helix.

Answer 17: Ribozymes are catalytic RNAs which cleave covalent bonds, generally degrading a target RNA.

Answer 18: The development of hybridoma technology and also protein engineering provides the ability to produce homogeneous, monoclonal antibodies and modified antibodies in the quantities necessary to reproducibly purify potential abzymes and characterize their properties.

Answer 19: Tissue engineering is the multidisciplinary field of varied strategies to regenerate natural or grow new human tissues and organs. Sometimes referred to as the more general term "regenerative medicine", tissue engineering has integrated biotechnology, clinical medicine, cell biology, developmental biology, and biomaterials engineering into an effort to overcome the challenges associated with conventional surgical approaches to tissue and organ repair or replacement.

Answer 20: Stem cells are cells that possess the ability to divide into daughter cells and multiple for infinite periods in culture giving rise to daughter cells with identical developmental potential and/or a cell with less potential.

Answer 21: Glycobiology may be defined as the study of the structure, synthesis and biological role of glycans and glycoconjugates in simple and complex systems.

Answer 22: High-throughput screening (HTS) provides for the bioassay of thousands of compounds in multiple assays at the same time. The process is automated with robots and utilizes multi-well microtiter plates.

Answer 23: There are two overall approaches to high-throughput synthesis. True combinatorial chemistry applies methods to substantially reduce the number of synthetic operations or steps needed to synthesize large numbers of compounds. Combichem, as it is sometimes referred to, is conducted on solid supports (resins) to facilitate the needed manipulations that reduce labor. Differing from combinatorial chemistry, parallel procedures apply automation to the synthetic process, but the number of operations needed to carry out a synthesis is practically the same as the conventional approach. Thus, the potential productivity of parallel methods is not as high as combinatorial chemistries. Parallel chemistries can be conducted on solid-phase supports or in solution.

7 Gene Therapy

Abraham Bout

General Introduction

Since the discovery that the genetic information of all living organisms is stored as DNA, the knowledge of genetics and molecular biology has been growing explosively. The genetic basis of a large number of inherited diseases has been identified, and it can be expected that the genes involved in major congenital disorders will be cloned and characterized within the coming years. Medicine has already benefited from the developments in molecular biology through the generation of biotechnological diagnostics and pharmaceuticals. Moreover, in the near future we can expect that a greater understanding of diseases at the molecular level will allow us to significantly improve the prognosis of, if not cure, these diseases by the introduction of gene(s) into cells of patients, which is called gene therapy, a rapidly growing discipline of medicine.

Gene therapy may be divided into germ-line gene therapy and somatic gene therapy. Germ-line gene therapy aims for the introduction of therapeutic genes into germ-cells or omnipotent embryonal cells (at the 4–8 cellular stage). As a result, all the cells of the individual derived from these cells will carry the therapeutic gene, including his or her germ cells. Further offspring will also carry the therapeutic gene. As the effect of expressing a therapeutic gene in both somatic and germ cells is not known, human germ-cell gene therapy is presently not accepted in our society. Somatic gene therapy, on the other hand, is the introduction of gene(s) into somatic cells. The ethical considerations of somatic gene therapy have been widely discussed and a consensus has emerged which allows genetic manipulation of a patient's somatic cells for the purpose of correcting severe disorders.

All current gene therapy protocols make use of gene addition, whereby an intact version of a gene is added to the chromosomal DNA of the target cell population of a patient. This chapter will deal with gene addition. However, before discussing the common gene transfer systems in use, a general overview of gene therapy strategies and diseases that are subject to gene therapy studies will be presented.

Ex Vivo Versus *In Vivo* Gene Therapy

Ex vivo Gene Therapy

Cells from a number of organs and tissues (e.g. skin, hematopoietic system, liver) or from tumors can be removed from the patient and cultured *ex vivo* in the laboratory. A therapeutic gene may be introduced during further culture of such cells. This introduction is then followed by re-infusion or re-implantation of these transduced cells into the patient (Figure 7.1A). In the majority of cases retroviral vectors are used to insert the therapeutic gene into the recipient's cells.

In vivo Gene Therapy

Other organs (e.g. lung, brain, and heart) are less suitable for *ex vivo* gene therapy, as culture of the cells or re-implantation

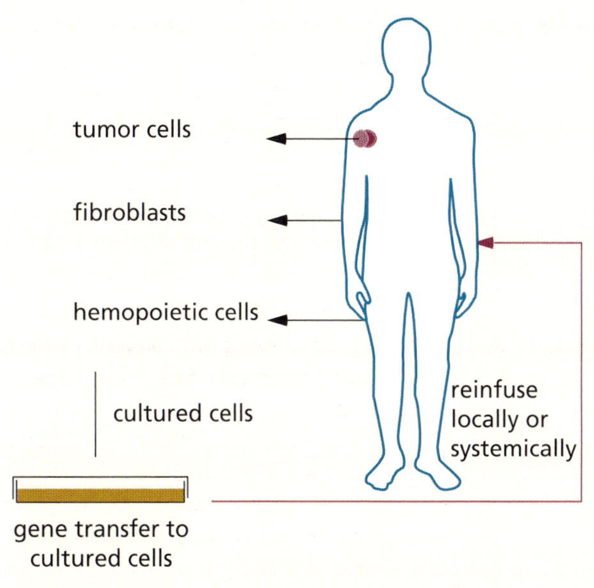

Figure 7.1a. Schematic outline of *ex vivo* (A) and *in vivo* (B) gene therapy strategies (courtesy of Crucell).

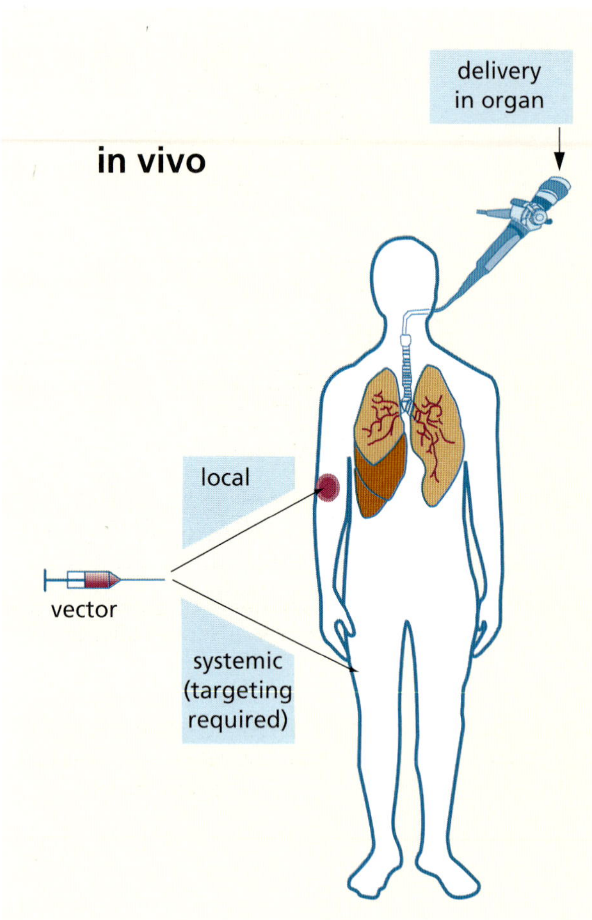

Figure 7.1b.

is not feasible. When this is the case, somatic gene therapy can only be attempted by *in vivo* gene transfer, in other words by administering the gene of interest either locally or systemically (Figure 7.1B).

Potential Target Diseases for Gene Therapy

Inherited Disorders

Somatic gene therapy of inherited disorders involves the introduction of an intact version of the affected gene into those cells where inadequate expression of the gene determines the major symptoms of the disease. Somatic gene therapy aims at the cells or organ where the disease is manifest, because in inherited disorders not all organs are involved or equally involved. Examples are the hematopoietic system in the case of adenosine deaminase (ADA) deficiency, the airway epithelium in cystic fibrosis (CF), muscle in Duchenne's muscular dystrophy and the liver in familial hypercholesterolemia (FH) and hemophilia. For inherited disorders, stable expression of the introduced genes is required (Figure 7.2). This may be achieved either by the integration of the therapeutic gene into the host cell's genome or by using episomal expression vectors. In the case of integration, the recombinant DNA is duplicated when chromosomal DNA is duplicated in the S-phase of the cell cycle. Episomal vectors carry an origin of replication, such as that derived from Epstein-Barr virus, which allows the vectors to replicate episomally (that is, not integrated into the host cell chromosome). The transfer of genes to cancer cells for the treatment of malignancies aims at killing the cancer cells. In such cases only short-term expression of the therapeutic gene is needed and therefore transient transfection systems (Figure 7.2) are sufficient.

Cancer

The most commonly employed approaches for cancer gene therapy include (see also Culver and Blaese, 1994):

1. The introduction of cytokine genes, such as GM-CSF, IFN-γ and interleukins (e.g. Il-2), into cancer cells. These cytokines induce a local inflammatory reaction in the tumor, which destroys a significant fraction of the treated tumor. The inflammation in turn induces an anti-tumor cell immune reaction, which destroys any surviving malignant cells in the primary tumor as well as in distant metastases (see Figure 7.3).
2. 'Suicide genes', such as the herpes simplex virus-thymidine kinase gene (HSV-tk). This enzyme is known to phosphorylate the systemically administered prodrug ganciclovir (a nucleotide analogue). Phosphorylated ganciclovir is incorporated into the DNA of dividing cells, which leads to the termination of DNA-chain elongation, resulting in the death of the cell. Not all cells within a tumor need to be transduced: cells surrounding a cell that expresses the HSV-tk are also killed after ganciclovir treatment. This is called the *bystander effect*. The bystander effect may be of different magnitude in different tumors. A current explanation for the bystander effect is that phosphorylated ganciclovir is transported from HSV-tk expressing cells to neighboring cells through gap-junctions (Figure 7.4).
3. Tumor suppressor genes such as p53, which are mutated in a large number of cancers, or antisense genes targeted at oncogenes (for example Ras) to reduce or abolish their expression.
4. Protection of hematopoietic stem cells (HSCs) from the toxic effects of chemotherapy by inserting a gene that confers drug resistance, e.g. multiple drug resistance gene MDR-1. The MDR-1 gene has been isolated from drug resistant tumor cells, where it pumps anticancer drugs out of the cell.

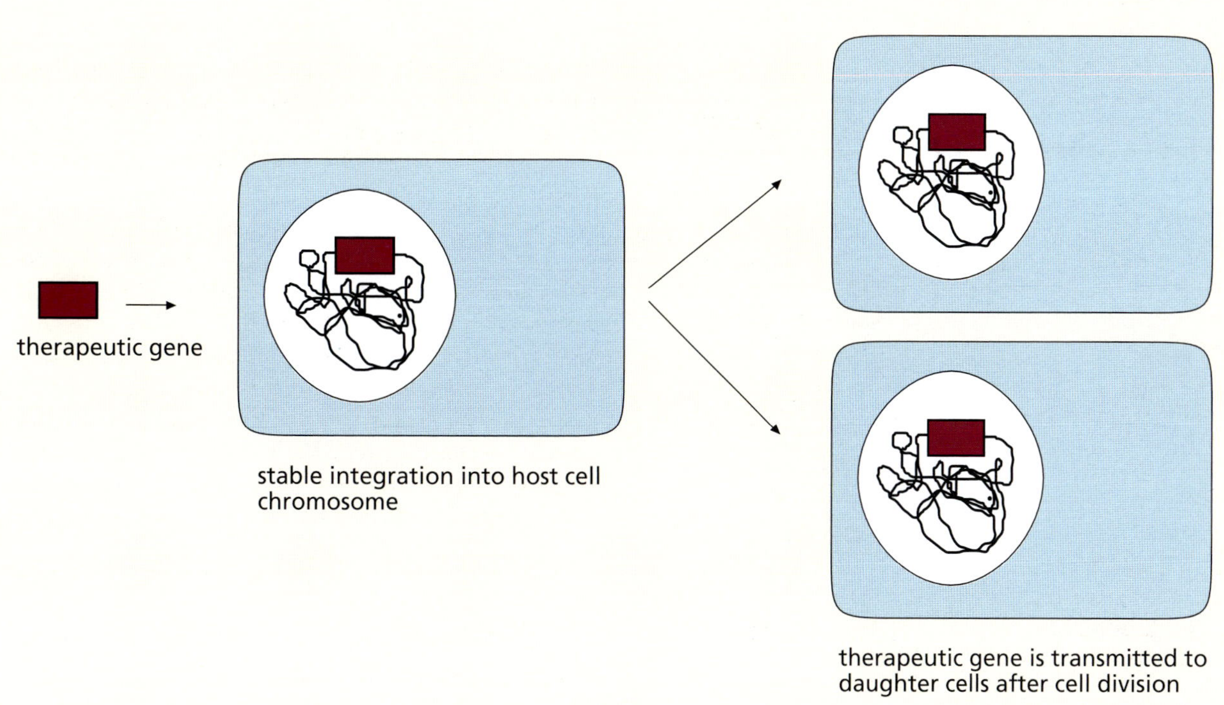
therapeutic gene
stable integration into host cell chromosome
therapeutic gene is transmitted to daughter cells after cell division

Figure 7.2a. Principles of stable and transient gene transfer. 2a: stable gene transfer is obtained when the therapeutic gene integrates into host cell chromosomal DNA (e.g. retrovirus or adeno-associated virus mediated gene transfer or at low efficiency after non-viral mediated DNA transfer). Therefore, the therapeutic gene is transmitted to progeny cells.

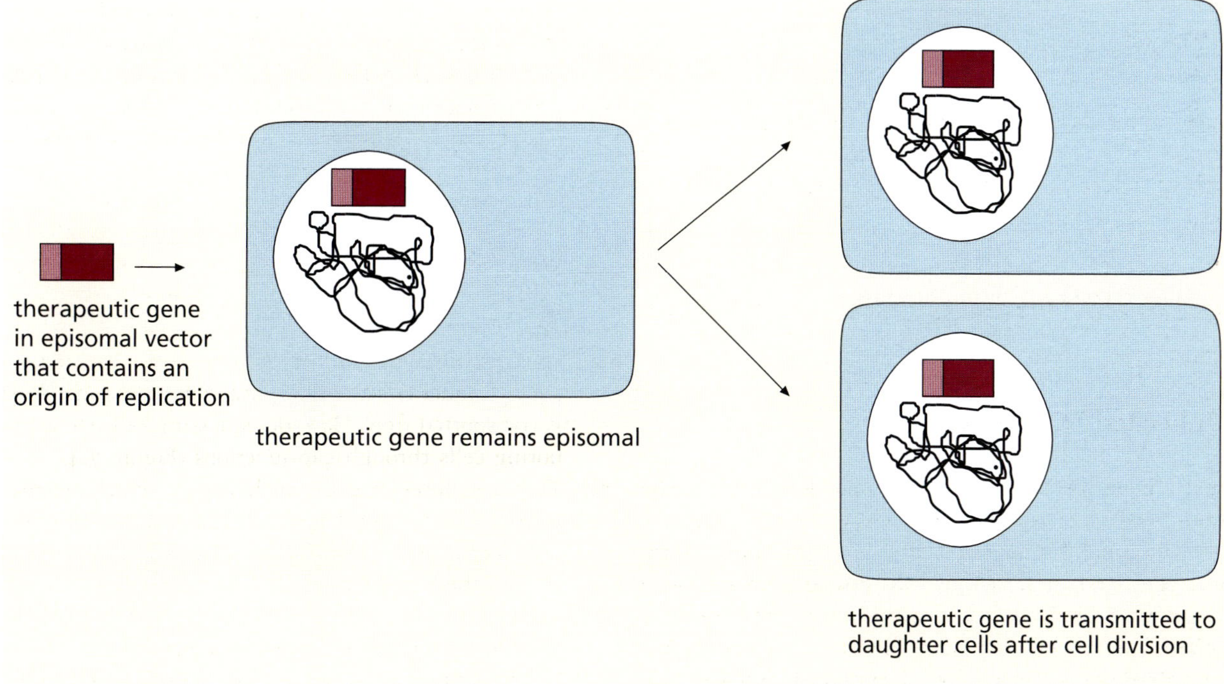
therapeutic gene in episomal vector that contains an origin of replication
therapeutic gene remains episomal
therapeutic gene is transmitted to daughter cells after cell division

Figure 7.2b. Principles of stable and transient gene transfer. 2b: stable gene transfer and transmittance to progeny cells also occurs when episomal vectors containing an origin of replication are used.

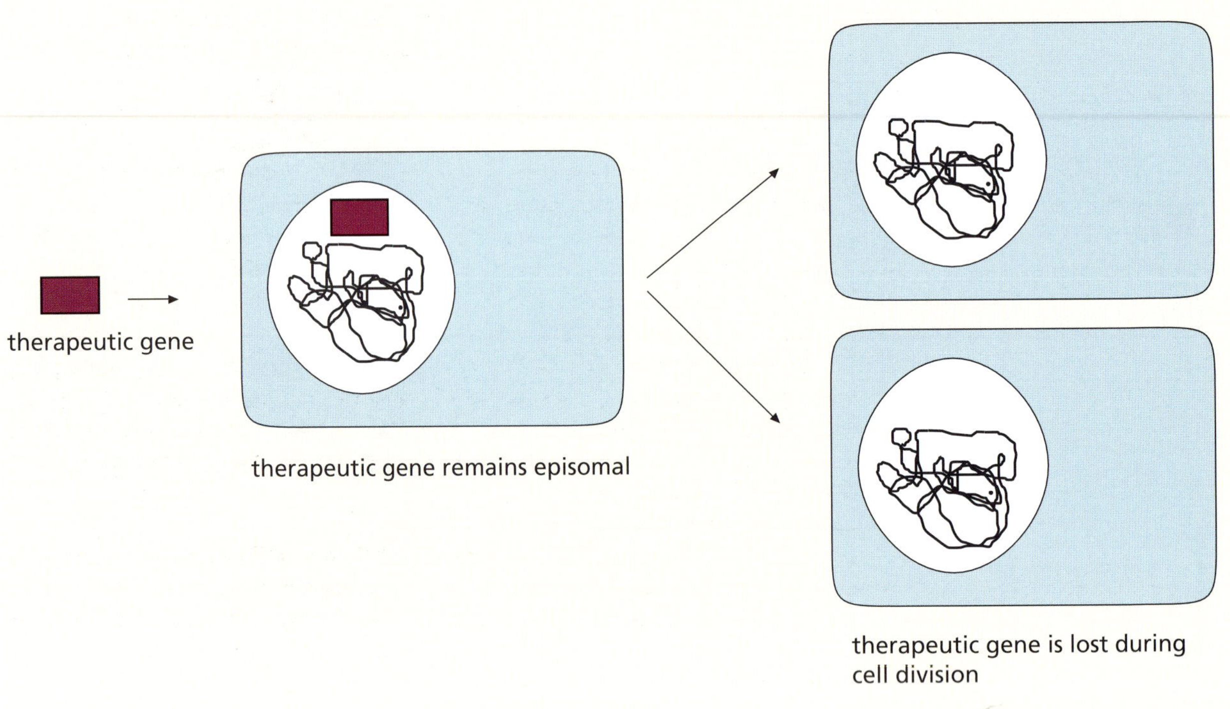
therapeutic gene
therapeutic gene remains episomal
therapeutic gene is lost during cell division

Figure 7.2c. Principles of stable and transient gene transfer. 2c: transient gene transfer occurs when the therapeutic gene remains episomal and is not integrated into the host cell chromosomal DNA. The episomal DNA is lost upon cell division.

Cytokine gene therapy is intended for treatment of both the primary tumor and distant metastases. Suicide and tumor suppressor genes have been designed to mediate direct cytotoxic or antiproliferative effects on the tumor cells, and are only effective for the treatment of localized tumors. MDR-1 gene therapy is expected to allow cancer patients to tolerate higher doses of chemotherapy, thereby increasing the efficacy of the therapy.

Gene Transfer Methods

The method to introduce the genetic material into the target cells of a patient is a key component of every gene therapy protocol. A variety of gene transfer systems are currently employed to insert therapeutic genes into somatic cells, and these can generally be divided into viral and non-viral gene transfer methods. The most important methods and their applications will be discussed. The examples of applications cited are limited to those that are currently being used in clinical studies. Table 7.1 summarizes the characteristics of the different gene transfer systems.

Non-Viral Gene Transfer

Non-viral Methods for Gene Transfer

Non-viral gene transfer systems include the injection of naked DNA, particle bombardment and entrapping DNA in liposomes (reviewed by Ledley, 1995, Li and Huang, 2000). The most straightforward procedure is the direct injection of naked plasmid DNA into tissue to allow cells of that tissue to take up the DNA, which works with reasonable efficiency in muscle and skin. The advantages of such a gene transfer system are clear: it is easy, safe and suitable for the transfer of large gene constructs (Table 7.1). Alternatively, naked DNA can be introduced with a 'gene-gun' or by electroporation. The gene-gun is a high pressure- or electrical discharge device, which forces microscopic gold- or tungsten particles, coated with DNA into tissues. Electroporation makes use of the change of permeability of the cell membrane that is induced when a strong electrical field is applied. As a result, large molecules including DNA molecules are taken up by the cells.

A common method of non-viral gene transfer is the administration of cationic (phospho)lipid associated DNA

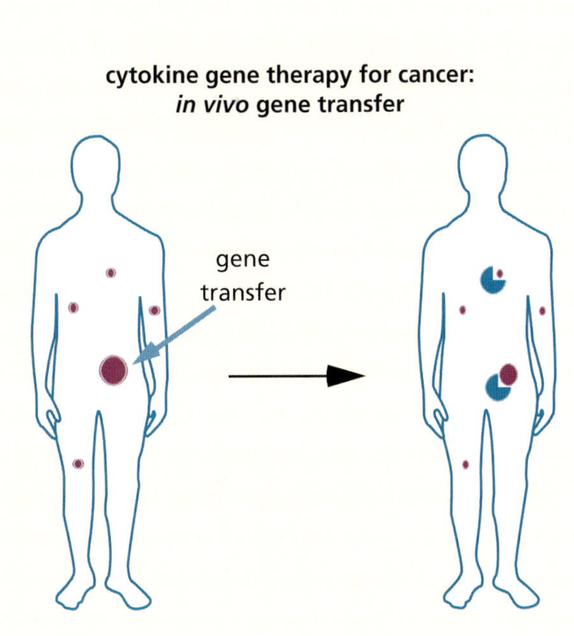

Figure 7.3a. Immuno-gene therapy of cancer (courtesy of Crucell). Gene therapy of cancer e.g. by in vivo gene transfer of cytokine genes (3a) or by the ex vivo 'vaccination' (3b). In the vaccination procedure, tumor cells are cultured and provided with e.g. a cytokine gene, and retransplanted. Both the in vivo and ex vivo procedure aim at eliciting an immune response (represented by the green dots) against the cancer cells, which should destroy both the cytokine bearing tumor cells as well as the other non-cytokine bearing cells.

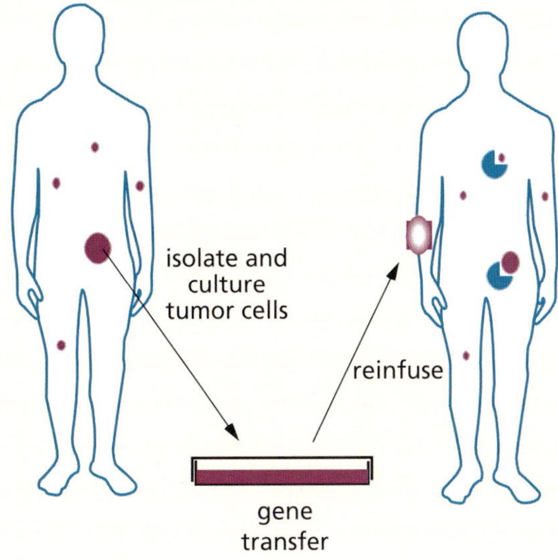

Figure 7.3b.

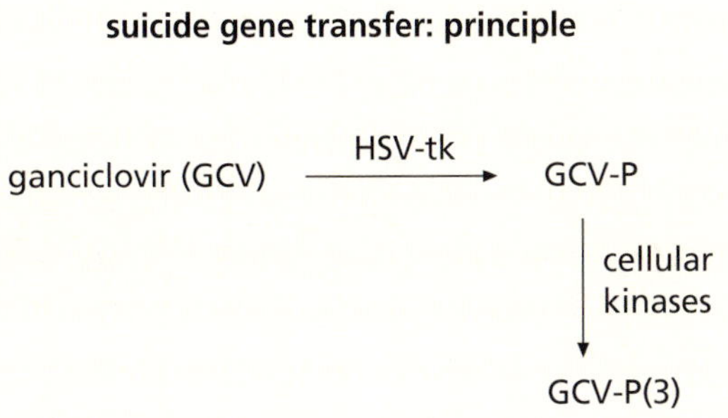

suicide gene transfer: principle

ganciclovir (GCV) —HSV-tk→ GCV-P

GCV-P —cellular kinases→ GCV-P(3)

Figure 7.4a. Suicide gene therapy of cancer (courtesy of Crucell). The reaction underlying suicide gene therapy is depicted in figure 4a.

complexes (Figure 7.5). DNA molecules have a negative charge at neutral pH and are complexed with cationic (phospho)lipids to form colloidal structures. These liposome/DNA complexes bind to the cellular membranes and, in most cases, are internalized into endosomes. However, relatively few DNA/plasmid molecules enter the nucleus and are expressed ($< 0.1\%$), which is probably due to the breakdown of DNA in the acidic environment of the endosomes. Several modifications of this system have been designed to disrupt the endosomes of the target cells to minimize breakdown of the DNA (endosomal escape strategies). Examples include the addition of specific endosome destabilizing peptides or virus shells to the DNA/liposome complex. These modifications have resulted in significant improvements in gene transfer efficacy. Finally, in order to achieve a measure of targeting towards a particular tissue or cell type, antibodies or proteins have been attached to the complexes.

Another class of non-viral vectors are cationic polymer-based gene delivery systems, such as cationic polymethacrylates, dendrimers and Poly-Ethylene Imines (PEI). The most promising among these can mediate efficient gene transfer by the intrinsic ability of this class of molecules to escape from the endosomes, thereby preventing breakdown of the encapsulated DNA in these organelles.

Application of Non-viral Gene Transfer Methods

The direct injection of naked DNA into pigskin results in the transient expression of the recombinant gene by epi-

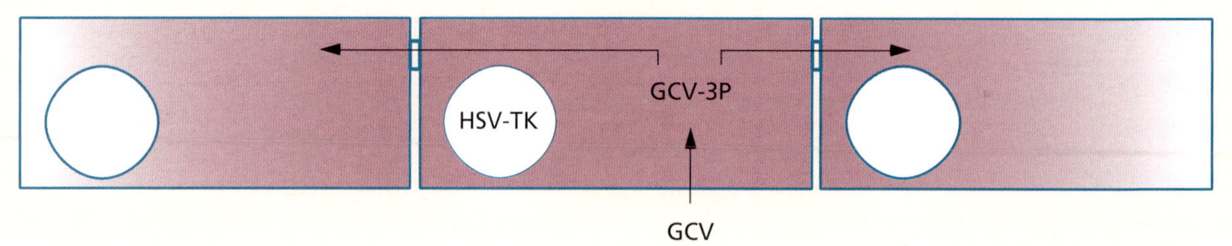

Figure 7.4b. The bystander effect is schematically represented in figure 4b. Three cells are presented, of which the middle one is transduced with the HSV-tk gene. When ganciclovir (GCV) is added, this is phosphorylated into the toxic product GCV-P. This GCV-P is transported to neighbouring cells through gap junctions.

	Retrovirus	Adenovirus	AAV	Naked DNA	Liposome-mediated
Genome transfer	RNA	DNA	DNA	DNA	DNA or RNA
Virus titers	$10^6 - 10^9$/ml	$10^{11} - 10^{12}$/ml	10^{10}/ml	n.a.	n.a.
Purification	difficult	yes	yes	yes	yes
Max. size recombinant gene	8 kb	7.5 kb	5 kb	at least 50 kb	at least 50 kb
In vivo use	no*	yes	yes	yes	yes
Integration	yes	no	yes	low	low
Efficiency	high	very high	moderate	moderate	low
Safety issues	insertional mutagenesis	immune reactions	no known	no known	no known
Non-dividing cells	no	yes	yes	probably	probably
Limitation	cell division needed	transient correction	production is difficult	efficiency is low	efficiency is low

Table 7.1. Characteristics of different methods of gene transfer. * = retrovirus producer cells are used *in vivo*.

dermal keratinocytes in the area surrounding the injection site. It has not been applied to humans yet, but potential applications may be the treatment of skin disorders and virus- and cancer vaccinations.

The gene-gun has been used only in pre-clinical studies (Yang and Sun, 1995) and gene transfer and transient transgene expression has been demonstrated in skin, liver and tumors of mice. Liposome-mediated gene transfer is currently being investigated in clinical trials with cystic fibrosis (CF) patients as well as for the treatment of cancer. In both cases, the *in vivo* gene transfer approach is used.

In summary, liposome-mediated gene transfer seems to be safe, but efficiencies are low and expression of the transferred genes is transient. Further work is underway to improve gene transfer efficiencies.

Gene Transfer Using Recombinant Viruses (Viral Vectors)

General Requirements

Viruses have a natural capacity to infect cells and deliver their genes very efficiently to the nucleus of the target

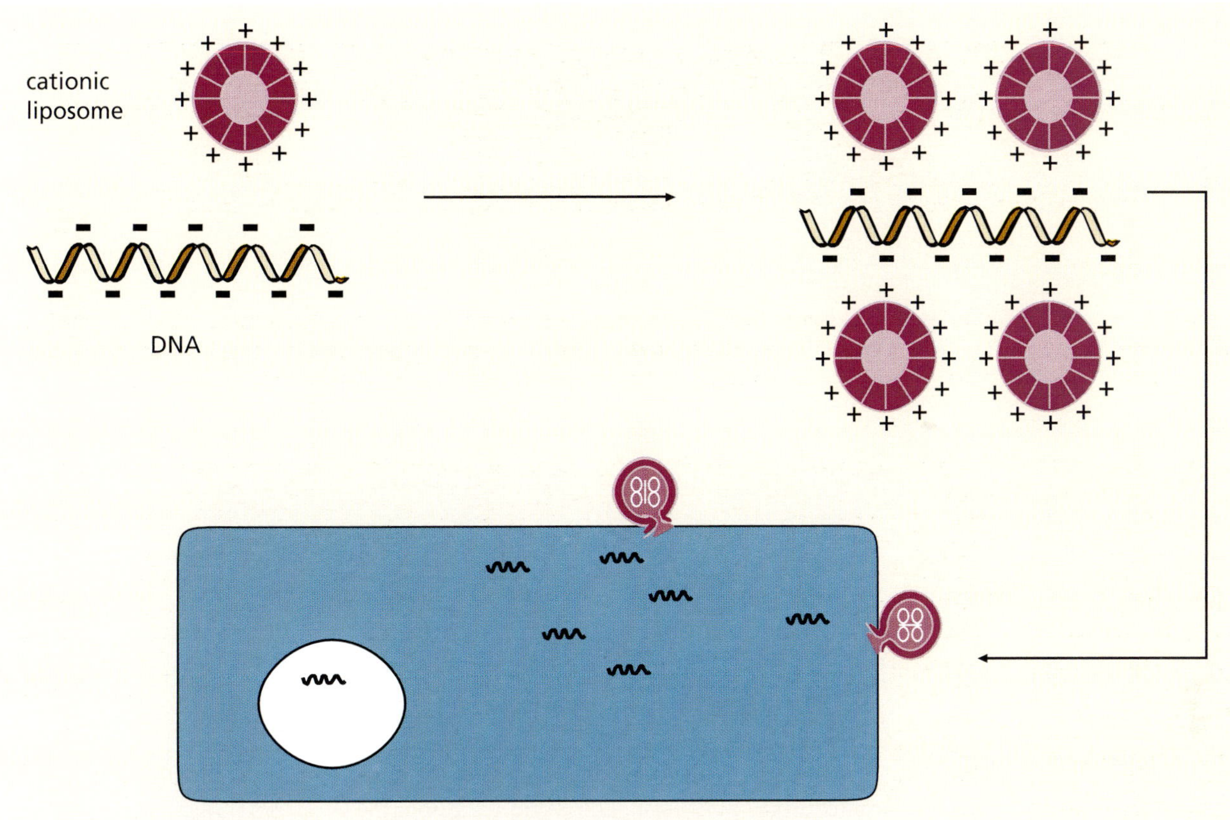

Figure 7.5. Hypothetical model for cationic-liposome mediated gene transfer. Liposomes (positive charge) and DNA (negative charge) form a complex and fuse with the membrane of the target cell, followed by release of DNA into the cell.

cells. In general, viruses have shown much more efficient gene transfer rates than non-viral gene delivery methods. When viruses are exploited as vehicles for therapeutic genes, they must meet the following criteria:

1. They must be replication defective to prevent uncontrolled spreading *in vivo* (unlike their wild-type variant);
2. The virus itself should not possess undesirable properties, and;
3. The viral genome must be able to accommodate the therapeutic gene (size constraints).

Three commonly used viral gene transfer systems (Smith, 1995; Jolly, 1995), namely those based on retrovirus, adenovirus and adeno-associated virus, are discussed in more detail below.

Retrovirus vectors

RETROVIRUS LIFE CYCLE

The most commonly employed retroviral vectors are derived from Murine Leukemia Virus (MuLV). When these viruses are injected into newborn rodents, leukemia develops after a latency period. They are not associated with any known pathology in humans.

The retrovirus particle consists of the retrovirus genome, present as two single copy RNA molecules, complexed to the viral core proteins, all of which is surrounded by a lipid envelope. The envelope consists of a cell membrane derived from the host cell and retroviral 'envelope' proteins.

The first step of the life cycle of retroviruses (Figure 7.6A) consists of the recognition of a receptor on the surface of the target cell. Such receptors are transmembrane proteins that in themselves have a function in normal cellular metabolism; for example amino acid or phosphate transport. Binding to the receptor triggers the fusion of the virus envelope with the host cell's plasma membrane. The viral envelope proteins bind to a receptor. After penetration of the cell membrane the viral core enters the cytoplasm of the host cell and the single-stranded viral RNA is converted into double-stranded DNA by the viral enzyme *reverse transcriptase*, which is also packaged within the viral core. Next, the retroviral DNA becomes integrated in the host cell genome. This integrated retroviral DNA is called the *provirus*. The provirus carries three genes

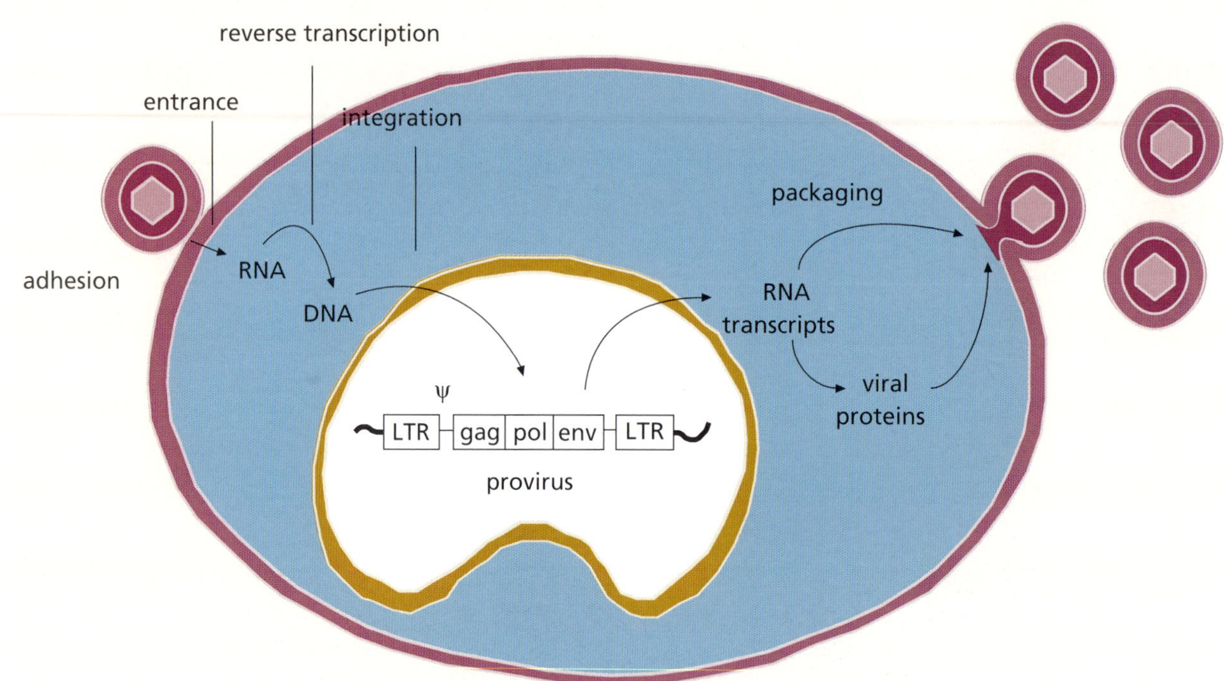

Figure 7.6a. The retrovirus life cycle (courtesy of Crucell). Following adhesion, the virion enters a cell and its RNA is reverse transcribed into a DNA molecule which is subsequently integrated into the cellular chromosome to form the provirus. Proviral DNA is transcribed and translated into viral proteins which encapsidate full length viral RNA molecules. The encapsidated viral RNA buds from the cell to give progeny virus particles.

designated *gag*, *pol* and *env*. The *gag* gene codes for the core proteins of the virus that are responsible for the encapsulation of viral genomic RNA and the assembly of the *virion.* The *pol* gene encodes reverse transcriptase that directs the synthesis of the DNA from the viral RNA. The *env* (envelope) proteins are located at the surface of the virions and interact with specific cell surface receptors on the target cell membrane. Both proviral termini consist of a non-coding sequence, called the Long Terminal Repeat (LTR). The LTR contains promoter sequences responsible for making RNA from the provirus and for integration of proviral DNA into the chromosomal DNA of the host. Downstream of the LTR, a stretch of sequences of approximately 300 bp. is present which is required for the packaging of the RNA genome into virions (so-called packaging sequence Ψ) (Figure 7.6A).

The provirus remains a stable part of the host cell's genome, with the consequence that the provirus is transferred to daughter cells following cell divisions. Transcription and translation of the provirus results in production of the retroviral proteins gag, pol and env. The env proteins are exposed on the host cell membrane. Part of the retroviral RNA is packaged into new particles. This is due to the packaging sequence Ψ (psi), which is present on this RNA molecule. Ψ is recognized by the retroviral gag proteins, which assemble into new infective retrovirus particles. The retrovirus particles bud from the host cell membrane, thereby surrounding the retroviral core with cellular membrane. This sheet of cellular membrane is also known as the retroviral envelope.

Recombinant retrovirus

The specific properties that render retroviruses suitable for foreign gene transfer are:

1. They can infect a wide variety of cell types with high efficiency;
2. The proviral copy integrates in a stable manner into the chromosomal DNA of the cell, thereby warranting life-long correction of the target cell type and its descendants, and;
3. The sequences required for viral replication can be physically separated into cis- and trans-acting elements (see also Figure 7.6B). This enables the generation of replication defective recombinant retroviruses.

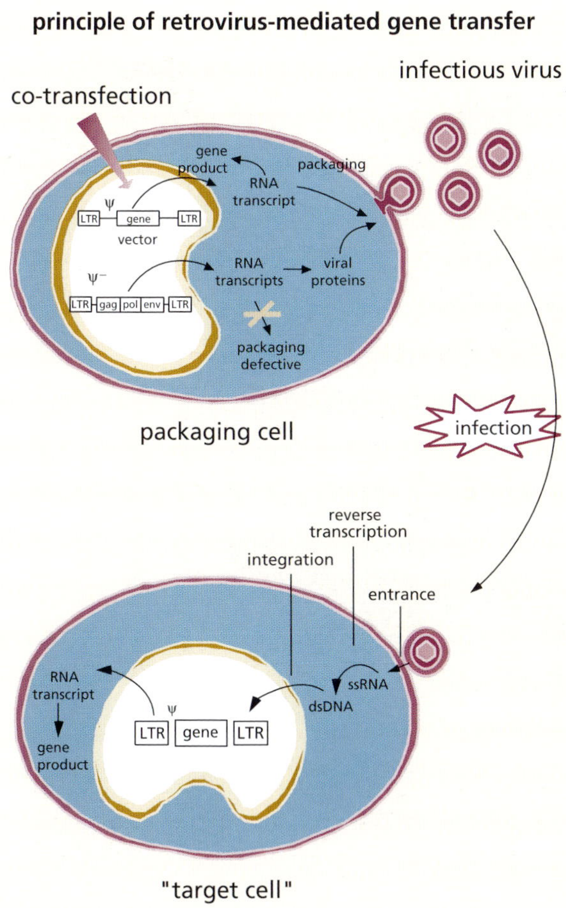

Figure 7.6b. A retrovirus packaging cell at work (courtesy of Crucell). The packaging cell by itself produces all of the viral proteins, but generates no viable virus particles. A retroviral shuttle vector carrying all of the in-cis requirements as well as the gene(s) of interest is introduced into the packaging cell, e.g. by physical transfection procedures. Transcripts from the shuttle vector can be packaged by the virus proteins present and form infectious virus. Virus stocks from such cells are therefore helper-free and the recombinant retroviruses are replication defective such that they can only undergo one cycle of infection.

Recombinant retrovirus production systems in essence consist of two building blocks, namely a retroviral vector, and a retrovirus packaging cell. Packaging cells are special cells. They contain the retroviral genes gag, pol and env, and hence these cells by themselves synthesize all retroviral proteins (Valerio, 1992). However, the packaging cells themselves do not contain the LTR and the packaging sequence. Thus, packaging cells only make retroviral proteins gag, pol and env, but are incapable of making retroviral particles.

Retroviral vectors are retroviral particles that have a retroviral RNA genome that contains, like wild-type retroviruses, the packaging signal Ψ and at each end a long terminal repeat (LTR). However, the retroviral genes gag, pol and env are replaced by a gene encoding a therapeutic protein.

When a retroviral vector infects a packaging cell (Figure 7.6B), a 'provirus' DNA is made which integrates into the host cell genome. The proviral DNA of the retroviral vectors does not contain the gag, pol and env genes. It contains the gene encoding the therapeutic protein. A packaging cell does make the gag, pol and env (the respective genes are present in the genome of the packaging cell, but not in the provirus) and the retroviral vector RNA is made and packaged into new particles similar to wild-type viruses. The newly generated virus particles are released into the culture medium. Using this procedure, virus producing cell lines can be derived that produce approximately 0.1 to 1 functional retrovirus particles per cell per hour, resulting in recombinant virus titers ranging from $\pm 10^3$ up to $\pm 10^8$ infectious particles per mL of culture medium. When the culture medium containing the virus particles is harvested and added to cells that have to be genetically corrected, the recombinant retrovirus is able to infect such cells, reverse transcribe its RNA into DNA and integrate as a provirus into the target cell's genome. Since the retroviral vector does not contain the viral genes, it can not replicate which, as mentioned, is considered a prerequisite in gene therapy procedures.

Application of retroviral vectors

Retroviruses are produced by packaging cells that have been transfected with a retroviral vector containing the therapeutic gene. The recombinant retroviruses are continuously produced by the cells and released into the culture medium. However, it is difficult to purify the viruses from the medium because of the instability of the retrovirus particles.

Therefore, retroviruses are used predominantly in *ex vivo* gene therapy protocols (Anderson, 1992; Miller, 1992). Cells requiring a therapeutic gene are isolated from a patient and exposed to culture medium containing the relevant transgene-containing retrovirus particles. Cells that have been used in the clinic include T-lymphocytes (for adenosine deaminase (ADA) deficiency), tumor infiltrating lymphocytes (TIL), bone marrow cells (for ADA deficiency, Gaucher's disease, gene marking studies), hepatocytes (for LDL-receptor deficiency) and tumor cells (such as melanoma). As cell division is needed for the integration of retroviral DNA into the host cell, growth factors are usually added to the medium to stimulate division of the target cells and hence increase gene transfer efficiency.

Retroviruses have been used in clinical gene marking protocols and gene therapy protocols (Anderson, 1992). Unlike gene therapy studies, gene marking studies have no therapeutic intent, but aim to demonstrate that an exogenous gene (such as an easily detectable non-human gene) can be safely transferred to a patient and how long this gene is detectable in the patient's target cells. Most of the marking protocols address additional specific questions.

A number of cancer vaccination protocols used retroviral vectors. Vaccination is most commonly attempted by surgically removing tumor cells from the patient, growing them *ex vivo* in tissue culture and inserting genes that stimulate inflammation and/or immunity. Vaccination with cells that produce cytokines has been shown to result in systemic immunity in mice, leading to the destruction of the tumor cells *in vivo*. Several gene therapy trials in humans have been approved, involving *ex vivo* retrovirus-mediated transfer of the IL-2, TNF-α or GM-CSF genes into melanoma, colorectal, renal cell carcinoma, neuroblastoma or breast cancer cells. Other protocols use insertion of the gene encoding IL-2 or IL-4 into autologous fibroblasts, which are then mixed with irradiated tumor cells from the patient and reinjected.

Recently, the first clinical success was reported. Three patients were cured from inherited severe combined immuno deficiency (SCID), which was caused by mutations in the gene encoding the γc cytokine receptor subunit (Cavazzana-Calvo *et al.*, 2000). A normal version of this gene was transferred to bone marrow cells of the patients, resulting in complete restoration of the immune functions.

In vivo gene transfer using retroviral vectors for suicide genes (see above) has been applied to the treatment of brain tumors. In this protocol, and not the retrovirus particles the actual retrovirus producing cells were injected into growing brain tumors (Culver and Blaese, 1994). The retroviruses produced by these cells harbor the HSV-tk gene. Since retrovirus-mediated gene transfer is limited to dividing cells, the HSV-tk gene is expected to integrate only into the proliferating tumor cells and not into normal brain tissue (which is mostly non-dividing tissue). When patients received intravenous infusions of ganciclovir (GCV), there was no evidence for toxicity related to the gene transfer and some patients showed a reduction in tumor size.

In general, *ex vivo* gene therapy is promising, although retroviral gene transfer efficiencies are still limiting. As retrovirus vectors need cell division for stable gene expression, such vectors will not transduce terminally differentiated cells and other non-dividing cells. A special group of retroviral vectors, the so-called lentiviral vectors to which retroviruses such as the human immunodeficiency virus (HIV) belong, are capable of integrating the proviral DNA into non-dividing cells (Trono, 2000). Replication defective lentiviral vectors were constructed and were demonstrated to efficiently deliver genes directly into the brain, muscle, lung, liver and islets.

In addition to the prototypic gag, pol and env genes found in all retroviruses, the lentiviral genome encodes six additional proteins that are essential for viral replication and pathogenesis, but are not essential for the transfer and expression of therapeutic genes by lentiviral vectors. A major drawback of lentiviral vectors is the highly pathogenic nature of the viruses from which they are derived (HIV viruses cause AIDS). Therefore, widespread clinical application of such vectors will only be allowed after rigorous safety testing.

Adenovirus vectors

ADENOVIRUS LIFE CYCLE

Adenoviruses are non-enveloped DNA viruses, the genome of which is a linear, double-stranded DNA molecule of about 36 kilobases (kb). The virion has icosahedral symmetry and a diameter of 88 nm. There are 51 distinct serotypes of adenoviruses, which are divided over six (A – F) different subgroups (for a review on human adenoviruses see Horwitz, 1990). Adenoviruses used for the construction of recombinants mainly belong to subgroup C, in particular serotypes 2 and 5. In humans, these viruses have only been associated with mild respiratory disease.

The structure of the adenovirus genome is described on the basis of the adenovirus genes expressed following infection of human cells (Figure 7.7A). Several regions can be distinguished on the adenoviral genome (see Figure 7.7A), including the Early (E) and Late (L) regions, so named according to whether transcription of these regions takes place prior or after the onset of DNA replication (see below). The extremities of the viral genome have a short sequence, the inverted terminal repeat (ITR), which is necessary for viral replication. Sequences required for replication and encapsidation (Ψ) of the virus are present in a region of 400 bp downstream of the left ITR.

Unlike retrovirus replication, where virions are released into the culture medium without affecting the viability of the cells, adenovirus replication causes lysis of the cells. The adenovirus lytic cycle is biphasic, comprising an early (E) phase that precedes viral DNA replication, and a late (L) phase, starting 6–8 hours later. The adenovirus particle is composed primarily of hexon, penton and fiber protein. The fiber protrudes from the surface of the virion. It binds to a receptor present on the cell surface, which is the first step in the infection process.

Following adhesion and the receptor-mediated uptake of adenovirus into the cell, the adenovirus particle enters the endosomes. These endosomes in turn fuse with primary lysosomes. The low pH in the endosomes probably induces a conformational change of the surface of the virion that

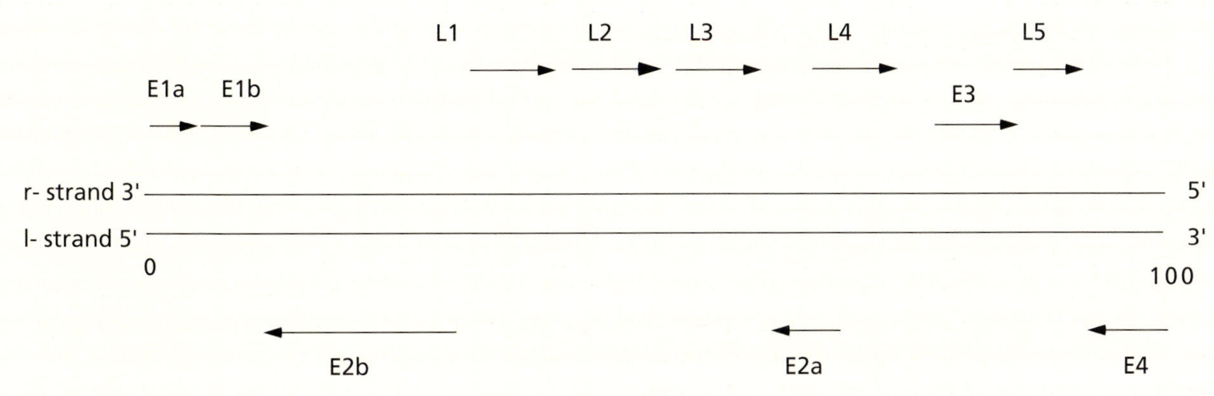

Figure 7.7a. Map of the adenovirus genome (courtesy of Crucell). The 36 kb double stranded adenovirus DNA molecule is usually divided into 100 map units (mu). The early (E) and late (L) regions are indicated on the map. Note that both DNA strands contain protein coding regions.

leads to the disruption of the endosomes. The adenovirus DNA is released into the cytoplasm and transported to the nucleus. The adenovirus DNA is not integrated into the host cell's chromosomal DNA, but remains *episomal* (extra-chromosomal). In the nucleus, the 'immediate early' E1 genes are expressed first, which trans-activate other early adenovirus genes (E2, E4) that cause the shutdown of host-cell protein synthesis and are involved in the replication of the adenoviral DNA. After the onset of DNA replication, the late genes L2–L5 are switched on. They encode structural adenovirus proteins that, in turn, form virion particles in the nucleus of the cell, in which the adenoviral DNA becomes entrapped. Depending on the serotype, approximately 10,000 progeny adenovirus particles can be generated in a single cell.

Recombinant adenoviruses

Gene-transfer vectors derived from adenoviruses (adenoviral vectors) have a number of features that make them particularly useful for gene transfer (Stratford-Perricaudet and Perricaudet, 1991). These features are:

1. The biology of adenoviruses is characterized in detail;
2. The adenovirus is not associated with severe human pathology;
3. The virus is extremely efficient in introducing its DNA into many different cell types;
4. The virus can be produced in large quantities with relative ease, and;
5. Unlike retroviruses, adenoviruses are able to transduce terminally differentiated cells.

Recombinant adenovirus production systems consist of two building blocks, namely a recombinant adenovirus (or adenoviral vector), and a packaging or complementation cell. As for all viral vectors, the recombinant adenovirus should be incapable of replicating in patients.

Vectors derived from human adenoviruses are deleted for at least the E1 region. E1 proteins are pivotal for replication (see above), because they are the first to be expressed after adenovirus infection and are needed to activate other adenovirus genes. Deletion of E1 therefore renders the adenovirus replication defective. Such vectors, where E1 is replaced by a gene of interest, have been used extensively for gene therapy study in both the pre-clinical and clinical phase.

In order to make or propagate E1 deleted adenoviruses, special cells have to be used that contain the E1 genes in their genome. Examples of such cells are 293 cells and PER.C6. Consequently, an adenovirus deleted for the E1 region can be grown in such cells (Figure 7.7B). The pharmaceutical application of adenoviral vectors is facilitated by the virus-particle stability. For example, adenoviral vectors can be purified and concentrated by cesium chloride density centrifugation or by chromatographic procedures and stored frozen until use. Titers of purified adenovirus up to 10^{11} – 10^{12} infectious particles/mL are routinely obtained.

Gene therapy using adenoviral vectors

Many studies with adenoviral vectors in laboratory animals, including rodents, rabbits, pigs and monkeys, have shown that the gene transfer to somatic cells is both effective and reasonably safe. Subsequently, many patients with hereditary (such as cystic fibrosis) or acquired (cancer, cardiovascular) diseases have been treated in a clinical trial setting. These trials have shown, with the exception of a few anecdotal reports, that adenoviral gene transfer to

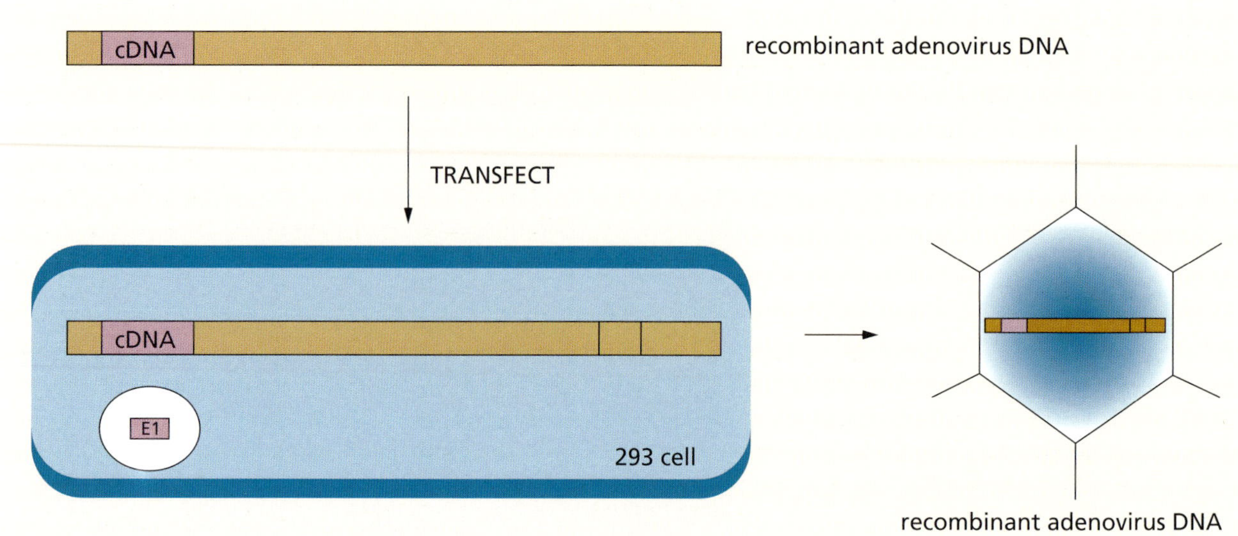

Figure 7.7b. Recombinant adenovirus (courtesy of Crucell). All replication defective recombinant adenoviruses that are nowadays available contain a deletion of 'immediate early' E1 sequences. As E1 sequences are pivotal for activation of other adenovirus genes, E1 deletion mutants are not able to replicate unless E1 proteins are provided by the cell in which the adenovirus is propagated. The cell line most widely used at this moment is the 293 cell line, a human embryonic kidney cell transfected with the E1 sequences of adenovirus. Replication of recombinant adenovirus is similar to wild-type virus and virions of recombinant virus and wild-type virus are identical. The deletion of E1 sequences from adenovirus DNA gives also room for cloning recombinant genes to be used in gene therapy protocols.

humans is as yet non-curative. In the majority of trials, adenoviral mediated gene transfer was found to be safe, although a fatal incident occurred after the administration of a very high-dose of vector to the liver.

Three issues may be responsible for the poor clinical results obtained with adenoviral vectors so far (Bout, 1999). Firstly, low gene transfer in humans may be caused by the fact that adenovirus types 2 and 5 are very common in the population. Hence, many people, as a result of exposure, have high titers of circulating neutralizing antibodies for these viruses. Neutralizing antibodies reduce gene transfer efficiency. The solution to this is to make novel adenoviral vectors that are not neutralized by human sera. Careful screening of the human population has indicated, for example, that adenovirus serotype 35 is neutralized at a low frequency and therefore could be the best basis for making novel adenoviral vectors.

Secondly, the infection of a cell by an adenovirus type 2 or 5 starts with the binding of the fiber to the Coxsackie adenovirus receptor (CAR) on the cell surface. However, CAR is expressed only on a limited number of human cells, and is low or absent on preferred target cells, such as lung cells, hepatocytes, smooth muscle cells and endothelial cells. As a result, these cells can only be infected when high concentrations of the adenoviral vectors are administered.

In order to reduce this dose, it is critical that adenoviral vectors bind to target cells independent of CAR. One way to achieve this is to exploit naturally occurring adenoviruses. It is known that some adenoviruses (e.g. B-type viruses) bind to cellular receptors other than CAR. Cloning of B-type fibers in adenovirus type 5 vectors has been shown to result in chimeras that transduce many cell types better than standard adenovirus type 5 vectors. Differences in infection efficacy of more than 3 logs between these vectors and standard vectors are no exception. Accordingly, the dose of adenovirus to be administered can be reduced accordingly.

Finally, the vast majority of clinical gene therapy studies have used E1-deleted adenoviral vectors. Consequently, the recombinant adenoviral DNA contains, in addition to the therapeutic gene of interest, all early and late genes of the adenovirus except for E1. Although E1 is the master gene that switches on all other adenoviral genes, significant expression of the adenoviral genes is observed despite the absence of E1 proteins. These adenoviral proteins are directly toxic to the target cells and/or cause the cells to be recognized by cytotoxic T lymphocytes, that lyse the target cells. The net result is the loss of the target cell expressing the therapeutic gene, accompanied by an undesirable inflammatory reaction.

Many attempts have been made to silence the adenoviral vector genome, including deletion of E2A, deletion of E4, mutation of E2B and deletion of all adenoviral genes (so-called minimal vectors) (Benihoud *et al.*, 1999). Many problems have yet to be solved, including efficient manufacturing (of minimal vectors), but significant improvements in expression duration and reduction of adenoviral toxicity have been reported.

APPLICATION OF ADENOVIRAL VECTORS

The vast majority of somatic cells in adults are non-dividing. Therefore, *in vivo* gene therapy should exploit strategies that are able to transduce non-dividing and even terminally differentiated cells. Thus far, adenoviruses have this property, and additionally have been shown to transfect cells *in vivo* in the intact organ.

Recombinant adenovirus is currently being explored for gene therapy of disorders of the lung (cystic fibrosis), muscle (Duchenne's muscular dystrophy), liver (e.g. for treatment of blood clotting disorders), central nervous system and heart.

A very promising area for the use of adenovirus is gene therapy of cancer. Gene therapy of cancer aims at the destruction of tumor cells, thereby requiring only the transient expression of 'therapeutic' genes. Adenovirus has proven to be very efficient in delivering genes *in vivo* to the tumors of animals. Clinical studies using adenovirus-mediated delivery of cytokine genes, p53 tumor suppressor genes or suicide genes are in progress.

To summarize, both *in vivo* (in experimental animals) and *in vitro* gene delivery by means of recombinant adenovirus is very efficient. This administrative efficiency is accompanied by the relative ease of production and purification. The major limitation of its clinical use is the immune response (antibodies and cellular immune response against adenovirus infected cells) elicited after *in vivo* delivery. To avoid these limitations, improved recombinant adenoviruses have been constructed.

Adeno-associated virus (AAV) vectors

AAV LIFE CYCLE

AAV is a member of the parvovirus family that is infectious for humans. They are icosahedral shaped viruses that lack an envelope. The virus particles are very heat-stable and resistant to a variety of chemicals such as chloroform and alcohol. Their genome is a single-stranded DNA molecule of approximately 5 kb. Wild-type AAV has thus far not been associated with human disease. AAV is a dependo virus, which means that the wild-type virus can not replicate on its own, but needs another virus, in this case adeno- or herpes virus, for efficient replication. In the absence of a helper virus, AAV establishes a latent infection in which its genome becomes integrated into the cellular chromosomal DNA. In human target cells, wild-type AAV integrates preferentially into a discrete region (19q13.3-qter) of chromosome 19. The AAV genome contains two large open reading frames. The left half of the genome encodes so-called *rep* proteins that are responsible for AAV DNA-*rep*lication during a lytic infection. The right half encodes the virus structural (*cap*) proteins that form the *cap*sid of the virus (Figure 7.8A). The protein coding region is flanked by inverted terminal repeats (ITR) of 145 bp each, which appear to contain all the *cis*-acting sequences required for virus replication and encapsidation.

RECOMBINANT AAV

In an AAV-vector, the entire protein-coding domain (±4.5 kb) can be replaced by the gene(s) of interest (Einerhand and Valerio, 1995; Flotte and Carter, 1995). The ITRs are the only *cis*-acting elements required for all steps of the AAV life cycle, including replication of viral DNA, chromosomal integration, and packaging of the viral genome. Such vectors are packaged into virions by supplying the AAV-proteins *in trans*. This supply is achieved by transfecting the vector plasmid and the packaging plasmid into adenovirus infected cells, generating a mixture of recombinant AAV and wild-type adenoviruses. (Figure 7.8B). Due to the stability of the AAV-virion, heat inactivation (one hour at 56 °C) clears the adenovirus contamination from the virus-preparation.

In the absence of helper virus, AAV will integrate into the host cell genome in a stable manner and remain latent. AAV-vectors do integrate with high efficiency into the host chromosomal DNA. However, thus far they do not share the integration site specificity of wild-type AAV. Site specific integration would be of great importance since it reduces the risk of transformation of the target cell through insertional mutagenesis. In contrast to adenoviral vectors, where the majority of viral genes are retained in the vector, the entire protein coding domain of AAV can be deleted and replaced by the sequences of interest, totally avoiding any immunity problems associated with viral proteins upon transduction of the target cell.

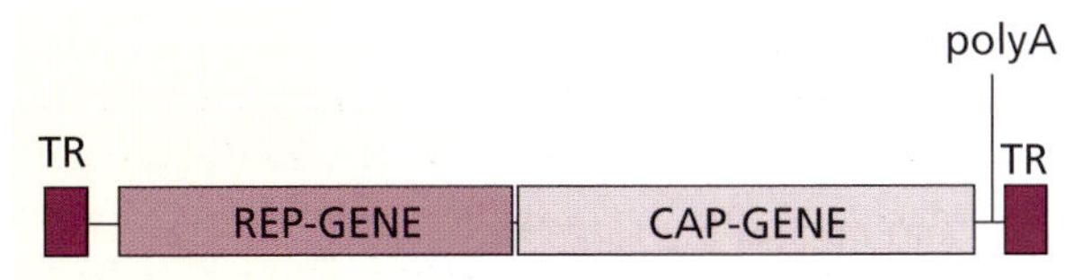

Figure 7.8a. Map of the adeno-associated virus genome (courtesy of Crucell). The positions of terminal repeats (TR) and the REP and CAP genes are indicated.

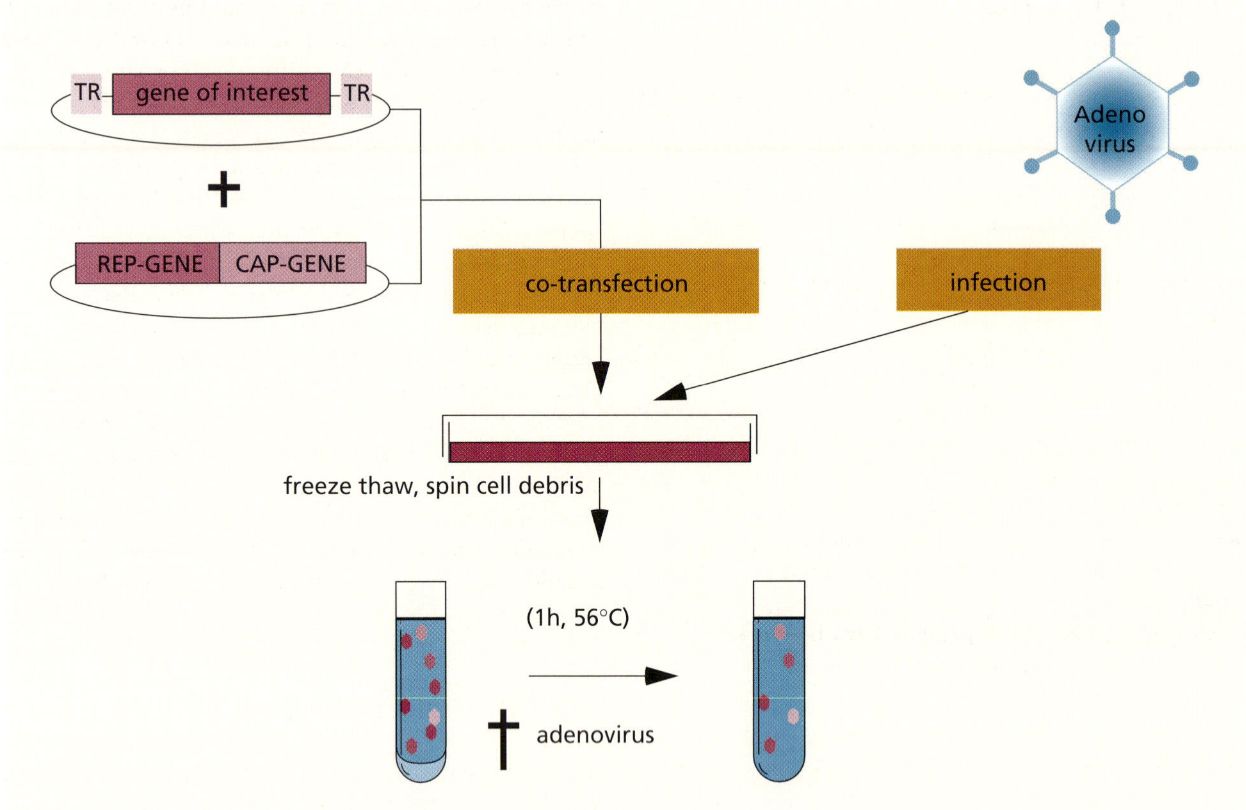

Figure 7.8b. Production of recombinant adeno-associated vector (courtesy of Crucell). DNA constructs containing the therapeutic gene in between TR sequences are cotransfected into a cell together with constructs harboring the AAV genes. After infection with adenovirus, recombinant AAV is made from the construct containing the therapeutic gene because it contains TR sequences which are sufficient for replication and packaging of DNA into virions. Also the adenovirus replicates, so a mixture of recombinant AAV and adenovirus is generated. Unlike adenovirus, AAV particles are stable at 56 °C so after heating at this temperature only viable AAV particles remain.

Application of AAV vectors

AAV-vector technology is under development for a number of different therapeutic purposes and target tissues. One application involves AAV-vector mediated gene transfer to lung cells. Gene transfer and expression for at least three months was reported following *in vivo* gene delivery to one lobe of the rabbit lung.

AAV-mediated gene transfer is also used for gene therapy for hemophilia B, a genetic disease that leads to improper blood clotting. It is caused by a defect in the gene coding for Factor IX. Animal studies have shown long-term gene expression of the Factor IX gene after AAV-mediated gene transfer. Clinical studies, where the vector is injected intramuscularly, are ongoing.

AAV-vector mediated gene transfer to hematopoietic stem cells is also under development for the treatment of ß-thalassemia and sickle cell anemia. Both diseases severely affect erythrocyte function: ß-thalassemic erythrocytes contain insufficient ß-globin chains, whereas sickle cell anemia makes mutant ß-globin chains. Both inherited diseases are recessive in nature, which indicates that one functional intact copy of the adult ß-globin gene would be sufficient to correct the defect. Expression vectors carrying the human ß-globin gene with its promoter and local enhancer elements can direct erythroid specific globin RNA expression.

The results obtained with AAV-vectors thus far indicate that AAV-vector mediated gene transfer into hematopoietic stem cells might become a valuable tool in gene therapy treatment protocols. Compared to retroviral and adenoviral vector technology, however, AAV-vector technology is still in its infancy. Although gene transfer into hematopoietic progenitor cells has been demonstrated using several functional assays, evaluation of the stability of vector integration into the host cell genome of primitive hematopoietic cells is still ongoing. Another open question is whether infection frequency is sufficient to elicit a therapeutic response.

Clinical Studies

The first approved clinical trial in patients using gene therapy began in 1990, with the objective of treating ADA deficiency, a rare immunodeficiency disorder (see above). Since that time, there has been substantial growth in the field of gene therapy, especially in the field of cancer gene therapy. More than 400 clinical studies have been approved worldwide. The protocols with a therapeutic intent include treatment of genetic disorders (13%), infectious disease (mainly HIV) (8%), cardiovascular disease (8%) and cancer (66%). Approximately one-third of the patients enrolled in clinical gene therapy studies were treated with retroviral vectors, mainly in *ex-vivo* studies. Non-viral gene transfer (approximately 25% of treated patients) and adenoviral vectors (16%) are becoming increasingly popular, in particular for *in vivo* gene transfer applications. The list of clinical studies is expected to continue to grow rapidly.

Altogether, over 3000 patients have been treated, and the preliminary conclusions that can be drawn from these studies are that gene transfer to humans is possible, although the levels are still low in most cases. Obviously, there is the need for the improvement of stable gene delivery for both *ex vivo* and *in vivo* purposes.

Pharmaceutical Production and Regulation

In general, drugs that have the potential to be used in humans must be tested for efficacy and safety in appropriate animal models before being tested in healthy volunteers or patients within the context of a clinical trial. Should an appropriate animal efficacy model not exist, rigorous safety testing in rodents and large animals such as monkeys has to be performed. When proven to be safe in such animal studies, clinical studies may be initiated after obtaining approval from the regulatory authorities and ethical committees. The objectives of such early phase clinical studies are, first and foremost, to assess safety and, potentially, the biological efficacy of the gene therapy product. When *in vivo* gene transfer is used, dose-related toxicity is assessed in dose escalation studies.

A fundamental prerequisite of gene therapy is that of safety, both for the patient and his environment. In addition, gene therapy raises scientific and ethical questions. All these issues have to be carefully reviewed when gene transfer experiments to humans are considered. The agents to be used in clinical studies have to be produced according to strict Good Laboratory Practice (GLP) and Good Manufacturing Practice (GMP) principles. Control of both biological sources (e.g. packaging cell lines) and end products (e.g. batches of recombinant virus) is mandatory. Such a safety program must ensure that the biopharmaceuticals are not contaminated with adventitious agents such as microbial or viral contaminants and toxins (Ostrove, 1994).

In the United States, proposals for experiments involving the transfer of recombinant DNA into humans require approval from the local Institutional Biosafety Committee and from the local Institutional Review Board. Then the proposal will be considered by the RAC (Recombinant DNA Advisory Committee of the National Institutes of Health (NIH)) and the FDA (Food and Drug Administration). The RAC deals with ethical and social concerns, scientific evaluation and public discussion. The FDA is the relevant authority with respect to safety of these biological products. Most European countries have a number of committees that must approve the clinical protocol, the production protocol, safety testing program and ethical considerations when gene transfer to protocol humans is considered.

Concluding Remarks

Although in the last decade gene therapy has evolved from 'possible in theory' to clinical testing in humans, we are still at the beginning of the gene therapy era. Despite encouraging results obtained to date in clinical studies, a number of scientific questions have to be answered to make gene therapy come of age. A few of the specific questions have already been addressed in the discussion of the different gene transfer systems. In general, retroviruses are used in *ex vivo* gene transfer protocols, where they are able to transduce the target cell population in a consistent and stable manner. The frequency of transduction depends on the cell type. *In vivo* gene transfer uses either cationic (phospho)lipid mediated gene transfer or recombinant adenoviruses. Recombinant adenoviruses are particularly effective. However, liposomes and adenoviruses either do not or only minimally integrate the transferred DNA into the host cell chromosome, necessitating the need for repeated deliveries. Stable integration and efficient *in vivo* gene transfer has been reported for recombinant AAV. When the encouraging results that have been obtained in animals can be extended to humans, AAV seem to be good candidates for future *in vivo* gene therapy for genetic disorders. AAV might be used in *ex vivo* protocols as well, because unlike retroviruses, AAV are able to infect non-dividing target cells. However, their main drawback is that large-scale production is difficult and poorly reproducible. A lot of research is necessary to increase efficiencies of non-viral gene delivery systems. As mentioned, the addition of proteins or peptides may improve gene delivery significantly.

The growth of medical interest in gene therapy is accompanied by increased commercial interest, which supports and propels research in this area. However, increased commercial interest should not lead to unrealistic expectations with respect to clinical applications of gene therapy. Although the medical potential is promising and potentially enormous, sound scientific research is needed to turn the modest clinical effects of current studies into real cures. ■

Further Reading

- **Ascadi G, Massie B, Jani A.** (1995). Adenovirus-mediated gene transfer into striated muscles. *J. Mol. Med.* 73, 165–180.
- **Crystal RG.** (1995). The gene as the drug. *Nature Medicine* 1, 15–17.
- **Crystal RG.** (1995). Transfer of genes to humans: early lessons and obstacles to success. *Science* 270, 404–410.
- **Mulligan RC.** (1993). The basic science of gene therapy. *Science* 260, 926–932.
- **Smith AE.** (1999). Gene therapy: where are we? *Lancet* 354 (suppl. 1), 1–4.
- **Spooner RA, Deonarain MP, Epenetos A.A.** (1995). DNA vaccination for cancer treatment. *Gene Ther.* 2, 173–180.
- **Verma IM.** (1990). Human Gene Therapy. *Sci. Am.* 263, 66–84.
- **Wilson JM.** (1993). Vehicles for gene therapy. *Nature* 365, 691–692.
- **Yu M, Poeschla E, Wong-Staal F.** (1994). Progress towards gene therapy for HIV infection. *Gene Ther.* 1, 13–26.

References

- **Anderson WF.** (1992). Human Gene Therapy. *Science*, 256, 808–813.
- **Bout A.** (1999) Towards safe and effective adenoviral vectors for human gene therapy. *Eur. Biopharm. Rev.*, December, 94–99.
- **Benihoud K, Yeh P, Perricaudet M.** (1999) Adenovirus vectors for gene delivery. *Current Opinion in Biotechnology*, 10, 440–447.
- **Cavazzana-Calvo M., Hacein-Bey S, Basile GS, Gross F, Yvon E, Nusbaum P, Selz F, Hue C, S. Certain S, Casanova J, Bousso P, Deist FL, Fischer A.** (2000) Gene therapy of human severe combined immunodeficiency (SCID)-X1 disease. *Science*, 288, 669–672.
- **Culver KW, Blaese RM.** (1994) Gene therapy for cancer. *Trends Genet*, 10, 174–178.
- **Einerhand MPW, Valerio D.** (1995) Viral vector systems for bone marrow gene therapy, in *Hematopoietic stem cells*, D. Levitt and R. Mertelsmann, Eds. New York: Marcel Dekker, 275–295.
- **Flotte TR, Carter BJ.** (1995) Adeno-associated virus vectors for gene therapy. *Gene Ther*, 2, 357–362.
- **Jolly D.** (1994). Viral vector systems for gene therapy. *Cancer Gene Ther*, 1, 51–64.
- **Ledley FD.** (1995). Nonviral gene therapy: the promise of genes as pharmaceutical products. *Human Gene Ther*, 6, 1129–1144.
- **Li S, Huang L.** (2000) Nonviral gene therapy: promises and challenges. *Gene Ther*, 7, 31–34.
- **Miller AD.** (1992). Human gene therapy comes of age. *Nature*, 357, 455–460.
- **Ostrove JM.** (1994). Safety testing programs for gene therapy viral vectors. *Cancer Gene Ther*, 1, 125–131.
- **Shenk T.** (1996). Adenoviridae: the viruses and their replication, in *Virology*, B.N. Fields, D.M. Knipe and P.M. Howley, Eds.: Lippincott-Raven Publishers, Philadelphia, 2111–2197.
- **Smith AE.** (1995). Viral vectors in gene therapy. *Ann Rev Microbiol*, 49, 807–838.
- **Stratford-Perricaudet L, Perricaudet M.** (1991). Gene Transfer into Animals: the promise of adenovirus; in *Human gene transfer*, O. Cohen-Adenauer and M. Boiron, Eds.: INSERM, 51–61.
- **Trono D.** (2000). Lentiviral vectors: turning a deadly foe into a therapeutic agent. *Gene Ther*, 7, 20–23.
- **Valerio D.** (1992). Retrovirus vectors for gene therapy procedures in *Transgenic Animals*, F. Grosveld and G. Kollias, Eds. London: Academic Press, pp. 211–246.
- **Yang NS, Sun WH.** (1995). Gene gun and other non-viral approaches for cancer gene therapy. *Nature Med.*, 1, 481–483.

Self-Assessment Questions

Question 1: *What is the approach for treatment of CF with gene therapy?*

Question 2: *What makes it possible to generate retrovirus packaging cell lines?*

Question 3: *Why are hematopoietic stem cells such an attractive target for cure of diseases in which blood cells are affected?*

Question 4: *What is the key determinant for successful stem cell gene therapy with retroviral vectors?*

Question 5: *In vivo liposome-mediated gene transfer was found to be relatively inefficient compared to virus-mediated gene delivery until recently. In order to improve non-virus mediated gene delivery, several components, often derived from viruses, have been added to liposome/DNA mixtures to improve their efficiency. Optimal non-viral gene delivery vehicles might look like 'artificial viruses' in the end: particles containing all the components that make virus mediated gene delivery efficient but not having the e.g. safety drawbacks associated with the use of recombinant viruses. Which steps might be subject to improvement for the efficacy of non-virus mediated gene delivery?*

Question 6: *The treatment of a certain inherited disorder in which a number of different organs are affected demands delivery of the therapeutic gene to a number of different locations in the body. It is impossible to deliver the genes to all affected organs separately. Therefore, delivery of the therapeutic gene by intravenous injection is considered. What are the possibilities for having the therapeutic gene expressed only in the affected tissues?*

Question 7: *For suicide gene therapy of malignant brain tumors, two different gene delivery procedures are being exploited: 1) introduction of retrovirus producing cells into the tumor; 2) injection of recombinant adenovirus into the tumor.*

Question A: *What is the basic mechanism of suicide gene therapy?*

Question B: *What is the 'bystander' effect?*

Question C: *What are the advantages and disadvantages of each of the two gene delivery systems mentioned above?*

Answers

Answer 1 To introduce a normal version of the CFTR gene into airway epithelium by *in vivo* gene transfer procedures.

Answer 2 Deletion of the packaging signal Ψ from the retroviral RNA prevents packaging of such an RNA molecule into a virus particle. However, synthesis of retroviral proteins from RNA molecules with a Ψ deletion is still possible.

Answer 3 Stem cells maintain at least one kg of bone marrow and blood cells in human adults. Therefore, correction of stem cells would result in life-long correction of the disease. Unlike stem cells, peripheral blood cells have a limited life span. Gene therapy of peripheral blood cells will therefore result only in a transient correction of the disease.

Answer 4 For retrovirus mediated gene delivery, cell division is a prerequisite. Therefore, the stem cells should be cycling when retroviral transduction is performed.

Answer 5 They should pass physical barriers (e.g. mucous layer should be passed for transfection of lung cells).
They should bind to (target cell specific) receptors (more efficient internalization)
Endosome disruption should be induced to prevent lysis of the DNA because of low pH in the endosomes/lysosomes.
They should transport the DNA to the nucleus.

Answer 6 1) Targeting to the cells or organs that were affected e.g. antibody mediated delivery.
2) Expression of the therapeutic gene is under the control of a tissue or cell-specific promoter, resulting in expression only in particular cell types.

Answer 7A Tumor cells are provided with a gene which encodes an enzyme that is able to convert a prodrug (e.g. ganciclovir) into a toxic compound.

Answer B The fact that not all tumor cells have to be provided with the suicide gene to accomplish eradication of the complete tumor.

Answer C Re retrovirus-producing cells

Advantages:

- They infect only dividing cells, thereby preferentially transducing tumor cells and not the surrounding normal brain cells.

Disadvantages:

- A strong immune response against the retrovirus producing cells is evoked, preventing efficient repeat deliveries.
- No efficient gene delivery occurs when a large fraction of the tumor is non-dividing.

Re advantages and disadvantages of the use of recombinant adenovirus:

Advantages:

- Efficient gene delivery to both dividing and non-dividing tumor cells.
- If gene transfer to cells of normal tissues occurs, the adenovirus DNA does not integrate into the host chromosome and expression of the therapeutic gene is transient in nature.

Disadvantages:

- Gene transfer to non-dividing normal (brain) cells is also possible.
- An immune response against adenovirus particles is evoked.

8 Hematopoietic Growth Factors

Jeanne Flynn, August J Salvado and MaryAnn Foote

Introduction

This chapter reviews the chemistry, pharmacology, pharmaceutical issues, and clinical aspects of hematopoietic growth factors. A review of the complete literature on these topics is beyond the scope of this paper and the reader is advised to consult the original research papers for further information. We suggest review articles and books that we have found useful and that summarize a given topic.

Hematopoietic (blood) cells are vital to life: they transport oxygen, contribute to host immunity, and facilitate blood clotting. An intricate, multistep process allows immature precursor cells in the bone marrow to mature and become functional blood cells. Ordinarily, this well-regulated process allows for replacement cells lost through daily physiologic activities. The process is also capable of producing adequate and appropriate cells for fighting infection and for replacing cell losses due to hemorrhaging or destruction. The process of production and maturation of blood cells is called "hematopoiesis." An excellent review of hematopoiesis can be found in Israels and Israels (1996).

In the early 1900s, scientists recognized the presence of circulating factors that regulate hematopoiesis. It took approximately 50 years, until cell culture systems were developed that could sustain cell colonies *in vitro*, to definitively prove the activity of these proteins. The growth and survival of early blood cells required the presence of specific factors, called "colony-stimulating factors (CSF)." However, "hematopoietic growth factor" (HGF) is the preferred term because it is more precise than the term based on laboratory observations of the effects of these factors.

Efforts to purify hematopoietic growth factors progressed throughout the 1970s and early 1980s. Blood and other materials (e.g. bone marrow and urine) contain extremely small amounts of growth factors. The presence of many growth factors confounded the search for a single growth factor with a specific activity. Scientific progress was slow until it became possible to purify sufficient quantities to fully evaluate the characteristics and biologic potential of the isolated materials. The introduction of recombinant DNA technology triggered a flurry of studies and an information explosion. More than 20 hematopoietic growth factors have been isolated; some have been studied extensively and a few have been made for clinical use. An excellent personal account of the race to find the hematopoietic growth factors is found in Metcalf (2000).

Hematopoiesis

Hematopoiesis is mediated by a series of growth factors that act individually and in various combinations involving complex feed-back mechanisms that stimulate the proliferation, differentiation, and function of hematopoietic cells.

Ten types of mature blood cells have been identified, each derived from primitive hematopoietic stem cells in the bone marrow. The most primitive pool of pluripotent stem cells comprises about 0.1% of the nucleated cells of the bone marrow, and 5% of these cells may be actively cycling at a given time. The stem cell pool maintains itself, seemingly without extensive depletion, by asymmetrical cell division. When a stem cell divides, one daughter cell remains in the stem cell pool and the other becomes a committed colony-forming unit (CFU). CFUs proliferate at a greater rate than the other stem cells and are more limited in self-renewal than pluripotent hematopoietic stem cells. The proliferation and differentiation are regulated by a number of things, including hematopoietic growth factors. These hematopoietic growth factors eventually convert the dividing cells into a population of terminally differentiated functional cells (Figure 8.1): cells committed to the myeloid pathway can develop into red blood cells (erythrocytes), platelets (thrombocytes), monocytes/macrophages, granulocytes (neutrophils, eosinophils, and basophils), or tissue mast cells. Cells committed to the lymphoid pathway give rise to lymphocytes (B or T lymphocytes and plasma cells).

This chapter focuses on growth factors that are produced by recombinant DNA technology (identified by the prefix "rh" which identifies a recombinant human form of the endogenous protein) and marketed in Europe, Canada, Australia, Japan, and/or the United States, although information about some other hematopoietic growth factors is included.

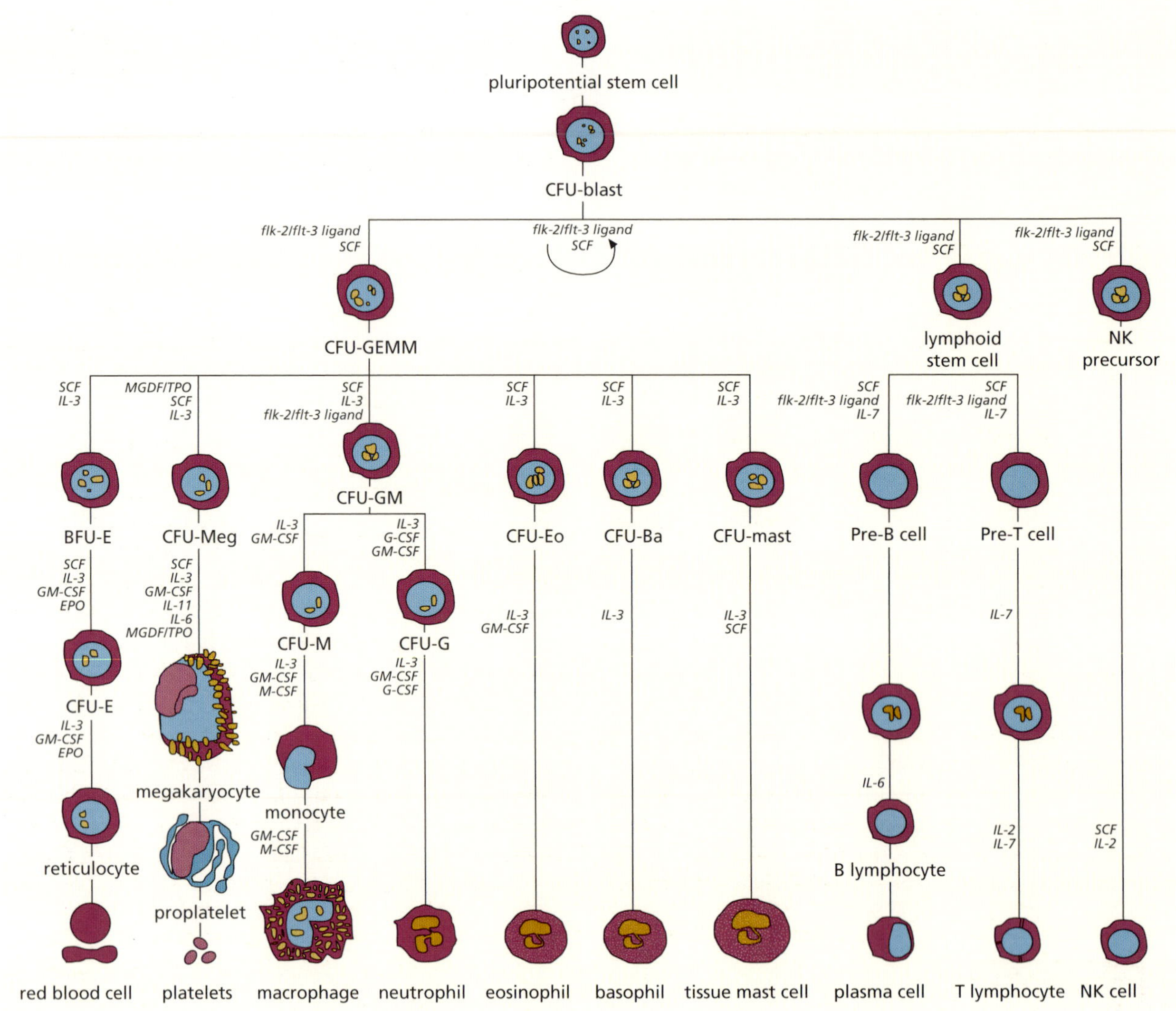

Figure 8.1. The hematopoietic tree. This cascade shows the pathways that give rise to mature blood cells and the sites of action of hematopoietic growth factors. Cell types are abbreviated; growth factors are abbreviated and in italics, (Figure courtesy of Amgen Inc. Thousand Oaks, CA.).

Chemical Description of Hematopoietic Growth Factors

Hematopoietic growth factors are generally glycoproteins, which can be distinguished by their amino acid sequence and glycosylation pattern (carbohydrate linkages). Recombinant hematopoietic growth factors are not necessarily glycoproteins. In spite of the lack of the carbohydrate moieties, they may still assume the structure necessary to exert the same biologic activity of the glycosylation form. Most hematopoietic growth factors are single-chain polypeptides with molecular weights of approximately 14 to 35 kDa. The carbohydrate content varies by growth factor and production method, which in turn affects the molecular weight but not necessarily the biologic activity.

Each hematopoietic growth factor is encoded by a specific gene. Production of the recombinant proteins is accomplished by first identifying the gene in question, isolating it by various techniques, inserting the gene of interest into a plasmid, and then expressing the protein of interest in a biologic system (e.g. bacteria, yeast, or mammalian cells) to produce recombinant growth factors. For a review of biotechnology basics, see Foote and Flynn (1993) and chapters 1 and 3 of this book.

The hematopoietic growth factors that will be discussed in detail include granulocyte colony-stimulating factor (G-CSF) and granulocyte-macrophage colony-stimulating factor (GM-CSF), two myeloid hematopoietic growth factors; and further, erythropoietin (EPO), the red cell factor; stem cell factor (SCF), an early-acting hematopoietic growth factor; and platelet-enhancing factors of thrombopoietin (TPO), megakaryocyte growth and development factor (MGDF), and interleukin-11 (IL-11).

Chemical Properties and Marketing Information for G-CSF and GM-CSF

The chemical properties of the myeloid hematopoietic growth factors, G-CSF and GM-CSF, have been characterized (Table 8.1). The gene that encodes for G-CSF is located on chromosome 17 and the mature G-CSF polypeptide has 174 amino acids. The gene that encodes for GM-CSF is located on chromosome 4 and the mature polypeptide has 127 or 128 amino acids. Filgrastim, a rhG-CSF, is marketed by several companies under several trade names throughout the world. More structural information on rhG-CSF can be found in Chapter 2. Lenograstim, another rhG-CSF, is not marketed in the United States but is marketed in other countries. Molgramostim and sargramostim are two versions of rhGM-CSF; the former is marketed in Europe and the latter, in the United States. For a review of rhG-CSF, see Welte *et al.* (1996); for a review of rhGM-CSF, see Armitage (1998).

Chemical Properties and Marketing Information for EPO

The gene that encodes EPO is located on chromosome 7. The mature polypeptide has 165 amino acids, two disulfide bonds, and three *N*- and one *O*-linked carbohydrate chains. Unlike G-CSF and GM-CSF, EPO requires glycosylation for its *in vivo* biologic activity. EPO is heavily glycosylated, which increases the molecular weight from 18.4 kDa for the unglycosylated molecule to approximately 34 kDa. Two rhEPO products are marketed and both are expressed in Chinese hamster ovary cells. In the United States, the proprietary name for recombinant erythropoietin is epoetin alfa; the international nonproprietary name is epoetinum alfa. Epoetin alfa is also available in Japan and China. The second recombinant erythropoietin is epoetin beta, which is available in Europe and Japan. Both recombinant products have the same primary amino acid sequence and almost identical glycosylation (Veys *et al.*, 1992). For a review of EPO and the role of the kidney in erythropoiesis, see Jacobson *et al.* (2000).

Chemical Properties and Marketing Information for SCF

The gene for SCF is located on chromosome 12. A longer form (SCF^{248}) and a shorter form (SCF^{220}) can be expressed, both of which are membrane bound. Soluble SCF^{165} is proteolytically released from SCF^{248}. SCF^{220} lacks the proteolytic cleavage site and tends to remain membrane bound. The approved rhSCF (ancestim), called Stemgen® in Canada, Australia, and New Zealand, corresponds to SCF^{165} plus an *N*-terminal methionine residue. It is recombinantly produced in *E coli* and is, therefore, non-glycosylated. Galli *et al.* (1994), Lacerna *et al.* (2000), and Broudy (1997) offer comprehensive reviews of rhSCF.

	G-CSF	GM-CSF
Proper names	filgrastim, lenograstim	molgramostim, sargramostim
Chromosome location	17	4
Amino acids	174[a]	127 or 128[b]
Glycosylation	*O*-linked (lenograstim)	*N*-linked (sargramostim)
Source of gene	bladder carcinoma cell line (filgrastim), squamous carcinoma cell line (lenograstim)	human monocyte cell line (molgramostim), mouse T lymphoma cell line (sargramostim)
Expression system	*E coli* (bacteria), filgrastim; Chinese hamster ovary cell line (mammalian), lenograstim	*E coli* (bacteria), molgramostim; *Saccharomyces cerevisiae* (yeast), sargramostim

[a] Native G-CSF has two forms, one with 177, which is less active than the other form with 174 amino acids; filgrastim has an N-terminal methionine.
[b] Molgramostim has 128 amino acids; sagramostim 127.

Table 8.1. Characteristics of the marketed myeloid growth factors, rhG-CSF an rhGM-CSF (Souza *et al.*, 1986; Nagata *et al.*, 1986; Gronski *et al.*, 1988).

Chemical Properties and Marketing Information for Thrombopoietins

Factors responsible for megakaryocyte development and platelet production, the thrombopoietins, include the Mpl ligands (TPO and MGDF) and interleukin (IL)-11. TPO and MGDF are Mpl ligands; IL-11 is not. For convenience, all three will be referred to as thrombopoietins, although it must be remembered that IL-11's receptor is different from those of TPO/MGDF and that IL-11 has other biological functions.

The existence of a thrombopoietin was suggested in 1958 and activity was demonstrated in the early 1960s. In 1990, studies investigating murine leukemia and oncogenes led to the recognition of a new hematopoietin receptor superfamily, Mpl, which was found to be the receptor of an important regulator of thrombopoiesis (Sheridan and Foote, 1998). Two forms of Mpl ligand were produced through recombinant DNA technology. The book edited by Kuter *et al.*, 1994a is a compilation of the biology, molecular, and cellular information about TPO, MGDF, and IL-11.

The gene for thrombopoietin is located on chromosome 3. Depending on the source, the mature polypeptide has between 305 and 355 amino acids, which may undergo cleavage to a smaller polypeptide that retains biological activity. A wide range of molecular weights (18 to 70 kDa) has been reported for active molecules (Kaushansky, 1995). At this time, no recombinant Mpl ligands are commercially available.

The gene for IL-11 is located on chromosome 19. IL-11 has multilineage effects. The precursor protein consists of 199 amino acids. IL-11 is rich in proline residues, and it lacks cysteine residues and disulfide bonds common to other hematopoietic growth factors (reviewed by Du and Williams, 1997).

Oprelvekin (rhIL-11) is a non-glycosylated polypeptide, 177 amino acids in length and approximately 19 kDa in molecular weight. Oprelvekin differs from endogenous IL-11 by a single amino acid – the amino terminal proline – but this difference does not affect bioactivity. Oprelvekin is marketed as Neumega™ in the United States.

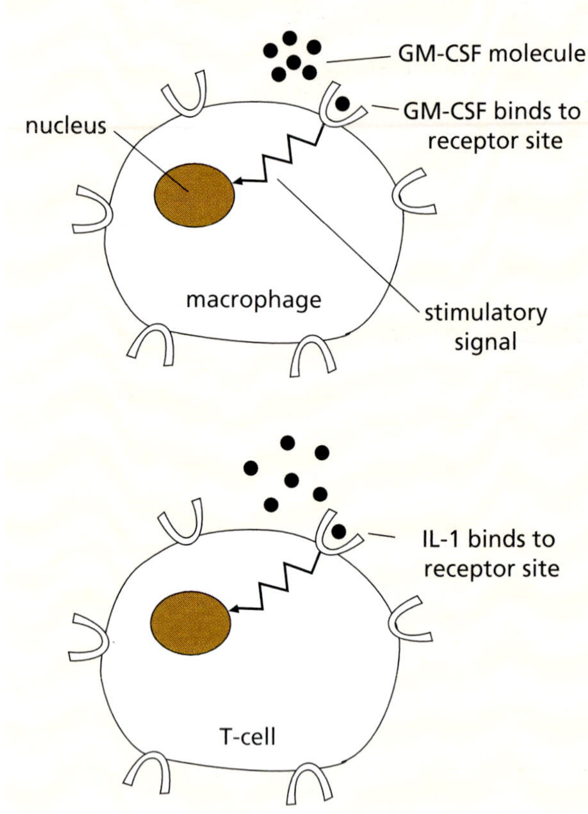

Figure 8.2. An example of a protein that acts both directly and indirectly on a cell. In this figure, GM-CSF binds to its receptor on a macrophage. GM-CSF may stimulate the macrophage to proliferate and differentiate. In addition, GM-CSF may induce the macrophage to produce and secrete a number of cytokines, including G-CSF, IL-1, and tumor necrosis factor (TNF). These cytokines leave the macrophage and bind to cells with specific receptors for them, such as neutrophils, T-cells, and fibroblasts (for G-CSF, IL-1 and TNF, respect ively). Thus, indirect acting CSFs may initiate a cytokine cascade (Figure courtesy of Amgen Inc., Thousand Oaks, CA.).

Pharmacology

Hematopoietic growth factors act by binding to specific cell surface receptors. Activation of these receptors results in a cascade of intracellular second messengers and altered gene expression, which in turn induce cellular proliferation, differentiation, or activation. A hematopoietic growth factor may also act indirectly by inducing the expression of a gene producing a different hematopoietic growth factor or cytokine, which in turn stimulates another target cell (Figure 8.2). This indirect activity has made it difficult to delineate the pharmacologic activity of individual hematopoietic growth factors and accounts for some of the differences between *in vitro* and *in vivo* results. Cell culture studies can be designed to exclude indirect effects, but animal and clinical studies generally reflect the full scope of direct and indirect biologic effects.

In Vitro Activity

As discussed in an earlier section (Hematopoiesis), the hierarchy for hematopoiesis involves many steps and pathways. By definition, the pluripotent stem cell is the progenitor or precursor for all hematopoietic cells.

Hematopoietic growth factor (normal range in serum)	Cellular source	Stimuli for release
G-CSF (9–51 pg/mL)	monocytes	lipopolysaccharide induction
	fibroblasts	TNF, IL-1
	endothelial cells	TNF, IL-1
	bone marrow stromal cells	cytokine activation
GM-CSF (0.4–2 pg/mL)	T cells	antigens, lectins, IL-1
	monocytes	lipopolysaccharide induction
	fibroblasts	TNF, IL-1
	endothelial cells	TNF, IL-1
EPO (3–7 mIU/mL)	kidney	hypoxia
	liver	hypoxia
TPO (20–300 pg/mL)	kidney	constitutively expressed
	liver	constitutively expressed
SCF (1200–1900 pg/mL)	fibroblasts	constitutively expressed
	bone marrow stroma	constitutively expressed

Table 8.2. Cellular sources, endogenous levels and stimuli for release of hematopoietic growth factors in humans (Groopman *et al.*, 1989; Kuter *et al.*, 1994; Lok *et al.*, 1994; Nichol *et al.*, 1995).

The complex interactions among progenitor cells and their mature progeny were determined by evaluating the effects of adding hematopoietic growth factors to cell cultures containing immature progenitor cells from the bone marrow.

In addition to their effects on progenitor cells, hematopoietic growth factors bind to and regulate the functional activity of mature cells. Whereas lineage-specific growth factors (e.g. G-CSF and EPO) predominantly affect one cell lineage, multilineage growth factors (e.g. GM-CSF and IL-3) affect more than one cell lineage. This phenomenon is concentration dependent. The GM-CSF concentrations that regulate monocytes and granulocytes (5 to 20 pg/mL) are lower than those for eosinophils and platelets (20 to 2000 pg/mL) (Metcalf, 1990).

In Vivo Activity

The *in vivo* activity of hematopoietic growth factors can be assessed by measuring endogenous levels under different conditions or by administering growth factors to animals or humans. Although the *in vivo* results are often consistent with those predicted by *in vitro* studies, differences can be observed and may be the result of interspecies variability. Other reasons for *in vivo* and *in vitro* variability include differences in clearance, pharmacokinetics, and glycosylation. Table 8.2 summarizes cellular sources, endogenous serum levels, and stimuli for release of growth factors.

Cellular Sources and Stimuli for Release

T lymphocytes, monocytes/macrophages, fibroblasts, and endothelial cells are the major cellular sources of most hematopoietic growth factors, excluding EPO and TPO. EPO is produced primarily (>90%) in the adult kidney (Jacobson *et al.*, 2000). The liver also produces some EPO (<10%), but the amount is insufficient to maintain normal red blood cell formation. TPO is produced in the liver and the kidney (Kuter, 1997).

Many inflammatory stimuli are capable of promoting the cellular release of hematopoietic growth factors (Table 8.2). Antigens, lectins, and IL-1 can signal T lymphocytes to produce GM-CSF and IL-3. Endotoxins such as lipopolysaccharides can induce monocytes/macrophages to release G-CSF and GM-CSF. IL-1 and tumor necrosis factor (TNF)-alpha, produced by activated monocytes, can trigger the release of G-CSF and GM-CSF by fibroblasts and endothelial cells. In addition, these findings suggest that hematopoietic growth factors play a major role in host response to infection or antigen challenge and may also play a limited role in maintaining normal hematopoiesis (Groopman *et al.*, 1989; Hartung *et al.*, 1999).

Physiologic Role of G-CSF and GM-CSF

G-CSF, but not GM-CSF, is usually detectable in the blood and increases during infection (Cebon *et al.*, 1994). Mice that lack endogenous G-CSF (i.e. 'knockout mice') have chronic neutropenia and impaired neutrophil mobilization (Lieschke *et al.*, 1994). The collective results of these *in vivo* studies, together with *in vitro* observations, suggest that the two myeloid growth factors have complementary roles. G-CSF may help maintain neutrophil production during steady-state conditions and increase production during acute situations such as infection. GM-CSF may be a locally active growth factor that remains at the site of infection to localize and activate neutrophils (Rapoport *et al.*, 1992).

In vivo definition of the physiologic role of GM-CSF in steady-state hematopoiesis has been further elucidated by a knockout mouse model (Stanley *et al.*, 1994). Both survival and fertility of GM-/- mice were found to be normal. The peripheral blood of six- to seven-week old GM-/- mice showed no significant difference from wild-type ('normal') in terms of hemoglobin, platelets, total white blood cells, neutrophils, lymphocytes, monocytes, or eosinophils. No other differences were noted in bone marrow cellularity, myeloid:erythroid ratios of marrow, or assayed progenitor cells from different lineages. These data suggest that steady-state hematopoietic pathways that might be affected by loss of GM-CSF are redundantly regulated. The most striking finding in the GM-CSF-/- mice was the development of pulmonary disease. At birth, knockout and wild-type mice have similar lung morphology, but by three weeks, knockout mice consistently showed focal peribronchovascular lymphoid aggregate. Older animals had alveoli with large foamy macrophages. The changes were histologically similar to those produced by pulmonary alveolar proteinosis. These changes were not seen in the wild-type animals.

rhG-CSF reduces neutrophil maturation time from five days to one day, leading to a rapid release of mature neutrophils from the bone marrow into circulation (Lord *et al.*, 1989; Lord *et al.*, 1992). rhGM-CSF does not reduce the mean maturation time. Neutrophils treated with rhG-CSF show normal intravascular half-life (Lord *et al.*, 1989); neutrophils treated with rhGM-CSF have an increased serum half-life of 48 hours (Lord *et al.*, 1989), which may be due to impaired maturation. rhG-CSF enhances chemotaxis by increasing the binding of fMLP (formyl-methionyl-leucyl-phenylalanine) (Colgan *et al.*, 1992). A short incubation (<30 minutes) with rhGM-CSF enhances neutrophil chemotaxis, but incubation >30 minutes results in the inhibition of neutrophil motility (Weisbart and Golde, 1989). Neutrophils treated with rhG-CSF have enhanced superoxide production in response to chemoattractants (Weisbart and Golde, 1989). rhGM-CSF also enhances superoxide production, but optimal priming requires a long incubation period. Clinical studies in patients receiving rhGM-CSF using the skin-window technique showed significantly reduced neutrophil migration compared with normal volunteers (Dale *et al.*, 1998).

$CD34^+$ hematopoietic cells harvested from bone marrow, umbilical cord blood, or peripheral blood can be co-cultured with TNF-alpha and GM-CSF to induce conversion of $CD34^+$ cells to dendritic cells. Dendritic cells are antigen-presenting cells capable of long-term activation of antibody/antigen complexes (Siena *et al.*, 1997; Hart, 1997). Peripheral blood monocytes co-cultured with IL-4 and GM-CSF can produce dendritic cells. The functional activity of dendritic cells generated using different culture methods can vary considerably (Hart, 1997).

Physiologic Role of EPO

EPO increases red blood cell count by causing committed erythroid progenitor cells to proliferate and differentiate into normoblasts (a nucleated precursor cell in the erythropoietic lineage). EPO also shifts reticulocytes (mature red blood cells) from the bone marrow into the peripheral circulation. EPO is ordinarily present in plasma in low, but detectable, quantities. Unlike some other hematopoietic growth factors, EPO release is not mediated by inflammatory stimuli. Tissue hypoxia resulting from anemia induces the kidney to increase its production of EPO by a magnitude of a hundred-fold or more. Patients with chronic renal failure are unable to produce adequate EPO levels because of the loss of renal function (Erslev, 1991).

rhEPO accelerates erythropoiesis in patients with chronic renal failure and has been used to enhance red cell production after chemotherapy and allogeneic bone marrow transplantation, and to increase red blood cell numbers for presurgical autodonation. Although rhEPO is a late-acting factor, it may synergize with thrombopoietins to stimulate the production of megakaryocyte colony-forming cells (Broudy *et al.*, 1997).

Physiologic Role of SCF

SCF is an early-acting hematopoietic growth factor that stimulates the proliferation of primitive hematopoietic and non-hematopoietic cells. *In vitro*, SCF alone has minimal colony-stimulating activity on hematopoietic progenitor cells; however, it synergistically increases colony-forming or stimulatory activity of other hematopoietic growth factors, including G-CSF, GM-CSF, EPO, MGDF, and IL-2. SCF is produced by bone marrow stroma and has an important role in steady-state hematopoiesis. Unlike most hematopoietic growth factors, SCF circulates in relatively high concentrations in normal human plasma (Langley *et al.*, 1993). The generation of dendritic cells from $CD34^+$ cells is enhanced 2.5-fold by the addition of SCF to the culture cocktail, and is enhanced five-fold if SCF and flt-3 ligand are added (Siena *et al.*, 1997).

Physiologic Role of Thrombopoietins

TPO/MGDF are hematopoietic growth factors that stimulate the production of megakaryocyte precursors, megakaryocytes, and platelets. Endogenous TPO is produced by the liver and enters the peripheral circulation. It eventually reaches the bone marrow and stimulates bone marrow megakaryocytes to produce platelets (Kuter, 1997). Platelet production is subject to a homeostatic regulation, similar to that observed for EPO.

IL-11 has pleiotropic effects on multiple tissues. In terms of thrombopoiesis, IL-11 works synergistically with IL-3, TPO, MGDF, or SCF to stimulate various stages of megakaryocytopoiesis and thrombopoiesis (Du and Williams, 1997). It is possible that IL-11's effects on platelet formation is mediated in part by TPO.

Pharmaceutical Issues

Pharmaceutical issues include the status and source, storage and stability, pharmacokinetics and pharmacodynamics of hematopoietic growth factors. Unless otherwise indicated, the information in this section is taken from the product package inserts for marketed products.

Commercially Available Hematopoietic Growth Factors for Clinical Use

Five hematopoietic growth factors are commercially available (Table 8.3):

- rhG-CSF (filgrastim and lenograstim)
- rhGM-CSF (molgramostim and sargramostim)
- rhEPO (epoetin alfa and epoetin beta)
- rhSCF (ancestim)
- rhIL-11 (oprelvekin)

Recombinant EPO, launched in 1989, was the first to be approved by governmental regulatory agencies in the United States. Filgrastim, lenograstim, and sargramostim followed in 1991. Molgramostim was introduced in 1992. Oprelvekin was approved in 1997 and ancestim in 1999. Soon after approval in the United States, most hematopoietic growth factors became available in Europe and other parts of the world.

Hematopoietic growth factors may be developed by one company, manufactured by another, and distributed by a third. These arrangements are dynamic, complex, and differ from country to country. Appropriate resources should be checked to determine the licensing and distribution agreements in a particular country. The pharmacist, physician, or other healthcare providers are responsible for reading the current package insert for each product before prescribing, preparing, or administering any recombinant hematopoietic growth factor discussed in this chapter.

Storage and Stability

Filgrastim is available as single-use prefilled syringes and as single-use vials for subcutaneous or intravenous administration. Filgrastim is stable in liquid form when kept at a suitable temperature. It should be stored in the refrigerator at 2° to 8 °C and should not be frozen, but accidental exposure to freezing temperatures does not adversely affect the stability. It can be left at room temperature (25 °C) for up to 24 hours. Filgrastim may be diluted in 5% dextrose/glucose, but it should never be diluted with saline, because saline may cause the product to precipitate.

Lenograstim is available as a lyophilized powder for reconstitution with Sterile Water for subcutaneous injection. If lenograstim will be administered as an intravenous injection, it must be reconstituted in 0.9% saline. Reconstituted lenograstim remains stable at room temperature (25 °C) for 24 hours. The lenograstim formulation contains human serum albumin.

Epoetin alfa is supplied as a sterile solution for intravenous or subcutaneous administration. Single-use vials have no preservative, whereas multiple-use vials contain 1% benzyl alcohol as a preservative. Prefilled syringes are available in some countries. Epoetin alfa should be stored at 2° to 8 °C and should not be shaken or frozen.

Epoetin beta is supplied as a powder for reconstitution with Sterile Water for Injection, USP, containing benzyl alcohol and benzalkonium chloride. Unreconstituted epoetin beta should be stored at 2° to 8 °C, but it can be stored for five days at room temperature (25 °C). The reconstituted solution should be used immediately and lack

	Proper name	Trade name	Country	Company
rhG-CSF	filgrastim	Neupogen	EU, USA, Canada, Australia	Amgen, Roche
		Granulokine	Italy	Dompe
		Granulokine	Spain	Esteve-Pensa
		Gran	Japan, Taiwan, Korea, China	Kirin, Sankyo
	lenograstim	Granocyte	EU	Rhône-Poulenc
		Euprotin	Australia	Amrad
		Euprotin	Spain	Almirall
		Neutrogin	Japan, China	Chugai
rhGM-CSF	molgramostim	Leucomax	EU, Canada	Schering, Sandoz
		Mielogen	Italy	Schering-Plough
	sargramostim	Leukine	USA	Immunex
		Leukine	Canada	Wyeth-Ayerst
rhEPO	epoetin alfa	Epogen	USA	Amgen
		Procrit	USA	Ortho
		Espo	Japan	Kirin, Sankyo
			China	Kirin
		Eprex	EU, Australia, Canada	Ortho
	epoetin beta	Epogin	Japan	Chugai
		NeoRecormon	EU	Boehringer Mannheim
rhSCF	ancestim	Stemgen	Canada, Australia	Amgen
rhIL-11	oprelvekin	Neumega	USA	Genetics Institute

Table 8.3. Status of commercially available hematopoietic growth factors as of September 2000. EU = European Union.

of refrigeration should be limited to the time needed to prepare the injection.

Ancestim is supplied as a lyophilized powder for reconstitution. Ancestim is reconstituted with Sterile Water for Injection, USP, and is always administered as a subcutaneous injection. Ancestim should not be administered as an intravenous injection under any circumstance. Ancestim can be reconstituted 36 hours in advance and stored at 2° to 8 °C.

Oprelvekin also is supplied as a lyophilized powder for reconstitution with Sterile Water for Injection, USP. The reconstituted material must be used within three hours of reconstitution whether refrigerated (2° to 8 °C) or kept at room temperature (25 °C).

Pharmacokinetics

The pharmacokinetic profiles of hematopoietic growth factors obtained in different studies should not be compared directly due to the clinically relevant differences in doses, administration routes, and study populations. For example, patients with advanced cancer typically receive chemotherapeutic agents, antibiotics, and other therapeutic interventions that may directly alter the disposition of hematopoietic growth factors or affect the organs that metabolize and eliminate these growth factors. Patients undergoing bone marrow transplantation are typically exposed to an even wider variety of therapeutic interventions.

Filgrastim and lenograstim exhibit first-order kinetics and increasing plasma concentrations with increasing doses (Roskos *et al.*, 1998). Both are rapidly absorbed after subcutaneous administration, achieving peak concentrations in two to eight hours. The elimination half-life of filgrastim is approximately 3.5 hours in both normal volunteers and cancer patients, and after intravenous as well as subcutaneous administration. The authors claim that the elimination half-life of lenograstim is three to four hours after subcutaneous administration and one to 1.5 hours after intravenous administration.

Pharmacokinetic parameters of sargramostim are similar between healthy individuals and patients (Armitage, 1998). In patients with advanced cancer, sargramostim is rapidly absorbed after subcutaneous administration, achieving peak concentrations in two hours. After intravenous infusion over two hours, serum concentrations initially decline rapidly ($t_{1/2\ alpha}$ = 12 to 17 minutes) and then gradually decline ($t_{1/2\ beta}$ = two hours). Elimination is primarily by non-renal means.

In pharmacokinetic studies with molgramostim, maximum serum concentration and area-under-the-concentration-versus-time curve increased with both subcutaneous and intravenous administration but serum concentration was higher for a longer period of time after intravenous dosing (Armitage, 1998). Immunoreactive molgramostim can be detected in the urine of patients, supporting a renal route of elimination. The reported half-life after intravenous administration is 0.24 to 1.18 hours; mean half-life after subcutaneous administration is 3.6 hours.

rhEPO follows first-order kinetics. Serum concentrations peak five to 24 hours after subcutaneous administration and are lower than after intravenous administration. The elimination half-life of intravenously administered rhEPO is four to 13 hours in patients with chronic renal failure and approximately 20% shorter in normal volunteers. The reported elimination half-life is longer after subcutaneous administration and results in more-sustained plasma concentrations (Erslev, 1991; Markham and Bryson, 1995).

Ancestim follows first-order kinetics after a single subcutaneous injection to normal healthy volunteers and to patients with cancer. After subcutaneous administration (dose range 5 to 15 µg/kg) to healthy men, ancestim was absorbed slowly, reaching peak concentrations between eight and 72 hours. The mean absorption half-life was 41 hours, with an initial lag time of approximately two hours. Elimination is also first-order, with a half life of five hours; hence, absorption is rate limiting. In patients with cancer, a single dose of 5 to 50 µg/kg produced a mean peak serum concentration approximately 15 hours after administration. Both absorption and elimination were first order with $T_{1/2}$ 36 and 2.6 hours, respectively. The pharmacokinetics of ancestim are very similar between healthy volunteers and patients with cancer.

Oprelvekin administered as a single, 50-µg/kg dose to men showed a terminal half-life of 6.9 ± 1.7 hours. Clearance of oprelvekin decreases with patient age and clearance in infants and children is 1.2- to 1.6-fold greater than in adults and adolescents.

Pharmacodynamics

Although there are no studies directly comparing different hematopoietic growth factors, a series of phase 1/2 studies provide insight (Figure 8.3) (Mertelsmann, 1991). In patients with advanced cancer not receiving chemotherapy, a hematopoietic growth factor was administered by subcutaneous injection and continued for approximately two weeks. rhG-CSF induced a rapid increase in neutrophil counts that was evident on day two and that gradually increased through day ten. Thereafter, the neutrophil count declined gradually, despite continued therapy, and quickly returned to baseline after therapy was stopped. rhGM-CSF gradually expanded white blood cell counts throughout the treatment period; this finding was attributable primarily to increases in neutrophils and bands and, less strikingly, to increases in eosinophils and monocytes. rhIL-3, not commercially available but used in a reported comparative study, promoted the expansion of all types of white blood cells, reticulocytes, and platelets.

In patients with anemia due to chronic renal failure, administration of rhEPO (three times weekly) increases reticulocyte counts within ten days. This reticulocyte increase is followed by increases in the red blood cell count, hemoglobin, and hematocrit within two to six weeks (Eschbach *et al.*, 1989).

In phase 1/2 studies in patients with cancer, ancestim administered over a range of 5 to 25 µg/kg/day, in combination with fixed doses of filgrastim, produced a dose-dependent increase in circulating peripheral blood progenitor cells (PBPCs), including $CD34^+$ cells, compared with the administration of ancestim alone (Glaspy *et al.*, 1995). Patients receiving the cytokine combination had increases in circulating PBPCs that resulted in apheresis yields

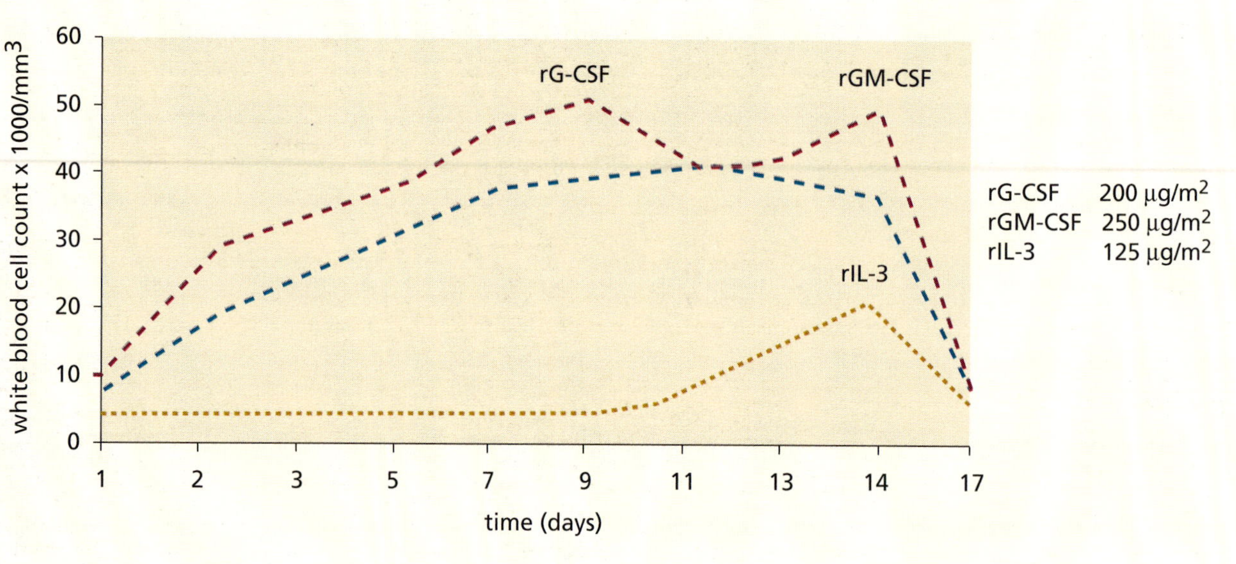

Figure 8.3. Effect of hematopoietic growth factors on white blood cell counts in patients with advanced cancer. rhG-CSF was administered at 200 μg/m^2; rhGM-CSF was administered at 250 μg/m^2; rhIL-3, not commercially available, was also used in this study and was administered at 125 μg/m^2. All drugs were administered by subcutaneous injection for approximately 14 days (Reproduced from Mertelsmann, 1991 with permission).

that were two- to three-fold greater than those of patients receiving filgrastim alone.

Oprelvekin administered daily for 14 days to patients who did not have myelosuppression from their chemotherapy caused platelet counts to increase in a dose-dependent manner (Orazi *et al.*, 1995). Platelet counts began to increase between five and nine days after the commencement of dosing; after the cessation of treatment, platelet counts continued to increase for another seven days. No change in platelet aggregation or activation was noted. Normal volunteers treated with oprelvekin had mean increases in plasma volume of >20%.

Clinical and Practice Aspects

Hematopoietic growth factors have been and continue to be evaluated in many clinical disorders involving different types of blood cells. This section focuses on established uses (Table 8.4) and introduces investigational uses.

Indications for biologics can become established through many mechanisms. In the United States, at least one randomized, pivotal study must be conducted before the Food and Drug Administration will consider a new indication for a biologic (Vincent-Gattis *et al.*, 1999). The official review and approval process can take many years, so biologics may be used for investigational indications before they receive official governmental approval. These uses may be considered established if they appear in major medical textbooks or other respected medical resources. The term "investigational uses" also has different meanings and, for the purpose of this section, will refer to two types of ongoing studies: commercially available hematopoietic growth factors being evaluated for purposes that have not yet been established, and growth factors that are not commercially available.

Established Uses

Not all uses discussed here have received regulatory approval in all countries. Check the current product package insert for licensed indications in the country of interest.

Neutrophil disorders are a logical therapeutic target for the myeloid hematopoietic growth factors. The disorder may be qualitative or quantitative. Abnormal neutrophil function may occur because of defective adhesion, movement, or phagocytosis and killing. Insufficient numbers of neutrophils (neutropenia) may result from accelerated destruction, maldistribution, or decreased production. In any case, patients generally have impaired host immunity and an increased risk of bacterial infection.

rhG-CSF is indicated for neutropenia associated with myelosuppressive cancer chemotherapy, bone marrow transplantation, chemotherapy for acute myeloid leukemia and severe chronic neutropenia, to mobilize PBPCs for stem cell transplantation, and for the reversal of clinically significant neutropenia and subsequent maintenance of adequate neutrophil counts in patients with advanced

Molecule	Proper Name	Approved/Investigational Uses
EPO	epoetin alfa, epoetin beta	treatment of anemia associated with chronic renal failure; treatment of symptomatic anemia in predialysis patients; increasing yield of autologous blood in presurgery donation programs; treatment of anemia due to zidovudine in HIV/AIDS patients; treatment of chemotherapy-induced anemia
G-CSF	filgrastim, lenograstim	treatment of chemotherapy-induced febrile neutropenia, severe chronic neutropenia, aplastic anemia; support of hematopoiesis after bone marrow transplantation; support of induction/consolidation chemotherapy for AML; mobilization of stem cells for transplantation; prevention of infections in HIV/AIDS patients
GM-CSF	molgramostim, sargramostim	support of hematopoiesis after induction chemotherapy for AML; mobilization of stem cells for transplantation; support of hematopoiesis after bone marrow transplantation; use in bone marrow transplantation failure or engraftment delay
IL-3	muplestim	support of hematopoiesis after high-dose chemotherapy or bone marrow failure, and for myelodysplastic syndromes
IL-6	sigosix	potential platelet stimulator
IL-11	oprelvekin	prevention of severe thrombocytopenia and reduction of platelet transfusions after chemotherapy
LIF[a]	emfilermin	hematopoietic reconstitution, particularly platelets
M-CSF[b]		treatment of myelosuppression
Oncostatin-M		treatment of cytopenias
SCF	ancestim	used in conjunction with filgrastim to increase mobilization of stem cells for autologous transplantation
TPO		treatment of thrombocytopenia

Table 8.4. Summary of approved and investigational uses for selected hematopoietic growth factors as of September 2000. Not all indications are approved for marketing in all countries. [a] leukemia inhibitory factor; [b] macrophage colony-stimulating factor.

HIV infection during treatment with antiviral and/or other myelosuppressive medications when other options to manage neutropenia are inappropriate. rhGM-CSF is indicated for neutropenia associated with myelosuppressive cancer chemotherapy in patients with acute myeloid leukemia, bone marrow transplantation, and antiviral therapy for AIDS-related cytomegalovirus, for failed bone marrow transplantation or delayed engraftment, and for use in mobilization and after transplantation of autologous PBPCs. rhEPO is indicated to treat anemia associated with chronic renal failure, zidovudine-induced anemia in HIV-infected patients, and chemotherapy-induced anemia, and to reduce the need for allogeneic blood transfusions and hasten erythroid recovery in surgery patients. Ancestim is indicated in combination with filgrastim to mobilize PBPCs in patients who are difficult to mobilize because of previous chemotherapy or radiation therapy.

Pivotal studies for each established use have been selected to illustrate the benefit of hematopoietic growth factors in patients with hematologic disorders.

CHEMOTHERAPY-INDUCED NEUTROPENIA

Neutropenia and infection are common dose-limiting effects of cancer chemotherapy. The risk of infection is directly related to the depth and duration of neutropenia. The severity of neutropenia depends on the intensity of the cancer chemotherapy regimen, as well as host- and disease-related factors. Fever may be the only manifestation of infection because underlying immunosuppression often obscures the classic signs and symptoms. Therefore, it is standard practice to administer broad-spectrum antibiotic therapy and even to hospitalize patients who have febrile neutropenia. Furthermore, oncologists may delay the start of subsequent cycles of chemotherapy until neutrophil recovery, decrease the dose of cancer chemotherapy, or both. Although this practice may be deemed necessary to prevent infectious complications, it may also compromise otherwise effective cancer chemotherapy.

The phase 3 pivotal trials for filgrastim demonstrated the beneficial effects of the hematopoietic growth factor on febrile neutropenia after standard-dose chemotherapy (Crawford *et al.*, 1991; Trillet-Lenoir *et al.*, 1993). In these two randomized, double-blind, placebo-controlled trials involving >300 patients with small-cell lung cancer, filgrastim significantly decreased the incidence, severity, and duration of neutropenia, days of hospitalization and duration of intravenous antibiotic use (Figure 8.4).

In a randomized, double-blind, placebo-controlled, multicenter, phase 3 trial of filgrastim, patients were treated with chemotherapy for *de novo* acute myeloid leukemia (Heil *et al.*, 1997). Treatment with filgrastim significantly reduced the median recovery time of neutrophil counts and the median duration of fever, antibiotic use, and hospitalization after induction chemotherapy. During consolidation chemotherapy, patients treated with filgrastim also had significant reductions in incidence of severe neutropenia, time to neutrophil recovery, incidence and duration of fever, and durations of intravenous antibiotic use and hospitalization.

In phase 3 studies, prophylactic administration of lenograstim shortened the duration of chemotherapy-induced neutropenia in patients with non-myelogenous cancers who received standard-dose chemotherapy or myeloablative chemotherapy followed by bone marrow transplantation (Chevallier *et al.*, 1993; Gisselbrecht *et al.*, 1993). The median neutrophil nadir was significantly higher in patients treated with lenograstim compared with placebo recipients. Incidences of culture-confirmed infections across all cycles were significantly reduced in the lenograstim group during the period of neutropenia. The incidence of all infections in lenograstim-treated patients was lower than in the placebo group, but the difference was not statistically significant.

Sargramostim is not indicated for the reduction of chemotherapy-induced neutropenia, but it is indicated for use after induction chemotherapy in adults aged >55 years with acute myeloid leukemia to shorten time to neutrophil recovery and to reduce the incidence of severe

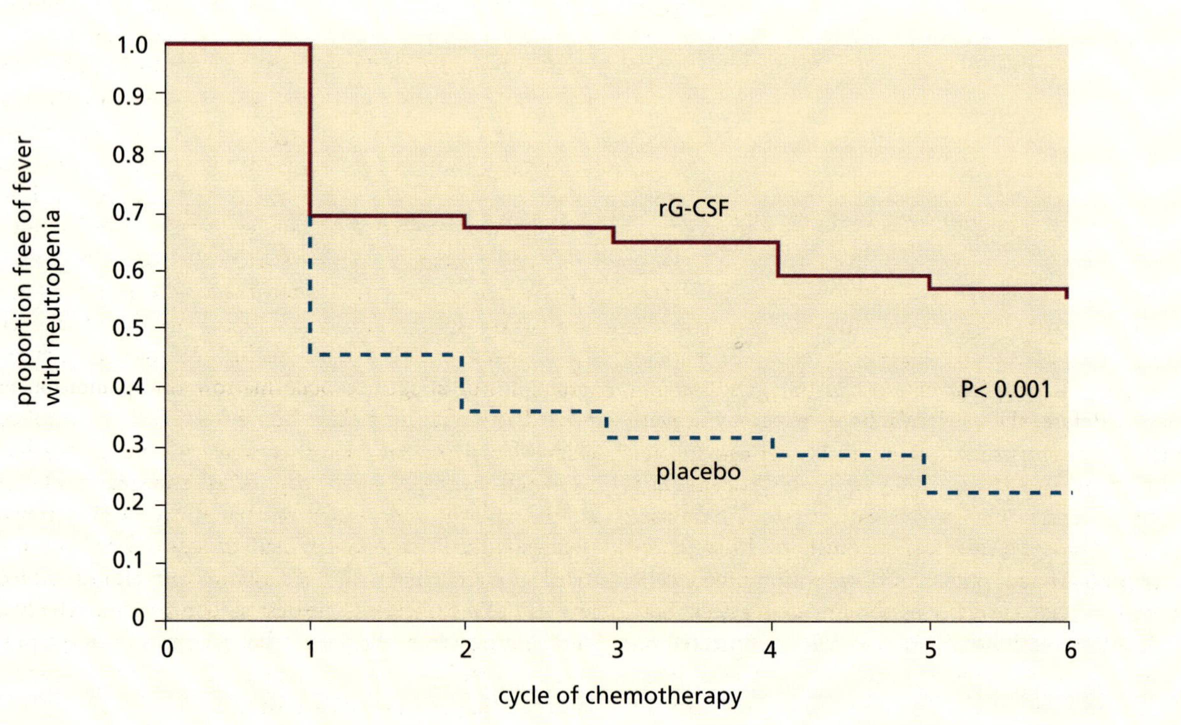

Figure 8.4. Effects of filgrastim on febrile neutropenia in a double-blind, randomized, placebo-controlled study of 194 evaluable patients (Adapted from Crawford *et al.*, 1991 with permission).

and life-threatening infections. In a phase 3 multicenter, randomized, double-blind, placebo-controlled study, sargramostim significantly shortened the median duration of neutropenia after induction chemotherapy compared with controls (Rowe *et al.*, 1995). During consolidation chemotherapy, however, the use of sargramostim did not shorten the median time to recovery of neutrophils compared with placebo. The incidence of severe infections and deaths associated with infections was significantly reduced in patients who received sargramostim compared with those who received placebo.

Contradictory evidence concerning the utility of sargramostim has been published. Steward *et al.* (1998) conducted a multicenter prospective trial in which patients with small-cell lung cancer were randomized to six cycles of chemotherapy administered every three weeks (intensified arm) or every four weeks (standard arm). A second double-blind randomization to sargramostim or placebo for 14 days between chemotherapy cycles was made. In 300 patients, no significant differences were reported in the incidence of febrile neutropenia, incidence of grade 4 neutropenia, duration of hospitalization, culture-confirmed infections, or use of antibiotics in any of the treatment groups.

In a phase 3 trial, patients with high-grade non-Hodgkin's lymphoma were administered molgramostim as a subcutaneous injection for seven days after chemotherapy (Gerhartz *et al.*, 1993). The frequency of infections, periods of neutropenia, days with fever, and days of hospitalization for infection were reduced significantly, and white blood cell counts increased.

Bone Marrow Transplantation

Bone marrow transplantation allows for the use of very high doses of chemotherapy, with or without radiotherapy, to eliminate malignant cells from patients with refractory tumors. The procedure involves administering ablative cancer chemotherapy and then infusing bone marrow progenitor cells that were harvested from the patient (autologous transplantation) or a donor (allogeneic transplantation). Before the patient's bone marrow recovers full function, the neutrophil count usually drops to zero and most patients experience profound pancytopenia and require multiple transfusions of blood and blood products. Allogeneic transplantation is more complicated than autologous transplantation because donor white blood cells may recognize host antigens as foreign and attack host tissues. Graft-versus-host disease can be life threatening and is manifested by epithelial damage in the skin, liver, and gastrointestinal tract. Consequently, recipients of allogeneic transplantation receive immunosuppressive therapy, which further increases the risk of infection. Regardless of the source of the bone marrow, the procedure may necessitate prolonged hospitalization, which increases the cost of treatment.

Two randomized, controlled trials have shown the utility of filgrastim in the autologous bone-marrow transplantation setting. In one study, filgrastim reduced the median number of days of severe neutropenia compared with placebo (Schmitz *et al.*, 1995). The other showed a statistically significant reduction in the median number of days of severe neutropenia in filgrastim-treated patients and the number of days of febrile neutropenia was reduced significantly, as well (Stahel *et al.*, 1994).

A phase 3 trial of 315 patients demonstrated the beneficial effects of lenograstim on neutrophil recovery in patients receiving either autologous or allogeneic bone marrow transplantation (Gisselbrecht *et al.*, 1994). The data suggested that lenograstim was beneficial for patients <15 years of age, as well as for the general population. No difference was seen between the lenograstim and placebo groups in the frequency of infections, culture-confirmed infections, or neutropenic fever, but the durations of infections and fever were shorter in lenograstim-treated patients. Use of lenograstim also shortened days of hospitalization, antibacterial use, and parenteral nutrition compared with placebo.

Sargramostim is indicated to accelerate myeloid recovery after autologous bone marrow transplantation in patients with non-Hodgkin's lymphoma, acute lymphoblastic leukemia, or Hodgkin's disease. It is also indicated in patients undergoing allogeneic transplantation from human leukocyte antigen (HLA)-matched related donors. In a double-blind, randomized, placebo-controlled study, 128 patients underwent autologous bone marrow transplantation for lymphoid cancer. Sargramostim administered by intravenous infusion over two hours was started within four hours after bone marrow infusion and continued for 21 days. Sargramostim shortened the duration of neutropenia, antibiotic therapy, and hospitalization (Nemunaitis *et al.*, 1991).

If engraftment is delayed or does not occur after bone marrow transplantation, the risk of infection and even death is considerable. Sargramostim's indication for failed autologous or allogeneic bone marrow transplantation or delayed engraftment is based on a historically controlled study of 243 patients. Patients were eligible if they had profound neutropenia 28 days after transplantation or infection plus profound neutropenia on day 21 after transplantation, or if the bone marrow graft failed after a transient engraftment. Use of sargramostim almost tripled survival. The benefit was greatest among patients who had autologous (versus allogeneic) bone marrow transplantation, no total body irradiation, non-leukemic malignancy, and fewer impaired organ systems.

The other rhGM-CSF product, molgramostim, is indicated to reduce the duration of neutropenia and its sequelae after bone marrow transplantation for non-myeloid malignancies. Molgramostim accelerated neutrophil recovery in a randomized phase 3 study in patients with delayed engraftment. Although molgramostim allowed recovery of neutrophil counts, some patients did not respond, and a few responded to treatment but subsequently died (Pedrazzini, 1993; Klingemann *et al.*, 1990; Brandwein *et al.*, 1991).

Peripheral Blood Progenitor Cell Mobilization for Harvesting and Transplantation

Stem (progenitor) cells found in the blood can be collected and concentrated for infusion after myelosuppressive cancer chemotherapy. PBPC harvesting (or collection) is attractive because it is less invasive than bone marrow harvesting. PBPC harvesting can be performed in the outpatient setting without anesthetizing the donor; it causes less morbidity and mortality, costs less, circumvents donor problems, and is suitable for a larger number of patients.

Hematopoietic growth factors expand the population of circulating hematopoietic progenitor cells and may be used to facilitate peripheral collection, which in turn can be used to supplement and/or replace autologous bone marrow collection. Hematopoietic growth factors can either be combined with chemotherapy to enhance the mobilizing effect of the latter or used alone to induce *de novo* mobilization. The optimal schedule is unknown. Hematopoietic growth factors can even be added to cultures containing hematopoietic progenitor cells to expand them *ex vivo.* These approaches are being investigated using commercially available hematopoietic growth factors alone and in combination with each other and investigational growth factors (Foote *et al.*, 2000).

In the United States, filgrastim is indicated to mobilize PBPCs for collection by leukapheresis in patients undergoing myelosuppressive or myeloablative therapy followed by transplantation. In Europe, filgrastim is indicated to mobilize PBPCs in patients undergoing myelosuppressive or myeloablative therapy followed by autologous PBPC transplantation with or without bone marrow transplantation.

Seventeen patients with non-myeloid malignancies who received filgrastim by continuous subcutaneous infusion had a 58-fold increase in the numbers of granulocyte-macrophage progenitor cells (CFU-GM) in peripheral blood (Sheridan *et al.*, 1992). Progenitor cells were collected by three leukapheresis procedures and infused after high-dose chemotherapy to augment autologous bone-marrow rescue and post-transplant filgrastim therapy. The time to platelet recovery was shorter in patients who received filgrastim-mobilized PBPCs compared with controls. A prospective randomized trial in lymphoma patients compared the effects of filgrastim-mobilized PBPCs or autologous bone marrow infused after high-dose chemotherapy. In this study, filgrastim-mobilized PBPCs significantly reduced the number of platelet transfusions and the time to platelet and neutrophil recovery. It also led to an earlier hospital discharge compared with patients receiving autologous marrow (Schmitz *et al.*, 1996).

Sargramostim is indicated to mobilize PBPCs in patients undergoing myelosuppressive or myeloablative therapy followed by autologous PBPC transplantation. It is also indicated to further accelerate myeloid recovery after PBPC transplantation. A trial of sargramostim alone, filgrastim alone, or the combination in normal donors showed a greater median $CD34^+$ cell yield with the combination or with filgrastim alone compared with sargramostim alone (Lane *et al.*, 1995).

A prospective, randomized, open-label trial directly compared the effects of filgrastim and sargramostim used prophylactically in hematologic recovery and resource utilization after myelosuppressive chemotherapy (Weaver *et al.*, 2000). One hundred fifty-eight patients with breast cancer, malignant lymphoma, or multiple myeloma were enrolled and received myelosuppressive chemotherapy. Starting the day after the completion of chemotherapy, patients received filgrastim or sargramostim or the combination of sargramostim followed by filgrastim. Patients treated with filgrastim alone had significantly faster neutrophil recovery, lower incidence of fever, less intravenous antibiotic use, and fewer hospital admissions compared with patients treated with sargramostim alone. Patients treated with sargramostim followed by filgrastim had significantly faster neutrophil recovery, lower incidence of fever, less intravenous antibiotic use, and fewer hospital admissions compared with patients treated with sargramostim alone. Patients treated with filgrastim alone did not have significant differences in clinical endpoints compared with patients treated with the growth factor combination, but did have a more rapid neutrophil recovery.

Molgramostim has been studied in combination and in sequence with rhG-CSF for mobilization of PBPCs (Winter *et al.*, 1996). The combination of the two growth factors resulted in dramatic and sustained increases in peripheral blood GM-CFUs. In patients receiving rhG-CSF with molgramostim, PBPC cell content increased nearly 80-fold.

A number of randomized, controlled studies, including a pivotal phase 3 trial, were done to evaluate the efficacy of ancestim plus filgrastim compared with filgrastim alone to mobilize PBPCs in patients who were chemotherapy naïve or who had received moderate to extensive prior chemotherapy or radiation therapy. Patients in these studies had tumors that are often treated with high-dose chemotherapy and PBPC support (i.e. breast cancer, non-Hodgkin's lymphoma, Hodgkin's disease, myeloma, and ovarian cancer). The phase 3 trial evaluated ancestim plus filgrastim in a cytokine-only mobilization regimen (Shpall *et al.*, 1999). The primary endpoint of this study was reduction in the number of leukaphereses. The combination of ancestim and filgrastim resulted in a statistically significant reduction in the number of leukaphereses needed to reach the $CD34^+$ cell target compared with mobilization with filgrastim alone. A median of four leukaphereses was needed in the ancestim plus filgrastim group compared with six or more in the filgrastim-alone group.

Severe Chronic Neutropenia

Severe chronic neutropenia may be present from birth (congenital), be periodic (cyclic), or have an unknown etiology (idiopathic). The condition is manifested by decreased neutrophil counts, recurrent fever, chronic oropharyngeal inflammation, and severe infection. Filgrastim is indicated to reduce the incidence and duration of these sequelae. In a phase 3 study, 123 patients were randomized to receive filgrastim immediately or after a four-months observation period (Dale *et al.*, 1993). Filgrastim was given by subcutaneous injection at doses of 3.45 μg/kg/day for idiopathic neutropenia, 5.75 μg/kg/day for cyclic neutropenia, and 11.50 μg/kg twice daily for congenital neutropenia. The dose was adjusted to maintain the median monthly absolute neutrophil count between 1500 and 10,000/mm^3. Hematologic responses were evident within a few days. Ninety percent of patients achieved complete responses: improved bone marrow morphology and a lower incidence and duration of infection-related events.

Several small studies have been published in Japanese and in English in abstract form concerning the use of lenograstim in severe chronic neutropenia. Lenograstim did improve neutrophil counts in this patient population (Griscelli and Donadieu, 1992).

AIDS

Patients infected with HIV often have neutropenia, anemia, and/or thrombocytopenia. These hematologic abnormalities may occur as a direct result of HIV infection, as secondary effects of comorbid conditions, or because of chronic myelosuppressive therapy. Antiviral therapy must be interrupted in up to half of the patients because of drug-induced neutropenia (Foote and Welch, 1999; Welch and Foote, 1999).

Filgrastim has been approved in Australia, Canada, the European Union, and Japan for use in patients with HIV infection for the reversal of clinically significant neutropenia and for the subsequent maintenance of adequate neutrophil counts during treatment with antiviral and/or other myelosuppressive medications when other options to manage neutropenia are inappropriate. A phase 3 study reported the effect of filgrastim on the incidence of severe neutropenia in patients with advanced HIV infection and its effect on the prevention of infectious morbidity (Kuritzkes *et al.*, 1998). Two hundred fifty-eight patients enrolled in the 24-week study, and 201 completed it. Filgrastim was administered daily at 1 μg/kg and adjusted up to 10 μg/kg/day or intermittently at 300 μg daily one to three days per week. Patients in a control group received filgrastim only if severe neutropenia (defined as a neutrophil count <500 cells/mm^3) developed. Both daily and intermittent administration of filgrastim lowered the incidence of bacterial infection rates compared with patients in the control group. Overall, filgrastim-treated patients developed 31% fewer bacterial infections than did control patients. Use of filgrastim produced significant reductions in the risk of severe bacterial infections and the number of days of hospitalization.

Various additional dosing regimens of filgrastim have been used alone or in combination with rhEPO to reverse the dose-limiting hematologic toxicity of ganciclovir or zidovudine (Miles *et al.*, 1991). For example, filgrastim permitted the use of higher doses of ganciclovir and improved the outcome of AIDS-related cytomegalovirus retinitis in a retrospective study of 28 patients (Morgan and Strickland, 1993). rhEPO may be useful in amelioration of anemia associated with HIV/AIDS in lieu of red blood cell transfusions. A study using quantitative polymerase chain reaction (PCR) to measure circulating HIV viral load indicated increased loads five days after transfusion (Mudido *et al.*, 1996). More information about the role of rhEPO in zidovudine-induced anemia is given in the section Anemia.

Lenograstim ameliorated the neutropenia associated with zidovudine treatment in patients with AIDS or AIDS-related complex (Vanderwouw *et al.*, 1991).

Sargramostim has been investigated in the setting of HIV/AIDS to determine its effects on the incidence and time to opportunistic infection or death, plasma HIV RNA, and CD34 cell count (Angel *et al.*, 2000). Three hundred nine patients with advanced HIV disease received at least one dose of sargramostim or placebo, and 70% completed 24 weeks of therapy. Sargramostim significantly increased CD34 cell and neutrophil counts and reduced the incidence of overall infection, as well as delayed time to first infection. Sargramostim did not appear to increase HIV RNA viral loads.

Molgramostim is indicated as adjuvant therapy for patients with AIDS-related cytomegalovirus retinitis to maintain the recommended dosage of ganciclovir (Hardy *et al.*, 1994). Fifty-three patients with AIDS and cytomegalovirus retinitis were randomized to receive ganciclovir with or without molgramostim by subcutaneous injection to maintain absolute neutrophil counts between 500 and 5000/mm^3. Molgramostim reduced the risk of neutropenia and interruptions in ganciclovir therapy, thereby resulting in a trend that delayed the progression of retinitis. Results of a study confirmed that this regimen did not alter the pharmacokinetic disposition of ganciclovir or promote HIV proliferation (Hardy, 1991).

Anemia

Anemia, a low number of red blood cells, a decreased volume of red blood cells, or a reduced hemoglobin concentration, has many causes. The symptoms of anemia may include fatigue, dizziness, headache, chest pain, shortness of breath, and depression. Anemia is associated with increases in illness and death in patients with chronic renal failure, cancer, or HIV infection. Like other hematopoietic cells, red blood cells originate in the bone marrow and undergo a series of steps that are regulated by hematopoietic growth factors (Figure 8.1).

In a phase 3 study of 333 patients with anemia and end-stage renal disease, epoetin alfa increased the hematocrit and eliminated the need for red blood cell transfusions in nearly all patients (Eschbach *et al.*, 1989) (Figure 8.5). The response was dose dependent, evident within two weeks, and maximal at six to ten weeks of dosing.

In patients with cancer receiving chemotherapy, rhEPO increases hemoglobin values and decreases the need for blood transfusions (Abels *et al.*, 1991). In patients with HIV/AIDS, rhEPO increased hemoglobin levels even when administered concomitantly with zidovudine therapy (Henry *et al.*, 1992).

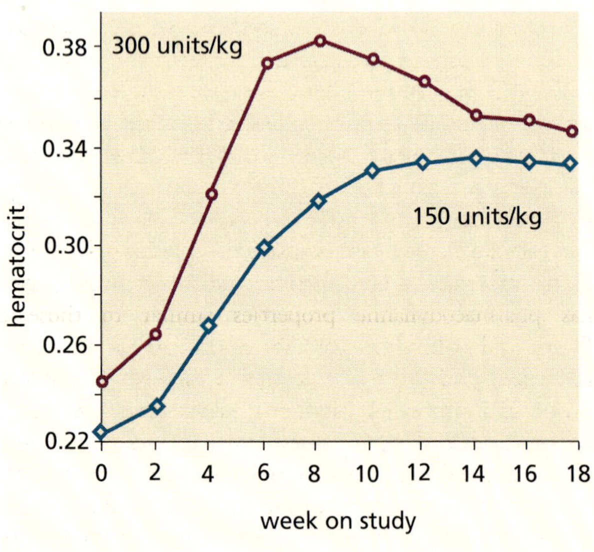

Figure 8.5. Effect of epoetin alfa on mean hematocrit in 236 evaluable patients with anemia and end-stage renal disease. Epoetin alfa 150 or 300 U/kg was given three times weekly by intravenous bolus injection (Reproduced from Eschbach *et al.* 1989, with permission).

Thrombocytopenia

Approximately 25% of patients receiving dose-intensive chemotherapy may develop grade 4 thrombocytopenia, and nearly 50% will require platelet transfusions (Sheridan and Foote, 1998). Almost all patients treated with chemotherapy for acute leukemia develop thrombocytopenia and require an average of 13 platelet transfusions during remission induction therapy and five platelet transfusions for each post-remission course of chemotherapy (Schiffer, 1996). Two forms of Mpl ligand have been produced through recombinant DNA technology: PEG-rhMGDF and rhTPO. Clinical studies with PEG-rhMGDF were stopped. Results from a few early trials with rhTPO have been published, but rhTPO is not currently available commercially.

Another non-Mpl-ligand, thrombopoietic factor, rhIL-11, is commercially available as oprelevkin, and is licensed for use for the prevention of severe thrombocytopenia and the reduction of platelet transfusions after chemotherapy. In a placebo-controlled trial of women receiving chemotherapy for breast cancer, oprelevkin 25 or 50 µg/kg produced dose-related increases in mean platelet counts and a reduction in chemotherapy-induced thrombocytopenia (Tepler *et al.*, 1996).

Toxicities

Many hematopoietic growth factors, especially multipotential factors that act on early progenitor cells, are associated with constitutional symptoms, such as fever, chills, rash, myalgia, injection-site reaction, and edema. The safety of individual hematopoietic growth factors depends on their receptor sites and the effects of secondary cytokine release.

Determination of the relative toxicity of hematopoietic growth factors is difficult because of the lack of comparative studies and confounding effects of different reporting methods and different cancer chemotherapy regimens. For example, patients who undergo bone marrow transplantation experience toxicity that may obscure hematopoietic growth factor-related adverse effects. Formulations with different levels of glycosylation may also play a role. Again, the healthcare provider is responsible for consulting the current product package insert of all medicines for precautions, warnings, and possible drug interactions. A summary of the most common adverse events is presented, as listed in the current package inserts, but it should not be considered to be comprehensive or inclusive.

rhG-CSF and rhGM-CSF

The most common adverse effect associated with filgrastim and lenograstim is mild-to-moderate bone pain, which occurs in 10% to 39% of patients receiving filgrastim

5 μg/kg/day, compared with 0% to 21% of control patients. Lenograstim is also associated with injection-site reaction. Loss of appetite, fever, and headache are mentioned in the Japanese package insert for lenograstim, but published information does not indicate whether the frequency is higher compared with controls. Other adverse events appear to be infrequent.

A long list of adverse effects has been attributed to the two rhGM-CSF products partly because of the use of high doses in early, uncontrolled trials. For example, much has been written about the capillary-leak syndrome because of its potential severity. This complication is manifested by fluid retention, pleural and/or pericardial effusions, peripheral edema, and hypoproteinemia. Fortunately, capillary-leak syndrome is rare and occurs at high doses (>15 μg/kg) of rhGM-CSF. Currently recommended doses of sargramostim were not associated with this syndrome and did not increase the incidence of most adverse events in a placebo-controlled study of bone marrow transplant recipients (Nemunaitis *et al.*, 1991). rhGM-CSF may also induce a first-dose reaction characterized by flushing, tachycardia, hypotension, musculoskeletal pain, dyspnea, nausea and vomiting, and leg spasms. This complication is much more common with molgramostim and with intravenous administration (Bennett *et al.*, 1996).

The results of non-comparative studies suggest differences among recombinant hematopoietic growth factors, but comparative studies are needed to confirm these perceptions. Fever may be more common with rhGM-CSF compared with rhG-CSF, but the clinical relevance is unknown (Bennett *et al.*, 1996). Glycosylation may be a factor and may prevent some adverse effects associated with rhGM-CSF. The results of independent studies (Rowe *et al.*, 1995; Stone *et al.*, 1995) suggest that glycosylated sargramostim may be less likely to cause adverse effects than non-glycosylated molgramostim. Differences in glycosylation may contribute to the higher incidence for sargramostim (3.6%) compared with molgramostim (1%).

Epoetin alfa, ancestim, and oprelvekin

rhEPO is generally well tolerated. Many adverse effects are indistinguishable from those of underlying diseases, such as chronic renal failure, AIDS, or cancer. Some patients experience flu-like symptoms, hypertension, or headaches. In patients with chronic renal failure, rhEPO may exaggerate pre-existing hypertension because the red blood cell count increases. Seizures and thrombotic events have been reported, but their relation to rhEPO is not clear or certain.

The most common event associated with ANCESTIM administration has been skin reaction at the injection site, which occurs in nearly all patients. These local skin reactions are generally mild to moderate, and manifest as edema or urticaria. They generally appear within 24 hours after a subcutaneous injection and persist for 24 to 48 hours. The reactions apparently are mast cell mediated (Costa *et al.*, 1996; Grinchnik *et al.*, 1995). A few patients have experienced severe life-threatening systemic allergic reactions. Based on available preclinical and clinical data, ancestim should not be administered to patients with a history of anaphylaxis, urticaria, or asthma requiring therapy, and all patients should receive premedication with cetirizine, ranitidine, and albuterol or salbuterol.

Administration of OPRELVEKIN is associated with several adverse effects (i.e., fluid retention, anemia, cardiac arrhythmias, and metabolic disturbances) that result from concomitant diuretic therapy (Sheridan and Foote, 1998). Co-administration of diuretics is apparently needed in many patients to limit the degree of expansion of plasma volume and extracellular fluid.

Other Uses and New Formulations

It is difficult to predict which investigational hematopoietic growth factor will reach the market next. Recombinant human macrophage colony-stimulating factor (rhM-CSF) has been under clinical evaluation nearly as long as rhG-CSF and rhGM-CSF, which may have implications for the likelihood of marketing. Fusion molecules of two cytokines theoretically having the advantages of both (particularly of interleukins and rhGM-CSF) have been developed and clinically tested. These fusion molecules are combinations of pleiotrophic molecules and, therefore, have the potential for more toxicities. Clinical development of most fusion molecules has been discontinued because of toxicities or lack of improved efficacy compared with a marketed hematopoietic growth factor. Some new molecules are in clinical trials.

Pegfilgrastim is a sustained-duration rhG-CSF that has been developed by covalent attachment of a polyethylene glycol molecule to the filgrastim molecule. Pegfilgrastim has pharmacodynamic properties similar to those of filgrastim but has the advantage of requiring only a single injection to achieve the same effect as several injections of filgrastim (Johnston *et al.*, 2000). Results of a randomized, dose-escalation study in patients with non-small-cell lung cancer showed that peak serum concentrations and the duration of elevated serum concentrations were dependent on the dose of pegfilgrastim. The effects of pegfilgrastim on neutrophil counts and PBPC mobilization were comparable to or greater than those achieved with daily filgrastim. The attachment of the polyethylene molecule to filgrastim to produce pegfilgrastim may result in one-per-chemotherapy-cycle administration, improve patient compliance, and lessen healthcare-related resources.

Novel erythropoiesis stimulating protein (NESP) was designed by introducing five amino acid changes into the primary sequence of EPO to create two extra consensus *N*-linked carbohydrate sites (Egrie *et al.*, 1997). Because of its increased carbohydrate content and sialic acid changes, NESP has a three-fold longer serum half-life in animal models compared with rhEPO, which was substantiated in a double-blind, randomized, crossover trial in humans (Macdougall *et al.*, 1999). The area-under-the-serum-concentration-time curve was significantly greater for NESP compared with rhEPO, and volume of distribution was similar for both products. The peak concentration of NESP administered subcutaneously was about 10% of that after intravenous administration, and bioavailability was approximately 37% by the subcutaneous route. The longer half-life of NESP may confer a clinical advantage over rhEPO by allowing less frequent dosing when treating patients for anemia of chronic renal failure or anemia associated with cancer and/or chemotherapy.

Many journals, websites, and drug-industry periodicals are good sources for information for the myriad of biotechnology/pharmaceutical products being developed, including new hematopoietic growth factors.

Concluding Remarks

Hematopoietic growth factors have had a significant impact on the ancillary treatment of cancer: prevention of infections associated with chemotherapy-induced neutropenia, chemotherapy-induced thrombocytopenia, and chemotherapy-induced anemia.

This review provides a brief introduction to commercially available and investigational hematopoietic growth factors. Appropriate resources should always be used for current and detailed information.

Basic understanding of hematopoietic growth factors and their clinical potential continues to grow, and the discovery of new factors and how all factors interact will undoubtedly be an area of research for some time.

Acknowledgements

Drs Flynn, Salvado, and Foote are employees of Amgen Inc., the manufacturer of epoetin alfa, filgrastim, ancestim, PEG-rhMGDF, SD/01, and NESP. We thank Dr Keith Langley and Jim Yuen for reviewing and editing this paper. ■

References

- **Abels RI, Larholt KM, Krantz KDA, Bryant EC.** (1991). Recombinant human erythropoietin (r-HuEPO) for the treatment of the anemia of cancer. In *Blood Cell Growth Factors*, edited by MJ Murphy, Dayton, Ohio, USA: Alpha Med Press; pp. 121–141.
- **Angel JB, High K, Rhame F, Brand D, Whitmore JB, Agosti JM, *et al.*** (2000). Phase III study of granulocyte-macrophage colony-stimulating factor in advanced HIV disease: effect on infections, CD4 cell counts and HIV suppression. *AIDS*, 14, 387–395.
- **Armitage JO.** (1998). Emerging applications of recombinant human granulocyte colony-stimulating factor. *Blood*, 92, 4491–4508.
- **Bennett CL, Smith TJ, Weeks JC, Bredt AB, Feinglass J, Fetting JH, *et al.*** (1996). Use of hematopoietic colony-stimulating factors: The American Society of Clinical Oncology Survey. *Journal of Clinical Oncology*, 14, 2511–2520.
- **Brandwein JM, Nayar R, Baker MA, Sutton DM, Scott JC, Sutcliffe SB, *et al.*** (1991). GM-CSF therapy for delayed engraftment after autologous bone marrow transplantation. *Experimental Hematology*, 19, 191–195.
- **Broudy VC.** (1997). Stem cell factor and hematopoiesis. *Blood*, 90, 1345–1364.
- **Broudy VC, Lin NL, Sabath DF, Papayannopoulou T, Kaushansky K.** (1997). Human platelets display high-affinity receptors for thrombopoietins. *Blood*, 89, 1896–1904.
- **Cebon I, Layton JE, Maher D, Morstyn G.** (1994). Endogenous haemopoietic growth factors in neutropenia and infection. *British Journal of Haematology*, 86, 265–274.
- **Chevallier B, Chollet P, Merrouche Y, Roche H, Maugard Louboutin C, Kerbrat P, *et al.*** (1993a). Glycosylated rhG-CSF (lenograstim) prevents morbidity from FEC-HD chemotherapy in inflammatory breast cancer. *Proceedings American Society of Clinical Oncology*, 12, 84 (abstract 137).
- **Colgan SP, Gasper PW, Thrall MA, Boone TC, Blancquaert AMB, Bruyninckx WJ.** (1992). Neutrophil function in normal and Chediak-Higashi syndrome cats following administration of recombinant canine granulocyte colony-stimulating factor. *Experimental Hematology*, 20, 1229–1234.
- **Costa JJ, Demetri GD, Harrris TJ, Dvorak AM, Hayes DF, Merica EA, *et al.*** (1996). Recombinant human stem cell factor (Kit ligand) promotes human mast cell and melanocyte hyperplasia and functional activation in vivo. *Journal of Experimental Medicine*, 183, 2681–2686.
- **Crawford J, Ozer H, Stoller R, Johnson D, Lyman C, Tabbara I, *et al.*** (1991). Reduction by granulocyte colony-stimulating factor of fever and neutropenia induced by chemotherapy in patients with small-cell lung cancer. *New England Journal of Medicine*, 325, 164–170.
- **Dale DC, Bonilla MA, Davis MW, Nakanishi AM, Hammond WP, Kurtzberg J, *et al.*** (1993). A randomized controlled phase III trial of recombinant human granulocyte colony-stimulating factor (filgrastim) for treatment of severe chronic neutropenia. *Blood*, 81, 2496–2502.
- **Dale DC, Liles WC, Llewellyn C, Price TH.** (1998). Effects of granulocyte-macrophage colony-stimulating factor (GM-CSF) on

neutrophil kinetics and function in normal human volunteers. *American Journal of Hematology*, 57, 7–15.

- **Du XX, Williams DA.** (1997). Interleukin-11: Review of molecular, cell biology, and clinical use. *Blood*, 89, 3897–3908.
- **Egrie JC, Dwyer E, Lykos M, Hitz A, Browne JK.** (1997). Novel erythropoeisis stimulating protein (NESP) has a longer serum half-life and greater in vivo biological activity compared to recombinant human erythropoietin (rhEPO). *Blood*, 90, 56a (abstract no.243).
- **Erslev AJ.** (1991). Erythropoietin. *New England Journal of Medicine*, 324, 1339–1344.
- **Eschbach JW, Abdulhadi MH, Browne JK, Delano BG, Downing MR, Egrie JC, *et al.*** (1989). Recombinant human erythropoietin in anemic patients with end-stage renal disease. Results of a phase III multicenter trial. *Annals of Internal Medicine*, 111, 992–1000.
- **Foote MA, Flynn J.** (1993). Biotechnology basics for medical writers. *AMWA Journal*, 8, 86–89.
- **Foote MA, Gringeri A, Mazanet R.** (2000). Cell therapy: use of hematopoietic growth factors and cell separation techniques. Oncology Nursing Press, Pittsburgh, PA, pp. 9.1–9.16.
- **Foote MA, Welch W.** (1999). Biopharmaceutical drug development: filgrastim (r-metHuG-CSF) use in patients with HIV infection. *Journal of Hematotherapy & Stem Cell Research*, 8, S3–S8.
- **Galli SJ, Zsebo KM, Geissler EN.** (1994). The kit ligand, SCF. *Advances in Immunology*, 55, 1–96.
- **Gerhartz HH, Englehard M, Meusers P, Brittinger G, Wilmanns W, Schlimok G, *et al.*** (1993). Randomized, double-blind, placebo-controlled, phase III study of recombinant human granulocyte-macrophage colony-stimulating factor as adjunct to induction treatment of high-grade malignant non-Hodgkin's lymphomas. *Blood*, 82, 2329–2339.
- **Gisselbrecht C, Lepage E, Haioun B, Coiffier B, Tilly H, Bosly A, *et al.*** (1993). Lenograstim (glycosylated recombinant human G-CSF) supported optimization in aggressive non-Hodgkin's lymphoma (NHL). *Proceedings American Society of Clinical Oncology*, 12, 363 (abstract 1226).
- **Gisselbrecht C, Prentice HG, Bacligalupo A, Biron P, Milpied N, Rubie H, *et al.*** (1994). Placebo-controlled phase III trial of lenograstim in bone marrow transplantation. *The Lancet*, 343, 696–700.
- **Glaspy JA, Shpall EJ, LeMaistre CF, Briddell RA, Menchaca DM, Turner SA, *et al.*** (1995). Peripheral blood progenitor cell mobilization utilizing stem cell factor in combination with filgrastim in breast cancer patients. *Blood*, 90, 2939–2951.
- **Grichnik JM, Crawford J, Jiminez F, Kurtzberg J, Buchanan M, Blackwell S, *et al.*** (1995). Human recombinant stem-cell factor induces melanocytic hyperplasia in susceptible patients. *Journal American Academy of Dermatology*, 33, 577–583.
- **Griscelli C, Donadieu J. European study of lenograstim in severe congenital agranulocytosis.** (1992). Congress of International Society of Hematology; abstract.
- **Gronski P, Badziong W, Habermann P, List W, Mullner H, Neurohr KJ, *et al.*** (1988). Escherichia coli derived human granulocyte-macrophage colony-stimulating factor (rh GM-CSF) available for clinical trials. *Behring Institute Mitteilungen*, 83, 246–249.
- **Groopman JE, Molina JM, Scadden DT.** (1989). Hematopoietic growth factors. Biology and clinical applications. *New England Journal of Medicine*, 321, 1449–1459.
- **Hardy WD.** (1991). Combined ganciclovir and recombinant human granulocyte-macrophage colony-stimulating factor in the treatment of cytomegalovirus retinitis in AIDS patients. *Journal of Acquired Immune Deficiency Syndrome*, 4, S22–S28.
- **Hardy W, Spector S, Polsky B, Crumpacker C, van der Horst C, Holland C, *et al.*** (1994). Combination of ganciclovir and granulocyte-macrophage colony-stimulating factor in the treatment of cytomegalovirus retinitis in AIDS patients. *European Journal of Clinical Microbiology and Infectious Diseases*, 13, S34–S46.
- **Hart D.** (1997). Dendritic cells: unique leukocyte populations which control the primary immune response. *Blood*, 90, 3245–3287.
- **Hartung T, Doecke WD, Bundschuh D, Foote MA, Ganter F, Hermann C, *et al.*** (1999). Effect of filgrastim treatment on inflammatory cytokines and lymphocyte functions. *Clinical Pharmacology & Therapeutics*, 66, 415–424.
- **Heil G, Hoelzer D, Sanz MA, Lechner K, Liu Yin JA, Papa G, *et al.*** (1997). A randomized, double-blind, placebo-controlled, phase III study of filgrastim in remission induction and consolidation therapy for adults with de novo acute myeloid leukemia. *Blood*, 90, 4710–4718.
- **Henry DH, Jemsek JG, Levin AS, Levine JD, Levine RL, Abels RI, *et al.*** (1992). Recombinant human erythropoietin and the treatment of anemia in patients with AIDS or advanced ARC not receiving ZDV. *Journal of Acquired Immune Deficiency Syndrome*, 5, 847–848.
- **Israels LG, Israels ED.** (1996). Mechanisms in Hematology. University of Manitoba. Manitoba, Canada.
- **Jacobson JO, Goldwasser E, Fried W, Plzak L.** (2000). Role of the kidney in erythropoiesis. *Journal of the American Society of Nephrology*, 11, 589–592.
- **Johnston E, Crawford J, Blackwell S, Bjurstrom T, Lockbaum P, Roskos L, *et al.*** (2000). Randomized, dose-escalation study of SD/01 compared with daily filgrastim in patients receiving chemotherapy. *Journal of Clinical Oncology*, 18, 2522–2528.
- **Kaushansky K.** (1995). Thrombopoietin: basic biology, clinical promise. *International Journal of Hematology*, 62, 7–15.
- **Klingemann HG, Eaves AC, Barnett MJ, Reece DE, Shepherd JD, Belch AR, *et al.*** (1990). Recombinant GM-CSF in patients with poor graft function after bone marrow transplantation. *Clinical and Investigative Medicine*, 13, 77–81.
- **Kuritzkes DR, Parenti D, Ward D, Rachlis A, Wong RJ, Mallon KP, *et al.*** (1998). Filgrastim prevents severe neutropenia and reduces infective morbidity in patients with

advanced HIV infection: results of a randomized, multicenter, controlled trial. *AIDS*, 12, 65–74.

- **Kuter DJ, Hunt P, Sheridan W, Zucker-Franklin D, editors.** (1994a). *Thromobopoiesis and Thrombopoeitin.* Totowa, New Jersey, USA: Humana Press Inc.; 412 pp.
- **Kuter DJ, Beeler DL, Rosenberg RD.** (1994b). The purification of megapoietin: a physiological regulator of megakaryocyte growth and platelet production. *Proceedings of the National Academy of Sciences of the United States of America*, 91, 11104–11108.
- **Kuter DJ.** (1997). The regulation of platelet production in vivo. In *Thrombopoiesis and Thrombopoietins*, edited by DJ Kuter, P Hunt, W Sheridan, D Zucker-Franklin, Totowa, New Jersey, USA: Humana Press Inc.; pp. 377–397.
- **Lacerna L, Sheridan WP, Basser R, Begley CG, Crawford J, Demetri G, *et al.*** (2000). Stem cell factor. In *Hematopoietic Stem Cell Transplantation*, edited by AD Ho, R Haas, RE Champlin, New York, NY, USA: Marcel Dekker, Inc.; pp. 31–46.
- **Lane TA, Law P, Maruyama M, Young D, Burgess J, Mullen M, *et al.*** (1995). Harvesting and enrichment of hematopoietic progenitor cells mobilized into the peripheral blood of normal donors by granulocyte-macrophage colony-stimulating factor (GM-CSF) or G-CSF: potential role in allogeneic marrow transplantation. *Blood*, 25, 275–282.
- **Langley KE, Bennett LG, Wypych J, Yancik SA, Liu XD, Westcott KR, *et al.*** (1993). Soluble stem cell factor in human serum. *Blood*, 81, 656–660.
- **Lieschke GJ, Grail D, Hodgson G, Metcalf D, Stanley E, Cheers C, *et al.*** (1994). Mice lacking granulocyte colony-stimulating factor have chronic neutropenia, granulocyte and macrophage progenitor cell deficiency, and impaired neutrophil mobilization. *Blood*, 84, 1737–1746.
- **Lok S, Kaushansky K, Holly RD. Kuijper JL, Lofton-Day CE, Oort PJ, *et al.*** (1994). Cloning and expression of murine thrombopoietin cDNA and stimulation of platelet production in vivo. *Nature*, 369, 565–568.
- **Lord BI, Bronchud MH, Owens S, Chang J, Howell A, Souza L, *et al.*** (1989). The kinetics of human granulopoiesis following treatment with granulocyte colony-stimulating factor in vivo. *Proceedings of the National Academy of Sciences of the United States of America*, 86, 9499–9503.
- **Lord BI, Gurney H, Chang J, Thatcher N, Crowther D, Dexter TM.** (1992). Haemopoietic cell kinetics in humans treated with rGM-CSF. *International Journal of Cancer*, 50, 26–31.
- **Macdougall IC, Gray SJ, Elston O, Breen C, Jenkins B, Browne J, *et al.*** (1999). Pharmacokinetics of novel erythropoiesis stimulating protein compared with epoetin alfa in dialysis patients. *Journal of the American Society of Nephrology*, 10, 2392–2395.
- **Markham A, Bryson HM.** (1995). Epoetin alpha. A review of its pharmacodynamic and pharmacokinetic properties and therapeutic use in nonrenal applications. *Drugs*, 49, 232–254.
- **Mertelsmann R.** (1991). Hematopoietins: biology, pathophysiology, and potential as therapeutic agents. *Annals of Oncology*, 2, 251–263.
- **Metcalf D.** (1990). The colony stimulating factors. Discovery, development, and clinical applications. *Cancer*, 65, 2185–2195.
- **Metcalf D.** (2000). Summon up the blood. In dogged pursuit of the blood cell regulators. AlphaMed Press, Dayton, Ohio, 214 pp.
- **Miles SA, Mitsuyasu RT, Moreno J, Baldwin G, Alton NK, Souza L, *et al.*** (1991). Combined therapy with recombinant granulocyte colony-stimulating factor and erythropoietin decreases hematologic toxicity from zidovudine. *Blood*, 77, 2109–2117.
- **Morgan KM, Strickland SR.** (1993). The use of granulocyte stimulating factor (GCSF) has improved the outcome in AIDS related CMV retinitis. *International Conference on AIDS*, 9, 413 (abstract PO-B16-1666).
- **Mudido PM, Georges D, Dorazio D, Yen-Lieberman B, Bae S, O'Brien WA, *et al.*** (1996). Human immunodeficiency virus type 1 activation after blood transfusion. *Transfusion*, 36, 860–865.
- **Nagata S. Tsuchiya M, Asano S, Kaziro Y, Yamazaki T, Yamamoto O, *et al.*** (1986). Molecular cloning and expression of cDNA for human granulocyte-colony stimulating factor. *Nature*, 319, 415–418.
- **Nemunaitis J, Rabinowe SN, Singer JW, Bierman PJ, Vose JM, Freedman AS, *et al.*** (1991). Recombinant granulocyte-macrophage colony-stimulating factor after autologous bone marrow transplantation for lymphoid cancer. *New England Journal of Medicine*, 324, 1773–1778.
- **Nichol JL, Hokom MM, Hornkohl A, Sheridan WP, Ohashi H, Kato T, *et al.*** (1995). Megakaryocyte growth and development factor. Analyses of in vitro effects on human megakaryopoiesis and endogenous serum levels during chemotherapy-induced thrombocytopenia. *Journal of Clinical Investigation*, 95, 2973–2978.
- **Orazi A, Cooper RJ, Tong J, Gordon MS, Battiato L, Sledge GW, *et al.*** (1996). Effects of recombinant interleukin-11 (Neumega rhIL-11 growth factor) on megakaryocytopoiesis in human bone marrow. *Experimental Hematology*, 24, 1289–1297.
- **Pedrazzini A.** (1993). Erythropoietin and GM-CSF following autologous bone marrow transplantation. *European Journal of Cancer*. 29A, S15–S17.
- **Rapoport AP, Abboud CN, DiPersio JF.** (1992). Granulocyte-macrophage colony-stimulating factor (GM-CSF) and granulocyte colony-stimulating factor (G-CSF): Receptor biology, signal transduction, and neutrophil activation. *Blood Reviews*, 6, 43–57.
- **Roskos LK, Cheung EN, Vincent M, Foote MA, Morstyn G.** (1998). Pharmacology of filgrastim (r-metHuG-CSF). In *Filgrastim (r-metHuG-CSF) in Clinical Practice*, edited by G Morstyn, TM Dexter, MA Foote, New York, New York, USA: Marcel Dekker, Inc; pp. 51–71.
- **Rowe JM, Andersen JW, Mazza JJ, Bennett JM, Paietta E, Hayes FA, *et al.*** (1995). A randomized placebo-controlled

phase III study of granulocyte-macrophage colony-stimulating factor in adult patients (>55 to 70 years of age) with acute myelogenous leukemia: a study of the Eastern Cooperative Oncology Group (E1490). *Blood*, 86, 457–462.

- **Schiffer CA,** (1997). Potential Clinical Applications of Thrombopoietic Growth Factors. In *Thrombopoiesis and Thrombopoietins*, edited by DJ Kuter, P Hunt, W Sheridan, D Zucker-Franklin, Totowa, New Jersey, USA: Humana Press Inc.; pp. 79–94.
- **Schmitz N, Dreger P, Zander AR, Ehninger G, Wandt H, Fauger AA, *et al.*** (1995). Results of a randomised, controlled, multicentre study of recombinant human granulocyte colony-stimulating factor (filgrastim) in patients with Hodgkin's disease and non-Hodgkin's lymphoma undergoing autologous bone marrow transplantation. *Bone Marrow Transplantation*, 15, 261–266.
- **Schmitz N, Linch DC, Dreger P, Goldstone AH, Boogaerts MA, Ferrant A, *et al.*** (1996). Randomised trial of filgrastim-mobilised peripheral blood progenitor cell transplantation versus autologous bone-marrow transplantation in lymphoma patients. *The Lancet*, 10, 353–357.
- **Shpall EJ, Wheeler CA, Turner SA, Yanovich S, Brown RA, Pecora AL, *et al.*** (1999). A randomized phase 3 study of peripheral blood progenitor cell mobilization with stem cell factor and filgrastim in high-risk breast cancer patients. *Blood*, 93, 2491–2501.
- **Sheridan WP, Begley CG, Juttner CA, Szer J, To LB, Maher D, *et al.*** (1992). Effect of peripheral-blood progenitor cells mobilised by filgrastim (G-CSF) on platelet recovery after high-dose chemotherapy. *The Lancet*, 339, 640–644.
- **Sheridan W, Foote MA.** (1998). Thrombopoietic growth factors. *Emerging Drugs*, 3:261–269.
- **Siena S, Nicola M, Mortorini R, Anichini A, Bregni M, Parmiani G, Gianni AM.** (1997). Expansion of immunostimulatory dendritic cells from peripheral blood of patients with cancer. *The Oncologist*, 2, 65–69.
- **Souza LM, Boone TC, Gabrilove J, Lai P, Zsebo KM, Murdock DC, *et al.*** (1986). Recombinant human granulocyte colony-stimulating factor: effects on normal and leukemic myeloid cells. *Science*, 232, 61–65.
- **Stahel RA, Jost LM, Cerny T, Pichert G, Honegger H, Tobler A, *et al.*** (1994). Randomized study of recombinant human granulocyte colony-stimulating factor after high-dose chemotherapy and autologous bone marrow transplantation for high-risk lymphoid malignancies. *Journal of Clinical Oncology*, 12, 1931–1938.
- **Stanley E, Lieschke GJ, Grail D, Metcalf D, Hodgson G, Gail JAM, *et al.*** (1994). Granulocyte/macrophage colony-stimulating factor-deficient mice show no perturbation of hematopoiesis but develop a characteristic pulmonary pathology. *Proceedings of the National Academy of Sciences, United States of America*, 91, 5592–5596.
- **Steward WP, von Pawel J, Gatzemeier U, Woll P, Thatcher N, Koschel G, *et al.*** (1998). Effects of granulocyte-macrophage colony-stimulating factor and dose intensification of VOICE chemotherapy in small-cell lung cancer: a prospective randomized study of 300 patients. *Journal of Clinical Oncology*, 16, 642–650.
- **Stone RM, Berg DT, George SL, Dodge RK, Paciucci PA, Schulman P, *et al.*** (1995). Granulocyte-macrophage colony-stimulating factor after initial chemotherapy for elderly patients with primary acute myelogenous leukemia. *New England Journal of Medicine*, 332, 1671–1677.
- **Tepler I, Elias L, Smith JW, Hussein M, Rosen G, Chang AY, *et al.*** (1996). A randomized placebo-controlled trial of recombinant human interleukin-11 in cancer patients with severe thrombocytopenia due to chemotherapy. *Blood*, 87, 3607–3614.
- **Trillet-Lenoir V, Green J, Manegold C, Von Pawel J, Gatzemeier U, Lebeau B, *et al.*** (1993). Recombinant granulocyte colony stimulating factor reduces infectious complications of cytotoxic chemotherapy. *European Journal of Cancer*, 29A, 319–324.
- **Vanderwouw PA, van Leeuwen R, van Oers RHJ, *et al.*** (1991). Effects of recombinant human granulocyte colony-stimulating factor on leucopenia in zidovudine-treated patients with AIDS and AIDS-related complex: a phase I/II study. *British Journal of Haematology*, 78, 319–324.
- **Veys N, Vanholder, R, Lameire N.** (1992). Pain at the injection site of subcutaneously administered erythropoietin in maintenance hemodialysis patients: a comparison of two brands of erythropoietin. *American Journal of Nephrology*, 12, 68–72.
- **Vincent-Gattis M, Webb C, Foote MA.** (1999). Clinical research strategies in biotechnology. In *Biotechnology Annual Review*, edited by MR El-Gewely, Elsevier Science, The Netherlands, pp. 259–267.
- **Weaver C, Schulman K, Wilson-Relyea B, Birch R, West W, Buchner CD.** (2000). Randomized trial of filgrastim, sargramostim, or sequential sargramostim and filgrastim after myelosuppressive chemotherapy for the harvesting of peripheral-blood stem cells. *Journal of Clinical Oncology*, 18, 43–53.
- **Weisbart RH, Golde DW.** (1989). Physiology of granulocyte and macrophage colony-stimulating factors in host defense. *Hematology and Oncology Clinics of North America*, 3, 401–409.
- **Welch W, Foote MA.** (1999). The use of filgrastim in AIDS-related neutropenia. *Journal of Hematotherapy & Stem Cell Research*, 8, S9–S16.
- **Welte K, Gabrilove J, Bronchud MJ, Platzer E, Morstyn G.** (1996). Filgrastim (r-metHuG-CSF): The first 10 years. *Blood*, 88, 1907–1929.
- **Winter JN, Lazarus HM, Rademaker A, Villa M, Mangan C, Tallman M, *et al.*** (1996). Phase I/II study of combined granulocyte colony-stimulating factor and granulocyte-macrophage colony-stimulating factor administration for the mobilization of hematopoietic progenitor cells. *Journal of Clinical Oncology*, 14, 277–286.

Self-Assessment Questions

Question 1: *What do hematopoietic factors do?*

Question 2: *What are the major lineages or types of mature blood cells?*

Question 3: *Generally, chemically describe the hematopoietic growth factors.*

Question 4: *How do hematopoietic growth factors function?*

Question 5: *Define the difference between multilineage growth factors and lineage-specific growth factors.*

Question 6: *What are the in vivo actions of rhG-CSF and rhGM-CSF in patients with advanced cancer?*

Question 7: *What is the physiologic role of EPO?*

Question 8: *What are the currently commercially available hematopoietic growth factors?*

Question 9: *What are the indications for rhG-CSF?*

Question 10: *What are the indications for rhGM-CSF?*

Question 11: *What are the indications for rhEPO?*

Question 12: *What are the indications for rhSCF?*

Question 13: *What are the indications for rhIL-11?*

Answers

Answer 1: Hematopoietic growth factors regulate both hematopoiesis and the functional activity of blood cells (including proliferation, differentiation, and maturation). Some hematopoietic growth factors mobilize progenitor cells to move from the bone marrow to the peripheral blood.

Answer 2: The myeloid pathway gives rise to red blood cells (erythrocytes), platelets, monocytes/macrophages, and granulocytes (neutrophils, eosinophils, and basophils). The lymphoid pathway gives rise to lymphocytes.

Answer 3: They are glycoproteins, which can be distinguished by their amino acid sequence and glycosylation (carbohydrate linkages). Hematopoietic growth factors have folding patterns that are dictated by physical interactions and covalent cysteine-cysteine disulfide bridges. Correct folding is necessary for biologic activity. Most hematopoietic growth factors are single-chain polypeptides weighing approximately 14 to 35 kDa. The carbohydrate content varies depending on the growth factor and production method, which in turn affects the molecular weight but not necessarily the biologic activity.

Answer 4: Hematopoietic growth factors act by binding to specific cell surface receptors. The resultant complex sends a signal to the cell to express genes, which in turn induce cellular proliferation, differentiation, or activation. A hematopoietic growth factor may also act indirectly if the cell expresses a gene that causes the production of a different hematopoietic growth factor or another cytokine, which in turn binds to and stimulates a different cell.

Answer 5: Multilineage growth factors (e.g. GM-CSF, IL-3, and SCF) affect multiple cell lineages and tend to act on early progenitor cells before they become committed to one lineage. Lineage-specific growth factors (e.g. G-CSF, M-CSF, EPO, and presumably thrombopoietin) predominantly affect one cell type and act later in the hematopoietic cascade.

Answer 6: Both growth factors cause a transient leukopenia that is followed by a dose-dependent increase in the number of circulating mature and immature neutrophils. Both growth factors enhance the *in vitro* function of neutrophils obtained from treated patients. rhGM-CSF, but not rhG-CSF, also increases the number of circulating monocytes/macrophages and eosinophils, as well as *in vitro* monocyte cytotoxicity and cytokine production.

Answer 7: EPO maintains a normal red blood cell count by causing committed erythroid progenitor cells to proliferate and differentiate into normoblasts. EPO also shifts marrow reticulocytes into circulation.

Answer 8: Five hematopoietic growth factors are commercially available, rhG-CSF (filgrastim and lenograstim), rhGM-CSF (molgramostim and sargramostim), rhEPO (Epoetin or epoetinum alpha, epoetin beta), rhSCF (ancestim), and rhIL-11 (oprelvekin).

Answer 9: Approval for marketing varies by country and not all countries have all labeled uses. rhG-CSF is indicated for neutropenia associated with myelosuppressive cancer chemotherapy, bone marrow transplantation, and severe chronic neutropenia; rhG-CSF is also indicated to mobilize peripheral blood progenitor cells (PBPC) for PBPC transplantation; rhG-CSF is indicated for the reversal of clinically significant neutropenia and subsequent maintenance or adequate neutrophil counts in patients with HIV infection during treatment with antiviral and/or other myelosuppressive medications.

Answer 10: rhGM-CSF is indicated for neutropenia associated with bone marrow transplantation and antiviral therapy for AIDS-related cytomegalovirus. rhGM-CSF is also indicated for failed bone marrow transplantation or delayed engraftment, and for use in mobilization and after transplantation of autologous PBPCs.

Answer 11: rhEPO is indicated to treat anemia associated with chronic renal failure, zidovudine-induced anemia in HIV-infected patients, and chemotherapy-induced anemia. rhEPO is also indicated to reduce allogeneic blood transfusions and hasten erythroid recovery in surgery patients.

Answer 12: rhSCF is used in combination with filgrastim to increase PBPC yield in hard-to-mobilize patients.

Answer 13: rhIL-11 is indicated to prevent thrombocytopenia and to reduce the need for platelet transfusions in patients with cancer receiving chemotherapy.

9 Interferons and Interleukins

Joseph Tami

Cytokine Introduction

Cytokines can generally be defined as soluble mediators or glycoproteins that aid in the communication between cells, primarily cells of the immunological, hematological, and neurological systems. Interleukins and interferons are groups of naturally occurring glycoproteins that belong to the overall category of cytokines. There are at least 60 different types of cytokines.

During the 1970s researchers began identifying molecules other than antibodies which were produced by the cells of the immune system. These molecules were involved in the communication network of the immune system. The released cytokines were found to bind to their target cells via specific receptors found on the cell surface. Many cytokines are produced during the effector phases of immunity or host defense.

Cytokines are not the same as hormones. Cytokines can be distinguished from hormones by various criteria. An individual cytokine can be secreted by a number of different types of cells while hormones are typically produced by just one or two very specialized cell types. Cytokines can also act on a variety of cell types. While cytokines are usually targeted to produce a local effect, hormones are targeted to affect cells at distant sites. The release of a cytokine is often a brief, self-limited event.

The soluble mediators classified as cytokines are made up of a wide array of glycoproteins including interleukins, interferons, colony stimulating factors (hematopoietic growth factors), chemokines, inflammatory cytokines, and anti-inflammatory factors. The classification of cytokines can be broken down into a number of sub-categories. For example, cytokines can be classified by their source. Lymphokines are produced by lymphocytes, primarily from T cells but also from B cells. Monokines are cytokines that are secreted from mononuclear cells.

Many of the cytokines are also grouped according to functional definitions. The term interleukin comes from inter-leukocyte, or a cytokine which communicates between white blood cells. The term interferon originally came from the ability of the cytokine to interfere with the viral infection of a cell.

In recent years it has been discovered that particular cells can be classified based on the typical types of cytokines that are produced by these cells. For example, CD4+ T cells are mainly cytokine-secreting helper cells, while CD8+ T cells are mainly cytotoxic killer cells. The CD4+ T cells can be further divided into Type 1 helper (TH1) T cells, and Type 2 helper (TH2) T cells, based upon their cytokine production pattern. TH1 cells typically secrete interleukin 2 and interferon gamma, but not interleukins 4, 5, or 6. TH2 helper T cells secrete interleukins 4, 5, 6, and 10, but not IL-2 or interferon gamma. In humans, this classification of TH1 and TH2 is not exclusive, but it can be used as a general rule of thumb (cf. Chapter 12).

A complete bibliography can be found at the conclusion of this Chapter.

The Interleukins

Terminology

Interleukins are often designated as IL-(number). The World Health Organization-International Union of Immunologic Societies (WHO-IUIS) gives official nomenclature status to the interleukins. At the present time, 18 different interleukins have been described, although not all these have been given official nomenclature status. Findings from the human genome project suggest that additional interleukin genes may be present. The IUIS recommendations for a molecule to be classified as an interleukin can be summarized in four guidelines:

1. The molecule must be purified, molecularly cloned, and expressed. It should be distinct from any previously described interleukin or other molecule.
2. The molecule must be a natural product of a cell of the immune system.
3. The molecule should not be part of a family of compounds that have a major function outside the immune system.
4. The molecule cannot be more suitably described by a descriptive designation.

A general description of the naturally occurring interleukins follows in the sections below. In general, once a unique interleukin has been identified, the protein sequence is determined in an attempt to further identify the gene encoding the protein. After the genetic sequence has been determined, recombinant DNA techniques are used to produce large quantities of the interleukin. This allows for the production of adequate supplies for basic and clinical studies. While many of the interleukins are in clinical studies, only two of the interleukins are currently approved by the FDA and commercially available for clinical use in the United States. These products are aldesleukin (rIL-2) and oprelvekin (rIL-11). Table 9.1 provides a list of interleukins that have been discovered to date.

Overview of the Interleukins

Interleukin 1

Interleukin 1 has been described by a variety of different names: lymphocyte activating factor (LAF), endogenous pyrogen, T cell replacing factor II, and B cell differentiation factor, as well as by several others. It can thus be deduced that IL-1 exhibits a large variety of activities.

Interleukin 1 represents at least two distinct polypeptides (IL-1 alfa and IL-1 beta). The molecular weights of the polypeptides are approximately 17 kDa. Differences in

Interleukin	MW (kDa)	Primary Cell Structure	Primary Activities	Commercial Product
IL-1α/IL-1β	17	macrophages, NK cells, B cells	Inflammation	
IL-2	15.5	T cells	Activates T cells	Aldesleukin
IL-3	28	T cells	Hematopoietic growth factor	
IL-4	20	T cells	B cell growth	
IL-5	50–60	T cells	Eosinophil and B cell growth	
IL-6	25	T cells and fibroflasts	Inflammation	
IL-7	25	stromal cells	B and T cell growth	
IL-8	8	macrophages	Chemoatracctant for neutrophils	
IL-9	30–40	activated T cells	T cell and erythroid growth	
IL-10	18	B cells, T cells	B cell growth/Inhibition of cytokine synthesis by T cells	
IL-11	23	bone marrow stromal cells	Hematopoietic co-factor	Oprelvekin
IL-12	70	macrophages, B cells	Induction of cell-mediated immunity	
IL-13	10	T cells	B cell growth	
IL-14				
IL-15	14	epithelial cells	T cell and NK cell growth	
IL-16	17	CD8+ T cells	CD4+ T cell chemoattractant	
IL-17		CD4+ T cells	Firoblast stimulation	
IL-18			Cell-mediated immunity, IFN gamma inducing activity	

Table 9.1. Interleukins

glycosylation are responsible for the wide variation of reported molecular weights. IL-1 alfa and IL-1 beta are encoded by two distinct genes. IL-1 alfa and IL-1 beta are synthesized as propeptides of approximately 30 kDa, and are then cleaved to produce products of 159 and 153 amino acids, respectively.

Both forms of IL-1 exert their effects by binding to two distinct types of IL-1 receptors. The first is IL-1 receptor type I which belongs to the immunoglobulin superfamily of receptors. The second IL-1 receptor is denoted type II and also belongs to the immunoglobulin superfamily. The two different forms of the IL-1 receptors bind IL-1 alfa and IL-1 beta with different affinities.

IL-1 has been associated with numerous activities. Some of these include:

1. Induction of the IL-2 receptor;
2. Stimulation of pre-B cell differentiation;
3. Augmentation of NK-cell cytotoxicity;
4. Induction of adhesion molecules on endothelial cells;
5. Induction of fever;
6. Stimulation of thymocyte proliferation;
7. Enhancement of collagen production, and;
8. Stimulation of the release of other cytokines involved in hematopoiesis.

Overall, it is believed that IL-1 is an important mediator of the body's response to infection, inflammation, and injury. IL-1 is released as part of the acute phase reaction of hepatocytes. The primary producers of IL-1 in the immune system are macrophages, B cells and neutrophils. Potential clinical uses of IL-1 are as a radioprotective agent due to its stimulatory effects on hematopoiesis, and its ability to accelerate wound healing.

A naturally occurring inhibitor of IL-1 has been cloned. This molecule is termed the IL-1 receptor antagonist, or IL-1ra. While it has limited sequence similarity to either IL-1 alfa or IL-1 beta, it does have the ability to bind to the IL-1 receptors. Lacking IL-1 activity, IL-1ra acts as a useful blocker of the receptor. A recombinant version of IL-1ra was investigated for its potential use in sepsis; however, the clinical trials were inconclusive as to the efficacy of the product in this setting. Recombinant IL-1ra has been used successfully in investigational studies for the treatment of rheumatoid arthritis. While not currently approved for human use by the FDA, there is a possibility that patients with rheumatoid arthritis will have this agent to select as an additional choice of immune modulating products in the future. An application for approval has been submitted to the FDA for use in patients with rheumatoid arthritis.

Interleukin 2

Interleukin 2 (IL-2) was originally described as T cell growth factor (TCGF). IL-2 is synthesized and secreted primarily by T cells. It has direct effects on a number of immunological cells. IL-2 can stimulate the growth, differentiation and activation of T cells, B cells, and NK cells. Aldesleukin, a recombinant form of interleukin 2, has been approved by the FDA for use in patients with renal cell carcinoma and metastatic melanoma.

IL-2 produces its immunological effects by binding to the cellular IL-2 receptor (IL-2R). There are various affinity forms of the IL-2R. Three chains are believed to comprise the cellular high affinity IL-2 receptor – the α, β and γ chains. A circulating form (also known as the soluble form) of the IL-2R has also been found in human serum. This circulating receptor is capable of binding IL-2. The circulating form of the IL-2R is a truncated version of the α chain, having no cytoplasmic tail. High levels of the circulating IL-2R have been found in patients with a wide variety of disorders, including HIV infection, cancer, solid organ transplant rejection, and arthritis. It is believed that the circulating form of the IL-2R binds released IL-2 prior to IL-2 binding to cells in an attempt to prevent overstimulation of the immune system. Several other cytokine and adhesion molecule receptors also have circulating forms. It is believed that this is one manner in which the immunological cascade maintains a checks and balance system.

Interleukin 3

IL-3 is a hematopoietic growth factor. The principle effects of IL-3 are on early hematopoietic progenitors in which IL-3 induces hematopoiesis and cell differentiation. Administration of IL-3 produces an increase in erythrocytes, neutrophils, eosinophils, monocytes and platelets. IL-3 can act synergistically or additively with other hematopoietic growth factors. IL-3 is believed to act early on in the hematological cascade.

Interleukin 4

Interleukin 4 is primarily derived from T cells. Its principle site of action is the B cell. IL-4 stimulates B cell proliferation and activation. It induces IgE and IgG1 expression from B cells, as well as class II Major Histocompatibility Complex (MHC) expression. In addition to its effects on B cells, IL-4 induces the differentiation of eosinophils and activity of T cytotoxic cells.

Interleukin 5

Interleukin 5 represents the compounds originally known as T cell replacement factor (TRF), eosinophil differentiation factor (EDF) and B cell growth factor (BCGFII). The primary effect of human IL-5 is on the eosinophilic lineage. It stimulates eosinophil chemotaxis, as well as eosinophil expansion. It also appears to have activity on basophils.

INTERLEUKIN 6

Interleukin 6 (IL-6) is produced by lymphoid and non-lymphoid cells. It exerts a multitude of effects on a wide variety of cells. It acts on T cells and B cells. IL-6 stimulates multilineage hematopoiesis, including the maturation of megakaryocytes. IL-6 was also formerly known as interferon-β2 for its weak antiviral activity.

INTERLEUKIN 7

Interleukin 7 acts primarily on pre-B cells to stimulate their differentiation. It can also stimulate the development of human T cells. Overall, it appears that IL-7 is important in B and T cell development.

INTERLEUKIN 8

IL-8 is a member of a group of glycoproteins known as chemokines. IL-8 is a potent chemoattractant for neutrophils. It also has a wide variety of pro-inflammatory effects, including the stimulation of neutrophil degranulation and the enhancement of neutrophil adherence to endothelial cells.

INTERLEUKIN 9 THROUGH INTERLEUKIN 18

Much more information will be needed in regards to the effects of the other interleukins before we see these interleukins used clinically on a routine basis. IL-9 appears to have effects on red blood cells; IL-10 is unique in that it appears to have immunosuppressive type activities, and; IL-13 is similar to IL-4 in its multiple inhibitory effects on monocytes and macrophages. IL-15 appears to be very similar to IL-2. Both stimulate T cells by binding to unique receptors that share common subunits (γ c chain). IL-17 is derived from helper T cells (CD4+). Its effects on cells include the induction of IL-6 production and IL-6 secretion from fibroblasts, the induction of ICAM-1 surface expression on fibroblasts, and costimulation of T cell proliferation. Recombinant versions of IL-10, IL-11, and IL-12 are currently in clinical trials for diseases such as hepatitis C, rheumatoid arthritis, asthma and Crohn's disease.

Commercially Available Interleukins

ALDESLEUKIN, RECOMBINANT IL-2

Interleukin 2 (IL-2) was originally referred to as T cell growth factor. IL-2 has a variety of immunoregulatory properties. IL-2 is produced primarily by activated T cells. The release of IL-2 results in increased T cell proliferation and differentiation. IL-2 has the ability to induce the activation of natural killer (NK) cells and lymphokine activated killer (LAK) cells. IL-2 can also stimulate the production and activity of B cells. Cells activated by IL-2 release a variety of other cytokines, such as tumor necrosis factor, IL-1, gamma interferon, and granulocyte-macrophage colony stimulating factor. Thus the activities attributed to IL-2 can be mediated by direct (T cell and NK cell stimulation) and indirect (release of secondary cytokines) mechanisms.

Activation of T cells by IL-2 occurs when the IL-2 molecule binds to a specific receptor (IL-2R) on the cell surface. The IL-2 receptor (IL-2R) is displayed on the surface of inactive T cells and B cells. The IL-2R consists of at least three different chains: α (p55), β (p75) and γ. The highest affinity receptor is comprised of all three chains. The IL-2R α chain is also referred to as T cell activating antigen (Tac). A circulating form of the IL-2 receptor (p40) has been described which is derived from the p55 α chain. The circulating or soluble form of the IL-2R is capable of binding IL-2. Therefore, the circulating form of the IL-2R may provide a mechanism for the down regulation of IL-2 effects.

Chemical description of aldesleukin

Recombinant human interleukin 2 (rIL-2), known generically as aldesleukin, is available as Proleukin. The chemical name is des-alanyl-1, serine-125-human interleukin-2. It is produced by a recombinant process involving genetically engineered *Escherichia coli*. Aldesleukin is not glycosylated. The molecule has no N-terminal alanine and has serine substituted for a cysteine at position 125. The molecular weight of the protein is approximately 15.3 kDa. The manufacturing process involves the use of tetracycline during fermentation, however, the presence of the antibiotic is not detectable in the final product.

Pharmacology of aldesleukin

The first approved indication for aldesleukin was in 1992 for the treatment of metastatic renal cell carcinoma, based on reports of objective remissions in some patients. Aldesleukin was also approved in 1998 for the treatment of metastatic melanoma in patients 18 years of age or older. The exact mechanism of action of the antineoplastic effects of aldesleukin is unknown, although the immunomodulatory properties of recombinant IL-2 are believed to be involved. The effects of aldesleukin on cellular immunity include lymphocytosis, eosonophilia and thrombocytopenia. Acitivation of T cells, NK cells and LAK cells are believed to play an important role in the immune-mediated destruction of tumor cells.

Greater than 80% of aldesleukin distributed to the plasma, cleared from the circulation, and presented to the kidney is metabolized to amino acids by the cells lining the proximal convoluted tubules of the kidney. Elimination is primarily from the kidney by glomerular filtration and peritubular extraction.

Pharmaceutical considerations of aldesleukin
Aldesleukin is provided in a 22 mIU vial containing 1.3 mg of drug. It is reconstituted by adding 1.2 mL of sterile water for injection to the vial. The injection of the diluent should be aimed at the side of the vial to prevent foaming and destruction of the protein. The reconstituted concentration is 18 mIU per mL. Undiluted vials should be stored refrigerated at 2–8 °C. As the vials contain no preservative, the solutions should be used within 48 hours.

Administration can be given by either the subcutaneous or intravenous routes. For administration by the intravenous route, the reconstituted solution should be further diluted into 50 mL of a 5% dextrose solution. Bacteriostatic water and 0.9% sodium chloride solutions should not be used for reconstitution because of aggregation.

The approved dosing regimen in metastatic renal cell carcinoma and metastatic melanoma is considered high dose therapy. Intravenous infusion of 600,000 International Units (IU) per kg of body weight is given over 15 minutes. This infusion is administered every eight hours for a total of 14 doses. Following nine days of rest, the schedule is repeated for another 14 doses, thereby fulfilling one course of a maximum of 28 doses. Two cycles constitute a treatment course. Plastic bags are recommended for infusion; in-line filters are not recommended due to the potential for protein adsorption.

Clinical and practice aspects of aldesleukin
The FDA-approved regimen for aldesleukin administration is a high dose regimen in which there is a high likelihood of adverse effects. The capillary leak syndrome often seen with this regimen is due to an increase in capillary permeability. Hypotension and reduced organ perfusion occur in this syndrome, manifested by a variety of clinical signs and toxicities. Dose modification in response to toxicity is accomplished by holding a dose or interrupting a dose. Permanent withdrawal of aldesleukin is required in some instances, such as sustained ventricular tachycardia, renal function impairment requiring dialysis for more than 72 hours, and toxic psychosis lasting more than 48 hours, among others. Due to the potential life threatening toxicities, it has been recommended (USP DI Advisory Panel) that one carefully considers the risk-benefit of aldesleukin therapy using the approved dosing regimen. This regimen causes frequent, often serious, and on occasion fatal toxicity.

Current investigation is examining the use of lower dose regimens of aldesleukin for the treatment of a variety of neoplastic diseases. The relative efficacy of these lower toxicity regimens will need to be carefully examined in comparison to the approved high dose regimen. Investigational use of aldesleukin in HIV infected individuals is also being examined further. One of the unique aspects of treatment of neoplastic diseases with aldesleukin is that significant responses have been seen in some individuals after a single course of therapy. These responses are in contrast to the traditional small molecule antineoplastic agents in which one does not typically see a significant response after several courses of treatment.

IL-2 Conjugated to Diphtheria Toxin

A fusion protein consisting of IL-2 conjugated to a portion of the diphtheria toxin has been approved for use in patients with persistent or recurrent cutaneous T cell lymphoma. This fusion protein is known as denileukin diftitox (Ontak). As T-cell lymphoma cells expresses high affinity IL-2 receptors, denileukin diftitox acts as a 'Trojan horse'. Ontak binds to the surface of the lymphoma cells via the IL-2 receptors and the molecule is then internalized. Once inside, the diphtheria portion of the conjugate kills the tumor cell. This fusion protein has also been used investigationally in T cell-mediated diseases, such as psoriasis.

Oprelvekin, recombinant IL-11
Interleukin eleven (IL-11) is a thrombopoietic growth factor that directly stimulates the proliferation of hematopoietic stem cells and megakaryocyte progenitor cells and induces megakaryocyte maturation, resulting in increased platelet production. IL-11 is a member of a family of human growth factors, which includes human growth hormone, granulocyte colony-stimulating factor (G-CSF), and other growth factors.

Chemical description of oprelvekin
Recombinant human interleukin 11 (rIL-11), known generically as oprelvekin, is available as the product Neumega. Oprelvekin is produced in *Escherichia coli*. The protein has a molecular mass of approximately 19 kDa, and is nonglycosylated. The polypeptide is 177 amino acids in length and differs from the 178 amino acid length of native IL-11 only in lacking the amino-terminal proline residue. This alteration has not resulted in measurable differences in bioactivity either *in vitro* or *in vivo*.

Pharmacology of oprelvekin
Oprelvekin is indicated for the prevention of severe thrombocytopenia. It is also indicated for the reduction of the need for platelet transfusions following myelosuppressive chemotherapy in patients with nonmyeloid malignancies who are at high risk of severe thrombocytopenia. Efficacy was demonstrated in patients who had experienced severe thrombocytopenia following the previous chemotherapy

cycle. Oprelvekin is not indicated following myeloablative chemotherapy. The primary hematopoietic activity of oprelvekin is the stimulation of megakaryocytopoiesis and thrombopoiesis. The mechanism of action of oprelvekin is due to the stimulation and proliferation of both hematopoietic stem cells and megakaryocyte progenitor cells, and the induction of megakaryocyte maturation, thus resulting in increased platelet production. Bone-forming and bone-resorbing cells are also potential targets of IL-11, as these cells express mRNA for the IL-11 receptor.

Based on animal studies, biotransformation of oprelvekin is extensive. Greater than 80% of oprelvekin is distributed to the plasma, cleared from the circulation, and presented to the kidney. The elimination half-life is approximately seven hours. Time to peak concentration is approximately three hours (3.2 ± 2.4 hrs) after a single subcutaneous 50 µg/kg dose. Elimination is primarily from the kidney. The amount of intact drug in the urine is low, indicating that the molecule was largely metabolized before excretion. In subjects with severe renal impairment, clearance was approximately 40% of the value seen in subjects with normal renal function. Pharmacokinetic studies suggest that clearance decreases with age.

Pharmaceutical considerations of oprelvekin

Oprelvekin is a sterile, white, preservative-free, lyophilized powder for subcutaneous injection upon reconstitution. Oprelvekin (5 mg vials) should be reconstituted aseptically with 1.0 mL of sterile water for injection, USP (without preservative). The injection of the diluent should be aimed at the side of the vial to prevent foaming and destruction of the protein. Excessive or vigorous agitation of the vial should be avoided. The reconstituted solution is clear, colorless, isotonic, with a pH of 7.0, and contains 5 mg/mL of oprelvekin. The single-use vial should not be re-entered or reused. Any unused portion should be discarded. Oprelvekin may be used within three hours of reconstitution when stored either at 2–8 °C (36–46 degrees F) or at room temperature up to 25 °C (77 degrees F). Do not freeze or shake the reconstituted solution.

Administration of oprelvekin is by the subcutaneous route. The recommended dose in adults is 50 µg/kg given once daily. Oprelvekin should be administered subcutaneously as a single injection in the abdomen, thigh, or hip (or upper arm if not self-injecting). Based upon a pharmacokinetic study, a dose of 75 to 100 µg/kg in the pediatric population will produce plasma levels consistent with those obtained in adults given 50 µg/kg.

Dosing should be initiated 6 to 24 hours after the completion of chemotherapy. Platelet counts should be monitored periodically to assess the optimal duration of therapy. Dosing should be continued until the post-nadir platelet count is 50,000 cells/µL. In controlled clinical studies, doses were administered in courses of 10 to 21 days. Dosing beyond 21 days per treatment course is not recommended. Treatment should be discontinued at least two days before starting the next planned cycle of chemotherapy.

Clinical and practice aspects of oprelvekin

The safety and efficacy of administration of oprelvekin prior to or concurrently with cytotoxic chemotherapy have not been established. The most common laboratory abnormality reported in patients in clinical trials was a decrease in hemoglobin concentration predominantly as a result of expansion of the plasma volume.

The increase in plasma volume is also associated with a decrease in the serum concentration of albumin and several other proteins (e.g. transferrin and gamma globulins). Patients receiving oprelvekin have commonly experienced mild to moderate fluid retention as indicated by peripheral edema or dyspnea on exertion. The fluid retention is reversible within several days following the discontinuation of oprelvekin. During dosing, fluid balance should be monitored.

A small proportion (1%) of patients in clinical studies developed antibodies to oprelvekin and transient rashes were occasionally observed at the injection site following administration. The presence of these antibodies or injection site reactions have not been correlated with clinical symptoms such as anaphylactoid reactions or a loss of clinical response.

Interferons

Introduction

The name interferon was coined prior to the identification of the actual compounds. The name was given to a substance that interfered with viral replication. There are currently three classes of interferons (IFN): interferon α (or α-interferon), interferon β (or β-interferon), and interferon γ (or γ-interferon). Products in all three classes have been approved for use by the FDA, with the most recent approval being interferon β-1b for use in patients with relapsing-remitting multiple sclerosis. Recombinant DNA versions of all three interferon classes exist.

Interferon α is the designation given to a group of substances that are of similar molecular weight and function. Interferons are produced by a large number of assorted cells. Leukocytes are the primary source of IFN α; IFN β is primarily produced by fibroblasts, and; IFN γ is produced by T lymphocytes. The antiviral actions of IFN are achieved through multiple mechanisms. The release of IFN by virally infected cells can prevent the infection of other cells. Interferon alfa has been approved for a wide variety of uses, including use in patients with genital warts, AIDS related Kaposi's sarcoma, hepatitis B and C, hairy cell leukemia and malignant melanoma. Interferon γ was approved for use in individuals with chronic granulomatous disease, a defect in phagocytic cells. Several interferon products are commercially available (described below).

Interferon α

There are a variety of systemic forms of α interferon commercially available. These can be broken down into recombinant versions of a specific α interferon subtype and purified blends of natural human α interferon. The natural family of human α interferon consists of at least 14 different subtypes. The recombinant cloning of a single α interferon gene allows for the production of one of the specific subtypes. The recombinant commercial versions of the subtypes include interferon α-2a and interferon α-2b, as well as a recombinant consensus α interferon (interferon αcon-1). The available purified mixture is interferon α-n3, which is manufactured from pooled units of human leukocytes that have been induced to release interferon by incomplete infection with the avian Sendai virus. Immunoaffinity chromatography with monoclonal antibodies is used to purify the released interferon. Another version of natural α interferons (interferon α-n1, lns) is not commercially available in the US. It is a mixture of natural α interferons, but in different proportions from that in human leukocyte interferon.

The different forms of interferon alfa are approved for a variety of different uses. The basic use of interferon α is the upregulation of the immune system, whether that is in the stimulation of immunological cells to fight cancer or to fight off viral infections such as hepatitis or genital warts. Accepted indications for the use of interferon α include use in hairy cell leukemia; intralesional treatment of condylomata acuminata (genital warts); active, chronic hepatitis C; AIDS-associated Kaposi's sarcoma; treatment (intravesically) of bladder carcinoma; cervical carcinoma therapy; renal cell carcinoma, chronic myelocytic leukemia; laryngeal papillomatosis; non-Hodgkin's lymphoma; malignant melanoma; multiple myeloma, and; mycosis fungoides. The various forms of the interferon α are FDA approved for different indications. It should be noted that while the efficacy of all α interferons for the various indications appears to be similar, there may be differences in the relative efficacy of a specific form for a particular indication. Very few comparative clinical studies exist to provide within-study efficacy data between one form of α interferon and another in a specific indication.

CHEMICAL DESCRIPTION OF INTERFERON α PRODUCTS

Recombinant interferon α-2a (Rofereron-A) is a version of interferon consisting of a protein chain of 165 amino acids. It is produced by genetically engineered *Escherichia coli*. It is, therefore, a non-glycosylated protein. The molecule has a lysine group at position 23. The purification process includes affinity chromatography with the use of murine monoclonal antibodies specific for the interferon. The final product contains a single α interferon subtype.

Interferon alfa-2a injection *(Roferon-A)*	Interferon alfa-2b *(Intron A)*	Interferon alfacon-1 *(Infergen)*
3 mU/mL (1 mL vials)*	3 mU vials (1 mL diluent)**	9 mcg per 0.3 mL*
6 mU/mL (3 mL vials, 18 mU vial)*	5 mU vials**	15 mcg per 0.5 mL*
10 mU/mL (0.9 mL, for Kaposi's sarcoma)*	10 mU vials (1 mL diluent for condylomata acuminata)**	
36 mU/mL (1 mL vials for Kaposi's sarcoma)*	18 mU vials (1 mL diluent for 18 mU/mL for malignant melanoma)**	
	25 mU vials (5 mLs diluent for 5 mU/ml)**	
18 mU vials** (3 mLs diluent)	50 mU vials (1 mL diluent for Kaposi's sarcoma)**	

* Liquid for injection
** Prepared for injection by addition of diluent

mcg = μg

Table 9.2. Recombinant interferon alfa dosage forms in the U.S.

Recombinant interferon α-2b (Intron A) is also a version of interferon α consisting of 165 amino acids. It is produced by genetically engineered *Escherichia coli*. It is, therefore, a non-glycosylated protein. It has an arginine group at position 23. The purification of the molecule is done by proprietary methods. The final product contains a single α interferon subtype.

Recombinant interferon alfacon-1 (Infergen) is a synthetic version of interferon α consisting of 166 amino acids, genetically engineered in *Escherichia coli*. The amino acid sequence of the product is derived by comparison of the sequences of several natural interferon α subtypes and assigning the most frequently observed amino acid in each corresponding position. Interferon αcon-1 shares 88% homology with interferon α-2, and is 30% identical to interferon beta. The manufacturing purification procedure includes sequential passages over a series of chromatography columns. Interferon αcon-1 was approved for use in 1997 for the treatment of chronic hepatitis C infection.

Interferon α-n3 (Alferon-N) is not a recombinant protein, but is a highly purified mixture of up to 14 natural human α subtypes. It consists of protein chains of approximately 166 amino acids. Sendai virus is used to infect pooled human white blood cells to produce the different subtypes of interferon α. The manufacturing process includes purification via immunoaffinity chromatography with a murine monoclonal antibody, acidification at a pH of 2 for five days at 4 °C, and gel filtration chromatography.

Interferon α-n1 (Wellferon) is not commercially available in the United States. It is a purified blend of natural human α interferons obtained from human lymphoblastoid cells following induction with Sendai virus.

Pegylated (PEG) versions of interferon α-2a and 2b are currently in investigational clinical trials for diseases such as hepatitis B and C. The addition of polyethylene glycol molecules to standard interferon α-2a results in substantial changes to the metabolism of the drug with a prolongation of the half-life. Dosing is performed once weekly. Studies comparing the activity of peginterferon α-2a versus interferon α-2a in patients with chronic hepatitis C, as well as in patients with chronic hepatitis C with cirrhosis or bridging fibrosis, have demonstrated greater efficacy with peginterferon. Combination treatment with ribavirin and peginterferon α-2a is under study. The approval of peginterferon α-2a is pending in the United States.

Pharmacology of interferon α products

α interferons have antiviral, antiproliferative, and immunomodulatory activities. Some of these activities are due to indirect effects. Most of the activities of α interferon are incompletely understood. Alterations in synthesis of RNA, DNA and proteins can be demonstrated after exposure to α interferon. These alteraftions are believed to be the mechanism of action for the antiproliferative and antiviral activities of the α interferons currently available.

Since these are proteins, they are, as yet, not delivered by the oral route due to destruction by the gastric acidity. Thus, the route for administration of the α interferons is typically intramuscular, subcutaneous, intralesional or intravesicular. Absorption from intramuscular and subcutaneous injection sites is typically greater than 80%. Although intralesional injections (genital warts) result in plasma concentrations, which are below detectable levels, systemic effects have been reported.

Subcutaneous injections, as compared to intramuscular injections, may result in a more delayed time to peak concentration for recombinant interferon α-2a after a single dose. Intramuscular injection peaks in 3.8 hours, while a subcutaneous injection peaks in 7.3 hours. For recombinant interferon α-2b after a single dose, the time to peak concentration for intramuscular or subcutaneous injection ranges from 3 to 12 hours. Plasma concentrations of interferon αcon-1 given by subcutaneous injection cannot be directly detected. However, analysis can detect significant increases of interferon-induced gene products, including 2'5' oligoadenylate synthetase and β-2 microglobulin.

α interferons are totally filtered through the renal glomeruli and undergo degradation during reabsorption in the renal tubules. Elimination occurs as only negligible amounts of unchanged α interferon reappear in the systemic circulation.

In hepatitis the normalization of serum alanine aminotransferase (ALT) concentrations may occur as early as two-weeks after the initiation of the interferon treatment. The time to peak effect in condylomata acuminata occurs in one to two months after the initiation of treatment.

Pharmaceutical considerations of interferon α products

The strengths and dosages of the available interferon α products are expressed in terms of Units. The Units are determined by a comparison of the antiviral activity of the particular interferon manufactured lot with the activity of the international reference preparation of human leukocyte interferon, which is established by the World Health Organization (WHO). As proteins, the various forms of α interferon should not be frozen. Storage should be between 2 and 8 °C. The solutions should not be shaken to prevent foaming and loss of protein.

Clinical and practice aspects of interferon α products

The doses for the different indications of the various α interferon products can vary greatly. For example, the dose for maintenance dosing of interferon α-2a in hairy cell leukemia is 3 million Units three times weekly. This does can be compared to dosing in the maintenance treatment of AIDS-associated Kaposi's sarcoma in which interferon α-2a is dosed at 36 million Units (1 mL) three times per week.

A selection of different strengths and vial volumes is available for the different recombinant products (see Table 9.1). In order to accurately dose, the higher concentration products should not be used to administer the lower doses. For example, the 36 million Unit per mL concentration of interferon α-2a should not be used for a 3 million Unit doses for a patient with hairy cell leukemia.

The interferon αcon-1 product (Infergen) is available as a 9 μg per 0.3 mL vial, as well as a 15 μg per 0.5 mL vial. Dosing in patients with chronic, active hepatitis C is initially 9 μg subcutaneously three times per week, at intervals of at least 48 hrs, for 24 weeks. Patients who relapse or don't respond, and who tolerated the initial dose, may be treated with 15 μg per dose. Dose reductions may be necessary in approximately a third of these patients.

The interferon α-n3 product (Alferon N) is available in the U.S. as a 5 mU/mL vial with a single-labeled indication for intralesional dosing in condylomata acuminata. Dosing is performed with a 30 gauge needle at the base of the wart using 250,000 Units two times a week for up to eight weeks.

It should be noted that the different recombinant products are dosed differently within the same disease. For example, in AIDS-associated Kaposi's sarcoma, interferon α-2a (Roferon-A) is recommended to be dosed via the intramuscular or subcutaneous route at 36 mU per day for 10–12 weeks, or to slowly increase the dose by starting at 3 mU per day on Days one to three, then 9 mU per day on Days four to six, then 18 mU per day on Days seven to nine, followed by 36 mU per day for the remainder of the 10–12 week induction period. This slow increase can help with the flu-like syndrome that is most pronounced during the first week of treatment as it is gradually reduced as a result of tachyphylaxis. In contrast, for the use of interferon α-2b (Intron A) in AIDS-associated Kaposi's sarcoma it is recommended to dose on a square meter regimen, at 30 mU per square meter three times a week. Interferon α-2b has been approved for use in combination with ribavirin (Rebetron) for the treatment of chronic hepatitis C in patients with compensated liver disease previously untreated with α interferon, as well as in patients who have relapsed following α interferon therapy.

Patients should be informed about some of the side-effects of interferon α administration in order to maximize therapy. The flu-like syndrome consists of aching muscles, fevers and chills, headaches, joint pain, back pain, and generalized malaise. This syndrome occurs in a majority of patients within the first week of therapy. Within continued treatment, the patient develops a 'tolerance' or tachyphylactic response to the interferon usually within two to four weeks after the start of therapy. The use of acetaminophen prior to dosing is also recommended, as is continued dosing for the treatment of subsequent fever and chills. If a patient is told to expect this reaction before the start of therapy it is more likely that the patient will continue dosing after the first week.

Other side- or adverse effects from interferon α administration include blurred vision, a change in taste, cold sores, diarrhea, dizziness, dry mouth, loss of appetite, nausea or vomiting, skin rash, and tiredness which can become more prominent with continued dosing and may necessitate a reduction in dosage. It can also be recommended to administer a dose at bedtime to minimize the inconvenience of fatigue. The more common adverse effects, which may require medical attention include anemia, cardiotoxicity such as supraventricular arrhythmia, leukopenia and thrombocytopenia. The incidence of peripheral neuropathy, altered thyroid status and hepatotoxicity is less frequent. Partial loss of hair also occurs, with prompt return of hair growth after withdrawal of interferon α dosing.

Patients will at times develop an antibody response to the administered interferons. Sometimes these antibodies can actually inhibit the activity of the interferon (the formation of neutralizing antibodies). If a patient develops neutralizing antibodies to a particular product, one can switch to another product. Cross-reactive antibodies may be produced to the recombinant products; it has been suggested that it is less likely that antibodies will be produced against the various subtypes found in the pooled interferon α-n3 product. For interferon αcon-1, antibody development has been reported, with the most frequently observed time to first antibody response occurring at week 16 of therapy. It should be noted that the interferon subtypes contained with the α-n3 product are glycosylated proteins. The recombinant versions are non-glycosylated proteins, having been produced by *E. coli*. It is theoretically possible that the recombinant versions are more immunogenic because they lack the sugars bound to the protein. The immune system could produce neutralizing antibodies to sites on the recombinant proteins, which were once covered by carbohydrates on the natural interferon.

Interferon β

Interferon β has been shown to possess both antiviral and immunoregulatory effects. By binding to specific cellular receptors, interferon β exerts its activity. The activities of β interferon are species specific, thus much of what is known about the effects of human β interferon come from *in vitro* studies using human cell lines.

Recombinant interferon β has shown activity in relapsing-remitting multiple sclerosis (MS). Recombinant interferon β-1b (Betaseron) was first to market, followed by recombinant interferon β-1a (Avonex). The exact mechanism of IFN-β activity in the treatment of MS is unknown, however it is presumed to be due to immunomodulatory activity. In a randomized, double-blind, placebo-controlled study recombinant interferon β-1b (Betaseron) was shown to have significant effects on exacerbation rates. There was a 31% reduction in the annual exacerbation rate in patients receiving Betaseron as compared to placebo at the two-year analysis. In the third year of analysis alone the difference between treatment groups was 28%, with a p value of 0.065, potentially due to a lower number of patients. Antibody formation to Betaseron was demonstrated, and 45% of patients were found to have serum-neutralizing activity at one point or more of the time points tested. The relationship between clinical efficacy of the drug and formation of antibody formation are not known.

Chemical description of interferon β-1b

Interferon β-1b is a purified, lyophilized, sterile protein commercially available as Betaseron. Interferon β-1b is produced by genetically engineered *E. coli*. The native gene was obtained from human fibroblasts and was altered in a way that substitutes serine for the cysteine residue found at position 17. Interferon β-1b consists of a protein with a molecular weight of 18.5 kDa, and is non-glycosylated.

Pharmacology of interferon β-1b

Interferon β-1b is indicated for use in ambulatory patients with relapsing-remitting multiple sclerosis to reduce the frequency of clinical exacerbations. Relapsing-remitting multiple sclerosis is characterized by recurrent attacks of neurologic dysfunction followed by complete or incomplete recovery. Interferon β-1b has not been evaluated in chronic progressive multiple sclerosis.

Pharmaceutical considerations of interferon β-1b

Each vial of interferon β-1b contains 0.3 mg (9.6 mIU). The specific activity of the interferon is approximately 32 mIU per mg interferon β-1b. It should be noted that a different analytical standard was used prior to 1993. This standard assigned a value of 54 mIU per 0.3 mg of interferon β-1b. This assessment should be remembered when reviewing articles and research dated prior to 1993 and comparing them to current dosing regimens.

Reconstitution of lyophilized product in vials is accomplished by adding 1.2 mL of the supplied diluent (0.54% sodium chloride solution). Vials should not be shaken. After reconstitution, vials contain 0.25 mg (8 mIU) per ml of solution. Administration is given by the subcutaneous route using a syringe with a 27 gauge needle. Vials are for single use only. Reconstituted product should be used with three hours.

Clinical and practice aspects of interferon β-1b

The recommended dose of interferon β-1b is 0.25 mg (8mIU) injected subcutaneously every other day in patients with relapsing-remitting MS. At this dose, many of the patients will experience the flu-like symptoms seen with other interferons, such as the α interferons. The median time to the first occurrence of flu-like symptoms was three days, although the median duration per patient was 10.4 days per year. Injection site reactions were common (85%) in patients receiving interferon β-1b, including inflammation, pain, hypersensitivity, necrosis and non-specific reactions. The median time to the first occurrence of an injection site reaction was seven days; patients with injection site reactions reported these events 183.7 days per year.

Laboratory tests to follow in these patients include hemoglobin, complete white blood cell count with differential, platelet counts, and blood chemistries with liver function tests. In the clinical trial, patients were monitored every three months. Mental status should also be observed as changes in mental status including confusion, depression, anxiety and depersonalization were observed in the study. One suicide and four attempted suicides were reported. Whether these mental status changes were induced by interferon β-1b or by the underlying neurological disease is unclear.

At this point, long term efficacy of interferon β-1b beyond-two years is unknown. More information needs to be gathered as patients continue on long-term therapy.

Recombinant interferon β-1a

In May of 1996, the FDA approved the use of Avonex, a recombinant human interferon β-1a product. It was approved for use in treating relapsing forms of multiple sclerosis. The approval was based upon the results obtained from a multi-center, placebo-controlled, double-blinded clinical trial. The study demonstrated that over two years the risk of significant progression of physical disability was reduced by 37% in people taking Avonex compared to those on placebo.

A study by Jacobs *et al.* (1996, 2000) has demonstrated that initiating treatment with interferon β-1a at the time of a first demyelinating event is beneficial for patients with brain lesions on MRI that indicate a high risk of clinically definite multiple sclerosis. This study in 383 patients provided evidence that early treatment with interferon β-1a was of benefit to patients, resulting in a reduction of the volume of brain lesions, as well as fewer new or enlarging lesions.

Recombinant interferon β-1a (Avonex) is administered by intramuscular injection once weekly (30 μg), in comparison to recombinant interferon β-1b (Betaseron) which is administered subcutaneously every other day. Recombinant interferon β-1a (Avonex) is provided as lyophilized powder, containing 33 μg (6.6 million International Units) in a vial to be reconstituted with 1.1 mLs of diluent. The solution should be held at 2–8 °C, and should not be frozen.

γ Interferon

Gramma interferon has antiviral, antiproliferative and immunomodulatory activities. The antiviral properties of γ interferon are probably less than that exerted by α interferon. γ interferon has a much more potent effect on phagocytic cells than α or β interferon. γ interferon is naturally produced by T cells which have been stimulated by antigen. It is usually released from T cells in conjunction with the release of IL-2. Natural killer (NK) cells can also secrete γ interferon.

By binding to cell surface receptors, γ interferon induces the activation of resting macrophages and monocytes. The stimulation increases the phagocytic activity of these cells, which is important in fighting off pathogens. One of the methods of killing engulfed pathogens by these cells is the intracellular production of toxic oxygen metabolites. γ interferon enhances the production of these toxic oxygen metabolites.

Antibody dependent cellular cytotoxicity (ADCC) and NK cell activity is increased by γ interferon. Increased expression of major histocompatibility (MHC) antigens is induced by γ interferon. Monocytes increase cell surface expression of immunoglobulin Fc receptors after exposure to γ interferon. The efficiency of macrophage-mediated killing of intracellular parasites is also increased upon exposure to γ interferon. Thus, an overall immunostimulation of phagocytic cells occurs with the release of γ interferon.

Natural γ interferon is a 143 amino acid protein that demonstrates little sequence homology to either the α or β interferons. Two different molecular weights of γ interferon have been described (20 kDa and 25 kDa) which vary in molecular weight due to differences in glycosylation.

Gramma interferon has shown efficacy in the treatment of chronic granulomatous disease (CGD). CGD is an inherited disorder, which is characterized by a deficiency in phagocytic oxidative metabolism. γ interferon increases the phagocytic function of granulocytes, such as neutrophils, and monocytes. After exposure to γ interferon these cells have an increased ability to produce superoxide anion, which helps eliminate phagocytosed pathogens. Early clinical trials in patients with CGD demonstrated the enhancement by γ interferon of phagocytic cell function, including the elevation of superoxide levels and improved killing of *Staphylococcus aureus*.

In a randomized placebo controlled trial in patients with CGD a recombinant version of γ interferon (Actimmune) significantly decreased the incidence of serious infection ($p = 0.0036$). CGD Patients receiving placebo had a significantly higher number of serious infections and longer length of hospitalizations. Placebo patients required three times as many inpatient hospitalization days as compared to those receiving Actimmune.

Chemical Description of interferon γ-1b

One recombinant version of γ interferon (interferon γ-1b) is currently available. Actimmune is a single-chain polypeptide that contains 140 amino acids. Interferon γ-1b is produced by genetically engineered *Escherichia coli*. Purification of the product is performed by column chromatography.

Pharmacology of interferon γ-1b

The accepted indications for interferon γ-1b are for reducing the frequency and severity of serious infections associated with chronic granulomatous disease, as well as for the treatment of osteoporosis. It appears that this product is effective in all genetic types of CGD. In patients with CGD, γ interferon-1b is believed to increase the activities of phagocytic cells.

The fraction of the dose absorbed is more than 89%. Absorption is slow. Time to peak plasma concentration for an intramuscular injection is four hours, while time to peak for a subcutaneous injection is seven hours. Via the subcutaneous route, the peak plasma concentration from a 100 μg per m2 of body surface is 0.6 nanograms per mL.

Pharmaceutical considerations of interferon γ-1b

The drug is available as a sterile clear solution containing 100 μg (3 mU) of interferon γ-1b in 0.5 mL. The vials are single use vials. The vials should not be shaken or frozen. They should be stored in a refrigerator at 2 – 8 °C. Prior to use, the unentered vials should not be left at room temperature for longer than 12 hours total.

Administration of the drug is by the subcutaneous route. The recommended dosage of interferon γ-1b for the treatment of patients with CGD is 50 mcg/m2 (1.5 mU/m2) in those whose body surface area is greater than 0.5 m2. For those patients equal to or less than 0.5 m2, the recommended dose is 1.5 μg/kg/dose. Injections are given three times weekly, typically on Monday, Wednesday and Friday. Because the vials do not contain a preservative they should be used for single use only.

CLINICAL AND PRACTICE ASPECTS OF INTERFERON γ-1B

As with the α interferons, the flu-like syndrome occurs in most patients receiving γ interferon-1b. Severity of the syndrome is dose related, while a decrease in the symptoms may occur with continued treatment. Acetaminophen can be given prior to dosing to reduce the fever, headaches and flu-like symptoms. Medical attention should be sought in patients developing leukopenia and, less frequently, in those patients developing hypotension, neurotoxicity, and thrombocytopenia.

The optimum sites for subcutaneous injection have been described as the right and left deltoids and the anterior portion of the thighs. No development of neutralizing antibodies has been reported in patients receiving γ interferon-1b. ■

References

- **Alderson MR, Tough TW, Zieger SF, Grabstein KH.** (1991). Interleukin-7 induces cytokine scretion and tumorcidal activity by human peripheral blood monocytes. *J Exp Med*; 173, 923–30.
- **Aldesleukin. Systemic. USP DI.** (1999).
- **Anonymous.** (1993). Interferon beta-1b is effective in relasping-remitting multiple sclerosis. I. Clinical results of a multicenter, randomized, double-blind, placebo-controlled trial. The IFNB Multiple Sclerosis Group. *Neurology*, 43, 655–61.
- **Anonymous.** (1995). Interferon beta-1b in the treatment of multiple sclerosis: final outcome of the randomized controlled trial. The IFNB Multiple Sclerosis Group and The University of British Columbia MS/MRI Analysis Group. *Neurology*, 45, 1277–85.
- **Anonymous.** (1998). Randomised double-blind placebo-controlled study of interferon beta-1a in relapsing/remitting multiple sclerosis. PRISMS (Prevention of Relapses and Disability by Interferon beta-1a Subcutaneously in Multiple Sclerosis) Study Group. *Lancet*. 352, 1498–504.
- **Bazan JF, Schall TJ.** (1996). Interleukin-16 or not? Letter. *Nature*, 381:29–30.
- **Bolinger AM, Taebul MA.** (1992). Recombinant interferon gamma for treatment of chronic granulomatous disease and other disorders. *Clin Pharm*, 11, 834–50.
- **Bresnihan B, Alvaro-Gracia JM, Cobby M, Doherty M, Domljan Z, Emery P; Nuki G, Pavelka K, Rau R, Rozman B, Watt I, Williams B, Aitchison R, McCabe D, Musikic P.** (1998). Treatment of rheumatoid arthritis with recombinant human interleukin-1 receptor antagonist. *Arthritis Rheum*. 41, 2196–204.
- **Cetus,** Inc, Proleukin package insert. Emeryville, CA: April 1992.
- **Davis GL, Esteban-Mur R, Rustgi V, Hoefs J, Gordon SC, Trepo C, Shiffman ML, Zeuzem S, Craxi A, Ling M-H, Albrecht J.** (1998). Interferon alfa-2b alone or in combination with ribavirin for the treatment of relapse of chronic hepatitis C. International Hepatitis Interventional Group. *N Engl J Med*. 339, 1493–9.
- **Davey RT jr, Murphy RL, Graziano FM, Boswell SL, Pavia AT, Cancio M, Nadler JP, Chaitt DG, Dewar RL, Sahner DK, Duiege A, Capra WB, Leong W-P, Giedlin MA, Lanr HC, Kahn JO.** (2000). Immunologic and virologic effects of subcutaneous interleukin 2 in combination with antiretroviral therapy: a randomized clinical trial. *JAMA*, 284, 183–9.
- **Dinarello CA, Mier JW.** (1986). Interleukins. *Ann Rev Med*, 37, 173–78.
- **Dinarello CA.** (1985). An update on human interleukin-1: from molecular biology to clinical relevance. *J Clin Immunol*, 5, 287–297.
- **Genentech**, Inc, Actimmune package insert. San Franciso, CA: 1990 December.
- **Gordon MS, McCaskill-Stevens WJ, Battiato LA, Loewy J, Loesch D, Breeden E, Hoffman R, Beach KJ, Kuca B, Kaye J, Sledge GW Jr.** (1996). A phase I trial of recombinant human interleukin-11 (neumega rhIL-11 growth factor) in women with breast cancer receiving chemotherapy. *Blood*, 87, 3615–24.
- **Heathcote EJ, Shiffman ML, Cooksley GE, Graham E, Dusheiko GM, Lee SS, Balart L, Reindollar R, Reddy RK, Wright TL, Lin A, Hoffman J, De Pamphilis J.** (2000). Peginterferon alfa-2a in patients with chronic hepatitis C and cirrhosis. *N Engl J Med*, 343, 1673–80.
- **Interferons**, Alfa. Systemic. USP DI. (1999).
- **Interferon**, Beta, Recombinant, Human. USP DI. (1999).
- **Interferon**, Gamma-1b, Recombinant. Systemic. USP DI. (1999).
- **Interleukin-2**, Recombinant, Human. Systemic. USP DI. (1999).
- **Isaacs C, Robert NJ, Bailey FA, Schuster MW, Overmoyer B, Graham M, Cai B, Beach KJ, Loewy JW, Kaye JA.** (1997). Randomized placebo-controlled study of recombinant human interleukin-11 to prevent chemotherapy-induced thrombocytopenia in patients with breast cancer receiving dose-intensive cyclophosphamide and doxorubicin. *J Clin Oncol*, 15:11, 3368–77.
- **Jacobs LD, Cookfair DL, Rudick RA, Herndon RM, Richert JR, Salazar AM, Fischer JS, Goodkin DE, Granger CV.** (1996). Intramuscular interferon beta-1a for disease progression in relapsing multiple sclerosis. The Multiple Sclerosis Collaborative Research Group (MSCRG). *Ann Neurol*, 39, 285–94.
- **Jacobs LD, Beck RW, Simon JH, Kinkel RP, Brownscheidle CM, Murray TJ, Simonian NA, Slasor PJ, Sandrock AW.** (2000). Intramuscular interferon beta-1a therapy initiated during a first demyelinating event in multiple sclerosis. CHAMPS Study Group. *N Engl J Med*. 343:898–904.
- **Jacobs L, Rudick R, Simon.** (2000). Extended observations on MS patients treated with IM interferon-beta1a (Avonex): implications for modern MS trials and therapeutics. *J Neuroimmunol*. 107: 167–73.
- **Jaffe HS, Sherwin SA.** (1991). Immunomodulators. In: Stites DP, Terr AI, eds. *Basic and clinical immunology*. East Norwalk, Conn: Appleton and Lange.

- **Jiang Y, Genant HK, Watt I, Cobby M, Bresnihan B, Aitchison R, McCabe D.** (2000). A multicenter, double-blind, dose-ranging, randomized, placebo-controlled study of recombinant human interleukin-1 receptor antagonist in patients with rheumatoid arthritis: radiologic progression and correlation of Genant and Larsen scores. *Arthritis Rheum.* 43, 1001–9.
- **Kintzel PE, Calis KA.** (1991). Recombinant interleukin-2: a biological response modifier. *Clin Pharm,* 10, 110–28.
- **Leutwyler K.** (1995). An inside job. IL-12 attacks tumors on two fronts, but can it win the battle. *Sci Am,* 273, 24.
- **Lublin FD, Whitaker JN, Eidelman BH, Miller AE, Arnason BG, Burks JS.** (1996). Management of patients receiving interferon beta-1b for multiple sclerosis: a consensus conference. *Neurology,* 46, 12.
- **Maciaszek JW, Parada NA, Cruikshank WW, Center DM, Kornfeld H, Viglianti GA.** (1997). IL-16 represses HIV-1 promoter activity. *J. Immunol,* 158, 5–8.
- **Male D, Champion B, Cooke A, Owen M.** (1991). *Advanced immunology.* JB Lippincott Co.Philadelphia.
- **McKenzie AN, Culpepper JA, de Waal Malefyt R, Briere F, Punnonen J, Aversa G, Sato A, Dang W, Cocks BG.** (1993). Interleukin 13, a T-cell-derived cytokine that regulates human monocyte and B-cell funtion. *Proc Natl Acad Sci USA,* 90, 3735–9.
- **Minty A, Chalon P, Derocq JM, Dumont X, Guillemot JC, Kaghad M, Labit C, Leplatois P, Liauzun P.** (1993). Interleukin-13 is a new human lymphokine regulating inflammatory and immune responses. *Nature.* 362, 248–50.
- **Neilly LK, Goodin DS, Goodkin DE, Hauser SL.** (1996). Side effect profile of interferon beta-1b in MS: results of an open-label trial. *Neurology,* 46, 552–4.
- **Opal SM, Fisher CJ Jr, Dhainaut JF, Vincent JL, Brase R, Lowry SF, Sadoff JC, Slotman GJ, Levy H, Balk RA, Shelly MP, Pribble JP, LaBrecque JF, Lookabaugh J, Donovan H, Dubin H, Baughman R, Norman J, DeMaria E, Matzel K, Abraham E, Seneff M.** (1997). Confirmatory interleukin-1 receptor antagonist trial in severe sepsis: a phase III, randomized, double-blind, placebo-controlled, multicenter trial. The Interleukin-1 Receptor Antagonist Sepsis Investigator Group. *Crit Care Med.* 25, 1115–24.
- **Opal SM, DePalo VA.** (2000). Anti-inflammatory cytokines. *Chest.* 117, 1162–72.
- **Patchen ML MacVitte TJ, Williams JL, Schwartz GN, Souza LM.** (1991). Administration of interleukin-6 stimulates multilineage hematopoiesis and accelerates recovery from radiation induced hematopoietic depression. *Blood,* 77, 472–80.
- **Paty DW, Li DK**. Interferon beta-1b is effective in relapsing-remitting multiple sclerosis. II. MRI analysis results of a multicenter, randomized, double-blind, placebo-controlled trial. UBC MS/MRI Study Group and the IFNB Multiple Sclerosis Study Group. *Neurology,* 43, 662–7.
- **Platanias LC, Vogelzang NJ.** (1990). Interleukin-1: biology,
- **pathophysiology**, and clinical prospects. *Am J Med,* 89, 621–629.
- **Roche Labs**, Roferon-A package insert. Nutely, NJ: 1990 November.
- **Roitt IM, Brostoff J, Male DK. eds.** (1989). *Immunology.* 2nd ed. St. Louis, Gower Medical Publishing.
- **Rosenberg SA, Lotze MT, Muul LM, Chang AE, Avis FP, Leitman S, Linehan WM, Robertson CN, Lee RE, Rubin JT.** (1987). A progress report on the treatment of 157 patients with advanced cancer using lymphokine-activated killer cells and interleukin-2 or high-dose interleukin-2 alone. *N Eng J Med,* 316, 889–97.
- **Rosenberg SA, Packard BS, Aebersold PM, Solomon D, Topalian SL, Toy ST, Simon P, Lotze MT, Yang JC, Seipp CA.** (1989). Use of tumor-infiltrating lymphocytes and interleukin-2 in the immunotherapy of patients with metastatic melanoma. *N Eng J Med,* 319, 1676–1680.
- **Sechler JM, Malech HL, White CJ, Gallin JI.** (1988). Recombinant human interferon-gamma reconstitutes defective phagocyte fucntion in patients with chronic granulomatous disease of childhood. *Proc Natl Acad Sci USA,* 85, 4874–8.
- **Sher A, Fiorentino D, Caspar P, Pearce E, Mosmann T.** (1991). Production of IL-10 by CD4+ T lymphocytes correlates with down regulation of TH1 cytokine synthesis in helminth infection. *J Immunol,* 147, 2713–16.
- **Sideras P, Noma T, Honjo T.** Structure and function of interleukin 4 and 5. Immunol Rev 1988;102:198–212.
- **Stern AS, Magram J, Presky DH.** (1996). Interleukin-12 an integral cytokine in the immune response. *Life Sci,* 58, 639–54.
- **Stites DP, Terr AI.** (1991). *Basic and clinical immunology.* 7th ed. Norwalk, Connecticut. Appleton and Lange.
- **Tami JA, Parr MD, Thompson JS.** (1986). The immune system. *Am J Hosp Pharm,* 43, 2483–93.
- **Tepler I, Elias L, Smith JW II, Hussein M, Rosen G, Chang AY-C, Moore JO, Gordon MS, Kuca B.** (1996). A randomized placebo-controlled trial of recombinant human interleukin-11 in cancer patients with severe thrombocytopenia due to chemotherapy. *Blood,* 87, 3607–14.
- **Vredenburgh JJ, Hussein A, Fisher D, Hoffman M, Elkordy M, Rubin P, Gilbert C, Kaye JA, Dykstra K, Loewy J, Peters WP.** (1998). A randomized trial of recombinant human interleukin-11 following autologous bone marrow transplantation with peripheral blood progenitor cell support in patients with breast cancer. *Biol Blood Marrow Transplant,* 4, 134–41 Weber JS. (1995). Clinical trials with IL-6. *Ann NY Acad Sci,* 762, 357–8.
- **Weening RS, Leitz GJ, Seger RA.** (1995). Recombinant human interferon-gamma in patients with chronic granulomatous disease – European follow up study. *Eur J Pediatr,* 154, 295–8.
- **WHO-ISUI Nomenclature Subcommittee on Interleukin Designation.** (1992). Nomenclature for secreted regulatory proteins of the immune system (interleukins). *Blood;* 79, 1645–1646.
- **Wong GC, Clark SC.** (1991). Multiple actions of IL-6 within a cytokine network. *Immunol Today;* 9, 137–143.
- **Yao Z, Painter SL, Fanskow WC, Ulrich D, Macduff BM, Spriggs MK, Armitage RJ.** (1995). Human IL-17: A novel cytokine derived from T cells. *J. Immunol,* 155, 5483–5486.
- **Zeuzem S, Feinman V, Rasenack J, Heathcote EJ, Lai M-Y, Gane E, O'Grady J, Reichen J, Diago M, Lin A, Hoffman J, Brunda MJ.** (2000). Peginterferon alfa-2a in patients with chronic hepatitis C. *N Engl J Med.* 343, 1666–72.

Self-Assessment Questions

Question 1: *What are cytokines?*
Question 2: *How do cytokines differ from hormones?*
Question 3: *What is a lymphokine?*
Question 4: *How many interleukins are approved for therapy in the U.S.?*
Question 5: *What is the physiological role of IL-1?*
Question 6: *What is IL-2R?*
Question 7: *How is IL-10 unique from the other ILs?*
Question 8: *How should undiluted vials of aldesleukin be stored?*
Question 9: *Where are interferons produced?*
Question 10: *What are the accepted indications for interferon α?*
Question 11: *What are the available forms of interferon α?*
Question 12: *What is/are the approved indication(s) of interferon β?*

Answers

Answer 1 Cytokines can generally be defined as soluble mediators or glycoproteins that aid in the communication between cells, primarily cells of the immunological, hematological, and neurological systems.

Answer 2 Cytokines can be distinguished from hormones by various criteria. An individual cytokine can be secreted by a number of different types of cells, while hormones are typically produced by just one or two very specialized cell types. Cytokines also can act on a variety of cell types. While cytokines are usually targeted to produce a local effect, hormones are targeted to affect cells at distant sites.

Answer 3 Lymphokines are cytokines produced by lymphocytes, primarily from T cells but also from B cells.

Answer 4 Aldesleukin (IL-2) and oprelvekin (rIL-11) are the only FDA-approved ILs that are commercially available in the U.S. However, a fusion protein consisting of IL-2 conjugated to a portion of the diphtheria toxin (denileukin diftitox) has also been approved for use in patients with persistent or recurrent cutaneous T cell lymphoma.

Answer 5 IL-l is an important mediator of the body's response to infection, inflammation, and injury.

Answer 6 IL-2 produces its immunological effects by binding to the cellular IL-2 receptor (IL-2R). There are various affinity forms of the IL-2R. The circulating form of the IL-2R is a truncated version of the α chain, having no cytoplasmic tail. High levels of the circulating IL-2R have been found in patients with a wide variety of disorders, including HIV infection, cancer, solid organ transplant rejection and arthritis. It is believed that the circulating form of the IL-2R binds release IL-2 prior to IL-2 binding to cells in an attempt to prevent overstimulation of the immune system. Several other cytokine and adhesion molecule receptors also have circulating forms. It is believed that this is one manner in which the immunological cascade maintains a checks and balance system.

Answer 7 IL-l0 is unique in that it appears to have immunosuppressive type activities.

Answer 8 Stored refrigerated at 2–8 °C.

Answer 9 Interferons are produced by a large number of assorted cells. Leukocytes are the primary source of IFN α, IFN β is primarily produced by fibroblasts, and IFN γ is produced by T lymphocytes.

Answer 10 Accepted indications for the use of interferon α include use in hairy cell leukemia; intralesional treatment of condylomata acuminata (genital warts); active, chronic hepatitis C; AIDS-associated Kaposi's sarcoma; treatment (intravesically) of bladder carcinoma; cervical carcinoma therapy; renal cell carcinoma, chronic myelocytic leukemia; laryngeal papillomatosis; non-Hodgkin's lymphoma; malignant melanoma; multiple myeloma; and mycosis fungoides.

Answer 11 Recombinant interferon α-2a, recombinant interferon α-2b, recombinant interferon αcon-1, and the non-recombinant products interferon α-n3 and interferon α-n1.

Answer 12 Recombinant interferon β has shown activity in relapsing-remitting multiple sclerosis.

10 Insulin

John M. Beals, Mark L. Brader, Michael R. DeFelippis, and Paul M. Kovach

Introduction

Insulin was discovered by Banting and Best in 1921 (Bliss, 1982). Soon afterward, manufacturing processes were developed to extract the insulin from porcine and bovine pancreas. From 1921 to 1980, efforts were directed at both increasing the purity of the insulin and providing different formulations for altering time-action for improved glucose control (Brange, 1987a; Brange, 1987b; Galloway, 1988). Purification was improved by optimizing the extraction and processing conditions and by implementing chromatographic processes (size exclusion, ion exchange, and reversed phase (Kroeff *et al.*, 1989)) to reduce the levels of both general protein impurities and insulin-related proteins, such as proinsulin and insulin polymers. Formulation development focused on improving the chemical stability by moving from acidic to neutral formulations and by modifying the time-action profile through the use of various levels of zinc and protamine. The evolution of recombinant DNA technology led to the unlimited availability of human insulin, which has eliminated issues with sourcing constraints while providing the patient with a natural exogenous source of insulin. Combining the improved purification methodologies and recombinant DNA technology, manufacturers of insulin are now able to provide the purest human insulin ever made, > 98%.

Chemical Description

Insulin, a 51-amino acid protein, is a hormone that is synthesized as a proinsulin precursor in the β-cell of the pancreas and is converted to insulin by enzymatic cleavage. The resulting insulin molecule is composed of two polypeptide chains that are connected by two inter-chain disulfide bonds (Figure 10.1) (Baker *et al.*, 1988). The A-chain is composed of 21 amino acids and the B-chain is composed of 30 amino acids. The inter-chain disulfide linkages occur between A^7–B^7 and A^{20}–B^{19}, respectively. A third intra-chain disulfide bond is located in the A-chain, between residues A^6 and A^{11}.

Bovine and porcine insulin preparations are also commercially available (Figure 10.1); however, the long-term availability of these products is uncertain. This uncertainty stems from sourcing issues. The amino acid sequence of porcine insulin differs from human insulin at the B^{30} position, where the Thr^{B30}→Ala^{B30}. The amino acid sequence of bovine insulin differs from human insulin at three positions, Thr^{A8}→Ala^{A8}, Ile^{A10}→Val^{A10}, and Thr^{B30}→Ala^{B30}.

The net charge on the insulin molecule results from the four glutamic acid residues, four tyrosine residues, two α-carboxyl groups, two α-amino groups, two histidine residues, a lysine, and an arginine residue. Insulin has an isoelectric point (pI) of 5.3 in the denatured state; thus, the insulin molecule is negatively charged at neutral pH (Kaarsholm *et al.*, 1990). This net negative charge-state of insulin has been used in formulation development, as will be discussed later.

In addition to the net charge, another important intrinsic property of insulin is its ability to readily associate into dimers and higher-order aggregates (Figure 10.2) (Pekar *et al.*, 1972). The driving force for dimerization appears to be the formation of favorable hydrophobic interactions at the C-terminus of the B-chain (Ciszak *et al.*, 1995). Insulin can associate into discrete hexameric complexes in the presence of various divalent metal ions (at 0.33 g-atom/monomer) (Goldman *et al.*, 1974). Physiologically, insulin is stored as a zinc-containing hexamer in the β-cells of the pancreas. As will be discussed later, the ability to form discrete hexamers in the presence of zinc has been used to develop therapeutically useful formulations of insulin.

Commercial insulin preparations also contain phenolic excipients (e.g. phenol, m-cresol, or methylparaben) as antimicrobial agents. As represented in Figure 10.2, these phenolic species also bind to specific sites on insulin hexamers, causing a conformational change that increases the chemical stability of insulin in commercial preparations (Brange and Langkjær, 1992). X-ray crystallographic data have identified the location of six phenolic ligand binding sites on the insulin hexamer and the nature of the conformational change that the binding of these ligands induces (Derewenda *et al.*, 1989). The phenolic ligands are stabilized in a binding pocket between monomers of adjacent dimers by hydrogen bonds with the carbonyl oxygen of Cys^{A6} and the amide proton of Cys^{A11}, as well as with numerous van der Waals contacts. The binding of these ligands stabilizes a conformational change that occurs at the N-terminus of the B-chain in each insulin monomer,

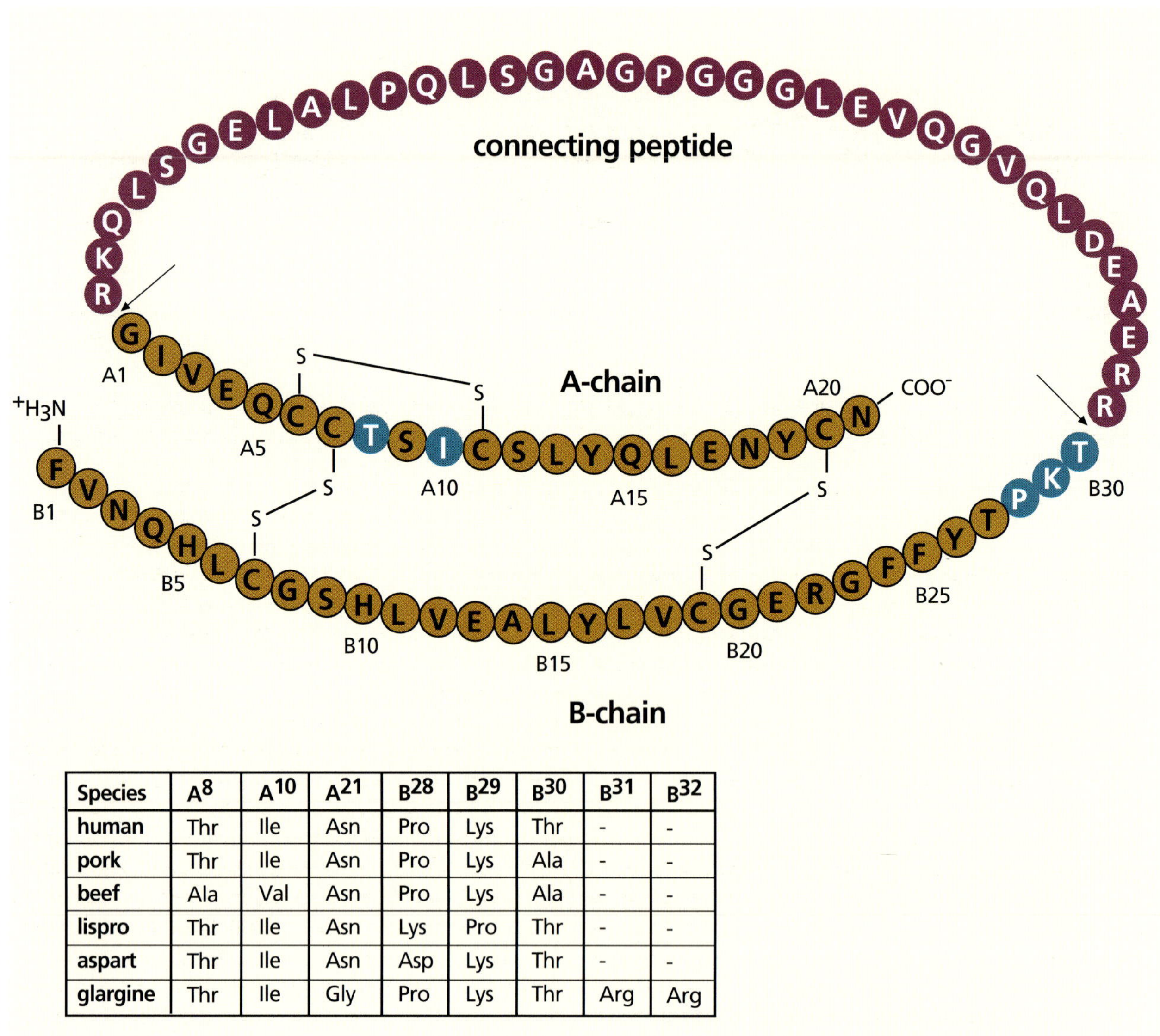

Species	A8	A10	A21	B28	B29	B30	B31	B32
human	Thr	Ile	Asn	Pro	Lys	Thr	-	-
pork	Thr	Ile	Asn	Pro	Lys	Ala	-	-
beef	Ala	Val	Asn	Pro	Lys	Ala	-	-
lispro	Thr	Ile	Asn	Lys	Pro	Thr	-	-
aspart	Thr	Ile	Asn	Asp	Lys	Thr	-	-
glargine	Thr	Ile	Gly	Pro	Lys	Thr	Arg	Arg

Figure 10.1. The primary structure of human proinsulin. The single-letter amino acid convention has been used to denote the amino acids (cf. Chapter 2). Insulin is represented by the brown/blue spheres. The connecting peptide that is excised by endopeptidase activity is represented by purple spheres. The blue spheres identify amino acids that are not conserved in other commercially available insulins.

shifting the conformational equilibrium of residues B1 to B8 from an extended structure (T-state) to an α-helical structure (R-state). This conformational change is referred to as the T↔R transition (Brader and Dunn, 1991).

In addition to the presence of zinc and phenolic preservatives, modern insulin formulations may contain an isotonicity agent (glycerol or NaCl) and/or a physiologic buffer (sodium phosphate). The former is used to minimize tissue damage and pain on injection. The latter is present to minimize pH drift in some pH-sensitive formulations.

Pharmacology and Formulations

Normal insulin secretion in the non-diabetic person falls into two categories: (i) insulin that is secreted in response to a meal, and; (ii) the background or *basal* insulin that is continually secreted between meals and during the night-time hours. The pancreatic response to a meal typically results in peak serum insulin levels of 60 to 80 microunits/mL, whereas basal serum insulin levels fall within the 5 to 15 microunits/mL range (Galloway and Chance, 1994). Due to these vastly different insulin

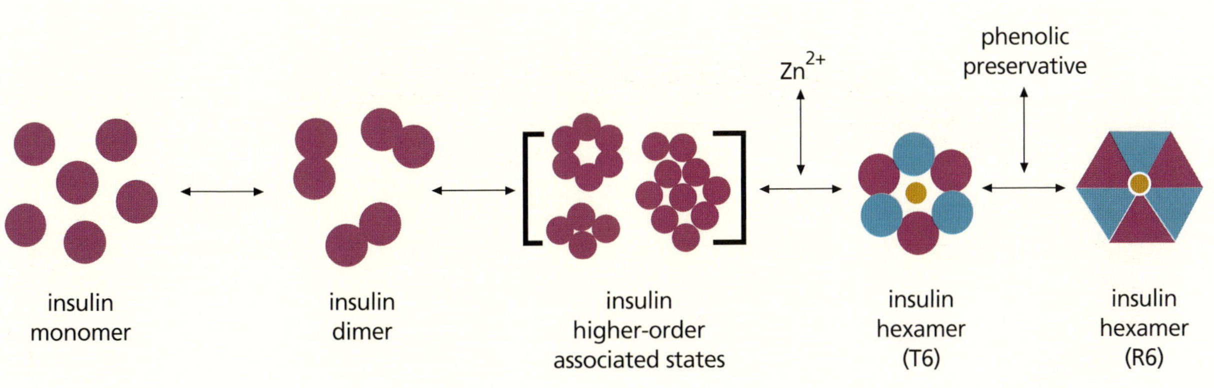

Figure 10.2. A schematic of the self-association of insulin. The hexamers are illustrated as a dimer of trimers. The monomers composing each trimer have been designated with either a blue or purple pattern. The small brown spheres represent zinc.

demands, considerable effort has been expended to develop insulin formulations that meet the pharmacokinetic and pharmacodynamic requirements of each condition. More recently, insulin analogs and insulin analog formulations have been developed to improve pharmacokinetic and pharmacodynamic properties.

Regular and Rapid-acting Soluble Preparations

Initial soluble insulin formulations were formulated under acidic conditions and were chemically unstable. In these early formulations, considerable deamidation was identified at Asn^{A21} and significant potency loss was observed during prolonged storage under acidic conditions. Efforts to improve the chemical stability of these soluble formulations led to the development of neutral, zinc-stabilized solutions.

The insulin in these neutral, regular formulations is chemically stabilized by the addition of zinc (~0.4%) and phenolic preservatives. As mentioned above, the zinc leads to the formation of discrete hexameric structures (containing 2 Zn atoms/hexamer) that can bind six molecules of phenolic preservatives, e.g. m-cresol (Figure 10.2). The binding of these excipients increases the stability of insulin by inducing the formation of a specific hexameric form (R_6), in which the B1 to B8 region of each monomer is in an α-helical conformation. This binding decreases the availability of residues involved in deamidation and high molecular weight polymer formation (Brange *et al.*, 1992a; Brange *et al.*, 1992b).

The pharmacodynamics of this soluble formulation is listed in Table 10.1. The neutral, regular formulations show peak insulin activity between two and three hours with a maximum duration of six to eight hours. As with other formulations, the variations in time-action can be attributed to factors such as dose, site of injection, temperature and the patient's physical activity. Despite the soluble state of insulin in these formulations, a delay in activity is still observed. This delay has been attributed to the time required for the hexamer to dissociate into the dimeric and/or monomeric substituents prior to absorption from the interstitium. This dissociation requires the diffusion of the preservative and insulin from the site of injection, effectively diluting the protein and shifting the equilibrium from hexamers to dimers and monomers (Figure 10.3) (Brange *et al.*, 1990). Recent studies exploring the relationship of molecular weight and cumulative dose recovery of various compounds in the popliteal lymph following subcutaneous injection suggest that lymphatic transport may account for approximately 20% of the absorption of insulin from the interstitium (Supersaxo *et al.* 1990; Porter and Charman, 2000). The remaining balance of insulin is predominately absorbed through capillary diffusion.

Monomeric insulin analogs were designed to achieve a more natural response to prandial glucose-level increases, while also providing more convenience to the patient. The development of monomeric analogs of insulin for the treatment of insulin-dependent diabetes mellitus has focused on shifting the self-association properties of insulin to favor the monomeric species and consequently minimizing the delay in time-action (Brange *et al.*, 1988; Brange *et al.*, 1990; Brems *et al.*, 1992). One such monomeric analog, $Lys^{B28}Pro^{B29}$-human insulin (Humalog® or Liprolog®; insulin lispro; Eli Lilly & Co.) has been developed and does have a more rapid time-action profile, with a peak activity of approximately one hour (Howey *et al.*, 1994).

Type [b]	Description	Appearance	Components	Action (hours) [a]		
				Onset	Peak	Duration
R [c]	Regular Soluble Insulin Injection	clear solution	metal: zinc (0.01–0.04 mg/100Units) buffer: none preservative: m-cresol isotonicity agent: glycerol	0.5	2–3	6–8
N	NPH Insulin Isophane Suspension	turbid or cloudy suspension	metal: zinc (0.01–0.04 mg/100Units) buffer: phosphate preservative: m-cresol and phenol isotonicity agent: glycerol modifying protein: protamine (0.32–0.44 mg/100Units)	1–2	6–12	18–24
L	Lente Insulin Zinc Suspension	turbid or cloudy suspension	metal: zinc (0.12–0.25 mg/100Units) buffer: acetate preservative: methylparaben isotonicity agent: glycerol modifying protein: none	1–3	6–12	18–24
U	Ultralente Extended Insulin Zinc Suspension	turbid or cloudy suspension	metal: zinc (0.12–0.25 mg/100Units) buffer: acetate preservative: methylparaben isotonicity agent: glycerol modifying protein: none	4–6	8–20	24–28
70/30 [d]	70% Insulin Isophane Suspension, 30% Regular Insulin Injection	turbid or cloudy suspension	metal: zinc (0.01–0.04 mg/100Units) buffer: phosphate preservative: m-cresol and phenol isotonicity agent: glycerol modifying protein: protamine (0.32–0.44 mg/100Units in NPH section)	0.5	2–12	14–24
50/50	50% Insulin Isophane Suspension, 50% Regular Insulin Injection	turbid or cloudy suspension	metal: zinc (0.01–0.04 mg/100Units) buffer: phosphate preservative: m-cresol and phenol isotonicity agent: glycerol modifying protein: protamine (0.32–0.44 mg/100Units in NPH section)	0.5	2–10	14–24

Table 10.1. A list of neutral human U100 insulin formulations. [a]The onset, peak and duration of insulin action depends on numerous factors, such as dose, injection site, presence of insulin antibodies, and physical activity. The action times listed below represent the generally accepted values in the medical community. [b]U.S. designation. [c] Another notable designation is S (Britain). Other soluble formulations have been designed for pump use and include Velosulin® and HOE 21PH®. [d]In Europe the ratio designation is inverted on the label, e.g., 30/70. In addition, other ratios are available in Europe and include 10/90, 20/80, and 40/60 (note: designation).

The sequence inversion at positions B28 and B29 yields an analog with reduced self-association behavior compared to human insulin (Figure 10.1). However, unlike some other monomeric analogs, insulin lispro can be stabilized in a preservative-dependent hexameric complex that provides the necessary chemical and physical stability required by insulin preparations. Despite the hexameric complexation of this analog, insulin lispro retains its rapid time-action. Based on the crystal structure of the insulin lispro hexameric complex, Frank and coworkers (Ciszak *et al.*, 1995) have hypothesized that the reduced dimerization properties of the analog, coupled with the preservative dependence, yields a hexameric complex that readily dissociates into monomers after rapid diffusion of the phenolic preservative into the

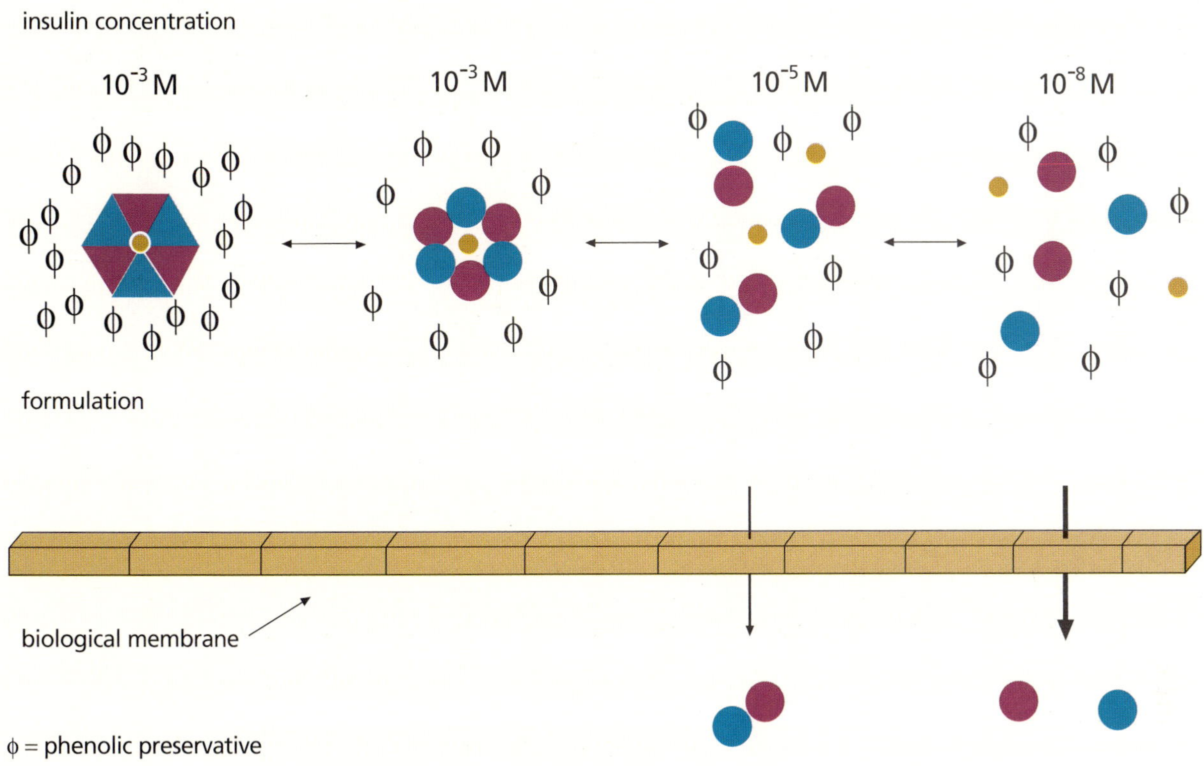

Figure 10.3. A schematic of the dissociation of human insulin after a subcutaneous injection. The hexamers are illustrated as a dimer of trimers. The monomers composing each trimer have been designated with either a blue or purple pattern. The small brown spheres represent zinc.

subcutaneous tissue at the site of injection (Figure 10.4). *Consequently, the substantial dilution (10^5) of the human insulin zinc hexamers is not necessary for the analog to dissociate from hexamers to monomers/dimers, which is required for absorption.*

Another rapid-acting insulin analog introduced to the market is Asp^{B28}-human insulin (NovoRapid® or NovoLog®; insulin aspart; Novo Nordisk A/S) and is shown in Figure 10.1 (Brange *et al.*, 1988; Brange *et al.*, 1990). Like $Lys^{B28}Pro^{B29}$-human insulin, Asp^{B28}-human insulin has been developed to have a more rapid time-action (Heinemann *et al.*, 1997). This rapid action is achieved through a reduction in the self-association behavior compared to human insulin (Brange *et al.*, 1990; Whittingham *et al.*, 1998).

In addition to the aforementioned rapid-acting formulations, manufacturers have designed soluble formulations for use in external or implanted pumps. In most respects, these formulations are very similar to Regular insulin (i.e. hexameric association state, preservative, and zinc); however, buffer and/or surfactants may be included in these formulations to minimize the physical aggregation of insulin that can lead to the clogging of the pump tubing. In early pump systems, gas-permeable tubing was used with the external pumps. Consequently, a buffer was added to the formulation in order to minimize pH changes due to dissolved carbon dioxide.

Intermediate-acting Insulin Preparations

There are two widely used types of intermediate acting insulin preparations: NPH and Lente. Both formulations achieve extended time-action by necessitating the dissolution of a precipitated and/or crystalline form of insulin. This dissolution is presumed to be the rate-limiting step in the bioavailability of intermediate- and long-acting insulin. Consequently, the time-action of the formulation is prolonged by further delaying the dissociation of the hexamer into dimers and monomers.

NPH refers to Neutral Protamine Hagedorn, named after its inventor H.C. Hagedorn (Hagedorn *et al.*, 1936), and is a neutral crystalline suspension that is prepared by the co-crystallization of insulin with protamine. Protamine consists of a closely related group of very basic proteins that are isolated from fish sperm. Protamine is heterogeneous in nature; however, four primary components have been identified and show a high degree of sequence homology

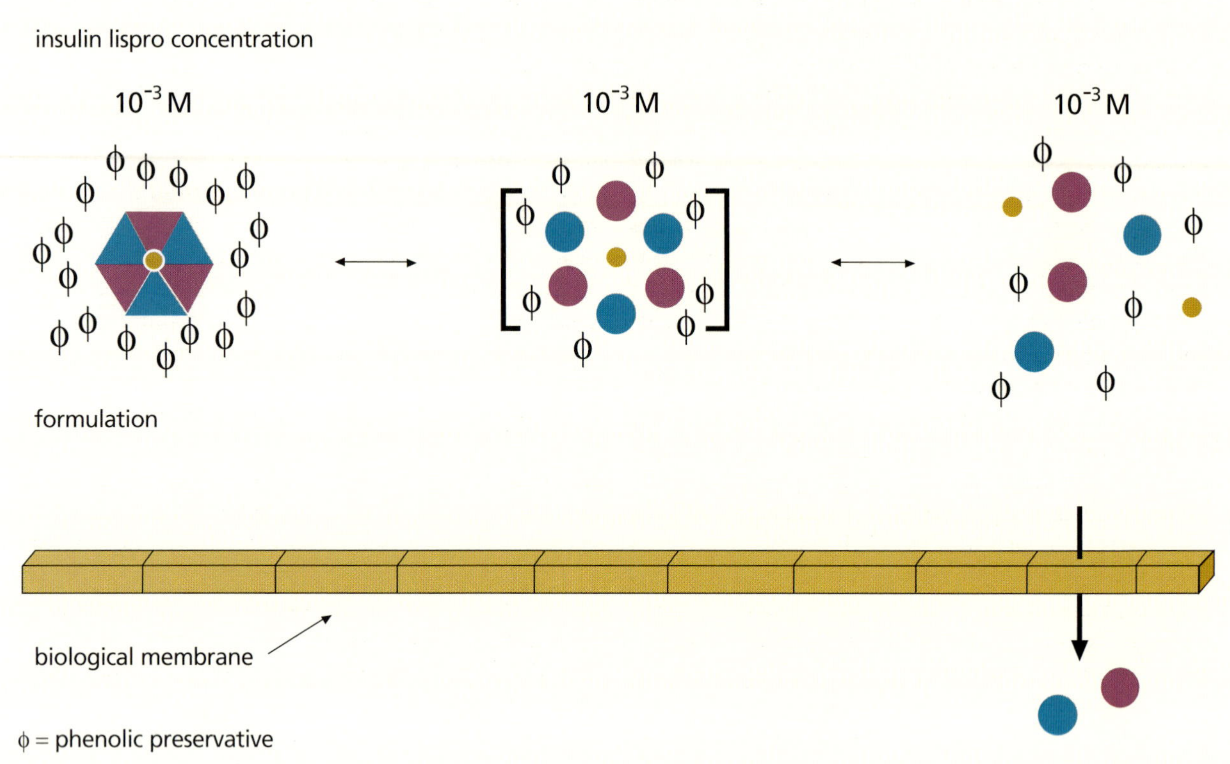

Figure 10.4. A schematic of the dissociation of insulin lispro after a subcutaneous injection. The hexamers are illustrated as a dimer of trimers. The monomers composing each trimer have been filled with blue or purple. The small brown spheres represent zinc.

(Hoffmann *et al.*, 1990). In general, protamine is ~30 amino acids in length and has an amino acid composition that is primarily composed of arginine, 65–70%. Using crystallization conditions identified by Krayenbühl and Rosenberg (Krayenbühl *et al.*, 1946), oblong tetragonal NPH insulin crystals with volumes between 1 and 20 μm^3 can be consistently prepared from protamine and insulin (Deckert, 1980). These formulations, by design, have very minimal levels of soluble insulin or protamine in solution. The condition at which no measurable protamine or insulin exists in solution after crystallization is referred to as the isophane point.

NPH has an onset of action from one to two hours, a peak activity from 6–12 hours, and a duration of activity from 18–24 hours (Table 10.1). As with other formulations, the variations in time-action are due to factors such as dose, site of injection, temperature, and the patient's physical activity.

NPH can be readily mixed with Regular insulin either extemporaneously by the patient or as obtained from the manufacturer in a premixed formulation. Premixed insulin, e.g. 30/70 or 50/50 Regular/NPH, has been shown to provide the patient with improved dose accuracy and consequently improved glycemic control (Bell *et al.*, 1991). In these preparations, a portion of the soluble Regular insulin will reversibly adsorb to the surface of the NPH crystals through an electrostatically-mediated interaction under formulation conditions (Dodd *et al.*, 1995); however, this adsorption is reversible under physiological conditions and consequently has no clinical significance (Galloway *et al.*, 1982; Hamaguchi *et al.*, 1990; Davis *et al.*, 1991). Due in part to the reversibility of the adsorption process, NPH/Regular mixtures are uniquely stable and have a two-year shelf life.

The rapid-acting insulin analog, insulin lispro, can be extemporaneously mixed with NPH; however, such mixtures must be injected immediately upon preparation due to the potential for exchange between the soluble and suspension components upon long-term storage. Exchange refers to the release of human insulin from the NPH crystals into the solution phase and concomitant loss of the analog into the crystalline phase. The presence of human insulin in solution could diminish the rapid time-action effect of the analog. One way to overcome the problem of exchange is to prepare mixtures containing the same insulin species in both the suspension and the solution phases, analogous to human insulin Regular/NPH preparations. However, this approach requires the availability of an NPH-like preparation of the rapid-acting analog.

An NPH-like suspension of Lys^{B28}, Pro^{B29}-human insulin has been prepared and its physicochemical properties relative to human insulin NPH have been described (DeFelippis *et al.*, 1998). In order to prepare the appropriate crystalline form of the analog, significant modifications to the NPH crystallization procedure are required. The differences between the crystallization conditions have been argued to result from the reduced self-association properties of Lys^{B28}, Pro^{B29}-human insulin.

Pharmacological studies have been reported for the Lys^{B28}, Pro^{B29}-human insulin NPH-like suspension commonly referred to as neutral protamine lispro (NPL) (DeFelippis *et al.*, 1998; Janssen *et al.*, 1997). The pharmacokinetic and pharmacodynamic properties of this analog suspension are analogous to human insulin NPH. As mentioned previously, the availability of analog NPH-like suspension allows the preparation of homogeneous biphasic mixtures containing intermediate and rapid acting components that are not impacted by exchange.

As with Lys^{B28}, Pro^{B29}-human insulin, premixed formulations of the Asp^{B28}-human insulin have been prepared in which rapid-acting soluble insulin aspart has been combined with a protamine-retarded crystalline preparation of insulin aspart (Balschmidt 1996). Clinical data on Lys^{B28}, Pro^{B29}-human insulin mixtures and those composed of Asp^{B28} insulin have been reported in the literature (Weyer *et al.*, 1997; Heise, *et al.*, 1998). The pharmacological properties of the rapid acting analogs are preserved in these stable mixtures. Premixed formulations of both rapid acting analogs are now commercially available in many countries.

Immunogenicity issues with protamine have been documented in a small percentage of diabetic patients (Kurtz *et al.*, 1983; Nell *et al.*, 1988). Individuals who show sensitivity to the protamine in NPH formulations are routinely switched to Lente or Ultralente preparations to control their basal glucose levels.

Lente insulin is a zinc insulin suspension that was designed for single daily injection (Hallas-Møller *et al.*, 1952). Lente insulin is a mixture of two insoluble forms of insulin, 70% rhombohedral zinc insulin crystals (Ultralente component) and 30% amorphous insulin particles (Semilente component). The pH of the formulation is neutral and contains acetate and excess zinc. The surplus zinc in the formulation presumably binds to weak metal sites on the insulin hexamer surface, reducing the solubility of the insulin, thus slowing the time-action of the insulin (Deckert, 1980). The volume of the crystalline Ultralente component is routinely between 200 and 1000 μm^3 (Deckert, 1980).

Lente has an onset of action of one to three hours, a peak activity from 6–12 hours, and a duration of action from 18–24 hours (Table 10.1). As with other formulations, the variations in observed time-action are due to factors such as dose, site of injection, temperature, and the patient's physical activity.

The mixability of Lente with Regular insulin is restricted to extemporaneous mixtures that are used immediately upon preparation (Deckert, 1980; Galloway *et al.*, 1982). Prolonged storage of Lente/Regular insulin mixtures leads to a change in the course of effect due to precipitation of the insulin from the Regular section (Deckert, 1980). The precipitation of Regular insulin is presumably due to binding of the surplus zinc found in the Lente formulation to weak binding sites on the insulin hexamer.

Long-acting Insulin Formulations

The normal human pancreas secretes approximately 1 unit of insulin (0.035mg) per hour to maintain basal glycemic control. Adequate basal insulin levels are a critical component of diabetes therapy because they regulate hepatic glucose output, which is essential for energy production by the brain. Consequently, a long-acting insulin must provide a very different pharmacokinetic profile than a meal time insulin.

There are two long-acting insulin preparations currently available: Ultralente, which was developed in the 1950s, and Lantus®, which is a new insulin analog that is commercially available. Each of these preparations derives their protracted time-action profiles from the slow and relatively constant dissolution of solid particles in the subcutaneous tissue. This slow dissolution precedes the dissociation of insulin into absorbable units, and thus the *rate of absorption* (units per hour) into the bloodstream is significantly decreased in comparison to that of a solution (mealtime) formulation.

Ultralente is analogous to NPH insulin in that they are both formulated as crystalline insulin suspensions. However, the preparations differ in their physical nature of the micro-crystals. Under microscopic examination, the larger rhombohedral Ultralente micro-crystals are notably different from the much smaller rod-shaped NPH micro-crystals. This difference originates from the different crystallization conditions employed to prepare these formulations. Ultralente contains no protamine and is crystallized at pH 5.5 in the presence of zinc, NaCl, and acetate buffer. The subsequent formulation process involves adjustment of the pH to a final value of 7.4, with the addition of excess zinc and methylparaben as an antimicrobial agent (preservative). The different formulation excipients used for Ultralente in comparison to NPH are a reflection of the different ways in which the insulin molecules are complexed into the respective crystal lattices. NPH crystals are believed to be composed of zinc insulin hexamers stabilized as a complex with protamine and preservative molecules (Balschmidt *et al.*, 1991), whereas Ultralente crystals incorporate zinc insulin hexamers only (Brange 1987a, Yip *et al.* 1998). A consequence of this composition is that methylparaben must be utilized as the preservative for Ultralente formulations because, unlike phenol and m-cresol, it does not interact with and destabilize the Ultralente crystal lattice.

Ultralente insulin should be uniformly resuspended prior to withdrawal of the dose from the vial to ensure accurate dosage. Ultralente has an onset of action of four to six hours, a peak activity between 8–20 hours, and a duration of action from 24–28 hours (Table 10.1). As with other formulations, the variations in time-action are due to factors such as dose, site of injection, temperature, and the patient's physical activity. Ultralente may be mixed with Regular insulin and Humalog, although its use in mixtures is constrained to extemporaneous mixing with immediate use for the reasons outlined for Lente.

Another long-acting insulin preparation is the insulin analog, Gly^{A21}, Arg^{B31}, Arg^{B32}-human insulin (Lantus®; insulin glargine; Aventis Pharma AG). It is shown in Figure 10.1. This analog differs from human insulin in that the amino acid asparagine is replaced with glycine at position A21 and two arginine residues have been added to the C-terminus of the B-chain. The impact of the additional arginine residues results in a shift in the isoelectric point from a pH of 5.4 to 6.7, thereby producing an insulin analog that is soluble at acidic pH values, but is less soluble at the neutral pH of subcutaneous tissue. Lantus® is a solution formulation prepared under acidic conditions, pH 4.0. The introduction of glycine at position A21 yields a protein with acceptable chemical stability under acidic formulation conditions, since the native asparagine is susceptible to acid-mediated degradation and reduced potency. Thus the changes to the molecular sequence of insulin have been made for pharmaceutical stability and to modulate absorption from the subcutaneous tissue, resulting in an analog that has approximately the same potency as human insulin. The Lantus® formulation is a clear solution that incorporates zinc and m-cresol (preservative) at a pH value of 4. This formulation approach obviates the need to administer preformed micro-crystals in order to achieve a protracted time-action. Consequently, Lantus® does not need to be resuspended prior to dosing. Immediately following injection into the subcutaneous tissue, the insulin glargine precipitates due to the pH change, forming a slowly dissolving precipitate. This results in a relatively constant rate of absorption over 24 hours with no pronounced peak. This profile allows once-daily dosing as a patient's basal insulin. As with all insulin preparations, the time course of Lantus®' action may vary in different individuals or at different times in the same individual and the rate of absorption is dependent on blood supply, temperature, and the patient's physical activity. Lantus® must not be diluted or mixed with any other solution or insulin.

Pharmaceutical Considerations

Chemical Stability of Insulin Formulations

Insulin is subject to two primary modes of chemical degradation upon storage and use: the hydrolytic transformation of amide to acid groups and the formation of covalent dimers and higher order polymers. Primarily the pH, the storage temperature, and the components of the specific formulation influence the rate of formation of these degradation products. The purity of insulin formulations is typically assessed by high performance liquid chromatography using reversed-phase and size exclusion separation modes (USPC) U.S. Pharmacopeia Convention, 2000). In acidic solution, the main reaction is the transformation of asparagine (Asn) at the terminal 21 position of the A-chain to aspartic acid. This reaction is relatively facile at low pH but is extremely slow at neutral pH (Brange *et al.*, 1992b). This reaction constituted the primary degradation route in early soluble (acidic) insulin formulations. However, the development of neutral solutions and suspensions has diminished the importance of this degradation route. Stability studies of neutral solutions indicate that the amount of A21 desamido insulin does not change upon storage. Thus, the relatively small amounts of this bioactive material present in the formulation arise either from the source insulin or from pharmaceutical process operations.

The deamidation of the Asn^{B3} of the B-chain is the primary degradation mechanism at neutral pH. The reaction proceeds through the formation of a cyclic imide that results in two products, aspartic acid (Asp) and iso-aspartic acid (iso-Asp) (Brennan and Clarke, 1994). This reaction occurs relatively slowly in neutral solution (approximately 1/10 the rate of A21 desamido formation in acid solution) (Brange *et al.*, 1992b). The relative amounts of these products are influenced by the flexibility of the B-chain, with approximate ratios of Asp:iso-Asp of 1:2 and 2:1 for solution and crystalline formulations, respectively. As noted earlier, the use of phenolic preservatives provides a stabilizing effect on the insulin hexamer that reduces the formation of the cyclic imide, as evidenced by reduced deamidation. The rate of formation also depends on temperature; typical rates of formation are approximately 2% per year at 5 °C. Studies have shown B3 deamidated insulin to be essentially fully potent (Chance, 1995).

High molecular weight protein (HMWP) products form at both storage and room temperatures. Covalent dimers that form between two insulin molecules are the primary condensation products in formulations. There is evidence that insulin-protamine heterodimers also form in NPH suspensions (Brange *et al.*, 1992a). At higher temperatures, the probability of forming higher order insulin oligomers increases. The rate of formation of HMWP is less than that of hydrolytic reactions; typical rates are less than 0.5% per year for soluble neutral Regular insulin formulations. The rate of formation can be affected by the strength of the insulin formulation or by the addition of glycerol as an isotonicity agent. The latter increases the rate of HMWP formation presumably by introducing impurities such as glyceraldehyde. HMWP formation is believed to also occur as a result of a reaction between the N-terminal B1 phenylalanine amino group and the C-terminal A21 asparagine of a second insulin molecule (Darrington and Anderson, 1995).

Disulfide exchange leading to polymer formation is also possible at basic pH; however, the rate for these reactions is very slow under neutral pH formulation conditions. The quality of excipients such as glycerol is also critical because small amounts of aldehyde and other glycerol-related chemical impurities can accelerate the formation of HMWP. The biopotency of HMWP is significantly less (1/10 to 1/5 of insulin) than of monomeric species (Chance, 1995).

Physical Stability of Insulin Formulations

The physical stability of insulin formulations is mediated by the non-covalent aggregation of insulin. Hydrophobic forces typically drive the aggregation although electrostatics play a subtle but important role. Aggregation typically leads to a loss in potency of the formulation, and should therefore be avoided. Extreme aggregation may lead to the formation of fibrils of insulin. The physical stability of insulin formulations is readily assessed by visual observation for macroscopic characteristics, as well as by instrumental methods such as light and differential phase contrast microscopy. Various particle-sizing techniques also may be used to characterize microscopic phenomena.

In general, insulin solutions have good physical stability. Physical changes in soluble formulations may manifest as color or clarity change or, in extreme situations, the formation of a precipitate. Insulin suspensions, such as NPH or Lente, are the most susceptible to changes in physical stability. These typically occur as a result of both elevated temperature and mechanical stress to the formulation. The increase in temperature favors hydrophobic interactions, while mechanical agitation serves to provide mixing and stress across interfacial boundaries. Nucleation of aggregation in suspensions can lead to conditions described as visible clumping of the suspension or 'frosting' of the glass wall of the insulin vial by aggregates. In severe cases, resuspension may be nearly impossible because of caking of the suspension in the vial. Temperatures above normal ambient (>25 °C) can accelerate the aggregation process, especially those at or above body temperature (37 °C). The normal mechanical mixing of suspensions prior to administration is not deleterious to physical stability. However, vigorous shaking or mixing should be avoided. Consequently, this latter constraint has, in part, led to the observation that patients do not place enough effort into resuspension. Thus, proper emphasis must be placed on training the patient in resuspension of crystalline, amorphous, and premixed formulations of insulin and insulin analogs. The necessity of rigorous resuspension may be the first sign of aggregation and should prompt a careful examination of the formulation to verify its suitability for use.

Clinical and Practice Aspects

Vial Presentations

Insulin is commonly available in 10-mL vials. In the U.S., a strength of U-100 (100 U/mL) is the standard, whereas outside the U.S. both U-100 and U-40 (40 U/mL) are commonly used. It is essential to obtain the proper strength and formulation of insulin in order to maintain glycemic control. In addition, species and brand/method of manufacture are important. Any change in insulin should be made cautiously and only under medical supervision (Galloway, 1988; Brackenridge, 1994). Common formulations, such as Regular, NPH, and Lente, are listed in Table 10.1. NPH/Regular mixtures, such as 70/30, are a popular choice for glycemic control. The ratio is defined as N/R 70/30 where 70% of a dose is available as NPH insulin and 30% as Regular insulin. Caution must be used in the nomenclature for NPH/Regular mixtures because it may vary depending on the country of sale and the governing pharmacopeial body. In the U.S., for example, the predominant species is listed first as in N/R 70/30, but in Europe the same formulation is described as R/N 30/70 (Soluble/Isophane) where the base ('normal') ingredient is listed first. Currently an effort is being made to standardize worldwide to the European nomenclature. Mixtures available in the U.S. include N/R 70/30 and 50/50 while Europe has R/N 10/90, 20/80, 30/70, 40/60, and 50/50.

Injectors

Insulin syringes should be purchased to match the strength of the insulin that is to be administered (e.g. for U-100 strength use 30- or 100-unit syringes designated for U-100). The needles available for insulin administration has been reduced to very fine gauges (28, 29, or 30 ga.) in order to minimize pain during injection. The use of a new needle for each dose maintains the sharp point of the needle and ensures a sterile needle for the injection.

In recent years the availability of insulin pen injectors has made dosing and compliance easier for the patient with diabetes. The first pen injector used a 1.5-mL cartridge of U-100 insulin. A needle was attached to the end of the pen, and the proper dose was selected and then injected by the patient. The cartridge was replaced when the contents were exhausted, typically after three to seven days. More recently, larger 3.0-mL cartridges are becoming available in U-100 strength for Regular, NPH, and the range of R/N mixtures for patients requiring larger doses. The advantages of the pen injectors are primarily better compliance for the patient through a variety of factors including more accurate and reproducible dose control, easier transport of the drug, more discrete dose administration, more timely dose administration, and greater convenience for the patient.

Storage

Insulin formulations should be stored in a cool place that avoids direct sunlight. Vials or cartridges that are not in active use should be stored under refrigerated (2–8 °C) conditions. Vials or cartridges in active use may be stored at ambient temperature. High temperatures, such as those found in non-air-conditioned vehicles in the summer, should be avoided. Insulin should not be frozen; if this occurs, the product should be disposed of immediately. Insulin should never be purchased or used past the expiration date on the package.

Usage

Resuspension

Insulin suspensions (e.g. NPH, Pre-mixtures, Lente, Ultralente) should be resuspended by gentle back-and-forth mixing and rolling of the vial between the palms to obtain a uniform, milky suspension. The patient should be advised of the resuspension technique for specific insoluble insulin and insulin analog formulations, which is detailed in the package insert. The homogeneity of suspensions is critical for obtaining an accurate dose. Any suspension that fails to provide a homogeneous dispersion of particles should not be used. Pen injectors may be suspended in the same manner. However, the smaller size of the container and shape of the injector device may require a slight modification of the resuspension method. A bead is added to cartridges to aid in the resuspension of NPH suspensions.

Dosing

Dose withdrawal should immediately follow the resuspension of any insulin suspension, especially Lente and Ultralente formulations because they settle relatively quickly. The patient should be instructed by his or her doctor or nurse educator in proper procedures for dose administration. Of particular importance are procedures for disinfecting the vial top and injection site. The patient is also advised to use a new needle and syringe for each injection. Reuse of these components, even after cleaning, may lead to contamination of the insulin formulation by microorganisms or by other materials, such as cleaning agents.

Extemporaneous Mixing

As discussed above in the section on "Intermediate- and Long-acting Insulin Preparations," Regular insulin can be mixed in the syringe with NPH, Lente, and Ultralente. However, only the Regular/NPH mixtures are stable enough to be stored for extended periods of time. The Lente/Regular and Ultralente/Regular formulations can be prepared but must be used immediately. Otherwise, the time-action of the Regular component can be affected. ■

Further Reading

- **Bliss, M.** (1982) *The Discovery of Insulin*, McClelland and Stewart Limited, Toronto.
- **Brange, J.** (1987) *Galenics of Insulin*, Springer-Verlag, Berlin.
- **Galloway, J.A., Potvin J.H., and Shuman, C.R.** (1988) *Diabetes Mellitus*, 9th, ed., Lilly Research Laboratories, Indianapolis, IN.

References

- **Baker, E.N., Blundell, T.L., Cutfield, J.F., Cutfield, S.M., Dodson, E.J., Dodson, G.G., Hodgkin, D.M.C., Hubbard, R.E., Isaacs, N.W., Reynolds, C.D., Sakabe, K., Sakabe, N. and Vijayan, N.M.** (1988) The structure of 2Zn pig insulin crystals at 1.5Å resolution. *Phil. Trans. R. Soc. Lond. B*, **319**, 369–456.
- **Balschmidt P, Benned Hansen F, Dodson EJ, Dodson GG, Korber F.** (1991) Structure of porcine insulin cocrystallized with clupeine-Z. *Acta Cryst.* **B47**, 975–986.
- **Balschmidt, P.** (1996) Asp^{B28} Insulin Crystals. United States Patent **5,547,930**.
- **Bell, D.S.H., Clements, R.S., Perentesis, G., Roddam, R. and Wagenknecht, L.** (1991) Dosage accuracy of self-mixed vs premixed insulin. *Arch. Intern. Med.*, **151**, 2265–2269.
- **Bliss, M.** (1982) Who discovered insulin. In *The Discovery of Insulin*, McClelland and Stewart Limited, Toronto, pp. 189–211.

- **Brackenridge, B.** (1994) Diabetes medicines: Insulin. In B. Brackenridge, (ed.), *Managing Your Diabetes*, Indianapolis, Eli Lilly and Company, pp. 36–50.
- **Brader, M.L. and Dunn, M.F.** (1991) Insulin hexamers: New conformations and applications. *TIBS*, **16**, 341–345.
- **Brange, J.** (1987a) Insulin Preparations. In *Galenics of Insulin,* Springer–Verlag, Berlin, pp. 17–39.
- **Brange, J.** (1987b) Production of bovine and porcine insulin. In *Galenics of Insulin*, Springer-Verlag, Berlin, pp. 1–5.
- **Brange, J., Havelund, S. and Hougaard, P.** (1992b) Chemical stability of insulin. 2. Formation of higher molecular weight transformation products during storage of pharmaceutical preparations. *Pharm. Res.*, **9**, 727–734.
- **Brange, J. and Langkjær, L.** (1992) Chemical stability of insulin. 3. Influence of excipients, formulation, and pH. *Acta Pharm. Nord.*, **4**, 149–158.
- **Brange, J., Langkjær, L., Havelund, S. and Vølund, A.** (1992a) Chemical stability of insulin. 1. Hydrolytic degradation during storage of pharmaceutical preparations. *Pharm. Res.*, **9**, 715–726.
- **Brange, J., Owens, D.R., Kang, S. and Vølund, A.** (1990) Monomeric insulins and their experimental and clinical applications. *Diabetes Care,* **13**, 923–954.
- **Brange, J., Ribel, U., Hansen, J.F., Dodson, G., Hansen, M.T., Havelund, S., Melberg, S.G., Norris, F., Norris, K., Snel, L., *et al.*** (1988) Monomeric insulins obtained by protein engineering and their medical implications. *Nature*, **333**, 679–82.
- **Brems, D.N., Alter, L.A., Beckage, M.J., Chance, R.E., DiMarchi, R.D., Green, L.K., Long, H.B., Pekar, A.H., Shields, J.E. and Frank, B.H.** (1992) Altering the association properties of insulin by amino acid replacement. *Prot. Eng.*, **6**, 527–533.
- **Brennan, T.V. and Clarke, S.** (1994) Deamidation and isoaspartate formation in model synthetic peptides. In D.W. Aswad, (ed.), *Deamidation and Isoaspartate Formation in Peptides and Proteins*, CRC Press, Boca Raton, pp. 65–90.
- **Chance, R.E.** (1995) Bioactivity data for insulin related substances. Personal Communication, Eli Lilly and Company, Indianapolis, IN.
- **Ciszak, E., Beals, J.M., Baker, J.C., Carter, N.D., Frank, B.H. and Smith, G.D.** (1995) The role of the C-terminal B-chain residues in insulin assembly: The structure of hexameric $Lys^{B28}Pro^{B29}$-human insulin. *Structure*, **3**, 615–622.
- **Darrington, R.T. and Anderson, B.D.** (1995) Effects of insulin concentration and self-association on the partitioning of its A-21 cyclic anhydride intermediate to desamido insulin and covalent dimer. *Pharm Res.*, **12**, 1077–84.
- **Davis, S.N., Thompson, C.J., Brown, M.D., Home, P.D. and Alberti, K.G.M.M.** (1991) A comparison of the pharmacokinetics and metabolic effects of Human Regular and NPH mixtures. *Diabetes Res. Clin. Pract.*, **13**, 107–118.
- **Deckert, T.** (1980) Intermediate-acting insulin preparations: NPH and Lente. *Diabetes Care*, **3**, 623–626.
- **DeFelippis, M.R., Bakaysa, D.L., Bell, M.A., Heady, M.A., Li, S., Pye, S., Youngman, K.M., Radziuk, and J., Frank, B.H.** (1998). Preparation and characterization of a cocrystalline suspension of [Lys^{B28},Pro^{B29}]-human insulin analogue. *J Pharm Sci*, **87**, 170–176
- **Derewenda, U., Derewenda, Z., Dodson, E.J., Dodson, G.G., Reynolds, C.D., Smith, G.D., Sparks, C. and Swenson, D.** (1989) Phenol stabilizes more helix in a new symmetrical zinc insulin hexamer. *Nature*, **338**, 594–596.
- **Dodd, S.W., Havel, H.A., Kovach, P.M., Lakshminarayan, C., Redmon, M.P., Sargeant, C.M., Sullivan, G.R. and Beals, J.M.** (1995) Reversible adsorption of soluble hexameric insulin onto the surface of insulin crystals cocrystallized with protamine: An electrostatic interaction. *Pharm. Res.*, **12**, 60–68.
- **Galloway, J.A.** (1988) Chemistry and clinical use of insulin. In J.A. Galloway, J.H. Potvin and C.R. Shuman, (eds.), *Diabetes Mellitus*, 9th, ed., Lilly Research Laboratories, Indianapolis, IN, pp. 105–133.
- **Galloway, J.A. and Chance, R.E.** (1994) Improving insulin therapy: achievements and challenges. *Horm. Metab. Res.* **26**, 591–598.
- **Galloway, J.A., Spradlin, C.T., Jackson, R.L., Otto, D.C. and Bechtel, L.D.** (1982) Mixtures of intermediate-acting insulin (NPH and Lente) with regular insulin: An update. In J.S. Skyler, (ed.), *Insulin Update: 1982,* Exerpta Medica, Princeton, pp. 111–119.
- **Goldman, J. and Carpenter, F.H.** (1974) Zinc binding, circular dichroism, and equilibrium sedimentation studies on insulin (bovine) and several of its derivatives. *Biochemistry,* **13**, 4566–4574.
- **Hagedorn, H.C., Jensen, B.N., Krarup, N.B. and Wodstrup, I.** (1936) Protamine Insulinate. *J.A.M.A.*, **106**, 177–180.
- **Hallas-Møller, K., Jersild, M., Petersen, K. and Schlichtkrull, J.** (1952) Zinc insulin preparations for single daily injection. *JAMA*, **150**, 1667–1671.
- **Hamaguchi, T., Hashimoto, Y., Miyata, T., Kishikawa, H., Yano, T., Fukushima, H. and Shichiri, M.** (1990) Effect of mixing short and intermediate NPH insulin or Zn insulin suspension acting Human insulin on plasma free insulin levels and action profiles. *J. Jpn. Diabetes Soc.*, **33**, 223–229.
- **Heinemann, L., Weyer, C., Rave, K., Stiefelhagen, O., Rauhaus, M., and Heise, T.** (1997) Comparison of the time-action profiles of U40- and U100-regular human insulin and the rapid-acting insulin analogue B28 Asp. *Exp Clin Endocrinol Diabetes*, **105**, 140–4.
- **Heise, T., Weyer, C., Serwas, A., Heinrichs, S., Osinga, J., Roach, P., Woodworth, J., Gudat, W., and Heinemann, L.** (1998). Time-action profiles of novel premixed preparations of insulin lispro and NPL insulin. *Diabetes* Care, **21**, 800–803.
- **Hoffmann, J.A., Chance, R.E. and Johnson, M.G.** (1990) Purification and analysis of the major components of chum salmon protamine contained in insulin formulations using high-performance liquid chromatography. *Protein Expression and Purification*, **1**, 127–133.

- **Howey, D.C., Bowsher, R.R., Brunelle, R.L. and Woodworth, J.R.** (1994) [Lys(B28),Pro(B29)]-human insulin: A rapidly-absorbed analogue of human insulin. *Diabetes*, **43**, 396–402.
- **Janssen, M.M.J., Casteleijn, S., Devillé, W., Popp-Snijders, C., Roach, P., and Heine, R.J.** (1997). Nighttime insulin kinetics and glycemic control in type 1 diabetic patients following administration of an intermediate-acting lispro preparation. *Diabetes Care*, **20**, 1870–1873.
- **Kaarsholm, N.C., Havelund, S. and Hougaard, P.** (1990) Ionization behavior of native and mutant insulins: pK Perturbation of B13-Glu in aggregated species. *Arch. Biochem. Biophys.* **283**, 496–502.
- **Krayenbühl, C. and Rosenberg, T.** (1946) Crystalline protamine insulin. *Rep. Steno Hosp. (Kbh.)*, **1**, 60–73.
- **Kroeff, E.P., Owen, R.A., Campbell, E.L., Johnson, R.D. and Marks, H.I.** (1989) Production scale purification of biosynthetic human insulin by reversed phase high performance liquid chromatography. *J. Chromatography*, **461**, 45–61.
- **Kurtz, A.B., Gray, R.S., Markanday, S. and Nabarro, J.D.N.** (1983) Circulating IgG antibody to protamine in patients treated with protamine–insulins. *Diabetologia*, **25**, 322–324.
- **Nell, L.J. and Thomas, J.W.** (1988) Frequency and specificity of protamine antibodies in diabetic and control subjects. *Diabetes*, **37**, 172–176.
- **Pekar, A.H. and Frank, B.H.** (1972) Conformation of proinsulin. A comparison of insulin and proinsulin self-association at neutral pH. *Biochemistry*, **11**, 4013–4016.
- **Porter, C.J. and Charman, S.A.** (2000) Lymphatic transport of proteins after subcutaneous administration. *J. Pharm. Sci.*, **89**, 297–310.
- **Supersaxo, A., Hein, W.R., and Steffen, H.** (1990) Effect of molecular weight on the lymphatic absorption of water-soluble compounds following subcutaneous administration. *Pharm Res*, **7**, 167–9
- **USPC** (2000) Official Monographs for USP 24. In *U.S. Pharmacopeia*, United States Pharmacopeia Convention, Inc., Rockville, pp. 880–887.
- **Weyer C., Heise T., Heinemann L.** (1997). Insulin aspart in a 30/70 premixed formulation. *Diabetes Care*, **20**, 1612–1614.
- **Whittingham, J.L., Edwards D.J., Antson, A.A., Clarkson, J.M., and Dodson, G.G.** (1998) Interactions of phenol and m-cresol in the insulin hexamer, and their effect on the association properties of B28 pro —> Asp insulin analogues. *Biochemistry*, 37, 11516–23.
- **Yip, C.M., DeFelippis, M.R, Frank, B.H., Brader, M.L., and Ward, M.D.** (1998) Structural and morphological characterization of Ultralente insulin crystals by atomic force microscopy: evidence of hydrophobically driven assembly. *Biophys. J.* **75**, 1172–1179.

Self-Assessment Questions

Question 1: *Which insulin formulations can be mixed and stored? Which insulin formulations can only be extemporaneously mixed? Why?*

Question 2: *What are the primary chemical and physical stability issues with insulin formulations?*

Answers

Answer 1: Mixtures of NPH/Regular can be prepared and have sufficient stability for long-term storage. NPH and Regular formulations can be mixed and stored because both formulations contain approximately the same level of zinc and consequently the soluble insulin will remain in solution after mixing. In addition, the adsorption of soluble insulin that occurs on the surface of NPH crystals is reversible under physiological conditions and therefore does not alter the bioavailability of the soluble insulin.

Mixtures of Lente/Regular and Ultralente/Regular should only be prepared by extemporaneous mixing and be used immediately; otherwise, the time-action of Regular will be blunted. The time-action of Regular is blunted by the binding of surplus zinc – present in the Ultralente and Lente formulations – to sites on the surface of the soluble insulin hexamer, present in Regular formulations, causing the soluble insulin to precipitate. Consequently, the rapid absorption of the monomeric/dimeric insulin species arising from the dissociation of the soluble insulin hexamer is delayed due to the requirement of an additional dissolution step for the newly formed insoluble precipitate.

Answer 2: The two primary modes of chemical degradation are Asn^{B3} deamidation and HMWP formation. These routes of chemical degradation occur in all formulations; however, they are generally slower in suspension formulations. Physical instability is most often observed in insulin suspension formulations and pump formulations. In suspension formulations, non-covalent aggregation can occur resulting in the visible clumping of the crystalline and/or amorphous insulin. The soluble insulin in pump formulations has also been observed to form non-covalent aggregates that precipitate.

11 Growth Hormones

Melinda Marian

Introduction

Human growth hormone (hGH) is a protein hormone essential for normal growth and development in humans. hGH affects many aspects of human metabolism, including lipolysis, the stimulation of protein synthesis and the inhibition of glucose metabolism. Human growth hormone was first isolated and identified in the late 1950s from extracts of pituitary glands obtained from cadavers and from patients undergoing hypophysectomy. The first clinical use of these pituitary-extracted hGHs for stimulation of growth in hypopituitary children occurred in 1957 and 1958 (Raben, 1958). From 1958 to 1985 the primary material used for clinical studies was pituitary-derived growth hormone (pit-hGH). Human growth hormone was first cloned in 1979 (Goeddel *et al.* 1979; Martial *et al.* 1979). The first use in humans of recombinant human growth hormone (rhGH) was reported in the literature in 1982 (Hintz *et al.*,1982). The introduction of rhGH coincided with reports of a number of cases of Creutzfeldt-Jakob disease, a fatal degenerative neurological disorder, in patients receiving pituitary-derived hGH. Concern over possible contamination of the pituitary-derived hGH preparations by the prion responsible for Creutzfeldt-Jakob disease led to the removal of pit-hGH products from the market in the US in 1985. The initial rhGH preparations were produced in bacteria (*E. coli*) and, unlike endogenous hGH, contained an N-terminal methionine group (met-rhGH). Natural sequence recombinant hGH products have subsequently been produced both in bacteria and mammalian cells.

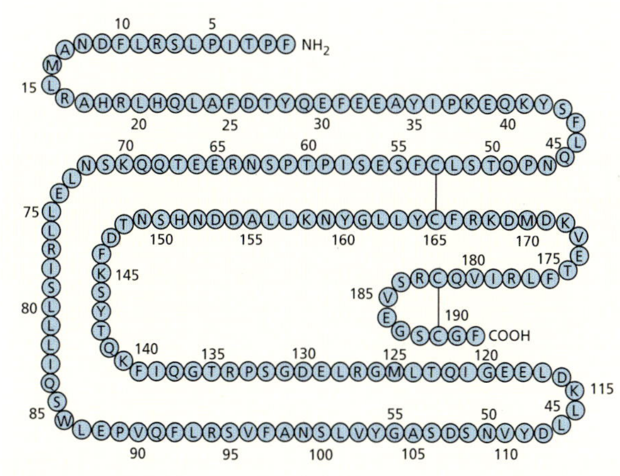

Figure 11.1. Primary structure of recombinant human growth hormone.

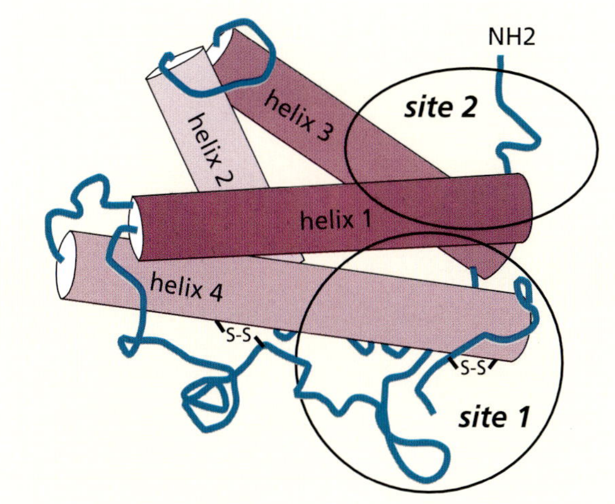

Figure 11.2. Schematic 3-D structure of hGH showing 4 anti-parallel α-helices and receptor binding sites 1 and 2. Approximate positions of the two disulfide bridges (S-S) are also indicated. Modified from Wells *et al.*, 1993.

hGH Structure and Isohormones

The major, circulating form of hGH is a non-glycosylated, 22 kDa protein composed of 191 amino acid residues linked by disulfide bridges in two peptide loops (Figure 11.1). The three dimensional structure of hGH includes four antiparallel alpha-helical regions (Figure 11.2). Helix 4 and Helix 1 have been determined to contain the primary sites for binding to the growth hormone receptor (Wells *et al.*, 1993). Endogenous growth hormone is comprised of approximately 85% 22 kDa monomer, 5–10% 20 kDa monomer, and 5% of a mixture of disulfide-linked dimers, oligomers and other modified forms (Baumann, 1991; Scanes and Campbell, 1995). The 20 kDa monomer, dimers, oligomers and other modified forms occur as a result of different gene products, different splicing of hGH mRNA and post-translational modifications. Glycosylated hGH forms less than 1% of pituitary hGH and appears to have biological effects comparable to non-glycosylated hGH.

There are two hGH genes in humans, the hGH-N gene and the hGH-V gene. The hGH-N gene is expressed in the pituitary gland and is responsible for the production of the 'normal' 22 kDa form of hGH. The hGH-V gene is expressed in the placenta and is responsible for the production of the 'variant' form of hGH found in high levels in pregnant women during the third trimester.

Pharmacology

Growth Hormone Secretion and Regulation

Growth hormone is secreted from somatotrophs in the anterior pituitary. Multiple feedback loops are present in normal regulation of hGH secretion (Casanueva, 1992; Harvey, 1995) (Figure 11.3). Growth hormone release from the pituitary is regulated by a 'short loop' of two coupled hypothalamic peptides – a stimulatory peptide, growth hormone releasing hormone (GHRH) and an inhibitory peptide, somatostatin. GHRH and somatostatin are, in

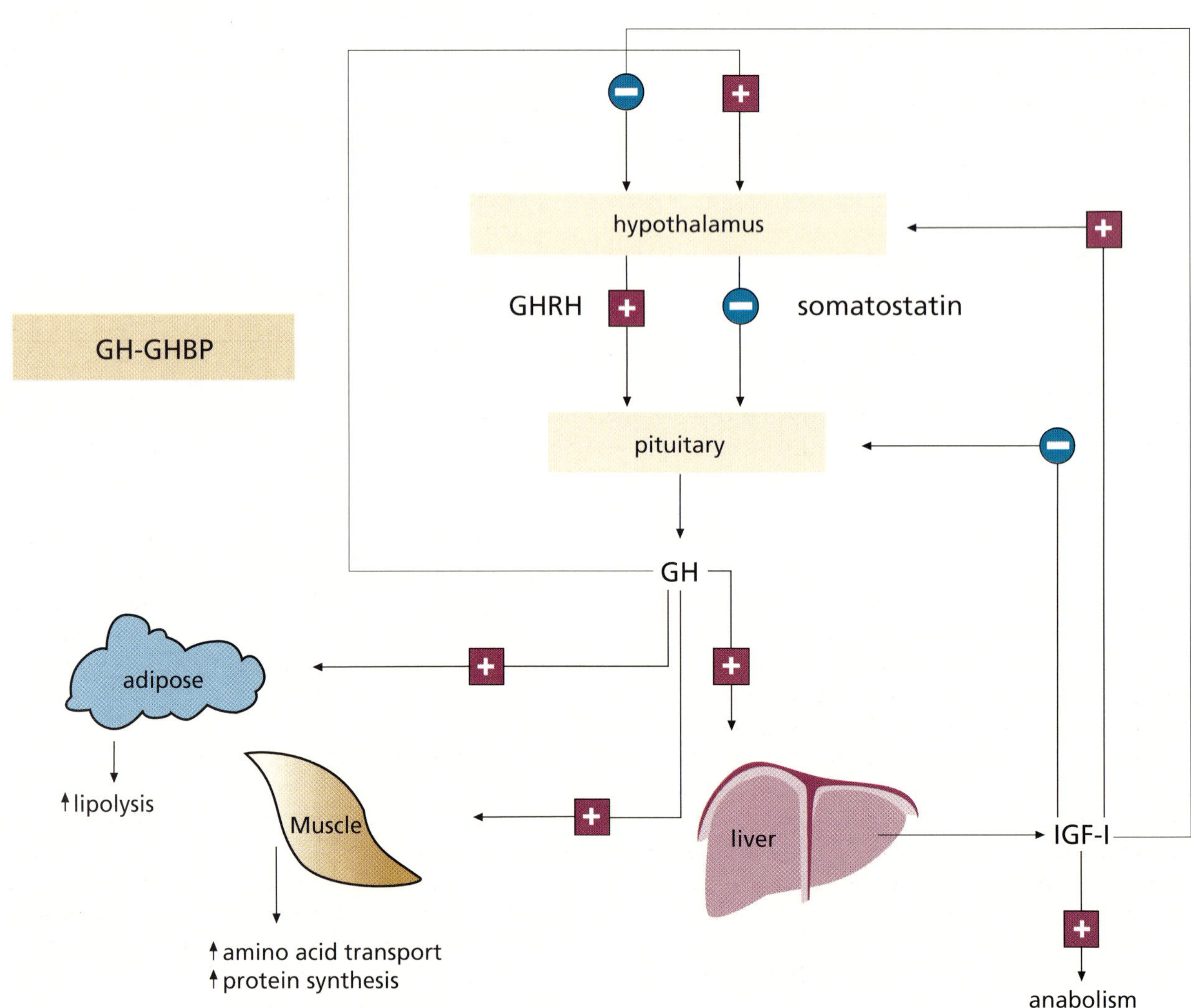

Figure 11.3. Schematic representation of hGH regulation and biologic actions in man. "Short loop" regulation of hGH secretion occurs between the hypothalamus and pituitary. "Long loop" of regulation of hGH secretion occurs through peripheral feedback signals, primarily from insulin-like growth factor I (IGF-I). hGH acts directly on muscle, bone and adipose tissue. Other anabolic actions are mediated through IGF-I.

turn, regulated by neuronal input to the hypothalamus. There is possibly also an 'ultrashort loop' in which hGH release is feedback-regulated by growth hormone receptors present on the somatotrophs of the pituitary themselves. Growth hormone secretion is also regulated by a 'long loop' of peripheral signals including, primarily, negative feedback via insulin-like growth factor (IGF-I). Growth hormone-induced peripheral IGF-I inhibits somatotroph release of hGH and stimulates somatostatin release.

Growth hormone secretion changes according to human development, with the highest production rates observed during gestation and puberty (Harvey and Daughaday, 1995; Brook *et al.*, 1992). Growth hormone production declines approximately 10–15% each decade from age 20 to 70. Endogenous hGH secretion also varies with sex, nutritional status, obesity, physical activity, and in a variety of disease states. Endogenous hGH is secreted in periodic bursts over a 24 hour period with great variability in burst frequency, amplitude and duration. There is little detectable hGH released from the pituitary between bursts. The highest endogenous hGH serum concentrations of 10–30 ng/mL usually occur at night when the secretory bursts are largest and most frequent

Growth Hormone Biologic Actions

hGH has well-defined growth promoting and metabolic actions. hGH stimulates the growth of cartilage and bone directly, through hGH receptors in those tissues, and indirectly, via local increases in IGF-I (Isaksson *et al.*, 1987; Bouillon, 1991). Metabolic actions, which may also be directly controlled by hGH, include the elevation of circulating glucose levels (diabetogenic effect) and acute increases in circulating concentrations of free fatty acids (lipolytic effect). Other hGH anabolic and metabolic actions believed to be mediated through increases in local or systemic IGF-I concentrations include: increases in net muscle protein synthesis (anabolic effect); modulation of reproduction in both males and females; maintenance, control and modulation of lymphocyte functions; increases in glomerular filtration rate and renal plasma flow rate (osmoregulation); influences on the release and metabolism of insulin, glucagon, and thyroid hormones (T3, T4); and possible direct effects on pituitary function and neural tissue development (Strobl and Thomas, 1994; Casanueva, 1992; LeRoith *et al.*, 1991).

hGH Receptor and Binding Proteins

The hGH receptor is a member of the hematopoietic cytokine receptor family. It has an extracellular domain consisting of 246 amino acids and a single transmembrane domain of 350 amino acids (Baumann, 1991; Bass *et al.*, 1991). The extracellular domain has at least six potential N-glycosylation sites and is usually extensively glycosylated. hGH receptors are found in most tissues in humans. However, the greatest concentration of receptors in humans and other mammals occurs in the liver.

As much as 40–45% of monomeric hGH circulating in plasma is bound to one of two binding proteins (GHBP) (Baumann, 1991; Harvey and Hull, 1995). Binding proteins decrease the clearance of hGH from the circulation (Baumann, 1991) and may also serve to dampen the biological effects of hGH by competing with cell receptors for circulating free hGH. The major form of GHBP in humans is a high affinity ($K_a = 10^{-9}$ to 10^{-8} M), low capacity form which preferentially binds the 22 kDa form of hGH (Baumann *et al.*, 1991; Herrington *et al.*, 1986). In humans, the high affinity GHBP is identical to the extracellular domain of the hGH receptor and arises by proteolytic cleavage of liver hGH receptors (Harvey and Hull, 1995). Another low affinity ($K_a = 10^{-5}$ M), high capacity GHBP is also present which binds the 20 kDa form with equal or slightly greater affinity than the 22 kDa form.

Molecular Endocrinology and Signal Transduction

X-ray crystallographic studies and functional studies of the extracellular domain of the hGH receptor suggest that two receptor molecules form a dimer with a single growth hormone molecule by sequentially binding to Site 1 on Helix 4 of hGH then to Site 2 on Helix 1 (Figure 11.4) (Wells *et al.*, 1993). Signal transduction may occur by activation/phosphorylation of JAK-2 tyrosine kinase followed by activation/phosphorylation of the extracellular signal-regulated kinase/mitogen-activated protein kinase (ERK/MAP) system (Scanes, 1995). The details of subsequent signalling events have not been elucidated, however, hGH receptor activation results in rapid induction of the c-fos, c-myc and c-jun genes, possibly through the activation of protein C kinase (Carter-Su *et al.*, 1996).

Dosing Schedules and Routes

The dosing levels and routes for exogenously administered growth hormone were first established for pit-hGH in growth hormone deficient (GHD) patients. This regimen, 0.05–0.1 mg/kg three times weekly by intramuscular (im) injection, was based on a number of factors including patient compliance and availability of hGH derived from cadaver pituitaries. A re-evaluation of subcutaneous (sc) administration of hGH (Russo and Moore, 1982; Albertsson-Wikland *et al.*, 1986) found a very strong patient preference for the sc route. Furthermore, increased growth rates were observed with daily sc injections compared to the previous two to three times weekly im

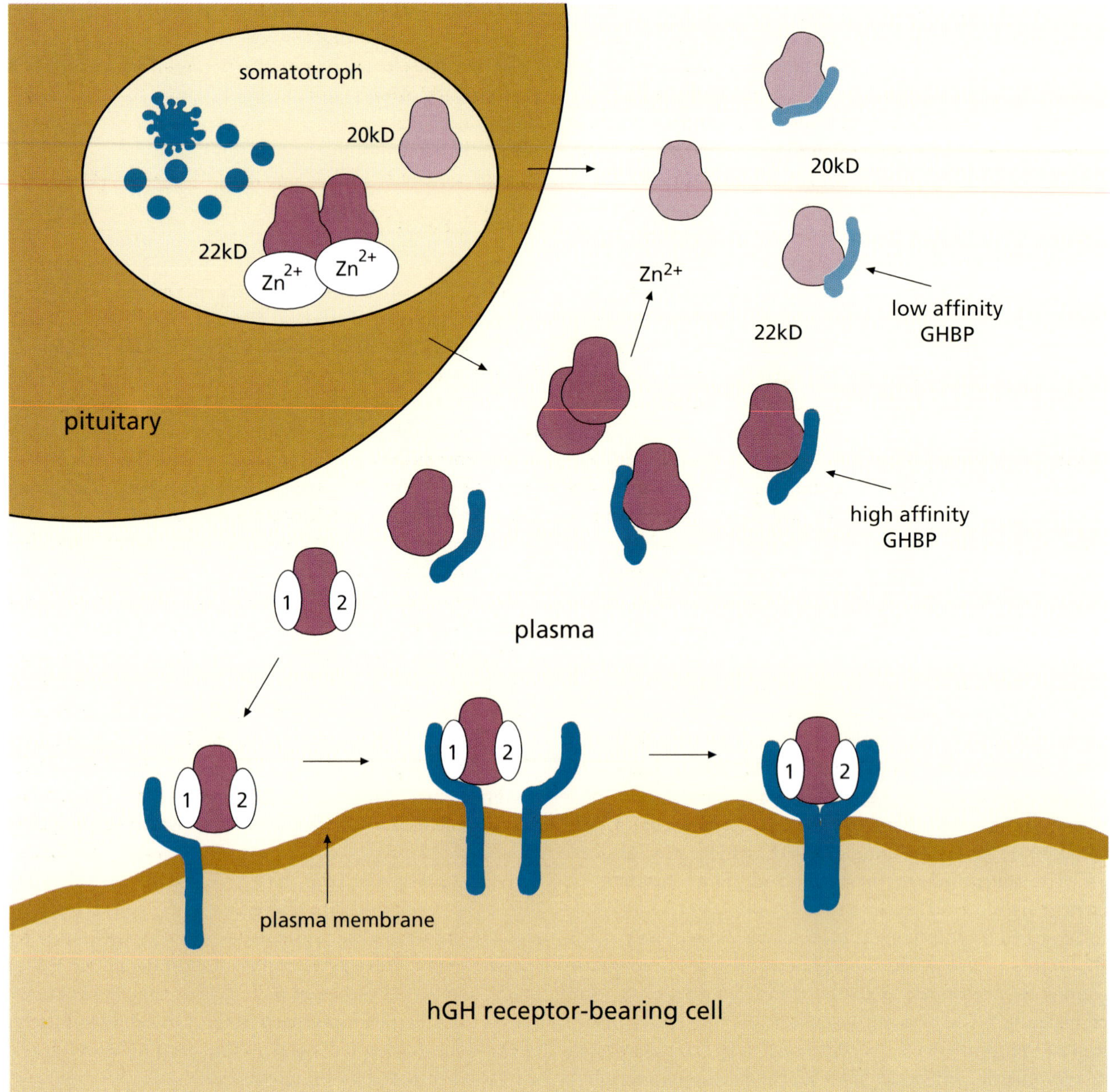

Figure 11.4. Growth hormone secreted isoforms, binding proteins and receptor interactions. Both 22kDa and 20kDa forms are secreted by the pituitary. Pituitary hGH is stored bound to zinc (Zn^{2+}) which is released upon secretion from the pituitary. Approximately 40% of secreted hGH is bound to either the low or high affinity GHBP in plasma. Receptor activation involves dimerization of two receptor molecules with one molecule of hGH. Modified from Wells *et al*., 1993.

injection schedule (Takano *et al*., 1988; Albertsson-Wikland *et al*., 1986). The abdomen, deltoid muscle, and thigh are commonly used subcutaneous injection sites. Current dosing schedules are usually daily sc injections, often self-administered. Some studies (Jorgensen *et al*., 1990; Christiansen *et al*., 1983) suggest that evening injections, which emulate the normal evening increases in endogenous secretion, are better than morning injections. The long-acting hGH product, Nutropin Depot® is administered by sc injection once or twice monthly.

Pharmacokinetics and Metabolism

The earliest pharmacokinetic studies were conducted with pituitary-derived hGH (pit-hGH). The pharmacokinetic profiles of pit-hGH, met-rhGH and rhGH have been compared (Takano *et al.*, 1983; Jorgenson *et al.*, 1987; Wilton *et al.*, 1987) and shown to be very similar. The pharmacokinetics of hGH have been studied in normal, healthy children and adults and a variety of patient populations.

Table 11.1 summarizes clearance and terminal half-life values reported from studies in normal subjects and various patient populations. Pit-hGH, met-rhGH and rhGH are rapidly cleared following intravenous (iv) injection with terminal half lives ranging from 8 to 31 minutes. Distribution volumes usually approximate the plasma volume. hGH clearance in normal subjects ranges from 90–222 mL/hr/kg. The majority of the data indicate that the clearance of hGH in children and adults are similar. Comparative analyses of hGH clearance have not shown consistent differences on the basis of age, gender or hGH secretory status.

Human growth hormone is slowly, but relatively completely, absorbed after both intramuscular (im) and subcutaneous (sc) injection. Time to peak concentration ranges from three to four hours following im bolus administration and four to six hours following sc bolus administration (Jorgensen, 1991). Subcutaneously administered rhGH is approximately 70–80% bioavailable (Wilton *et al.*, 1988). Elimination half-lives following extravascular administration (two to five hours) are usually longer than the iv terminal half-lives indicating absorption rate-limited kinetics. Daily or thrice weekly dosing does not influence absorption or elimination (Kearns *et al.*, 1991). The extent of subcutaneous absorption appears to be independent of needle type, concentration of the injection solution or injection volume (Blok *et al.*, 1991; Laursen *et al.*, 1993).

The absorption and elimination in GHD patients are similar to published reports in healthy adults (Table 11.1). Changes in hGH pharmacokinetics due to the presence of diabetes, or diseases of the thyroid, liver and kidney, have been investigated. Results suggest disposition is not significantly altered compared with normal subjects except in severe liver or kidney dysfunction (Haffner *et al.*, 1994; Owens *et al.*, 1973; Cameron *et al.*, 1972; Taylor *et al.*, 1969; Navalesi *et al.*, 1975; Refetoff and Sonksen, 1970). The reduction in clearance observed in severe liver (30%) or kidney dysfunction (40–75%) is consistent with the role of the liver and kidney as major organs of hGH elimination.

hGH is rapidly metabolized *in vivo*. Both the kidney and the liver have been shown to be important in the clearance of hGH in humans (Bennett *et al.*, 1979; Cameron *et al.*, 1972; Carone *et al.*, 1979; Maack *et al.*, 1979; Owens *et al.*, 1973; Taylor *et al.*, 1969). The relative contribution of each organ has not been definitively determined in humans, but the preponderance of studies in laboratory animals and in isolated perfused organ systems, suggest a dominant role for the kidney at pharmacologic dose levels of hGH. Renal handling of hGH appears to involve filtration, re-absorption and intracellular catabolism (Maack *et al.*, 1979; Bennett *et al.*,1979; Carone *et al.*, 1979). Little intact hGH (0.01% of serum concentrations) is normally excreted in human urine (Walker *et al.*, 1990; Sohmiya and Kato, 1992).

Protein Manufacture, Formulation and Stability

Commercially available hGH preparations are summarized in Table 11.2.

All recombinant growth hormones except Serostim®/Saizen® are produced in *E. coli*. Met-rhGH is produced by direct cytoplasmic expression of the protein. Natural sequence rhGH is produced either by enzymatic cleavage of the methionine during the purification procedures or by periplasmic secretion of rhGH into refractile bodies. The rhGH is then released from the refractile bodies by osmotic shock and the protein recovered and purified. rhGH synthesized in mammalian cells is transported across the endoplasmic reticulum and secreted directly into the culture medium from which it is recovered and purified.

Historically, the potency of hGH products has been expressed in International Units per mg (IU/mg). The initial standard, established in 1982 for pit-hGH preparations, was 2 IU/mg. The standard for rhGH products was 2.6 IU/mg until September 1994. The current WHO standard, established in September 1994, is 3.0 IU/mg. Dosages are usually expressed as IU/kg or IU/m^2 in Europe and Japan and as mg/kg in the US. However, the use of IU dosages may no longer be necessary due to the high level of purity and consistent potency of recombinant hGH products.

Most current formulations are lyophilized preparations, which are reconstituted prior to injection. Lyophilized formulations usually include 5 or 10 mg of protein in a glycine and mannitol or sucrose-containing phosphate buffer excipient. The materials are usually reconstituted with sterile water for injection for single use or with bacteriostatic water or bacteriostatic saline for multiple injection use. Two liquid formulations of rhGH (Nutropin AQ® and Norditropin® cartridge) are also available for use. The liquid formulations contain mannitol/histidine or citrate buffer with either poloxamer 188 or polysorbate 20 and phenol. Product stability has been very good with shelf lives of approximately two years at 2–8 °C. A long-acting dosage form of rhGH (Nutropin Depot®) was approved for use in 1999. Nutropin Depot® consists of micronized particles of rhGH embedded in biocompatible, biodegradable polylactide-coglycolide (PLGA) microspheres. The formulation is a free-flowing powder, which is suspended in diluent containing carboxymethylcellulose, sodium chloride, polysorbate 20 and sterile water for sc injection (cf. Chapter 4).

Population	CL (mL/hr/kg)[a]	Terminal $t_{1/2}$ (min)[a]	References
Normal adults	90–222	8–31	Haffner *et al.*, 1994 Rosenbaum and Gertner, 1989 Taylor *et al.*, 1969 Thompson *et al.*, 1972 Owens *et al.*, 1973 Navalesi *et al.*, 1975 Sohmiya and Kato, 1992 Wilton *et al.*, 1988 Holl *et al.*, 1993 Parker *et al.*, 1962 Takano *et al.*, 1983
GHD children	125–245	8–13	Rosenbaum and Gertner, 1989 Albertsson-Wikland *et al.*, 1989
GHD adults	239	9–38	Hindmarsh *et al.*, 1989 Retetoff and Sonsken, 1970 Parker *et al.*, 1962 Hendricks *et al.*, 1985
CRI children	47–109	25–32	Haffner *et al.*, 1994
CRI adults	68–175	19–48	Haffner *et al.*, 1994 Owens *et al.*, 1973 Cameron *et al.*, 1972
Normal elderly	138	14	Sohmiya and Kato, 1992
Diabetes	87–175	22	Navalesi *et al.*, 1975 Taylor *et al.*, 1969 Owens *et al.*, 1973
Liver disease	86–124	29	Owens *et al.*, 1973 Cameron *et al.*, 1972
Acromegaly	46–190	33	Retetoff and Sonsken, 1970 Taylor *et al.*, 1969
Hyperthyroid	240	nr	Taylor *et al.*, 1969
Hypothyroid	122	nr	Taylor *et al.*, 1969
Thyrotoxicosis	201	16	Owens *et al.*, 1973
Myxedema	153	24	Owens *et al.*, 1973

Table 11.1. Intravenous pharmacokinetic parameters for hGH in various populations. [a] Values have been converted from units reported in the original publications for ease of comparison. Where specific activity of GH was not stated in the original publication, values of 2.6 IU/mg for rhGH and 2.0 IU/mg for pit-hGH were used. 70 kg/1.73 m^2 and 40 kg/1 m^2 were used as adult and child body weight/body surface values, respectively. Listed values are means or ranges of means. nr = not reported.

Growth hormone type	Source	Brand names	Product Form	Supplier
Pituitary-derived human growth hormone (pit-hGH)	cadaver pituitaries	Crescormon®	no longer marketed	KabiVitrum AB (now Pharmacia Corp.)
		Nanormon®	no longer marketed	Novo Nordisk A/S
Somatrem, methionyl human growth hormone (met-rhGH)	recombinant protein produced in bacteria *(E. coli)*	Somatonorm®	no longer marketed	KabiVitrum AB (now Pharmacia Corp.)
		Protropin®	lyophilized powder for injection	Genentech, Inc.
Somatropin, natural sequence human growth hormone (rhGH)	recombinant protein produced in bacteria *(E. coli)*	Genotropin®	lyophilized powder in two chamber cartridge for use with Genotropin® Pen	Pharmacia Corp.
		Genotropin® Miniquick	single-use syringe device containing lyophilized powder in two chamber cartridge	
		Norditropin®	lyophilized powder for injection	Novo Nordisk
		Norditropin® cartridge	liquid for injection in cartridges for use with NordiPen™	
		Nutropin®	lyophilized powder for injection	Genentech, Inc.
		NutropinAQ®	liquid for injection	
		Nutropin Depot®	lyophilized, sustained-release microspheres for injection	
		Humatrope®	lyophilized powder for injection in cartridges for use with HumatroPen ™	Eli Lilly & Co.
		Bio-Tropin™ Sci Tropin® Zomacton® Growject®	lyophilized powder for injection	Bio-Technology General Corp.
	recombinant protein produced in mammalian cells (C127 mouse cell line-derived)	Serostim® (growth inadequacy)	lyophilized powder for injection	Serono S.A.
		Saizen® (AIDS wasting)	cool.click injection device	

Table 11.2. Human growth hormone preparations.

Clinical Usage

Recent clinical usage has been reviewed by Vance and Mauras (1999), Tritos and Mantzoros (1998) and Meling and Nylen (1996). Investigations of clinical usage of hGH have focused, generally, on two major areas of hGH biologic action: 1) linear growth promotion, and 2) modulation of metabolism. Growth promoting indications which have been approved for market include treatment of growth hormone insufficiency in children, growth failure associated with chronic renal failure in children, short stature in Prader-Willi syndrome and short stature in Turner's syndrome. Growth hormone products are also approved for long term replacement therapy in adults with GH deficiency of either childhood- or adult-onset and for AIDS wasting or cachexia. Additional indications for which hGH has been investigated as a possible therapeutic are summarized in Table 11.3 and detailed in the references contained within the reviews cited above. The following sections summarize observations from studies in the approved indications and selected indications under current investigation. Specific references for the investigated indications can be found in the cited review articles.

Growth Hormone Deficiency/Idiopathic Short Stature in Children

The major indication for therapeutic use of hGH is the long-term replacement treatment for children with classic growth hormone deficiency (GHD) in whom growth failure is due to a lack of adequate endogenous hGH secretion. Diagnosis of hGH deficiency is usually defined based on an inadequate response to two hGH provocation tests implying a functional deficiency in the production or secretion of hGH from the pituitary gland. Usual doses range from 0.08–0.35 mg/kg/week administered as daily sc injections in prepubertal children. Doses up to 0.7 mg/kg/week have been used for adolescent subjects to improve final height (Mauras *et al.,* 2000). The long-acting growth hormone formulation, Nutropin Depot®, is approved for use in GH-deficient children and is administered by sc injection once or twice a month. hGH treatment results in increased growth velocity and, at least in some populations, enhancement in final adult height. The growth response correlates positively with hGH dose and frequency of injections and negatively with chronological age at onset of treatment. hGH therapy in children is usually continued until growth has been completed, as evidenced by epiphyseal fusion. Partial GHD and idiopathic short stature (ISS) comprise a heterogeneous group of growth failure states due to impaired spontaneous hGH secretion, hGH resistance due to low levels of hGH receptors or possible other defects in either secreted hGH or hGH receptors. hGH treatment in these groups has resulted in acceleration of growth and improvement of final height.

Turner Syndrome

Turner syndrome is a disease of females caused by partial or total loss of one sex chromosome and is characterized by decreased intrauterine and postnatal growth, short final adult height, incomplete development of the ovaries and secondary sexual characteristics, and other physical abnormalities. Although serum levels of hGH and IGF-I are not consistently low in this population, hGH treatment, alone or in combination with oxandrolone, significantly improves growth rate and final adult height in this patient group.

Prader-Willi Syndrome

Prader-Willi syndrome is a pediatric disease caused by the functional deletion of the paternal allele of chromosome 15. Clinical manifestations include obesity, hypotonia, short stature, hypogonadism and behavior abnormalities. Growth hormone treatment has been shown to improve growth, body composition, physical strength and agility (Carrel *et al.*, 1999) in children with Prader-Willi syndrome.

Chronic Renal Insufficiency (CRI)

Children with renal disease grow slowly, possibly related to defects in metabolism and/or defects in the IGF-I/hGH axis. Basal serum hGH concentrations and IGF-I responses to hGH stimulation are usually normal. However, there are reported abnormalities in the IGF-binding protein levels in renal disease patients suggesting possible problems with GH/IGF-I action. Growth hormone therapy in children with chronic renal insufficiency has resulted in significant increases in height velocity. Increases were best during the first year of treatment for younger children with stable renal disease. Responses were less for children on dialysis or children post-transplant receiving corticosteroids.

Growth Hormone Deficient Adults and the Elderly

Early limitations in hGH supply severely limited treatment of adults with GHD. However, with rhGH abundantly available, replacement therapy for adults has received renewed clinical interest. Growth hormone has been used in three growth hormone deficient adult populations: a) adults with childhood onset GHD; b) adults with adult onset GHD usually due to pituitary tumors and subsequent hypophysectomy, and; c) elderly normal adults, 60 years of age or older. Adults with GHD show a predisposition to cardiovascular disease, have increased body fat and decreased lean muscle mass and strength. The elderly

Growth hormone biologic actions	Clinical indications
Promotion of linear growth	classic GHD partial GHD/Idiopathic short stature Turner syndrome Down's syndrome Prader-Willi syndrome Noonan's syndrome intrauterine growth retardation (IUGR) Silver-Russel syndrome thalassemia hypochondroplasia spina bifida myelomeningocele chronic renal insufficiency (CRI) growth impairment in chronic steroid therapy
Modulation of metabolism Stimulation of lipolysis Stimulation of protein synthesis	GHD in adults aging obesity weight training in athletes
Anabolism Stimulation of protein synthesis Improved nitrogen retention Prevention of starvation-induced hypoglycemia	catabolic states due to chronic disease, infections, surgery, trauma, burns, chronic obstructive pulmonary disease (COPD), short bowel syndrome (SBS), acquired immunodeficiency syndrome (AIDS)
Lipolysis Muscle anabolism	cardiovascular dysfunction
Stimulation of collagen formation	burns wound healing
Stimulation of bone formation	osteoporosis fractures
Stimulation of conversion of thyroxine (T4) to triiodothyronine (T3)	hypothyroidism
Osmoregulation Increased GFR, increased renal plasma flow	chronic renal disease
Maintenance of immune function	immune dysfunction
Enhancement of gonadotropin action	female and male infertility
Stimulation of lactation	lactational failure in women

Table 11.3. Growth hormone biologic actions and related clinical investigations.

are considered growth hormone deficient due to the progressive decline in hGH secretion with ageing which results in substantial decreases in serum IGF-I levels. The elderly also show changes in body composition which are consistent with partial hGH deficiency (decreases in lean body mass and strength, increases in visceral fat, decreases in skin thickness and organ volumes).

Growth hormone treatment reduced body fat, increased lean body mass, increased exercise capacity and muscle strength in the elderly and adult GHD patients. Increases in bone density were observed in some bone types although treatment duration greater than six months may be necessary to see significant effects. hGH treatment consistently elevated both serum IGF-I and insulin levels. However, consistent reductions in serum cholesterol and/or LDL levels were not seen in all studies. Women have also been shown to require higher doses to normalize IGF-I levels than men, especially women taking oral estrogens (Cook *et al.*, 1999; Span *et al.*, 2000).

Clinical Malnutrition and Wasting Syndromes

The use of hGH therapy to ameliorate the catabolism seen in patients following surgery and/or infections have been investigated in a number of studies. Treatment with hGH alone improved nitrogen and phosphorous retention and increased body weight. Improvements in nitrogen balance were even greater with co-administration of hGH and IGF-I. Growth hormone has also shown benefit, when used with controlled diets, in increasing body weight and nitrogen retention in wasting associated with AIDS.

Other Indications

A number of studies have investigated the use of hGH in osteoporosis. Growth hormone was not successful in reducing the bone loss associated with osteoporosis, and use of this therapy must await further studies in which hGH is co-administered with inhibitors of bone reabsorption. Studies on hGH effects in wound healing and burns have been modestly successful with hGH showing significant effectiveness in mild injuries and in acceleration of healing in skin graft sites.

Several studies have demonstrated improved bone mineral density (BMD) with hGH administration in GH-deficient adults. Positive effects are best demonstrated with long term administration (>1 year), as short term (<3 months) therapy can produce apparent decreases in BMD due to increased bone re-modeling.

Growth hormone has recently been shown to significantly reduce multiple disease symptoms and improve well-being in Crohn's disease, a chronic inflammatory disorder of the bowel (Slonim *et al.*, 2000). Growth hormone has also shown benefit in cardiovascular recovery and function in congestive heart failure (Osterziel *et al.*, 1998, 2000).

Safety Concerns

hGH has been widely used for many years and has been proven to be remarkably safe in pediatric indications (Blethen and MacGillivray, 1997). Adverse events have been reported in a small number of children and include intracranial hypertension, glucose intolerance and the development of anti-hGH antibodies. The antibodies have not been positively correlated with a loss in efficacy. Leukemia has been reported in children receiving hGH therapy but a definite correlation with hGH treatment has not been established (Blethen, 1998). Growth hormone therapy is also not associated with increased risk of solid tumors or tumor recurrence (Blethen, 1998; Vance and Mauras, 1999). However, growth hormone treatment should generally not be initiated in children until one year or more after completion of anti-neoplastic therapy.

Growth hormone has caused significant, dose-limiting, fluid retention in adult populations resulting in increased body weight, swollen joints and arthralgias and carpal tunnel syndrome. Symptoms were usually transient and resolved upon reduction of hGH dosage or upon the discontinued hGH treatment. Growth hormone administration has been associated with increased mortality in clinical trials in critically ill, intensive-care patients with acute catabolism (Takala *et al.*, 1999). Growth hormone is, therefore, contraindicated for use in the treatment of acute catabolism in critically ill patients.

Concluding remarks

The abundant supply of hGH, made possible by recombinant DNA technology, has allowed enormous advances to be made in understanding the basic structure, function and physiology of hGH over the past 15 years. As a result of those advances, recombinant hGH has been developed into a safe and efficacious therapy for growth hormone deficiency, chronic renal insufficiency, Turner's syndrome, Prader-Willi syndrome and AIDS wasting. Additional clinical studies in osteoporosis, Crohn's disease and congestive heart failure hold promise for additional future uses for this versatile hormone. ■

Further Reading

- **Baumann G.** (1991). Growth hormone heterogeneity: genes, isohormones, variants and binding proteins. *Endoc. Re.*, 12, 424–449.
- **Casanueva F.** (1992). Physiology of growth hormone secretion and action. *Endocrinl. Metab Clin N Am*,21, 483–517.
- **Harvey S, ScaneCG and Daughaday, WH.** (1995). *Growth Hormone*, CRC Press, Inc, Boca Raton, Florida.
- **Meling TR, Nylen ES.** (1996). Growth hormone deficiency in adults: a review. *Am J Med Sci,* 311, 153–166.
- **Tritos NA, and Mantzoros CS.** (1998). Recombinant growth hormone: old and novel uses. *Am J Med,* 105, 44–57.
- **Vance ML and Mauras N.** (1999). Drug therapy: growth hormone therapy in adults and children. *New Engl J Med,* 341, 1206–1216.
- **Wells JA, Cunningham BC, Fuh G, Lowman HB, Bass SH, Mulkerrin MG, Ultsch M and DeVos, AM.** (1993). The molecular basis for growth hormone-receptor interactions. *Rec Prog Horm Res,* 48, 253–275.

References

- **Albertsson-Wikland K, Rosberg S, Libre E, Lundberg L-O and Groth, T.** (1989). Growth hormone secretory rates in children as estimated by deconvolution analysis of 24–h plasma concentration profiles. *Am J Physiol (Endocrinol Metab 20)*, 257, E809–E814
- **Albertsson-Wikland K, Westphal O, and Westgren, U.** (1986). Daily subcutaneous administration of human growth hormone in growth hormone deficient children. *Acta Pediatr Scand*, 75, 89–97
- **Bass SH, Mulkerrin MG and Wells JA.** (1991). A systematic mutational analysis of hormone-binding determinants in the human growth hormone receptor. *Proc Natl Acad Sci USA*, 88, 4498–4502
- **Bennett HPJ and McMartin C.** (1979). Peptide hormones and their analogues: distribution, clearance from the circulation and inactivation *in vivo*. *Pharmacol Rev*, 30, 247–292
- **Beshyah SA, Anyaoku V, Niththyananthan R, Sharp P and Johnston DG.** (1991). The effect of subcutaneous injection site of absorption of human growth hormone: abdomen versus thigh. *Clin Endocrinol*, 35, 409–412
- **Blethen S.** (1998). Leukemia is children treated with growth hormone. *Trends Endocrinol Metab*, 9, 367–370
- **Blethen SL and MacGillivray MH.** (1997). A risk-benefit assessment of growth hormone use in children. *Drug Safety*, 5, 303–316
- **Blok GJ, van der Veen EA, Susgaard S and Larsen F.** (1991). Influence of concentration and injection volume on the bioavailability of subcutaneous growth hormone: comparison of administration by ordinary syringe and by injection pen. *Pharmacol Toxicol*, 68, 355–359
- **Bouillon R.** (1991). Growth hormone and bone. *Horm Res*, 36 (suppl 1), 49–55
- **Brook CGD and Hindmarsh PC.** (1992). The somatotropic axis in puberty. *Endocrinol Metab Clin N Am*, 21, 767–782
- **Cameron DP, Burger HG, Catt KJ, Gordon E and Watts JMcK.** (1972). Metabolic clearance of human growth hormone in patients with hepatic and renal failure, and in the isolated perfused pig liver. *Metab*, 21, 895–904
- **Carone FA, Peterson DR, Oparil S and Pullman TN.** (1979). Renal tubular transport and catabolism of proteins and peptides. *Kidney Int*, 16, 271–278
- **Carrel AL, Myers SE, Wlhitman BY and Allen DB.** (1999). Growth hormone improves body composition, fat utilization, physical strength and agility, and growth in Prader-Willi syndrome: a controlled study. *J Ped*, 134, 215–221
- **Carter-Su C, Schwartz J, Smit LS.** (1996). Molecular mechanisms of growth hormone action. *Ann Rev Physiol*, 58, 187–207
- **Christiansen JS, Orskov H, Binder C and Kastrup KW.** (1983). Imitation of normal plasma growth hormone profile by subcutaneous administration of human growth hormone to growth hormone deficient children. *Acta Endocrinol*,102, 6–10
- **Cook DM, Ludlam WH, Cook MB.** (1999). Route of estrogen administration helps to determine growth hormone (GH) replacement dose in GH-deficient adults. *J Clin Endocrinol Metab*, 84, 3956–3960
- **Goeddel DV, Heyreker HL, Hozumi T, Arentzen R, Itakura K, Yansura DG, Ross MJ, Miozarri G, Crea R and Seeburg PH.** (1979). Direct expression in *Escherichia coli* of a DNA sequence coding for human growth hormone. *Nature*, 281, 544–548
- **Haffner D, Schaefer F, Girard J, Ritz E and Mehls O.** (1994). Metabolic clearance of recombinant human growth hormone in health and chronic renal failure. *J. Clin Invest*, 93,1163–71
- **Harvey S.** (1995). Growth hormone release: feedback regulation. In *Growth Hormone*, edited by S. Harvey, C.G. Scanes, and W.H. Daughaday, pp163–184. Boca Raton, Florida: CRC Press, Inc.
- **Harvey, S. and Daughaday, W.H.** (1995). Growth hormone action: clinical significance. In *Growth Hormone*, edited by S. Harvey, C.G. Scanes, and W.H. Daughaday, pp 476–504. Boca Raton, Florida: CRC Press,Inc.
- **Harvey, S. and Hull, K.** (1995). Growth hormone transport. In *Growth Hormone*, edited by S. Harvey, C.G. Scanes, and W.H. Daughaday, pp 257–284. Boca Raton, Florida: CRC Press, Inc.
- **Hendricks CM, Eastman RC, Takeda S, Asakawa K and Gorden P.** (1985). Plasma clearance of intravenously administered pituitary human growth hormone: gel filtration studies of heterogeneous components. *J Clin Endocrinol Metab*, 60, 864–867
- **Herington AC, Ymer S and Stevenson J.** (1986). Identification and characterization of specific binding proteins for growth hormone in normal human sera. *J Clin Invest*, 77, 1817–1823
- **Hindmarsh PC, Matthews DR, Brain CE, Pringle PJ, DiSilvio L, Kurtz AB and Brook CGD.** (1989). The half-life of exogenous growth hormone after suppression of endogenous growth hormone secretion with somatostatin. *Clin Endocrinol*, 30, 443–450
- **Hintz RL, Rosenfeld RG, Wilson DM, Bennett A, Finno J, McClellan B and Swift R.** (1982). Biosynthetic methionyl human growth hormone is biologically active in adult man. *Lancet*, 1, 1276–1279
- **Holl RW, Schwarz U, Schauwecker P, Benz R, Veldhuis JD and Heinze E.** (1993). Diurnal variation in the elimination rate of human growth hormone (GH): the half-life of serum GH is prolonged in the evening, and affected by the source of the hormone, as well as by body size and serum estradiol. *J Clin Endocrinol Metab*, 77, 216–220
- **Isaksson OG, Lindahl A, Nilsson A and Isgaard J.** (1987). Mechanism of the stimulatory effect of growth hormone on longitudinal bone growth. *Endocr Rev*, 8, 426–438

- **Jorgensen JOL, Moller N, Lauritzen T, Alberti KGMM, Orskov H and Christiansen JS.** (1990). Evening versus morning injections of growth hormone (GH) in GH-deficient patients: effects on 24-hour patterns of circulating hormones and metabolites. *J Clin Endocrinol Metab*, 70, 207–214
- **Jorgensen JOL.** (1991). Human growth hormone replacement therapy: pharmacological and clinical aspects. *Endocr Rev*, 12,189–207
- **Jorgensen JOL, Flyvbjerg A, Dinesen J, Lund H, Alberti KGMM, Orskov H and Christiansen JS.** (1987). Serum profiles and sort-term metabolic effect of pituitary and authentic biosynthetic human growth hormone in man. *Acta Endocrinol*,116, 381–386
- **Kearns GL, Kemp, SF and Frindik JP.** (1991). Single and multiple dose pharmacokinetics of methionyl growth hormone in children with idiopathic growth hormone deficiency. *J Clin Endocrinol Metab*, 72, 1148–1156
- **Laursen T, Jorgensen JOL, Susgaard S, Moller J and Christiansen JS.** (1993). Subcutaneous absorption kinetics of two highly concentrated preparations of recombinant human growth hormone. *Ann Pharmacother*, 27, 411–415
- **Le Roith D, Adamo M, Werner H and Roberts CT Jr.** (1991). Insulin-like growth factors and their receptors as growth regulators in normal physiology and pathologic states. *Trends Endocrinol Metab*, 2, 134–139
- **Maack T, Johnson V, Kau ST, Figueiredo J and Sigulem D.** (1979). Renal filtration, transport and metabolism of low-molecular weight proteins: a review. *Kidney Int*, 16, 251–270
- **Martial JA, Hallewell RA and Baxter JD.** (1979). Human growth hormone: complementary DNA cloning and expression in bacteria. *Science*, 205, 602–607
- **Mauras N, Attie KM, Reiter EO, Saenger P, Baptista J and the Genentech Inc Cooperative Study Group.** (2000). High dose recombinant human growth hormone (GH) treatment of GH-deficient patients in puberty increases near-final height: a randomized, multicenter trial. *J Clin Endocrinol Metab*, 85, 3653–3660
- **Navalesi R, Pilo, A and Vigneri R.** (1975). Growth hormone kinetics in diabetic patients. *Diabetes*, 24, 317–327
- **Osterziel KJ, Ranke MB, Strohm O and Rainer D.** (2000). The somatotrophic system in patients with dilated cardiomyopathy: relation of insulin-like growth factor-1 and its alterations during growth hormone therapy to cardiac function. *Clin Endocrinol* 53, 61–68
- **Osterziel KJ, Strohm O, Schuler J, Friedrich M, Hanlein D, Willenbrock R, *et al.*** (1998). Randomised, double-blind, placebo-controlled trial of human recombinant growth hormone in patients with chronic heart failure due to dilated cardiomyophathy. *Lancet*, 351, 1233–37
- **Owens D, Srivastava MC, Tompkins CV, Nabarro JDN and Sonksen PH.** (1973). Studies on the metabolic clearance rate, apparent distribution space and plasma half-disappearance time of unlabelled human growth hormone in normal subjects and in patients with liver disease, renal disease, thyroid disease and diabetes mellitus. *Europ J Clin Invest*, 3, 284–294
- **Parker ML, Utiger RD and Daughaday WH.** (1962). Studies on human growth hormone II. The physiological disposition and metabolic fate of human growth hormone in man. *J Clin Invest*, 41, 262–268
- **Raben MS.** (1958). Treatment of a pituitary dwarf with human growth hormone. *J Clin Endocrinol Metab*, 18, 901–903
- **Refetoff S and Sonksen PH.** (1970). Disappearance rate of endogenous and exogenous human growth hormone in man. *J Clin Endocr*, 30, 386–392
- **Rosenbaum M and Gertner JM.** (1989). Metabolic clearance rates of synthetic human growth hormone in children, adult women, and adult men. *J Clin Endocrinol Metab*, 69, 821–824
- **Russo L and Moore WV.** (1982). A comparison of subcutaneous and intramuscular administration of human growth hormone in the therapy of growth hormone deficiency. *J Clin Endocrinol Metab*, 55, 1003–1006
- **Scanes CG.** (1995). Growth hormone action: intracellular mechanisms. In *Growth Hormone*, edited by S. Harvey, C.G. Scanes, and W.H. Daughaday, pp 337–346. Boca Raton, Florida: CRC Press,Inc.
- **Scanes CG and Campbell RM.** (1995). Growth hormone: chemistry. In *Growth Hormone*, edited by S. Harvey, C.G. Scanes, and W.H. Daughaday, pp 1–24. Boca Raton, Florida: CRC Press,Inc.
- **Slonim AE, Bulone L, Damore MB, Goldberg T, Wingertzahn MA and McKinely MJ.** (2000). A preliminary study of growth hormone therapy for Crohn's disease. *New Engl J Med*, 342, 1633–1637
- **Sohmiya M and Kato Y.** (1992). Renal clearance, metabolic clearance rate, and half-life of human growth hormone in young and aged subjects. *J Clin Endocrinol Metab*, 75, 1487–90
- **Span JPT, Pieters GFFM, Sweep CGJ, Hermus ARMM and Smals AGH.** (2000). Gender difference in insulin-like growth factor I response to growth hormone (GH) treatment in GH-deficient adults: role of sex hormone replacement. *J Clin Endocrinol Metab*, 85, 1121–1125
- **Strobl JS and Thomas MJ.** (1994). Human growth hormone. *Pharm Rev*, 46, 1–34
- **Takala J, Ruokonen E, Webster NR, Nielsen MS, Zandstra DF, Vundelinckx G, *et al.*** (1999). Increased mortality associated with growth hormone treatment in critically ill adults. *New Engl J Med*, 341, 785–792
- **Takano K, Hizuka N, Shizume K, Asakawa K and Kogawa M.** (1983). Short-term study of biosynthesized hGH in man. *Endocrinol Japon*, 30, 79–84
- **Takano K, Shizume K, Hibi I and Members of Committee for the Treatment of Pituitary Dwarfism in Japan.** (1988). A comparison of subcutaneous and intramuscular administration of

human growth hormone (hgh) and increased growth rate by daily injection of hGH in GH deficient children. *Endocrinol Japon*, 35, 477–484

- **Taylor AL, Finster JL and Mintz DH.** (1969). Metabolic clearance and production rates of human growth hormone. *J Clin Invest*, 48, 2349–2358
- **Thompson RG, Rodriguez A, Kowarski A and Blizzard RM.** (1972). Growth hormone: metabolic clearance rates, integrated concentrations, and production rates in normal adults and the effect of prednisone. *J Clin Invest*, 51, 3193–3199
- **Walker JM, Wood PJ, Williamson S, Betts PR and Evans AJ.** (1990). Urinary growth hormone excretion as a screening test for growth hormone deficiency. *Arch Dis Child*, 65, 89–92
- **Wilton P, Widlund L and Guilbaud O.** (1987). Bioequivalence of genotropin and somatonorm. *Acta Paediatr Scand (Suppl)*, 337, 118–121
- **Wilton P, Widlund L and Guilbaud O.** (1988). Pharmacokinetic profile of an iv and sc dose of recombinant human growth hormone. *Pediatr Res*, 23, 117

Self-Assessment Questions

Question 1: *One molecule of hGH is required to sequentially bind to two receptor molecules for receptor activation. What consequences might the requirement for sequential dimerization have on observed dose-response relationships?*

Question 2: *Growth hormone is known or presumed to act directly upon which tissues?*

Question 3: *You are investigating the use of hGH as an adjunct therapy for malnutrition/wasting in a clinical population which also has severe liver disease. What effects would you expect the liver disease to have on the observed plasma levels of hGH after dosing and on possible efficacy (improvement in nitrogen retention, prevention of hypoglycemia, etc.)?*

Answers

Answer 1 Sequential dimerization will potentially result in a 'bell-shaped' dose response curve, i.e. response is stimulated at low concentrations and inhibited at high concentrations. The inhibition of responses at high concentrations is due to blocking of dimerization caused by the excess hGH saturating all the available receptors. Inhibition of *in vitro* hGH binding is observed at high hGH (mM) concentrations. Reductions in biological responses (Total IGF-I increase and weight gain) have also been seen with increasing hGH doses in animal studies. However, inhibitory effects of high concentrations of hGH are not seen in treatment of human patients since hGH dose levels are maintained within normal physiological ranges and never approach inhibitory levels.

Answer 2 Growth hormone is known to act directly on both bone and cartilage and possibly also on muscle and adipose tissue. Growth hormone effects on other tissues appear to be mediated through the IGF-I axis or other effectors.

Answer 3 Severe liver disease may reduce the clearance of the exogenously administered hGH and observed plasma levels may be higher and persist longer compared to patients without liver disease (Table 11.1). However, the increased drug exposure may not result in increased anabolic effects. The desired anabolic effects require the production/release of IGF-I from the liver. Both IGF-I production and the number of hGH receptors may be reduced due to the liver disease. To understand the results (or lack of results) from the treatment, it is important to monitor effect parameters (i.e. IGF-I and possibly IGF-I binding protein levels, liver function enzymes, etc) in addition to hGH levels.

12 Vaccines

Wim Jiskoot, Gideon F.A. Kersten, and E. Coen Beuvery

Introduction

Vaccination aims to prevent infectious diseases. Considered one of the most successful medical strategies of the twentieth century, conventional vaccines routinely administered are very effective in preventing a number of infectious diseases. This prevention is illustrated by the fact that mass vaccination has resulted in the worldwide eradication of smallpox during the 1970s. Moreover, diphtheria, pertussis, tetanus, poliomyelitis, measles, mumps, and rubella are under control in developed countries, as well as in an increasing number of developing countries, because of the application of childhood vaccines.

In the rapidly evolving field of new vaccine technologies one can discern (1) the improvement of existing vaccines, and (2) the development of vaccines for diseases against which there are no vaccines currently available. Modern biotechnology has an enormous impact on current vaccine development. The elucidation of the molecular structures of pathogens and the tremendous progress made in immunology during the past few decades have led to the identification of protective antigens. Together with technological advances, the advances in biotechnology has caused a shift from empirical vaccine development to more rational approaches. A major goal of modern vaccine technology is to fulfill all requirements of the ideal vaccine, as summarized in Figure 12.1, by expressing antigen epitopes (the smallest molecular structures recognized by the immune system) and/or isolating those antigens that confer an effective immune response, and eliminating structures that cause deleterious effects. Thus, 'cleaner', well-defined products can be obtained, resulting in improved safety and efficacy. In addition, modern methodologies may provide simpler production processes for selected vaccine components.

The following section summarizes immunological principles that are important for vaccine design. Conventional vaccines, those products that are not a result of modern genetic or chemical engineering technologies, will be addressed in a separate section. Conventional and modern vaccines are listed in Table 12.1. Current strategies used in the development and manufacture of new vaccines are discussed in the section "Modern Vaccine Technologies." This chapter does not intend to provide a comprehensive review of all possible vaccine options for all possible diseases. Rather, it explains modern approaches to vaccine development and illustrates these approaches with representative examples. The last two sections deal with the pharmaceutical and the regulatory and clinical aspects of vaccines.

The ideal vaccine

- is 100% efficient in all individuals of any age
- provides lifelong protection after single administration
- does not evoke an adverse reaction
- is stable under various conditions (temperature, light, transportation)
- is easy to administer, preferably orally
- is available in unlimited quantities
- is cheap

Figure 12.1. Characteristics of the (hypothetical) ideal vaccine.

Immunological Principles

Introduction

After most natural infections a healthy immune system launches an immunological response to the particular pathogen. After recovery from the disease, the immunological response indeed protects us from that disease forever in the ideal case. This phenomenon is called immunity and is due to the presence of circulating antibodies, activated cytotoxic cells and memory cells (see below). Memory cells become active when the same type of antigenic material enters the body on a later occasion. Unlike the primary response after the first infection, the response after repeated infection is very fast and usually sufficiently strong to prevent reoccurrence of the disease.

Vaccination mimics an infection in such a way that the natural specific defense mechanism of the host against the pathogen will be activated, while the host remains free of

Category	Technology	Live/non-living	Characteristics
Attenuated vaccines	conventional	live	bacteria or viruses attenuated in culture; empirically developed
Inactivated vaccines	conventional	non-living	heat-inactivated or chemically inactivated bacteria or viruses; empirically developed
Subunit vaccines	conventional	non-living	extracts of pathogens; combination of purified proteins with killed suspension; purified single components (proteins, polysaccharides); combination of purified components with adjuvant; purified components in a suitable presentation form; polysaccharide-protein conjugates
Genetically improved live vaccines	modern	live	genetically attenuated micro-organisms; live viral or bacterial vectors
Genetically improved subunit vaccines	modern	non-living	genetically detoxified proteins; proteins expressed in host cells; recombinant peptide vaccines
Anti-idiotype vaccines	modern	non-living	antigen-mimicking antibodies
Synthetic peptide-based vaccines	modern	non-living	linear or cyclic peptides; multiple antigen peptides; peptide-protein conjugates
Nucleic acid vaccines	modern	non-living	DNA or mRNA coding for antigen

Table 12.1. Categories of conventional vaccines and vaccines obtained by modern technologies.

the disease that normally results from a natural infection. This process is effectuated by the administration of antigenic components that consist of, are derived from, or are related to the pathogen. The success of vaccination relies on the induction of a long-lasting immunological memory. Vaccination is also referred to as active immunization, because the host's immune system is activated to respond to the 'infection' through humoral and cellular immune responses (see below), resulting in acquired immunity against the particular pathogen. The immune response is generally highly specific: it discriminates not only between pathogen species, but often also between different strains within one species (e.g. meningococci, poliovirus, influenza virus). Although this is sometimes a hurdle for vaccine development, the high specificity of the immune system allows for an almost perfect balance between response to foreign antigens and tolerance with respect to self-antigens. Apart from active immunization, the administration of specific antibodies can be utilized for short-lived immunological protection of the host. This administration technique is termed passive immunization (Figure 12.2).

Traditionally, active immunization has primarily served to prevent infectious diseases, whereas passive immunization has been applied for both the prevention and therapy of infectious diseases. Through recent developments new potential applications of vaccines for active immunization have emerged, such as the prevention of pregnancy as well as noninfectious diseases such as cancer. Furthermore, the use of vaccines in the treatment of chronic diseases, such as cancer, autoimmune diseases and AIDS, is being explored; such vaccines are referred to as therapeutic vaccines. The difference between passive and active immunization for preventive and therapeutic applications is outlined in Figure 12.2. Since antibody preparations for passive immunization do not fall under the strict definition of a vaccine, they are not discussed here. Monoclonal antibodies for passive immunization will be addressed later in this book (Chapter 13).

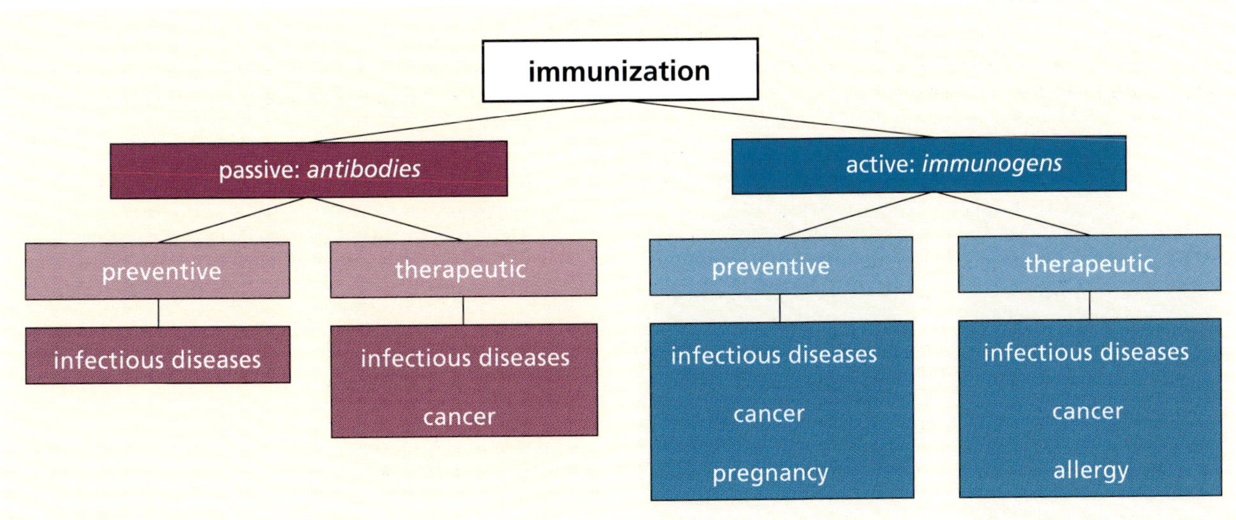

Figure 12.2. Scheme of active immunization (= vaccination) and passive immunization and examples of their fields of application.

Humoral and Cell-Mediated Immunity

Main stage players in the generation of an immune response are phagocytes (macrophages, dendritic cells, Langerhans cells) and lymphocytes (B- and T-cells). These cells communicate and stimulate each other by direct contact between surface bound receptors, as well as by soluble lymphokines (interleukins and interferons). An extremely complicated network emerges from these interactions. Lymphocytes are classified by the presence or absence of certain receptors (CD molecules) and the secretion of lymphokines. It should be emphasized that cells can have different functions at different stages in the immune response (e.g. antigen presentation versus antibody production; cytotoxicity versus help functions). Furthermore, a similar action of an effector mechanism may lead to different, sometimes even opposite results under different circumstances (for example, at the start or at the end of a response).

Specific acquired immunity to infectious diseases can be divided into humoral and cell-mediated immunity (CMI) (see Figure 12.3 and Table 12.2). The humoral response results in antibody formation (but contains cell mediated events, see Figure 12.3, panels A and B); CMI results in the generation of cytotoxic cells (see Figure 12.3, panels A and C). The action of antibodies and of T-cells is dependent on accessory factors, some of which are mentioned in Table 12.2. In general, after infection with a pathogen or a protective vaccine, both humoral and cellular responses

Immune response	Immune product	Accessory factors	Infectious agents
Humoral	IgG	complement, neutrophils	bacteria and viruses
	IgA	alternative complement pathway	micro-organisms causing respiratory and enteric infections
	IgM	complement, macrophages	(encapsulated) bacteria
	IgE	mast cells	parasites
Cell-mediated	CTL	cytolytic proteins	viruses and mycobacteria
	T_{DTH}	macrophages	viruses, mycobacteria, treponema (syphilis), fungi

Table 12.2. Immune products protecting against infectious diseases (adapted from Sell and Hsu, 1993).

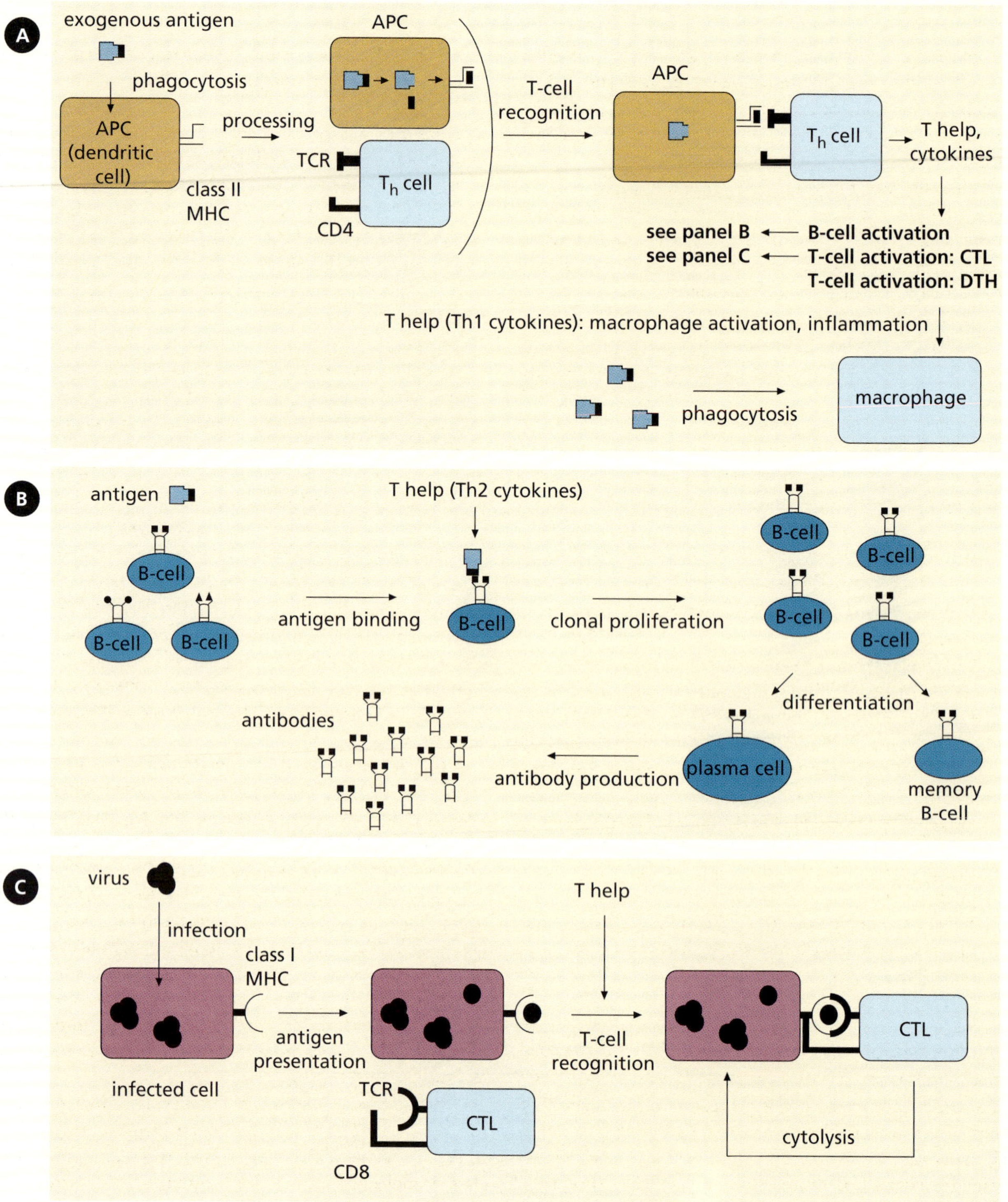

Figure 12.3. Schematic representation of antigen-dependent immune responses. (A) Activation of T-helper cells (Th-cells). An antigen-presenting cell (APC), e.g., a dendritic cell phagocytozes exogenous antigens (bacteria or soluble antigens) and degrades them partially. Antigen fragments are presented by MHC class II molecules to a CD 4 positive Th-cell; the MHC-antigen complex on the APC is recognized by the T-cell receptor (TCR) and CD 4 molecules on the Th-cell. The APC-Th-cell interaction leads to activation of the Th-cell. The activated Th-cell produces cytokines, resulting in the activation of macrophages (Th1 help), B-cells (Th2 help; panel B) or cytotxic T-cells (panel C). (B) Antibody production. The presence of antigen and Th2-type cytokines cause proliferation and differentiation of B-cells. Only B-cells specific for the antigen become activated. The B-cells, now called plasma cells, produce and secrete large amounts of antibody. Some B-cells differentiate into memory cells. (C) Activation of cytotoxic T-lymphocytes (CTLs). CTLs recognize non-self antigens expressed by MHC class I molecules on the surface of virally infected cells or tumor cells. Cytolytic proteins are produced by the CTL upon interaction with the target cell.

are generated, indicating that both are needed for efficient protection. The balance between humoral and cellular responses, however, can differ widely between pathogens, and may have consequences for the design of a particular vaccine.

Antibodies are the typical representatives of humoral immunity, and belong to one of four immunoglobulin classes (IgM, IgG, IgA or IgE). Upon immunization, B-cells expressing specific antibodies on their cell surface (representing a fifth immunoglobulin class, IgD) are activated. The surface-bound antibodies recognize antigenic structures of the vaccine called epitopes. Upon contact with the vaccine, and in close cooperation with T-helper cells (T_h-cells), B-cells activate and massive clonal proliferation occurs. The proliferated B-cells are called plasma cells and excrete large amounts of soluble antibodies (Figure 12.3, panel B). Antibodies are able to prevent infection or disease by several mechanisms:

1. Binding of antibody covers the antigen with Fc (constant fragment), the 'rear-end' of immunoglobulins. Phagocytic cells, like macrophages express surface receptors for Fc. This allows targeting of the opsonized (antibody-coated) antigen to these cells, followed by enhanced phagocytosis.
2. Immune complexes (antibodies bound to target antigens) can activate complement, a system of proteins which then becomes cytolytic to bacteria, enveloped viruses or infected cells.
3. Phagocytic cells may express receptors for complement factors associated with immune complexes. Binding of these activated complement factors enhances phagocytosis.
4. Viruses can be neutralized by antibodies through binding at or near receptor binding sites on the virus surface. This neutralization may prevent binding to and entry into the host cell.

Antibodies are effective against certain but not all infectious microorganisms; they may have limited therapeutic value when CMI is the major protective mechanism. CMI refers to the induction of cytotoxic cells (see above). Of the cell types that are known to exhibit cytotoxicity, two are antigen-sensitized. Because of their specificity, they are of special importance with respect to vaccine design:

1. Cytotoxic T-lymphocytes (CTLs) react with target cells and kill them by releasing cytolytic proteins like perforin. Target cells express non-self antigens like viral proteins or tumor antigens, by which they are identified. CTL responses, as antibody responses, are highly specific.
2. T-cells involved in delayed type hypersensitivity (T_{DTH}) are able to kill target cells as CTLs do, but also have helper (T_{h1}-type, see below) functions that enable them to activate macrophages.

Macrophages, which can be activated as accessory factors in humoral as well as cellular immune responses (Table 12.2), engulf infected cells and foreign particulate material. Other less specific cells involved in cytotoxic immune responses are natural killer cells (NK-cells). These play a role in antibody-dependent cellular cytotoxicity (ADCC), and recognize opsonized (antibody coated) cells with their Fc-receptors.

Besides plasma cells and cytotoxic cells, memory B- and T-cells may develop. Memory B-cells do not produce soluble antibody, but on repeated antigen contact their response time is shorter compared to naïve B-cells. Currently, it is not clear how immunization can result in immunity for decades. Induction of a long-lasting (preferably lifelong) memory is nevertheless one of the main objectives in vaccinology (see Figure 12.1).

The occurrence of different types of immune responses to vaccines is the result of the differences by which antigen-presenting cells (APCs) process the vaccine. One of the results is the activation of T_h-cells (Figure 12.3). Major histocompatibility complex (MHC) molecules play an important role in the presentation of processed antigens to T-cells. Cells expose either MHC class I or II molecules on their surface.

APCs carrying class II molecules process soluble, exogenous (extracellular) proteins or more complicated structures such as microorganisms (see Figure 12.3, panel A). After their endocytosis, the proteins are subject to limited proteolysis before they return as peptides to the surface of the APC, in combination with the class II molecules, for presentation to a T-cell receptor of CD4 positive T_h-cells. The T_h-cells provide type 2 help necessary for the effector function of B-cells. This type 2 help is characterized by the lymphokine pattern produced: interleukin 4 (IL-4), IL-5, IL-6, IL-10 and IL-13. These lymphokines trigger B-cells, which eventually results in the production of IgM and IgG antibodies.

Cells carrying MHC class I molecules process endogenous (intracellularly produced) antigens like viral and tumor antigens, and present them in combination with class I molecules on the cell surface (see Figure 12.3, panel C). The class I-antigen combination on the APC is recognized by the T-cell receptor of CD8 positive CTLs. T_h-cells provide help for the CTLs. For the induction of CMI (Figure 12.3, panels A and C), type 1 help is needed (production of IL-2 and IL-12, interferon-γ, and tumor necrosis factor). T_h-cells are CD4 positive, regardless of whether they have T_{h1} or T_{h2} functions. There is increasing evidence that the T_{h1}/T_{h2} balance is an important immunological parameter since some diseases coincide with T_{h1} (autoimmunity) or T_{h2} (allergy) type responses.

Vaccine Design in Relation to the Immune Response

For the rational design of a new vaccine, understanding the mechanisms of the protective immunity to the pathogen against which the vaccine is developed is crucial. For instance, to prevent tetanus a high blood titer of antibody against tetanus toxin is required; in mycobacterial diseases such as tuberculosis a macrophage-activating CMI is most effective; in the case of an influenza, virus infection CTLs probably play a significant role. The immune effector mechanisms are triggered by a vaccine and, hence, the success of immunization not only depend on the nature of the protective components but also on their presentation form, the presence of adjuvants, and the route of administration (see below).

The response by B-cells is dependent upon the nature of the antigen; two types of antigens have been distinguished. (1) Thymus-independent antigens include certain linear antigens that are not readily degraded in the body and have a repeating determinant, such as bacterial polysaccharides. They are able to stimulate B-cells without the T_h-cell involvement. Thymus-independent antigens do not induce immunological memory. (2) Thymus-dependent antigens provoke little or no antibody response in animals with few T-cells. Proteins are the typical representatives of thymus-dependent antigens. A prerequisite for thymus-dependency is that a physical linkage exists between the sites recognized by B-cells and those by T_h-cells. When a thymus-independent antigen is coupled to a carrier protein containing T_h-epitopes, it becomes thymus-dependent. As a result, these conjugates are able to induce memory.

When the vaccine is a protein, the epitopes can be continuous or discontinuous. Continuous epitopes involve linear peptide sequences (usually consisting of up to ten amino acid residues) of the protein (see Figure 12.7, panel A). Discontinuous epitopes comprise amino acid residues sometimes far apart in the primary sequence, which are brought together through the unique folding of the protein (see Figure 12.7, panel B). Antibody recognition of B-cell epitopes, whether continuous or discontinuous, is usually dependent on the conformation (= three-dimensional structure). T-cell epitopes, on the other hand, are continuous peptide sequences, whose conformation does not seem to play a role in T-cell recognition.

Route of Administration

The immunological response to a vaccine is also dependent on the route of administration. Most current vaccines are administered intramuscularly, with some exceptions, such as live polio vaccine and live typhoid vaccine, which are administered orally. Parenteral immunization usually induces systemic immunity. However, local immunization may be preferred, because mucosal surfaces are the common entrance of many pathogens. The induction of a local humoral response of secretory IgA may prevent the attachment and entry into the host. For example, antibodies against cholera need to be in the gut lumen to inhibit adherence to and colonization of the intestinal wall. Moreover, local (oral, intranasal, or intravaginal) immunization is attractive because it may induce not only mucosal immunity, but also systemic immunity. For example, orally administered *Salmonella typhi* not only invades the mucosal lining of the gut, but also infects cells of the phagocytic system throughout the body, thereby stimulating the production of both secretory and systemic antibodies, as well as CMI. Additional advantages of local immunization are the ease of administration and the avoidance of systemic side-effects (Walker, 1994; Shalaby, 1995). Up to now, however, successful local immunization has only been achieved with a limited number of oral vaccines. The formulation of the antigens is probably crucial for the success of local immunization.

Conventional Vaccines

Classification

Conventional vaccines originate from viruses or bacteria and can be divided into live attenuated vaccines and non-living vaccines. In addition, three vaccine generations can be distinguished for non-living vaccines. The *first generation* vaccine consists of an inactivated suspension of the pathogenic microorganism. Little or no purification is applied. For *second generation* non-living vaccines purification steps are applied, varying from the purification of a pathogenic microorganism, such as improved non-living polio vaccine, to the complete purification of the protective component like the polysaccharide vaccines. The *third generation* is either a well-defined combination of protective components like the pertussis vaccine, or the protective component with the desired immunological properties as in polysaccharides conjugated with carrier proteins. Table 12.3 provides an overview of the various groups of conventional vaccines and their generations.

Live Attenuated Vaccines

Before the introduction of recombinant-DNA (rDNA) technology, a first step towards improved live vaccines was the attenuation of virulent microorganisms by serial passage and selection of mutant strains with reduced virulence or toxicity. Examples of this approach are vaccine strains for oral polio vaccine, measles-rubella-mumps (MMR) combination vaccine, and tuberculosis vaccine consisting of bacille Calmette-Guérin (BCG). An alternative approach

Type	Example	Marketed	Characteristics[a]
Live			
Viral	Adenovirus	yes	oral vaccine, USA military services only
	Poliovirus (Sabin)	yes	oral vaccine
	Hepatitis A virus	no	
	Measles virus	yes	
	Mumps virus	yes	
	Rubella virus	yes	whole organisms
	Varicella zoster virus	yes	
	Vaccinia virus	yes	
	Yellow fever virus	yes	
	Rotavirus	no	
	Influenza virus	no	
Bacterial	Bacille Calmette-Guérin	yes	whole organism
	Salmonella typhi	yes	whole organism, oral vaccine
Non-living (first generation products)			
Viral	Poliovirus (Salk)	yes	
	Influenza virus	yes	inactivated whole organisms
	Japanese B encephalitis virus	yes	
Bacterial	Bordetella pertussis	yes	
	Vibrio cholerae	yes	inactivated whole organisms
	Salmonella typhi	yes	
Non-living (second generation products)			
Viral	Poliovirus	yes	
	Rabies virus	yes	purified, inactivated whole organisms
	Hepatitis A virus	yes	
	Influenza virus	yes	subunit vaccine
	Hepatitis B virus	yes	plasma-derived hepatitis B surface antigen
Bacterial	Bordetella pertussis	yes	bacterial protein extract
	Haemophilus influenzae type b	yes	capsular polysaccharides
	Neisseria meningitidis	yes	capsular polysaccharides
	Streptococcus pneumoniae	yes	capsular polysaccharides
	Vibrio cholerae	yes	bacterial suspension + B subunit of cholera toxin
	Corynebacterium diphtheriae	yes	diphtheria toxoid
	Clostridium tetani	yes	tetanus toxoid
Non-living (third generation products)			
Viral	Measles virus	no	subunit vaccine, ISCOM formulation
Bacterial	Bordetella pertussis	yes	mixture of purified protein antigens
	Haemophilus influenzae type b	yes	polysaccharide-protein conjugates
	Neisseria meningitidis	no	polysaccharide-protein conjugates
	Streptococcus pneumoniae	no	polysaccharide-protein conjugates

Table 12.3. Conventional vaccines (source: Plotkin and Mortimer, 1994). [a] Unless mentioned otherwise, the vaccine is administered parenterally. ISCOMS: Table 12.6.

is chemical mutagenesis. For instance, by treating *Salmonella typhi* with nitrosoguanidine, a mutant strain lacking some enzymes responsible for the virulence can be isolated (Germanier and Furer, 1975).

Live attenuated organisms have a number of advantages as vaccines over non-living vaccines. After administration, live vaccines may replicate in the host similarly to their pathogenic counterparts. This replication confronts the host with a larger and more sustained dose of antigen, which means that fewer and lower doses are required. In general, these vaccines give long-lasting humoral and cell-mediated immunity.

Live vaccines also have drawbacks. Live viral vaccines bear the risk that the nucleic acid is incorporated into the host's genome. Moreover, reversion to a virulent form may occur, although this is unlikely when the attenuated seed strain contains several mutations. For diseases such as viral hepatitis, AIDS and cancer, this drawback makes the use of conventional live vaccines virtually unthinkable. Furthermore, it is important to recognize that immunization of immunodeficient children with live organisms can lead to serious complications. For instance, a child with T-cell deficiency may become overwhelmed with BCG and die.

Non-Living Vaccines: Whole Organisms

An early approach for preparing vaccines is the inactivation of whole bacteria or viruses. A number of reagents (e.g. formaldehyde, glutaraldehyde) and heat are commonly used for inactivation. Examples of this first generation approach are pertussis, cholera, typhoid fever, and inactivated polio vaccines. These non-living vaccines have the disadvantage that little or no CMI is induced. Moreover, they cause adverse effects more frequently than live attenuated vaccines and second and third generation non-living vaccines.

Non-Living Vaccines: Subunit Vaccines

Diphtheria and tetanus toxoids

Some bacteria such as *Corynebacterium diphtheriae* and *Clostridium tetani* form toxins. Antibody-mediated immunity to the toxins is the main protection mechanism against infections with these bacteria. Both toxins are proteins. Around the beginning of the twentieth century, a combination of toxin and antibodies to diphtheria toxin was used as diphtheria vaccine. This vaccine was far from ideal and was replaced in the 1920s with formaldehyde-treated toxin. The chemically treated toxin was devoid of toxic properties and was called toxoid. The immunogenicity of this preparation was relatively low and was improved after adsorption of the toxoid to a suspension of aluminum salts. This combination of an antigen and an adjuvant is still used in existing combination vaccines. Similarly, tetanus toxoid vaccines have been developed.

Diphtheria toxin has also been detoxified by chemical mutagenesis of *Corynebacterium diphtheriae* with nitrosoguanidine. These diphtheria toxoids are referred to as cross-reactive materials (e.g. CRM_{197}).

Acellular pertussis vaccines

The relatively frequent occurrence of side-effects of whole-cell pertussis vaccine was the main reason to develop subunit vaccines in the 1970s. These vaccines are referred to as acellular pertussis vaccines. These vaccines are prepared by either extraction of the bacterial suspension followed by purification steps, or purification of the cell-free culture supernatant. Although their composition is variable, they all contain detoxified pertussis toxin. These second generation vaccines show relatively large lot-to-lot variations as a result of their poorly controlled production processes.

The development of third generation acellular pertussis vaccines during the 1980s exemplifies how a better insight into factors that are important for pathogenesis and immunogenicity can lead to an improved vaccine. It was conceived that a subunit vaccine consisting of a limited number of purified immunogenic components and devoid of (toxic) lipopolysaccharide would significantly reduce undesired effects. Four protein antigens important for protection have been identified. However, there currently exists no consensus about the optimal composition of an acellular pertussis vaccine. Candidate vaccines typically contain different amounts of two to four of these proteins.

Polysaccharide vaccines

Bacterial capsular polysaccharides consist of pathogen-specific multiple repeating carbohydrate epitopes, which are isolated from cultures of the pathogenic species. Plain capsular polysaccharides (second generation vaccines) are thymus-independent antigens that are poorly immunogenic in infants and show poor immunological memory when applied in older children and adults. The immunogenicity of polysaccharides is highly increased when they are chemically coupled to carrier proteins containing T_h-epitopes. This coupling makes them T-cell dependent, due to the participation of T_h-cells activated during the response to the carrier. Examples of such third generation polysaccharide conjugate vaccines include *Haemophilus influenzae* type b polysaccharide vaccines recently introduced in many national immunization programs. Four different conjugated polysaccharide structures are presently available, chemically linked to either tetanus toxoid, diphtheria toxoid, CRM_{197} (mutagenically detoxified diphtheria toxin, see above), or meningococcal outer membrane complexes. Apart from the carrier, the four structures vary in the size of the polysaccharide moiety, the nature of the spacer group, the ratio of polysaccharide-to-protein, and the molecular size and aggregation state of the conjugates. As a result, they induce different immunological responses, illustrating not only the nature of the antigen, but also its presentation form that determines the immunogenicity of a vaccine. Therefore, the determination of optimal conjugation procedures, the standardization of conjugation, as well as the separation of conjugates from free proteins and polysaccharides are of the utmost importance.

Modern Vaccine Technologies

Genetically Improved Live Vaccines

GENETICALLY ATTENUATED MICROORGANISMS

Emerging insights into the molecular pathogenesis of many infectious diseases now make it possible to attenuate microorganisms very efficiently. By making multiple deletions the risk of reversion to a virulent state during production or after administration can be virtually eliminated. A prerequisite for attenuation by genetic engineering is that the factors responsible for virulence and the life cycle of the pathogen are known in detail. It is also obvious that the protective antigens should be known: attenuation must not result in reduced immunogenicity.

An example of an improved live vaccine obtained by homologous genetic engineering is an experimental, oral cholera vaccine. An effective cholera vaccine should induce a local, humoral response in order to prevent colonization of the small intestine. Initial trials with *Vibrio cholerae* cholera toxin (CT) mutants caused mild diarrhea, most likely induced by the expression of accessory toxins. A natural mutant was isolated that was negative for these toxins. Next, CT was detoxified using rDNA technology. The resulting vaccine strain, called CVD 103, is well tolerated by children (Suharyono *et al.*, 1992) and challenge experiments with adult volunteers showed protection (Tacket *et al.*, 1992).

Genetically attenuated live vaccines have the same general drawbacks as conventionally attenuated live vaccines. For these reasons, it is not surprising that homologous engineering is mainly restricted to pathogens that are used as starting materials for the production of subunit vaccines (see the section "Genetically Improved Subunit Vaccines," below).

LIVE VECTORS

One way to improve the safety or efficacy of vaccines is using live, harmless (i.e. non-pathogenic or attenuated) viruses or bacteria as carriers for antigens from other pathogens. These are called vectors. Potentially useful vectors are listed in Table 12.4.

Most of the knowledge about vectors has been acquired from the vaccinia virus by using the principle that is schematically shown in Figure 12.4. Advantages of vaccinia virus as a vector include: (1) its proven safety in humans as a smallpox vaccine; (2) the possibility for multiple immunogen expression; (3) its ease of production; (4) its relative heat-resistance, and; (5) its various routes of administration. A multitude of live recombinant vaccinia vaccines with viral and tumor antigens have been constructed (Flexner and Moss, 1997), and several have been tested in clinical settings. It has been demonstrated that the products of genes coding for viral envelope proteins

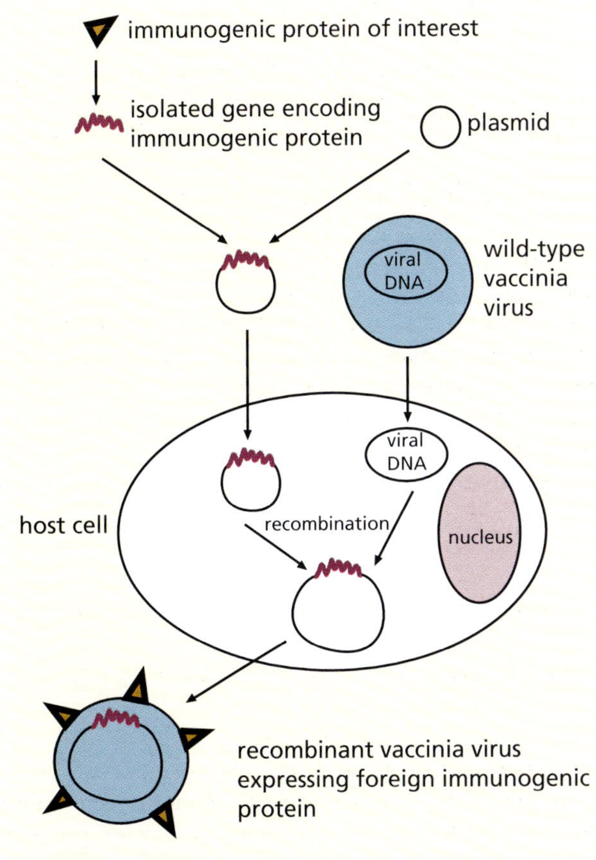

Figure 12.4. Construction of recombinant vaccinia virus as a vector of foreign protein antigens. The gene of interest encoding an immunogenic protein is inserted into a plasmid. The plasmid containing the protein gene and wild-type vaccinia virus are then simultaneously introduced into a host cell line to undergo recombination of viral and plasmid DNA, after which the foreign protein is expressed by the recombinant virus.

Vector	Antigens from	Advantages of vector	Disadvantages of vector
Viral			
Vaccinia	RSV, HIV, VSV, Rabies virus, HSV, Influenza virus, EBV, Plasmodium spp. (malaria)	widely used in man (safe); large insertions possible (up to 41 kB)	sometimes causing side effects; very immunogenic: repeated use difficult
Avipox viruses (canary-pox, fowlpox)	Rabies virus, Measles virus	abortive replication in man low immunogenicity	
Poliovirus	Vibrio cholerae, Influenza virus, HIV, Chlamydia	widely used in man (safe) live/oral and inactivated/parenteral forms possible	small genome
Adenoviruses	RSV, HBV, EBV, HIV, CMV	oral route applicable	small genome
Herpes viruses (HSV, CMV, varicella virus)	EBV, HBV	large genome	
Bacterial			
Salmonella spp.	B. pertussis, HBV, Plasmodium spp., E. coli, Influenza virus, Streptococci, Vibrio cholerae, Shigella spp.	strong mucosal responses	
Mycobacteria (BCG)	Borrelia burgdorferi (lyme disease)	widely used in man (safe)	
E. coli	Bordetella pertussis, Shigella flexneri		

Table 12.4. Recombinant live vaccines. BCG = bacille Calmette-Gurin; CMV = cytomegalovirus; EBV = Epstein-Barr virus; HBV = hepatitis B virus; HIV = human immunodeficiency virus; HSV = herpes simplex virus; RSV = respiratory syncytial virus; VSV = vesicular stomatitis virus.

can be correctly processed and inserted into the plasma membrane of infected cells. Problems related to the side-effects or immunogenicity of vaccinia may be circumvented by the use of attenuated strains or poxviruses with a non-human natural host.

Genetically Improved Subunit Vaccines

Genetically detoxified proteins

A biotechnological improvement of the acellular pertussis vaccine has been the switch from chemically to genetically inactivated pertussis toxin. The principle of both chemical and genetic inactivation is schematically illustrated in Figure 12.5. Chemical treatment with formaldehyde results in a crippled protein molecule with partial loss of conformational and antigenic properties (Figure 12.5, panel B). This crippling reduces its immunogenicity, and potential reversal to a biologically active toxin is a major concern. Variations in the extent of detoxification can affect both the immunogenicity and the toxicity of the product. In contrast, genetic detoxification by site-directed mutagenesis warrants the reproducible production of a non-toxic mutant protein that is highly immunogenic because the integrity of immunogenic sites is fully retained (Figure 12.5, panel C). In the pertussis toxin example, codons for two amino acids were mutated in the cloned pertussis gene, abolishing the toxicity of the protein without changing its immunological properties. The altered gene was then substituted in *Bordetella pertussis* for the native gene (Nencioni *et al.*, 1990). Other candidates for genetic detoxification are diphtheria toxin, tetanus toxin, and cholera toxin. Alternatively, proteins can be detoxified by the genetic deletion of active sites or subunits.

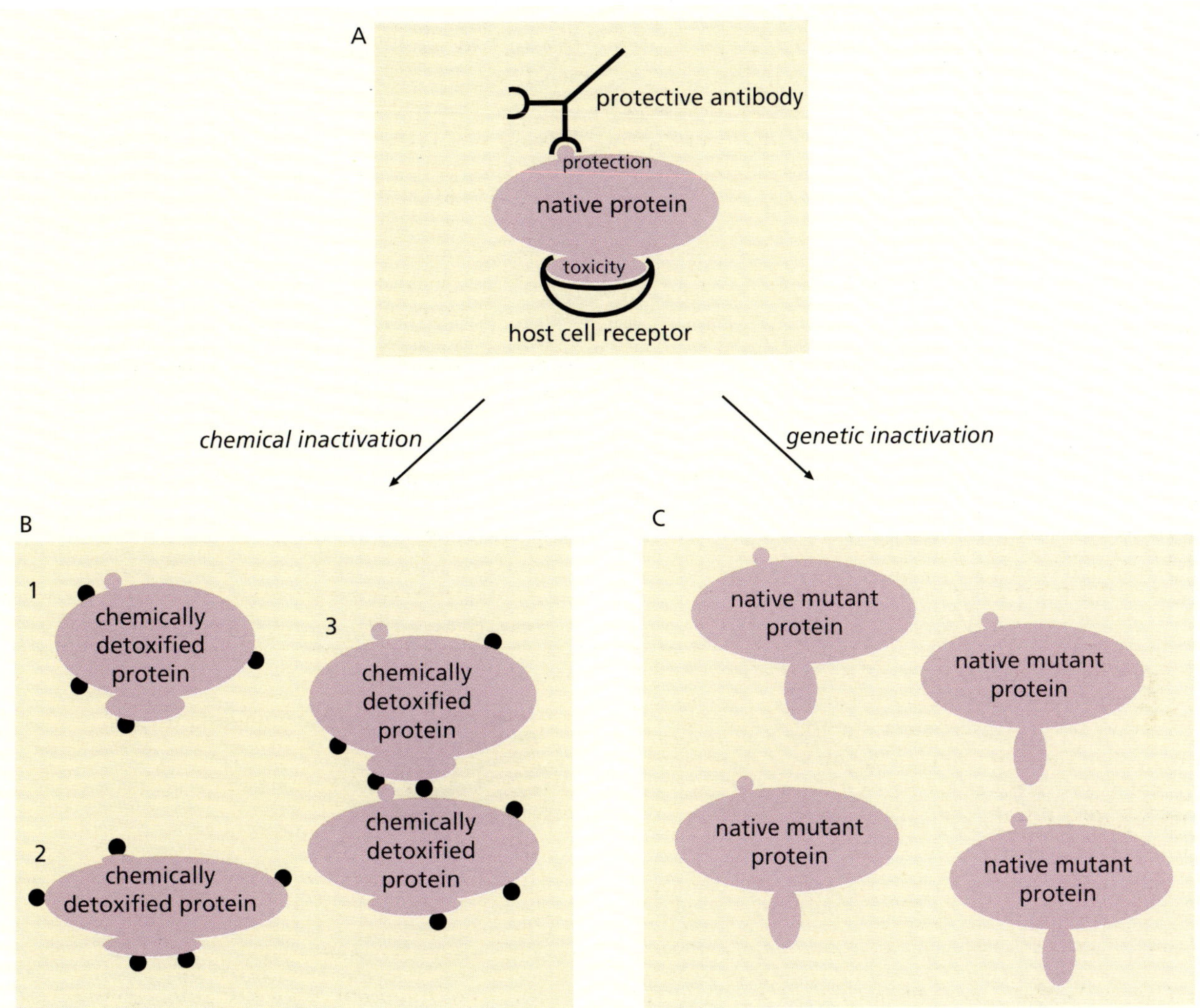

Figure 12.5. Schematic representation of chemical and genetic detoxification of immunogenic toxins. A hypothetical toxin contains an epitope recognized by protective antibodies and a site responsible for toxicity through interaction with a host cell receptor (panel A). Toxins can be chemically inactivated by treatment with (usually) formaldehyde, resulting in a heterogeneous population of chemically detoxified proteins that carry covalently bound formaldehyde residues on their surface (represented by black spheres in panel B). Chemically detoxified proteins preferably retain protective epitopes while the toxicity-related site is blocked (B1). However, part of the protein population may contain epitopes that are no longer recognized by protective antibodies (B2). Formaldehyde treatment may also lead to the formation of covalent multimers (B3) and slight perturbations of the three-dimensional protein structure (B2, B3). Apart from chemical inactivation, toxins can be genetically detoxified by selectively changing the amino acid sequence in the site responsible for toxicity without affecting the protective epitope, resulting in a homogeneous toxoid population (panel C).

PROTEINS EXPRESSED IN HOST CELLS

To improve yield, facilitate the production, and/or improve the safety of protein-based vaccines, protein antigens are sometimes expressed by host cells of the same (homologous) species or of different (heterologous) species that are safe to handle and/or allow high expression levels.

Heterologous hosts used for the expression of immunogenic proteins include yeasts, bacteria, and mammalian cell lines. Hepatitis B surface antigen (HBsAg), which was obtained previously from the plasma of infected individuals, has been expressed in bakers' yeast (*Saccharomyces cerevisae*; Valenzuela *et al.*, 1982) and in mammalian cells (Chinese Hamster Ovary cells; Burnette *et al.*, 1985) by transforming the host cell with a plasmid containing the HBsAg-encoding gene. Both expression systems yield 22-nm HBsAg particles (also referred to as virus like particles or VLPs) that are identical to those excreted by the native virus. Their advantages are safety, consistent quality, and high yields. The yeast-derived vaccine has become available worldwide and appears to be as safe and efficacious as the classical plasma-derived vaccine.

The experimental multivalent meningococcal vesicle vaccine is an example of the expression of multiple antigens in homologous host cells (Van der Ley *et al.*, 1995). The vaccine is prepared by extraction of vesicles from the meningococcal outer membrane. These vesicles serve as a natural carrier for immunogenic outer membrane proteins (OMPs), incorporated into the vesicle membrane. Each wild-type meningococcus strain expresses strain-specific OMPs. Taking a wild-type strain as starting point, mutant strains expressing OMPs specific for three strains have been made through transformation with plasmid constructs in *E. coli* and their recombination into the meningococcal chromosome. Outer membrane vesicles of two trivalent strains have been prepared and combined to a hexavalent vaccine, shown to be immunogenic in infants (Cartwright *et al.*, 1999).

An interesting development is the exploration of transgenic plants for their potential as a heterologous expression system for antigenic components (Richter and Kipp, 1999). This approach aims to express antigenic components in edible (parts of) plants, such as bananas. Advantages of edible vaccines include: (1) no need for purification; (2) ease of immunization; (3) built-in protection of antigens by cell walls and cellular membranes, and; (4) the possibility of local production in developing countries. Problems related to the production of edible vaccines are the low expression levels and the control of the level and quality of the antigen. Examples of candidate vaccine components are VLPs, such as HBsAg and Norwalk virus capsid protein.

Recombinant peptide vaccines

After the identification of a protective epitope, it is possible to incorporate the corresponding peptide sequence into a carrier protein containing T_h-epitopes through genetic fusion (Francis, 1991). The peptide-encoding DNA sequence is synthesized and inserted into the carrier protein gene. Such fusion proteins comprise HBsAg, hepatitis B core antigen, and β-galactosidase. An example of the recombinant peptide approach is a malaria vaccine based on a 16-fold repeat of the Asn-Ala-Asn-Pro sequence of a *Plasmodium falciparum* surface antigen. The gene encoding this peptide was fused with the HBsAg gene and the fusion product was expressed by yeast cells (Vreden *et al.*, 1991). Genetic fusion of peptides with proteins offers the possibility of producing protective epitopes of toxic antigens derived from pathogenic species as part of non-toxic proteins expressed by harmless species. Furthermore, the product obtained is uniform compared to the variability of chemical conjugates (see the section "Synthetic Peptide-Based Vaccines," below).

Anti-Idiotype Antibody Vaccines

Antibodies can be elicited against any antigenic structure on almost any molecule, including antibodies themselves. The concept of anti-idiotype vaccines is to elicit antibodies against the antigen-binding site of protective antibodies (Figure 12.6). First, a monoclonal antibody (Mab-1) that recognizes a protective epitope of a particular immunogen is selected. Next, a monoclonal antibody (Mab-2) is generated against the idiotype, such as the three-dimensional structure of the antigen-binding site of Mab-1. Hence, Mab-2 immunologically mimics the protective epitope of the immunogen and may thus be used as a vaccine component. The original epitope is not necessarily of protein origin, implying that immunological mimicry is not always present at the atomic level (Pan *et al.*, 1995). This latter fart makes the approach especially attractive for non-protein epitopes.

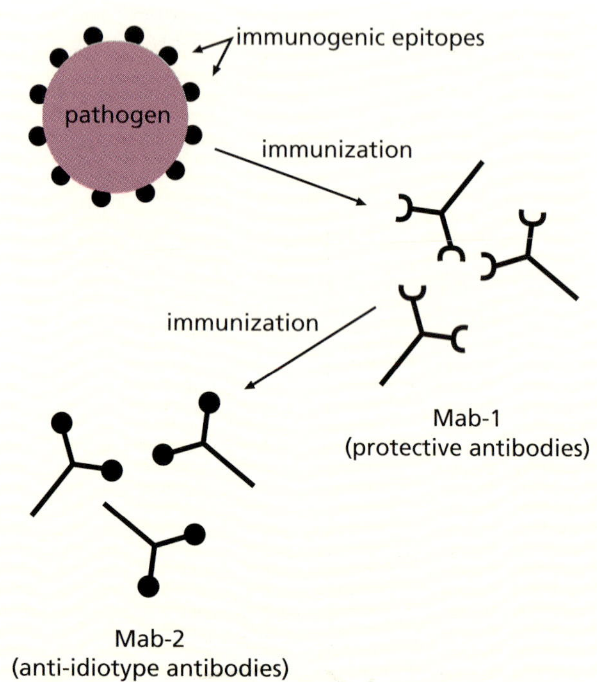

Figure 12.6. The anti-idiotype vaccine concept. Immunization of animals with a pathogen elicits antibodies against immunogenic epitopes on that pathogen. Antibodies are screened for protection and a protective monoclonal antibody (Mab-1) is selected. Subsequently, a different animal species is immunized with Mab-1. A selected monoclonal antibody (Mab-2) recognizing the antigen-binding site (the idiotype) of Mab-1 mimics the immunogenic epitope of the pathogen and can thus serve as vaccine component.

For instance, anti-idiotype antibodies carrying the 'internal image' of carbohydrates that are difficult to produce and/or isolate in large quantities, or of immunogenic carbohydrate residues of toxic lipopolysaccharides or glycoproteins, may serve as vaccine components.

Large quantities of monoclonal antibodies are easy to produce using modern hybridoma technology. Experimental anti-idiotype vaccines that have been studied in animals include a *Streptococcus pneumoniae* vaccine based on phosphorylcholine-mimicking antibodies (McNamara *et al.*, 1984) and a vaccine consisting of anti-idiotype antibodies resembling lipopolysaccharide from *Pseudomonas aeruginosa* (Schreiber *et al.*, 1991). The clinical applicability of anti-idiotype antibodies, however, remains to be established. A drawback is that the major structural part of the anti-idiotype antibody molecule does not have any relationship with the structure of the original antigen and may give rise to unwanted (immunological) reactions, unless human, humanized, and/or single-chain Mabs are used, (discussed later in Chapter 13).

Synthetic Peptide-Based Vaccines

Another form of molecular mimicry is synthetic peptides, which are vigorously being explored for immunization. With recent improvements in solid-phase peptide synthesis, large quantities of oligopeptides that are capable of eliciting an immune response toward the native protein can be readily prepared. Primarily, peptide-based vaccines have been designed based on antibody recognition. Two approaches are used, as outlined in Figure 12.7, depending on whether the epitope is continuous or discontinuous.

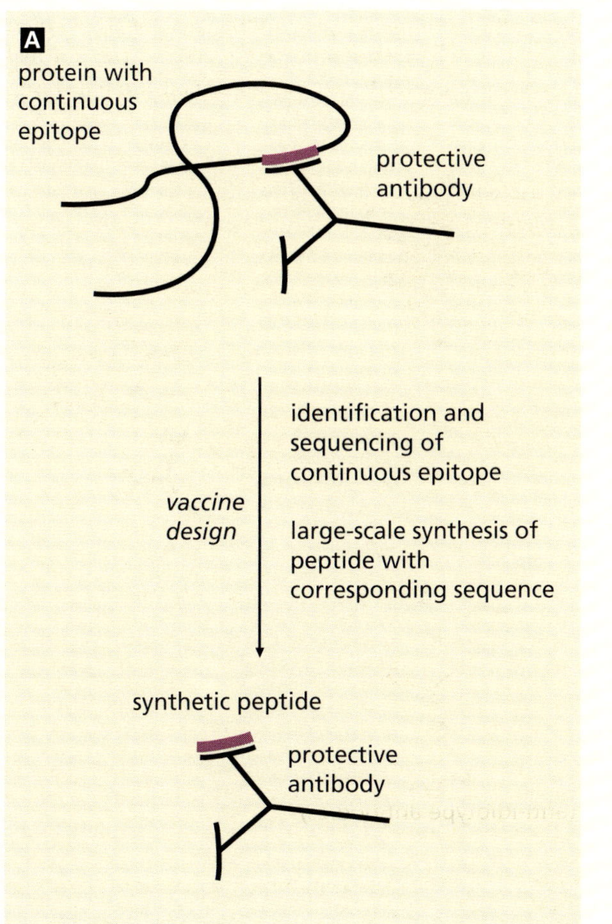

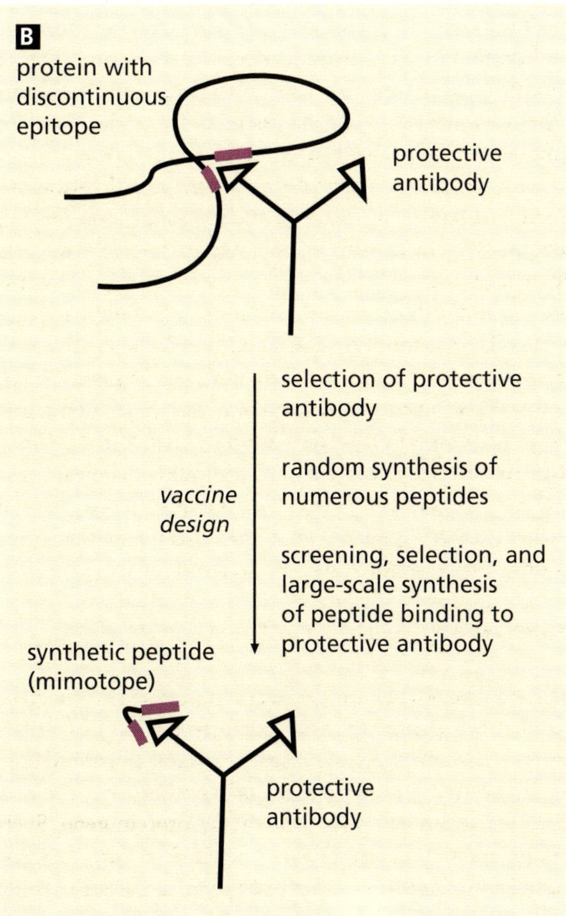

Figure 12.7. Two approaches for the design of synthetic peptide vaccines. Panel A: identification and sequencing of a continuous epitope on an immunogenic protein is followed by the synthesis of peptides with the amino acid sequence corresponding to that of the epitope. Panel B: synthesis of peptides mimicking discontinuous epitopes that are determined by the three-dimensional structure of the immunogenic protein; a peptide that strongly binds to a protective antibody recognizing the discontinuous epitope is selected. The peptide (mimotope) does not necessarily contain the exact amino acid sequence of the constituent fragments that form the epitope.

In the first approach (Figure 12.7, panel A) immunogenic epitopes are determined by DNA cloning and nucleotide sequencing of protein antigens and serology studies. The small linear peptide sequence is chemically synthesized and can be used as a vaccine component. A limitation of this concept is that it is only applicable to continuous epitopes that are solely determined by the primary amino acid sequence and not by the conformation of the epitope. Many B-cell epitopes, however, are conformationally determined and/or discontinuous. For continuous conformational epitopes, synthetic peptides can be forced to adopt the proper conformation by cyclization (see below).

The second approach (Figure 12.7, panel B) is particularly useful for discontinuous epitopes. In this case, the optimal sequence of a synthetic peptide is not easy to determine *a priori*. With current technology, however, thousands of peptides are rapidly synthesized at random and screened for optimal binding to protective antibodies. The sequence of a specific peptide can, if necessary, be optimized for antibody binding by selectively substituting one or more amino acid residues. Such peptides approximating the native epitope – but not necessarily containing the exact (linear or non-linear) sequence of the epitope – are referred to as mimotopes. In theory, analogous with anti-idiotype antibodies, mimotopes may be useful as an internal image not only of peptide epitopes but also of non-protein structures.

Similar to B-cell epitope peptides, T-cell epitope peptide vaccines can also be designed. T-cell epitopes usually have a continuous, non-conformational nature and are relatively easy to mimic after their sequence has been identified, analogous to the approach for continuous B-cell epitopes.

Synthetic peptide vaccines have the following advantages:

1. they can be prepared in unlimited quantities using solid-phase technology;
2. they are easily purified by HPLC methods;
3. they do not contain infectious or toxic material.

The use of synthetic peptides as vaccines has two main complications regarding their immunogenicity. First, plain short peptide antigens are usually poorly immunogenic. This trait can be alleviated by (1) synthesizing them as multiple antigen peptides (MAPs; Tam, 1988) or (2) by coupling them to a carrier protein (Francis, 1991). MAPs consist of branched multimers with a small oligolysine core at the center. Apart from MAPs containing multiple copies of a single epitope, multivalent peptides consisting of different covalently linked epitopes can be constructed, including combinations of B-cell and T-cell epitopes. Examples of increased immunogenicity of synthetic MAPs are experimental malaria vaccines consisting of combined B-cell and T-cell epitopes (Tam *et al.*, 1990) or a multimeric tetrapeptide with the sequence of a repetitive *Plasmodium falciparum* surface antigen epitope (Pessi *et al.*, 1991). A convincing success of a synthetic peptide-carrier protein vaccine *in vivo* was reported by Langeveld *et al.* (1994). Peptides with the sequence of the amino-terminal region of protein VP2 of canine parvovirus were synthesized and chemically coupled to a protein (keyhole limpet hemocyanin). This vaccine induced full protection against virulent virus in dogs.

A second concern about synthetic peptide analogs is that they can adopt various conformations, which upon immunization may give rise to antibodies that recognize the peptide but not the native antigen. This is especially true for conformational epitopes. This problem may be overcome by the cyclization of peptides using chemical linkers (usually oligopeptides). Thus, the conformation of the peptide is constrained to that of the native epitope. The nature of the peptide, as well as the length and conformation of the cyclic construct, determine the success of cyclization, as illustrated in Figure 12.8. One of the first examples of the successful induction of the proper conformation through cyclization was reported by Muller *et al.* (1990). Antibodies raised to ovalbumin conjugates of cyclic peptide analogs of the influenza virus hemagglutinin reacted with native hemagglutinin. The immunogenicity of the peptides was strongly dependent on the loop conformation and on the orientation of the peptide on the carrier protein. Hoogerhout *et al.* (1995) showed that the ring size and the cyclization chemistry are of crucial importance for the immunogenicity of cyclic peptide analogs (coupled to tetanus toxoid) of a meningococcal OMP epitope.

Nucleic Acid Vaccines

A revolutionary application of rDNA technology in vaccinology has been the introduction of nucleic acid vaccines (Davis and Whalen, 1995). In this approach plasmid DNA or messenger RNA encoding the desired antigen is directly administered into the vaccinee. The host cells then express the foreign protein that generates an immune response.

Plasmid DNA is produced by the replication in *E. coli* or other bacterial cells and purification occurs by established methods (e.g. density gradient centrifugation, ion-exchange chromatography). Until now plasmid DNA has been administered to animals and humans mostly via intramuscular injection. The favorable properties of muscle cells for DNA expression are probably due to their relatively low turnover rate, preventing plasmid DNA from being rapidly dispersed in dividing cells. After the intracellular uptake of the DNA, the encoded protein is expressed on the surface of host cells. After a single injection, the expression can last for more than one year. Besides intramuscular injection, subcutaneous, intradermal, and intranasal administrations also seem to be effective.

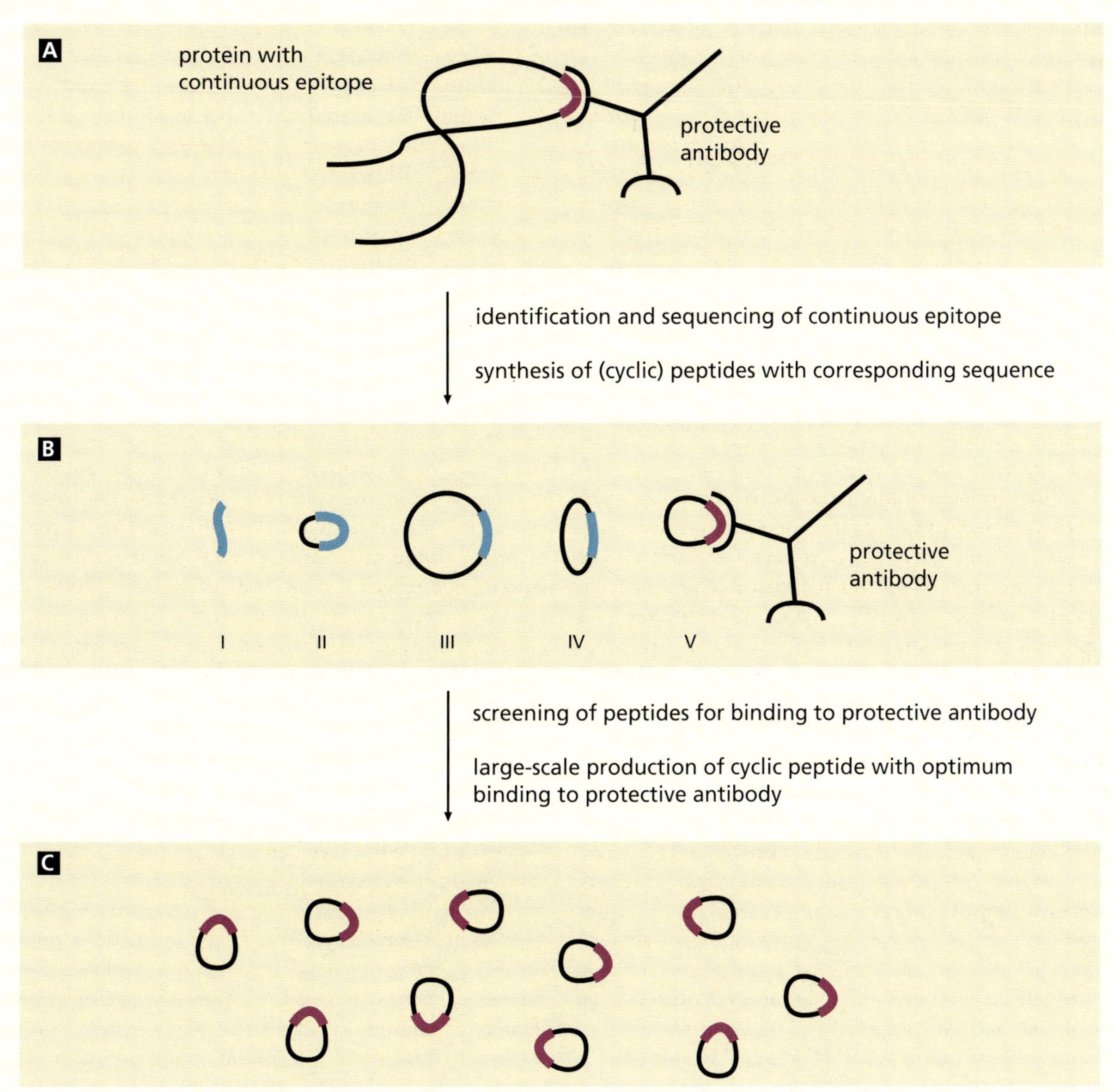

Figure 12.8. Design of synthetic peptide vaccines by cyclization of continuous, conformational epitopes. First, a continuous epitope that evokes protective antibodies is identified and sequenced (panel A). Next, peptides with the amino acid sequence corresponding to that of the epitope are synthesized (whether or not with a linker to form a loop structure) and are screened for binding to protective antibody (panel B). In this example, immunization with peptides I-IV would induce non-protective antibodies to the misfolded epitope. Linear peptide I does not have the proper conformation corresponding to that on the native protein. Loops for cyclization in peptides II-IV are too short (II), too long (III) or improperly folded (IV), thereby inducing incorrect peptide conformations. Cyclic peptide V has the correct native conformation and is likely to induce protective antibody formation upon immunization. Therefore, cyclic peptide V is produced for vaccine purposes (panel C).

Needleless injection into the skin of DNA-coated gold nanoparticles via a gene gun has been reported to require up to 1000-fold less DNA when compared to intramuscular administration.

Nucleic acid vaccines offer the safety of subunit vaccines and the advantages of live recombinant vaccines. Possible disadvantages of nucleic acid immunization concern acceptability issues. In particular, the long-term safety of nucleic

Advantages	Disadvantages
Low intrinsic immunogenicity of nucleic acids	effects of long-term expression unknown
Induction of long-term immune responses	formation of anti-nucleic acid antibodies possible
Induction of both humoral and cellular immune responses	possible integration of the vaccine DNA into the host genome
Possibility of constructing multiple epitope plasmids	concept restricted to peptide and protein antigens
Heat-stability	
Ease of large-scale production	

Table 12.5. Advantages and disadvantages of nucleic acid vaccines.

acid vaccines remains to be established. The main pros and cons of nucleic acid vaccines are listed in Table 12.5. An advantage of RNA over DNA is that it is not able to incorporate into host DNA. A drawback of RNA, however, is that it is less stable than DNA. Nucleic acids coding for a variety of antigens have shown to induce protective, long-lived humoral and cellular immune responses in various species, including man. Examples of DNA vaccines that have been tested in clinical trials comprise plasmids encoding HIV-1 antigens and malaria antigens.

Pharmaceutical Considerations

Production

Except for synthetic peptides, vaccines are derived from microorganisms or animal cells. For optimal expression of the required vaccine component(s), these microorganisms or animal cells can be genetically modified. Animal cells are used for the cultivation of viruses and for the production of some subunit vaccine components. Animal cells also have the advantage of releasing the vaccine components into the culture medium.

Three stages can be discerned in the manufacture of cell-derived vaccines: (1) cultivation; (2) downstream processing, and; (3) formulation. In this section the first two stages (cf. Chapters 3 and 4) will be presented briefly, whereas the formulation is addressed in the next section.

The development of the seed strain is a crucial part in the development of vaccines. The strain has to be characterized well in order to insure its genetic stability (e.g. with regard to the synthesis of the antigens) during cultivation. Next, the master and working seed lots are prepared. The development of the strain as well as the production and control of the seed lots must be performed under "good manufacturing practice" (GMP) conditions.

Bacteria and yeasts are relatively easily cultivated in bioreactors (cf. Chapter 3). The cultivation of animal cells is more complicated, because they are very sensitive to environmental factors such as shear and oxygen concentration, and the composition of the culture media is complex. The seed culture, the medium composition, the cultivation conditions (such as pH, dissolved oxygen), and the criteria for harvesting should be well defined. The cultivation conditions are chosen in such a way that scaling up to production scale does not affect the quality of the vaccine component.

After cultivation, the vaccine component is separated from the bacteria, yeasts, or animal cells, and from other unwanted cell suspension components. The applied downstream processing procedures depend on several factors, such as the cell type, the localization (cellular or released) of the vaccine component, and the physico-chemical characteristics of the component. If the component is linked to a microorganism or a cell, the microorganisms or cells have to be collected; if the component is secreted, the cell-free culture liquid has to be collected. Filtration and centrifugation techniques are most commonly applied for the separation of cells and the cell-free culture liquid. For the release of cell-associated vaccine components, the cells are to be extracted or disrupted by physical, chemical or enzymatic methods, and the cellular mass must be removed by filtration or centrifugation. Subsequently, the cell-free component is processed in a series of purification steps (e.g. column chromatography, extraction with organic solvents, precipitation techniques) and a viral inactivation step, if necessary. After this stage the purified vaccine component –referred to as bulk product– is ready for formulation.

In modern vaccine production, consistency of production is a major issue; lot-to-lot variations of bulk products should be minimal. This goal is realized by applying rigorous GMP rules, including the control and validation of each production step, well-written standard operating procedures, collection of all relevant production data including results of the controls of intermediate and bulk products, and comparison of these data with those of previous lots. The implementation of automated production steps, in-process controls, as well as data analysis and collection, is currently becoming common practice in production lines.

Formulation

Additives

Vaccine formulations may include buffer components, salts, preservatives, and stabilizers. These additives should not adversely affect vaccine components upon addition, storage, and application. Preservatives used include thimerosal, phenoxyethanol, phenol, and antibiotics. Stabilizers may be proteins or other (bio)polymers, carbohydrates, sugar alcohols or any other substances that can serve to prolong the vaccine shelf life and/or to minimize deleterious effects of freeze-drying (cf. Chapter 4). Formaldehyde, used as an inactivating agent of toxins and poliovirus, is often present in final products where it serves as a stabilizer of vaccine components. An alternative approach for vaccine stabilization is the encapsulation of vaccine components in biodegradable microspheres. This approach may prevent their degradation by low pH and lytic enzymes in the gastrointestinal tract upon oral administration (Morris *et al.*, 1994).

Adjuvants and delivery systems

The success of immunization is not only dependent on the nature of the immunogenic components, but also on their presentation form. Therefore, the search for effective and acceptable adjuvants and delivery systems (Gupta *et al.*, 1993) is an important issue in modern vaccine development. Adjuvants are defined as any material that can increase the humoral and cellular response against an antigen. Colloidal aluminum salts (hydroxide, phosphate) are widely used in many classical vaccine formulations. Other adjuvants are in experimental testing or are sometimes used in veterinary vaccines. Delivery systems are injectable devices that allow the multimeric presentation of antigens and may also contain adjuvants. Table 12.6 shows a list of some well-known adjuvants and delivery systems.

Unfortunately, the mode of action of adjuvants has not yet been fully unraveled. Better insight into adjuvant action would aid in the rational design of vaccine formulations. Mechanisms proposed for adjuvant action include:

1. slow release of the antigen;
2. attraction and stimulation of macrophages and lymphocytes;
3. delivery of the antigen to regional lymph nodes.

Combination vaccines

Since oral immunization is not possible for most available vaccines (see the section "Route of Administration," above), mixing individual vaccines in order to limit the number of injections has long been common practice. Traditional examples are diphtheria-tetanus-pertussis (DTP) vaccines and DTP with non-living (inactivated) polio vaccine (IPV) as a fourth component. Recently, a combination of DTP-IPV and *Haemophilus influenzae* type b vaccine has become available. Another example is the measles-mumps-rubella (MMR) vaccine, alone or in combination with varicella vaccine.

Combining vaccine components may face pharmaceutical as well as immunological problems. For instance, formaldehyde-containing components may chemically react with other components; thimerosal (e.g. in DTP vaccine) is incompatible with IPV and can therefore not be added to combination vaccines containing the polio component. Components that are not compatible can be mixed prior to injection if there is no short-term incompatibility. For this purpose dual-chamber syringes have been developed, e.g. for the *H. influenzae*-DTP vaccine (Hoppenbrouwers *et al.*, 1998).

From an immunological point of view, the immunization schedules of the individual components of combination vaccines should match. Even when this condition is fulfilled and the components are pharmaceutically compatible, the success of a combination vaccine is not guaranteed, because vaccine components in combination vaccines may exhibit a different behavior *in vivo* compared to separate administration of the components. For instance, enhancement (Paradiso *et al.*, 1993) as well as suppression (Gold *et al.*, 1994) of humoral immune responses have been reported in field trials.

The use of live vectors such as vaccinia to express multiple antigens would technically facilitate the pharmaceutical formulation of combination vaccines. This technical facilitation may also hold true for nucleic acid vaccines, which can simply be mixed. Peptide or polysaccharide conjugate vaccine components can be combined after or perhaps during conjugation with a carrier protein.

Characterization

Second and third generation conventional vaccines and modern vaccines are well-defined products in terms of immunogenicity, structure, and purity. This means that the products can be characterized with a combination of appropriate biochemical, physico-chemical, and immunochemical techniques (cf. Chapter 2). Vaccines are considered drugs and have to meet the same standards as other (biotechnological) pharmaceuticals. The use of modern analytical techniques for the design and release of new

Adjuvant	Characteristics
Aluminum salts	antigen adsorption is crucial
Lipid A and derivatives	fragment of lipopolysaccharide, a bacterial endotoxin
Muramyl peptides	active fragments of bacterial cell walls
Saponins	plant triterpene glycosides
NBP	synthetic amphiphiles
DDA	synthetic amphiphile
CpG	non-methylated DNA-sequences containing CpG-oligodinucleotides
Cytokines	interleukins (1, 2, 3, 6, 12), interferon-γ, tumor necrosis factor
Cholera toxin, B subunit	mucosal adjuvant
Delivery system	**Characteristics**
Emulsions	both water-in-oil and oil-in-water emulsions are used; often contain amphiphilic adjuvants
Liposomes	phospholipid membrane vesicles; aqueous interior as well as lipid bilayer may contain antigens and/or adjuvants
ISCOMs	micellar lipid-saponin complex; not suitable for soluble antigens
Microspheres	biodegradable polymeric spheres, often poly(lactide-co-glycolide)

Table 12.6. Adjuvants and antigen delivery systems. DDA = dioctadecyldimethylammoniumbromide; ISCOM = immune stimulating complex; NBP = non-ionic block copolymers.

vaccines is currently becoming more important. These analytical techniques may eventually partly substitute for preclinical tests *in vivo*. During the development of the production process of a vaccine component, a combination of suitable assays can be defined. These assays can be subsequently applied during its routine production.

Column chromatographic (HPLC) and electrophoretic techniques (e.g. gel electrophoresis and capillary electrophoresis) provide information about the purity, molecular weight, and electric charge of the vaccine component. For instance, formation of covalent bonds during the inactivation of toxins or viruses with formaldehyde is easily detected. Physico-chemical assays include mass spectrometry, nuclear magnetic resonance spectroscopy, and light spectroscopy, both circular dichroism and fluorescence spectroscopy. Information is obtained mainly about the molecular weight and the conformation of the vaccine component. Immunochemical assays, such as enzyme-linked immunoassays and radioimmunoassays, are powerful methods for the quantification of the vaccine component. By using well-defined monoclonal antibodies (preferably with the same specificity as those of protective human antibodies) information can be obtained about the conformation of the epitope to which the antibodies are directed. Moreover, the use of biosensors makes it possible to measure antigen-antibody interactions momentarily, allowing accurate determination of binding kinetics and affinity constants.

Storage

Depending on their specific characteristics, vaccines are stored as solution or as a freeze-dried formulation, usually at 2–8 °C. Their shelf life depends on the physico-chemical characteristics of the vaccine formulation and on the storage conditions, and typically is in the order of several years. The quality of the container can also influence the long-term stability of vaccines. For instance, adsorption or pH changes resulting from contact with the vial is a concern; evaporation or sorption of water through the stopper should be avoided. The use of pH indicators or temperature or time sensitive labels ('vial vaccine monitors', which change color when exposed to excessively high temperatures or after the expiration date) can avoid unintentional administration of inappropriately stored or expired vaccine.

Regulatory and clinical Aspects

Vaccine manufacturers need a license to produce and to distribute a vaccine. This license is issued by the national control authority after inspection of the production facilities and review of the production process documentation, as well as efficacy and safety data.

The quality requirements that conventional vaccines have to meet (e.g. sterility, absence of adventitious agents, antigen content, immunogenicity) have been formulated by WHO, and published in its Technical Report Series. Tests to assess whether vaccine lots and their intermediate products meet these requirements are performed in a quality control department independently of the production department. The vaccine lot is released for application in humans if both production data and the data of the controls are in accordance with the required specifications.

The licensing of a vaccine is preceded by a premarketing stage. Clinical studies in humans are crucial in this stage. First, all relevant information about the production and the control of the candidate vaccine is collected and described. This documentation and a detailed description of the proposed clinical study are submitted for permission to the responsible national authority. Local authorities (e.g. ethical committees) are linked to the clinical center in which the study is performed. Clinical studies are divided into phase I, II, and III trials. In phase I trials, the major side-effects of a new vaccine are studied in a small number of healthy subjects. In phase II trials, the desired immune response and relative safety are investigated in a larger group of people. In phase III trials, the efficacy and safety of the vaccine are evaluated and documented in official reports. After successfully completing the clinical studies, the licensing stage of the vaccine begins.

Most vaccines manufactured according to one of the strategies discussed in the section "Modern Vaccine Technologies" are still in the stage of clinical or preclinical testing. As yet, the only commercially available biotechnological vaccine is the yeast-derived hepatitis B vaccine, whereas the genetically improved acellular pertussis vaccine is in the process of being licensed. Although classical whole-cell and chemically detoxified vaccines are poorly defined pharmaceutically, and may exhibit fairly large lot-to-lot variations, they have proven their safety and efficacy in many national immunization programs for several decades. For instance, there is a great deal of reluctance to replace the classical whole-cell pertussis vaccine with the acellular pertussis vaccine. Also, the safety of recombinant live vaccinia as a vector for foreign antigens has yet to be determined, although extensive information about the safety of vaccinia is available. Because of uncertainty about the safety of nucleic acid vaccines, target groups for future clinical trials usually include chronically, severely ill people such as cancer patients, for which the possibility of cure may outweigh risk factors.

On the other hand, there are still many viral and parasitic diseases for which no effective vaccine exists. In addition, the growing resistance to the existing arsenal of antibiotics increases the need to develop vaccines against common bacterial infections. As novel vaccines against several of these diseases become available, technologies described in this chapter have great promise. ■

Further Reading

- **Davis HL and Whalen RG.** (1995). Genetic immunization. In *Molecular and Cell Biology of Human Genetic Therapeutics*, edited by G. Dickson. London: Chapman & Hall, pp. 368–387
- **Dintzis RZ.** (1992). Rational design of conjugate vaccines. *Pediatr Res*, 32, 376–385
- **Hasan UA, Abai AM, Harper DR, Wren BW and Morrow WJW.** (1999). Nucleic acid immunization: concepts and techniques associated with third generation vaccines. *J Immunol Methods*, 229, 1–22
- **Levine MM, Woodrow GC, Kaper JB and Cobon GS.** (1997). *New Generation Vaccines*, 2nd edn. New York, NY: Marcel Dekker
- **Liljeqvist S and Ståhl S.** (1999). Production of recombinant subunit vaccines: protein immunogens, live delivery systems and nucleic acid vaccines. *J Biotechnol*, 73, 1–33
- **Plotkin SA and Mortimer EA.** (1994). *Vaccines*, 2nd edn. Philadelphia, PA: WB Saunders Company
- **Roitt I.** (1994). *Essential Immunology*, 8th edn. London: Blackwell Scientific Publications
- **Roitt I, Brostoff J and Male D.** (1993). *Immunology*, 3rd edn. St. Louis, MO: Mosby
- **Sing M and O'Hagan D.** (1999). Advances in vaccine adjuvants. *Nature Biotechnol*, 17, 1075–1081

References

- **Burnette WN, Samai B, Browne J and Ritter GA.** (1985). Properties and relative immunogenicity of various preparations of recombinant DNA-derived hepatitis B surface antigen. *Dev Biol Stand,* 59, 113–120
- **Cartwright K, Morris R, Rümke H, Fox A, Borrow R, Begg N, *et al.*** (1999). Immunogenicity and reactogenicity in UK infants of a novel meningococcal vesicle vaccine containing multiple class 1 (PorA) outer membrane proteins. *Vaccine,* 17, 2612–2619
- **Davis HL and Whalen RG.** (1995). Genetic immunization. In *Molecular and Cell Biology of Human Genetic Therapeutics,* edited by G. Dickson. London: Chapman & Hall, pp. 368–387
- **Flexner C and Moss B.** (1997). Vaccinia virus as a live vector for expression of immunogens. In *New Generation Vaccines,* 2nd edn, edited by MM Levine, GC Woodrow, B Kaper and GS Cobon. New York, NY: Marcel Dekker, Inc, pp. 297–314
- **Francis MJ.** (1991). Enhanced immunogenicity of recombinant and synthetic peptide vaccines. In *Vaccines: Recent Trends and Progress,* edited by G Gregoriadis, AC Allison and G Poste. New York, NY: Plenum Press, pp. 13–23.
- **Germanier R and Furer E.** (1975). Isolation and characterization of gal E mutant Ty21a of *Salmonella typhi*: A candidate strain for a live oral typhoid vaccine. *J Infect Dis,* 114, 553–558
- **Gold R, Scheifele D, Barreto L, Wiltsey S, Bjornson G, Meekison W, *et al.*** (1994). Safety and immunogenicity of *Haemophilus influenzae* vaccine (tetanus toxoid conjugate) administered concurrently or combined with diphtheria and tetanus toxoids, pertussis vaccine and inactivated poliomyelitis vaccine to healthy infants at two, four and six months of age. *Pediatr Infect Dis J,* 13, 348–355
- **Gupta RK, Relyveld EH, Lindblad EB, Bizzini B, Ben-Efraim S and Gupta CK.** (1993). Adjuvants – a balance between toxicity and adjuvanticity. *Vaccine,* 11, 293–306
- **Hoogerhout P, Donders EMLM, Van Gaans-van den Brink JAM, Kuipers B, Brugghe HF, Van Unen LMA, *et al.*** (1995). Conjugates of synthetic cyclic peptides elicit bactericidal antibodies against a conformational epitope on a class 1 outer membrane protein of *Neisseria meningitidis. Infect Immun,* 63, 3473–3478
- **Hoppenbrouwers K, Lagos R, Swennen B, Ethevenaux C, Knops J, Levine MM and Desmyter J.** (1998). Safety and immunogenicity of an Haemophilus influenzae type b – tetanus toxoid conjugate (PRP-T) and diphtheria-tetanus-pertussis (DTP) combination vaccine administered in a dual-chamber syringe to infants in Belgium and Chile. *Vaccine,* 16, 921–927
- **Langeveld JPM, Casal JI, Osterhaus ADME, Cortés E, De Swart R, Vela C, *et al.*** (1994). First peptide vaccine providing protection against viral infection in the target animal: studies of canine parvovirus in dogs. *J Virol,* 68, 4506–4513
- **McNamara MK, Ward RE and Kohler H.** (1984). Monoclonal idiotope vaccine against *Streptococcus pneumoniae* infection. *Science,* 226, 1325–1326
- **Muller S, Plaué S, Samana JP, Valette M, Briand JP and Van Regenmortel MHV.** (1990). Antigenic properties and protective capacity of a cyclic peptide corresponding to site A of influenza virus haemagglutinin. *Vaccine,* 8, 308–314
- **Nencioni L, Pizza M, Bugnoli M, De Magistris T, Di Tommaso A, Giovannoni F, *et al.*** (1990). Characterization of genetically inactivated pertussis toxin mutants: candidates for a new vaccine against whooping cough. *Infect Immun,* 58, 1308–1315
- **Pan Y, Yuhasz SC and Amzel LM.** (1995). Anti-idiotypic antibodies: biological function and structural studies. *FASEB J,* 9, 43–49
- **Paradiso PR, Hogerman DA, Madore DV, Keyserling H, King J, Reisinger KS, *et al.*** (1993). Safety and immunogenicity of a combined diphtheria, tetanus, pertussis and *Haemophilus influenzae* type b vaccine in young infants. *Pediatrics,* 92, 827–832
- **Pessi A, Valmori D, Migliorini P, Tougne C, Bianchi E, Lambert P-H, *et al.*** (1991). Lack of H-2 restriction of the *Plasmodium falciparum* (NANP) sequence as multiple antigen peptide. *Eur J Immunol,* 21, 2273–2276
- **Plotkin SA and Mortimer EA.** (1994). *Vaccines,* 2nd edn, Philadelphia, PA: WB Saunders Company
- **Richter L and Kipp PB.** (1999). Transgenic plants as edible vaccines. *Curr Top Microbiol Immunol,* 240, 159–176
- **Schreiber JR, Nixon KL, Tosi MF, Pier GB and Patawaran MB.** (1991). Anti-idiotype-induced, lipopolysaccharide-specific antibody response to *Pseudomonas aeroginosa. J Immunol,* 146, 188–193
- **Shalaby WSW.** (1995). Development of oral vaccines to stimulate mucosal and systemic immunity: barriers and novel strategies. *Clin Immunol Immunopathol,* 74, 127–134
- **Suharyono, Simanjuntak C, Witham N, Punjabi N, Heppner DG, Losonsky G, *et al.*** (1992). Safety and immunogenicity of single-dose live oral cholera vaccine CVD 103-HgR in 5–9-year-old Indonesian children. *Lancet,* 340, 689–694
- **Tacket CO, Losonsky G, Nataro JP, Cryz SJ, Edelman R, Kaper JB and Levine MM.** (1992). Onset and duration of protective immunity in challenged volunteers after vaccination with live oral cholera vaccine VCD 103-HgR. *J Infect Dis,* 166, 837–841
- **Tam JP.** (1988). Synthetic peptide vaccine design: synthesis and properties of a high-density multiple antigenic peptide system. *Proc Natl Acad Sci USA,* 85, 5409–5413
- **Tam JP, Clavijo P, Lu Y, Nussenzweig V, Nussenzweig R and Zavala R.** (1990). Incorporation of T and B epitopes of the circumsporozoite protein in a chemically defined vaccine against malaria. *J Exp Med,* 171, 299–306

- **Valenzuela P, Medina A, Rutter WJ, Ammerer G and Hall BD.** (1982). Synthesis and assembly of hepatitis B virus surface antigen particles in yeast. *Nature*, 298, 347–350
- **Van der Ley P, Van der Biezen J and Poolman JT.** (1995). Construction of *Neisseria meningitidis* strains carrying multiple chromosomal copies of *porA* gene for use in the production of a multivalent outer membrane vesicle vaccine. *Vaccine*, 13, 401–407
- **Vreden SGS, Verhave JP, Oettinger T, Sauerwein RW and Meuwissen JHE.** (1991). Phase I clinical trial of a recombinant malaria vaccine consisting of the circumsporozoite repeat region of *Plasmodium falciparum* coupled to hepatitis B surface antigen. *Am J Trop Med Hyg*, 45, 533–538
- **Walker RI.** (1994). New strategies for using mucosal vaccination to achieve more effective immunization. *Vaccine*, 12, 387–400

Self-Assessment Questions

Question 1: *What are the characteristics of the ideal vaccine? Which aspects should be addressed in the design of a vaccine in order to approach these characteristics?*

Question 2: *How do antibodies neutralize antigen activity?*

Question 3: *How do T-cells discriminate between exogenous (extracellular) and endogenous (intracellular) antigens? What is the eventual result of these differences in responsiveness?*

Question 4: *Which categories of conventional vaccines exist and what are their characteristics?*

Question 5: *Which technological approaches for modern vaccine development can be discerned? Mention at least one example of each category.*

Question 6: *Mention two main problems related to the immunogenicity of peptide-based vaccines. How are these problems dealt with?*

Question 7: *Mention at least three advantages and three disadvantages of nucleic acid vaccines. Give one advantage and one disadvantage of RNA vaccines over DNA vaccines.*

Question 8: *Which stages are discerned in the manufacture of cell-derived vaccines?*

Question 9: *Mention two or more examples of currently available combination vaccines. Which pharmaceutical and immunological conditions have to be fulfilled when formulating combination vaccines?*

Answers

Answer 1: The characteristics of the ideal vaccine are listed in Figure. 12.1. The first step in vaccine development is the identification of protective antigens. These antigens form the basis of the vaccine. Structures that cause deleterious effects should be eliminated. The antigens should be expressed by a safe expression system with high expression levels. The desired immunological effect, as well as the route of administration, are pivotal factors in the choice of a formulation form. The antigens may either be formulated as part of a live vaccine (either attenuated bacteria or viruses or live vectors), or isolated and formulated as a subunit vaccine, by using one of the modern strategies (including anti-idiotype, synthetic peptide, and nucleic acid vaccines) discussed in this chapter. An adjuvant is usually added to enhance the immune response. The immunogenicity of subunit vaccines can be improved by proper presentation forms, e.g. by incorporation of protein antigens into carrier systems such as liposomes or ISCOMs, or by the chemical conjugation of peptide or polysaccharide antigens to carrier proteins. The physico-chemical stability of the vaccine components should also be addressed. The overall production process should be easy, consistent and cheap.

Answer 2: Antibodies are able to neutralize antigen activity by at least four mechanisms:

(a) Fc mediated phagocytosis;
(b) complement activation resulting in cytolytic activity;
(c) complement mediated phagocytosis;
(d) competitive binding on sites that are crucial for the biological activity of the antigen.

Answer 3: T-cells are able to distinguish exogenous from endogenous antigens by the type of self-antigen (MHC antigen) that is associated with processed antigen on the surface of the antigen-presenting cell. Processed antigen binds to MHC molecules, resulting in a cell surface located antigen/MHC complex. The complex is recognized by the T-cell receptor/CD4 or CD8 complex. A cell infected with a virus presents partially degraded viral antigen (i.e. endogenous antigen) complexed with class I MHC. The complex is recognized by CD8 positive T-cells, resulting in the induction of cytotoxic T-cells. Professional antigen-presenting cells like macrophages phagocytose exogenous antigen and present it in conjunction with class II MHC. CD4 positive T-cells bind to the MHC-antigen complex. Subsequent B-cell or macrophage activation leads to antibody or inflammatory responses, respectively.

Answer 4: Conventional vaccines consist of either live attenuated vaccines or non-living vaccines. For non-living vaccines we discern three generations. The first generation comprises suspensions of inactivated, pathogenic organisms. Second generation vaccines contain purified components, varying from whole organisms or extracts of organisms to purified single components. Third generation vaccines are either well-defined mixtures of purified components or protective components formulated in an immunogenic presentation form. Examples of these categories are given in Table 12.3.

Answer 5: Improved live vaccines are obtained by genetic engineering. The two main strategies are (a) genetic attenuation of organisms (e.g. oral cholera vaccine) and (b) use of live vectors expressing proteins from pathogenic species (e.g. live recombinant vaccinia vaccines carrying viral or tumor antigens).

Subunit vaccines can be improved by rDNA technology as follows: (a) genetic detoxification of proteins (e.g. genetically detoxified pertussis toxin); (b) expression of proteins in host cells (e.g. recombinant hepatitis B vaccine), and; (c) genetic fusion of peptide epitopes with carrier proteins (e.g. experimental malaria vaccines based on epitopes genetically fused with hepatitis B surface antigen). Strategy (b) can be combined with (a) or (c).

Subunit vaccines can also be based on molecular mimicry according to two strategies: (a) anti-idiotype antibodies (e.g. experimental Pseudomonas and Streptococcus vaccines) and (b) synthetic peptides (e.g. experimental influenza vaccine).

Most recently, nucleic acids coding for pathogen-derived antigens have emerged as potential vaccine candidates. In particular, plasmid DNAs coding for viral antigens (e.g. hepatitis B, influenza, HIV) are being explored.

Answer 6: The first problem concerns the low immunogenicity of plain peptide vaccines. The immunogenicity can be improved by constructing multiple antigen peptides or by chemical coupling of peptides to carrier proteins. Alternatively, peptide epitopes can be incorporated into carrier proteins through genetic fusion of the peptide DNA with that of the carrier protein. The second problem of peptide antigens is that their conformation does not necessarily correspond to that of the epitope in the native protein, which may lead to poor immune responses or responses to irrelevant peptide conformations. Solutions to this problem are sought in constraining the conformation of the synthetic peptide by chemical cyclization methods.

Answer 7: The advantages and disadvantages of nucleic acid vaccines are listed in Table 12.5. An advantage of RNA is that there is no risk of incorporation into the host DNA. On the other hand, RNA is less stable than DNA.

Answer 8: The three production stages are (a) cultivation of cells and/or virus, (b) purification of the desired components,
and (c) formulation of the vaccine.

Answer 9: Examples of combination vaccines include diphtheria-tetanus-pertussis-(polio) vaccines and measles-mumps-rubella-(varicella) vaccines. Prerequisites for combining vaccine components are:

(a) pharmaceutical compatibility of vaccine components and additives;
(b) compatibility of immunization schedules;
(c) no interference between immune responses to individual components.

13 Monoclonal Antibody-Based Pharmaceuticals

Marc A. van Dijk and Gestur Vidarsson

Introduction

Antibodies, or immunoglobulins, were first identified in 1890. At that time, Behring and Kitasato discovered that rabbits immune to tetanus have substances in their blood capable of destroying tetanus toxins. They called the fraction containing this activity "antitoxin." This fraction contains immunoglobulins. The first therapeutic application of antibodies followed in 1891, when Behring and Kitasato successfully treated children with diphtheria with antitoxin isolated from diphtheria toxin-immunized rabbits. Although vaccination and antibiotics have replaced immunoglobulins in the treatment of diphtheria, preparations containing total immunoglobulin from immune animals or humans are still in use today. At present, they are being used for two purposes. Firstly, preparations of total immunoglobulin from normal human donors are used for chronic treatment of people unable to produce sufficient immunoglobulin by themselves. Secondly, immunoglobulin preparations from immune animals are used for diseases for which there is no alternative treatment, such as snake or spider bites, where the snake or spider toxins are neutralized.

Around 1900, Paul Ehrlich coined the phrase 'magic bullets'. He saw antibodies as therapeutic agents that could target and neutralize their antigens and developed the first theoretical principles describing antibody-antigen interactions. However, it was not until the advent of hybridoma and molecular cloning techniques in the 1970s that the molecular intricacies of antibody biology became accessible for detailed analysis.

Immunoglobulins in blood can recognize many different antigens, but individual immunoglobulin molecules are highly specific and normally recognize only one antigen. It was not until 1975, when Kohler and Milstein first described the principles of hybridoma technology, that virtually unlimited quantities of antibody of uniform specificity, so-called monoclonal antibodies, could be produced. Antibodies are produced by B-cells. Upon immunization with an antigen, many B-cells producing antibodies are formed. Each B-cell isolated from the immunized animal produces antibodies of one unique specificity. However, these cells can not by themselves be grown outside an animal. For this reason, Köhler and Milstein fused the B-cells of an immunized mouse with immortal tumor cells derived from a mouse myeloma. The resulting 'hybridoma' is immortal and still produces the same antibody as the original B-cell. For this discovery they were awarded the Nobel Prize in 1984. A schematic outline of the original approach using hybridoma technology for the production of (murine) monoclonal antibodies is presented in Figure 13.1.

Despite a promising start, it has taken nearly two decades of struggle for the technology to reach a level at which monoclonal antibodies and their derivatives can be developed into safe and efficient therapeutics. Currently, nearly 25% of pharmaceutical biotech products in development for therapy are antibodies or antibody derivatives and several therapeutic monoclonal antibody products have reached the market (Table 13.1). This chapter aims to give a basic introduction into the biology of antibodies, and the development of antibodies and their derivatives for therapeutic and diagnostic purposes.

Antibody Biology

Antibody Structure

Antibodies are produced by B-cells as soluble molecules to specifically recognize foreign extracellular antigens and subsequently trigger appropriate action from the host immune system. Each B-cell produces its own unique antibody. The most abundant type of antibodies found in blood, IgG, are 150 kDa glycoproteins consisting of four polypeptide chains: two identical so-called 'heavy chains' with a molecular mass of approximately 50–55 kDa, and two identical so-called 'light chains' (~ 25 kDa). These chains are held together by intra-molecular disulfide bridges. The heavy chain molecules contain N-linked sugar moieties at specific locations, which are important for the biological function of the molecule. A schematic view of an IgG molecule is depicted in Figure 13.2 (cf. Figure 4.27). The antibody molecule contains separate molecular modules dedicated to perform the different functions of antigen recognition and to trigger the immune system. The antibody molecule can be divided into several parts: the antigen-binding fragment, also called F(ab), and the

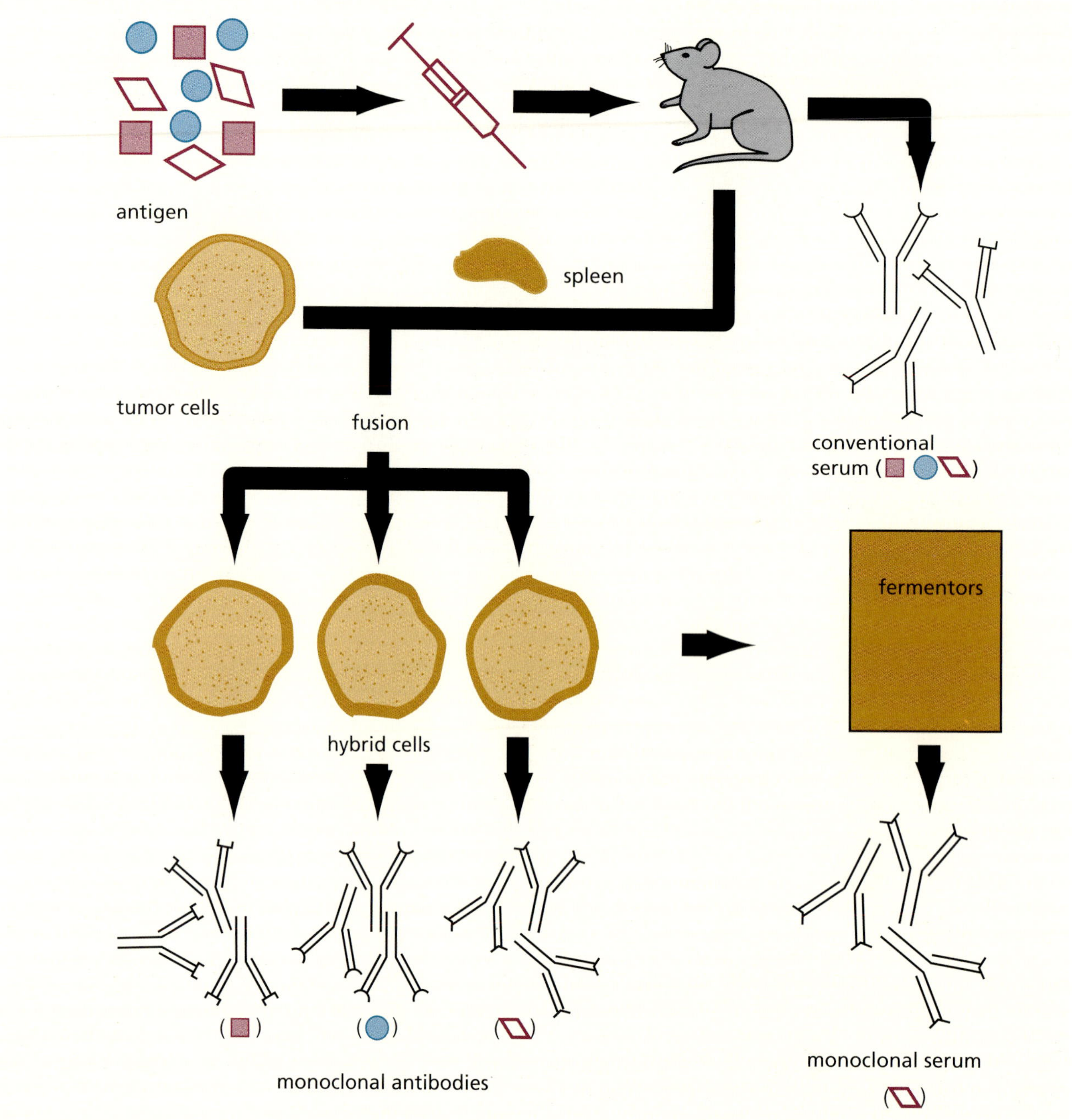

Figure 13.1. Schematic outline of hybridoma technique for production of murine monoclonal antibodies.

constant region, called Fc ("Fc" stands for "Fragment crystalline"). The F(ab) can be divided into a constant part and a variable domain, called Fv. As the name implies, the constant regions are common to each immunoglobulin class, while the variable domains are unique for every immunoglobulin. How B-cells/immunoglobulins achieve their specificity is outlined below.

Antigen Recognition: Generation of Diversity

Every nucleated human cell contains non-rearranged gene segments that can potentially encode functional antibodies. The locus containing gene segments needed for heavy chain formation are located on chromosome 14. The locus

Product name (substance name)	Target antigen	Therapeutic use	Molecule	Registered (country)	Company
gemtuzumab ozogamicin (Mylotarg)	CD33	treatment of acute myeloid leukemia	human mAb conjugated to calichaemicin	2000 (US)	Celltech group PLC/American Home products
mabthera/ rituxan (Rituximab)	CD20 surface antigen of B lymphocytes	treatment of Non-Hodgkin's lymphoma	chimeric mAb	1997 (US) 1998 (EU)	Genentech/ IDEC (US), Hoffmann La-Roche (EU)
+ Herceptin (Trastuzumab)	human epidermal growth factor-like receptor 2 (HER 2)	treatment of metastatic breast cancer overexpressing HER2 protein	humanized mAb	1998 (US)	Genentech
Synagis (Palivizumab)	undisclosed epitope on the surface of respiratory syncytial virus	prophylaxis of lower respiratory tract disease caused by respiratory syncytial virus in children	humanized mAb	1998 (US) 1999 (EU)	MedImmune (US) Abbott (EU)
Remicade (Infliximab)	TNF-alfa	1: treatment of Crohn's disease 2: treatment of rheumatoid arthritis	chimeric mAb	1:1998 (US) 1999 (EU) 2:1999 (US) 2000 (EU)	Centocor
+ Simulect (Basiliximab)	alfa-chain of the IL-2 receptor (CD25)	prophylaxis of acute organ rejection in allogeneic renal transplantation	chimeric mAb	1998 (EU)	Novartis
+ Zenapax (Daclizumab)	alfa-chain of the IL-2 receptor (CD25)	prevention of acute kidney transplant rejection	humanized mAb	1997 (US) 1999 (EU)	Hoffmann La-Roche
Panorex (Edrecolomab)	17-1a, EpCAM	treatment of Dukes' C stage colorectal cancer	murine mAb	1995 (DE)	Centocor/ Glaxo Wellcome
+ ReoPro (Abciximab)	platelet surface receptor GPIIb/IIIa	prevention of blood clots	Fab derived from chimeric mAb	1994 (US)	Centocor
Orthoclone OKT3 (Muromomab)	T-lymphocyte surface antigen CD3	reversal of acute kidney transplant rejection	murine mAb	1986 (US)	Ortho Biotech

Table 13.1. Monoclonal antibody-based therapeutics on the market.
+ Discussed in appendices

containing gene segments needed for kappa light chain formation are located on chromosome 2, and those needed for the formation of a second class of light chains (lambda) are located on chromosome 1. These gene segments are in 'germ line' configuration, which means they will have to be rearranged to create a functional gene. The rearrangement process is depicted in Figure 13.3a.

The Ig loci of developing B-cell goes through several reshuffling or rearrangement steps, which can be divided into two phases. In phase I, the heavy chain locus on chromosome 14 is reshuffled. When this process has produced a functional heavy chain gene, phase II is initiated in which the light chain gene is reshuffled. Products of functionally rearranged heavy and light chain genes are expressed as

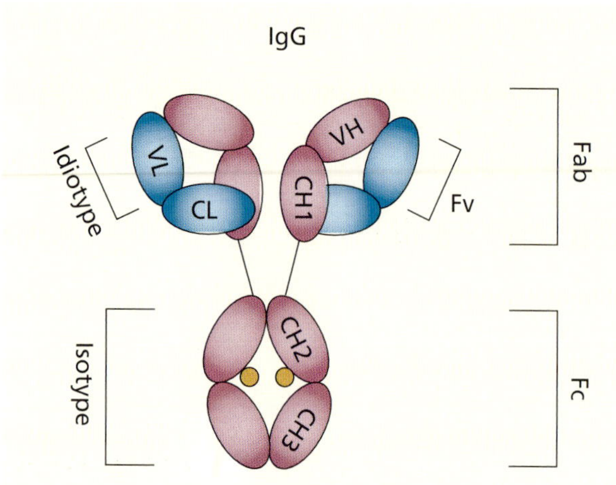

Figure 13.2. **Antibody structure.** Cartoon of IgG antibody structure. Antibodies bind antigen via their variable region (VL and VH), encoded by the V-genes. The CH2 and CH3 domains of heavy chains make up the Fc part and determine the biological activity. N-linked glycosylation sites are indicated in brown. L stands for light chain, H for heavy chain.

cell surface receptors and exposed to antigens. This exposure is a crucial selection step. Only those B-cells expressing surface Ig that bind a foreign antigen are allowed to progress. Those recognizing so-called 'self' antigens are removed. B-cells that recognize a foreign antigen are induced to proliferate and secrete antibodies. During proliferation, a process called "affinity maturation" is initiated. During this process random mutations are introduced in specific parts of the variable domains (CDRs, see below). B-cells producing mutated antibodies with higher affinity for the same antigen are favored over those which produce lower affinity antibodies. This process is highly efficient and enables the immune system to develop antibodies against virtually any molecule. The final result is an antibody molecule with a unique combination of somatically mutated heavy and light chain variable regions. This unique assembly of variable regions is called the antibody "idiotype."

Antigen Recognition: Affinity and Avidity

As variable regions from antigen-specific heavy and light chain genes have been studied in more detail, it has been discovered that only small sub-regions are highly variable between different antibody genes. Large parts of the variable regions remain relatively unchanged; the highly variable sub-regions are largely responsible for the observed antigen specificity and affinity of antibodies. These regions are therefore called "complementarity-determining regions" (CDR, Figure 13.4). The variable regions from heavy and light chain each contain three CDRs. The relatively unchanged parts of the variable regions function as a framework allowing proper orientation of the CDRs. This orientation is critical for positioning of the amino acids in the CDR in such a way that they can make close contacts with the epitope on the antigen (the specific region of antigen contacted by an antibody is called "epitope").

CDR1 and 2 are encoded in germ-line V-segments. However, as depicted in Figure 13.4, CDR3 is not pre-formed; most of its sequence is generated *de novo* upon joining the V and J segments of the light chain, and V, D and J segments of the heavy chain. The affinity of antibodies for their target antigens usually ranges from $\sim 10^7$ M^{-1} to $\sim 10^{12}$ M^{-1}.

A second property called "avidity" plays an important role in determining the strength with which an antibody binds to its target. As depicted in Figures 13.2 and 13.5, antibodies contain at least two antigen-binding regions, located on separate 'arms'. The pentameric structure of IgM even contains ten antigen-binding regions. When a target contains many copies of the same epitope (such as a bacterial cell wall) the antibody can bind with two (or more) arms at the same time. This phenomenon, called avidity, greatly increases the binding strength of the antibody. The overall binding strength of an antibody is therefore determined by two properties: affinity and avidity. However, avidity can only come into play when the target contains multiple binding sites (epitopes).

Class Switching

While the molecular class of antibody depicted in Figure 13.2 (IgG) is the most abundant antibody class found in blood, B-cells can produce nine different antibody classes, also called "isotypes." The arrangement of heavy chain gene segments encoding the different isotypes is depicted in Figure 13.3b. While the idiotype is determined by the antibody's unique combination of somatically mutated heavy and light chain variable regions, the antibodies isotype is determined by the constant regions of the heavy chain (Fc).

The isotypes found in humans and their genomic organisation are depicted in Fig. 13.5 (Figure 13.3b). The function of the immunoglobulin isotype is to determine which immune response will be activated upon encountering the antigen. Upon the first encounter, B-cells are stimulated to secrete IgM. In addition to affinity maturation and proliferation, a process called "class switching" is induced. This process also involves the gene rearrangement of constant regions (Figure 13.3b). The final isotype is determined by the nature of the encountered antigen. For instance, B-cells that have switched to IgA will be favored

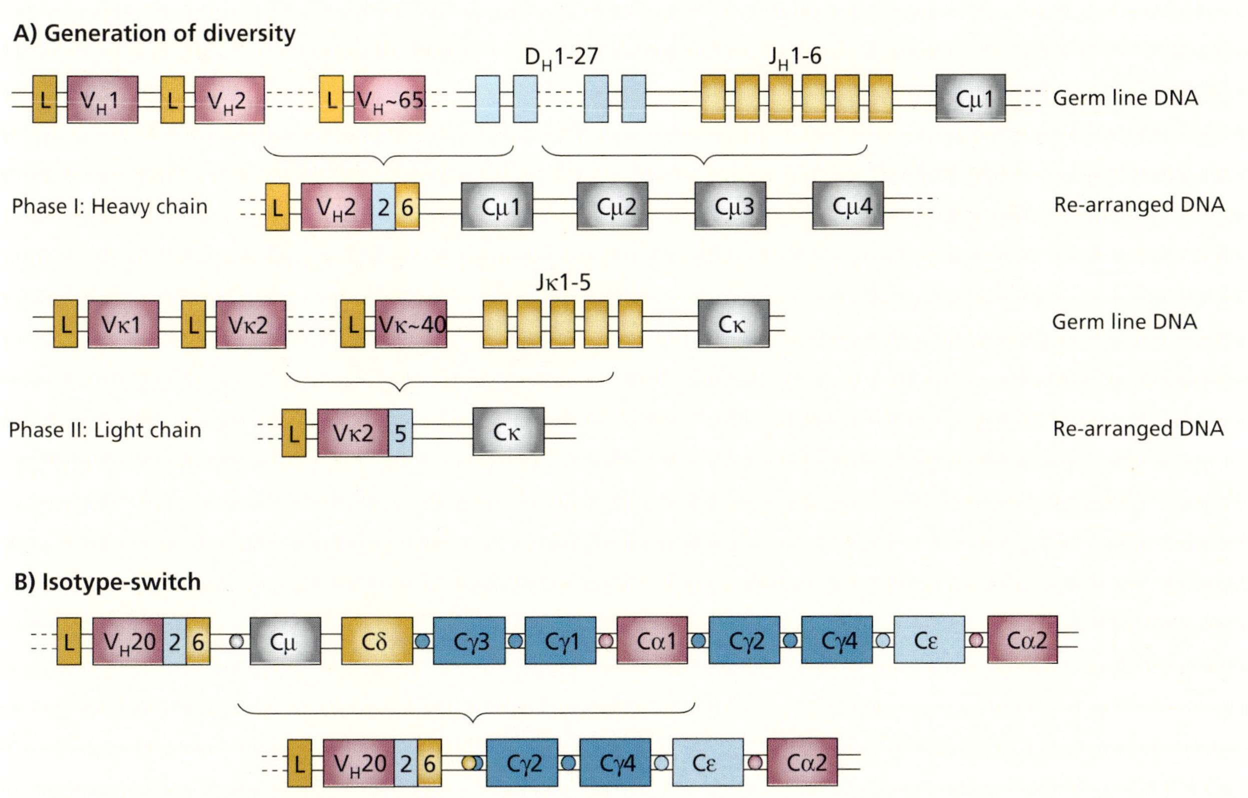

Figure 13.3. **Somatic DNA recombination in B-cells determines antibody specificity and functions.**
A) B-cell precursors undergo highly regulated recombination in both light chain (κ and λ, for simplicity, only the κ-locus is shown) and heavy chain genes (H), where the Variable genes (V) associate with Diversity gene fragments (D, only for the heavy chains), and with Joining (J) genes. A functionally rearranged product shuts down further rearrangements. The resulting rearranged genes (one from each allele), a κ or λ, with one heavy chain gene), are expressed on the surface of the mature B-cells with their corresponding Constant (C) regions, as IgM (μ) and IgD (not shown). L stands for Leader peptide, and the number in or above V (1-65), D (1-27), or J (1-6) indicates the number of known segments in the human genome.
B) If a B-cell encounters a specific antigen for its surface expressed antibody, and receives the proper stimulus from T-cells, it becomes activated and starts secreting IgM. Subsequently, the heavy-chain locus may undergo further rearrangements, which occurs between signal sequences located upstream of the IgM constant region (Cμ) and other constant regions. The end result is that the same rearranged V-gene is expressed now with a different constant region (in the example shown it is Cγ2, which encodes for IgG2). Thus, the antigen specificity has not changed, but the antibody function has.

in immune responses to microorganisms located at mucosal surfaces (e.g. gut and lungs). B-cells that have switched to IgG2 are favored in response to polysaccharide antigens in immune responses. The specific molecular properties of the individual isotypes are described in Table 13.2.

Pharmacokinetics

The Fc part of antibodies is also largely responsible for its pharmacokinetic properties. The relative long half-life of immunoglobulins in general (several days to weeks) results from several properties of antibody molecules as a whole. The first property is their size (>150 kDa), which prevents excretion through the filtering system of the kidney. Another property is the relative resistance to proteases. Also, in purified form many isotypes are exquisitely stable, and can be safely kept in solution at 4 °C for months to years.

These properties are shared between most isotypes. However, IgG is protected from breakdown by an additional mechanism not available for other isotypes. *In vivo*, all serum proteins are taken up by endothelial cells in a process called "pinocytosis." The Fc part of IgG contains a region that is recognized by a specialized Fc receptor, called

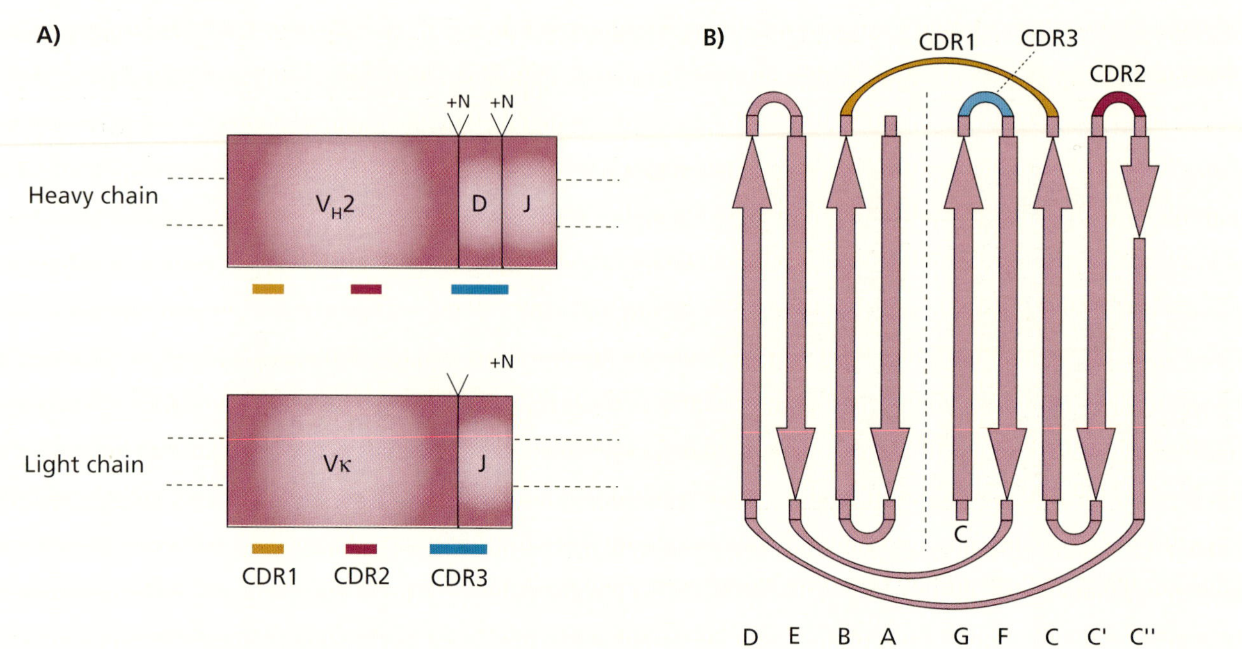

***Figure 13.4.* CDR regions are involved in antigen binding.**
A) Certain areas in immunoglobulin genes are highly variable as a result of imprecise splicing (of V, D and J genes) in combination with high somatic mutation rates. These areas, called "Complementarity Determining Regions" or CDR's, are encoded by three nonlinear stretches. In the folded antibody these regions are located on the tip of the variable region.
B) The folding of the V-genes follows the general pattern of immunoglobulin superfamily domain building blocks, and is very similar for both heavy and light chains (only light chain is shown here). Each domain is composed of two anti-parallel β sheets (arrows), which fold as indicated by the broken line. The location of the CDR regions at the "top" of the immunoglobulin molecule is indicated.

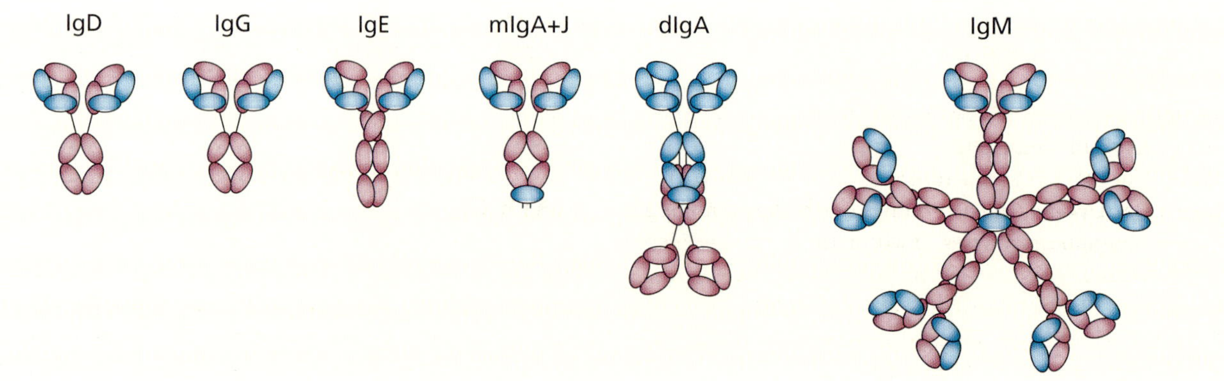

***Figure 13.5.* Antibody classes.** IgG, IgD, IgE molecules are monomeric, while IgA can be monomeric (mIgA), dimeric (dIgA) or polymeric (pIgA, not shown). IgM is predominantly present in pentameric form. A prerequisite for polymerization is the joining (J) chain, which need the tail-piece only found in IgM and IgA. IgM and IgE have longer Fc-tails (4 CH domains vs 3 in other cases) but do not have hinge regions (located between CH1 and CH2 in other isotypes).

	IgG1	IgG2	IgG3	IgG4	IgM	IgA1	IgA2	IgD	IgE
Molecular weight (kDa)	146	146	165	146	970	160	160	184	188
Adult serum level (mg/ml)	9	3	1	0.5	1.5	3	0.5	0.03	$5E^{-5}$
Serum half life (days)	21	20	7	21	10	6	6	3	2
Activation of classical complement pathway	++	+	+++	+	+++	–	–	–	–
Placental transfer	+++	+	++	+/–	–	–	–	–	–
Mucosal transfer	+/–	+/–	+/–	+/–	+	+++	+++	–	–
Binding to phagocytes	+++	++*	+++	–	–	++	++	–	+
Binding to mast cells and basophils	–	–	–	–	–	(+)	(+)	–	+++

Table 13.2. Characteristics and functional properties of human antibody isotypes.
* IgG2 binds only to one of two known functionally expressed FcγRIIa alleles (FcγRIIa-H131).

the Brambell receptor or FcRN. When taken up by endothelial cells, IgG encounters FcRN in the endosomal compartment. FcRN binds Fc under the acidic conditions prevalent in endosomes. Subsequently, FcRN recycles bound IgG to the cell surface. At the physiological pH of blood Fc dissociates from FcRN and resumes its place in circulation. The binding to FcRN is the cause for the long half-life (21 days) of IgG molecules in blood. Other proteins (and other isotypes) cannot bind to this receptor and are broken down in endothelial cells.

Immune complexes (Ig+antigen) are cleared by a different mechanism; they are transported to the liver and spleen, where they are taken up and broken down by fixed tissue macrophages.

Effector Functions

The antibody classes all have a different capacity in triggering the immune system.

Some of these characteristics are summarized in Table 13.2. Upon antigen binding, antibodies can trigger different immune responses. Two of these are considered the most relevant for immunotherapeutic approaches in cancer. These are antibody-dependent cellular cytotoxicity (ADCC) and antibody-mediated complement activation or complement dependent cytotoxicity (CDC). These effector mechanisms are schematically depicted in Figure 13.6.

Complement-Dependent Cytotoxicity (CDC)

The complement system is an important part of the 'innate' (i.e. non-adaptive) immune system (B-cells are part of the adaptive immune system). It consists of many protein enzymes that form a cascade; each enzyme acts as a catalyst for the next. The classical pathway for complement activation is initiated by the binding of C1q to a complex consisting of many antibodies bound to an antigen (e.g. a bacterium). C1q consists of five polypeptides. C1q binds specifically to a part of the constant region of IgG1-3 and IgM. This binding is partially dependent on the glycosylation status of the CH2 domain. Upon binding to immune complexes, C1q undergoes a conformational change leading to autocatalytic self-cleavage. The resulting activated complex initiates an enzymatic cascade involving complement proteins C2 to C9 and several other factors. This cascade spreads rapidly and ends in the formation of the membrane attack complex (MAC). This is a hydrophobic protein complex that inserts into the membrane of the target and causes osmotic disruption and lysis of the target.

Antibody-Dependent Cellular Cytotoxicity (ADCC)

Antibody-dependent cellular cytotoxicity represents another immune defense mechanism. When many antibodies are bound to a target such as a bacterium, this antibody-coated (or opsonized) bacterium can be captured by Fc-receptors abundantly expressed on immune cells of the myeloid lineage (cf. Chapter 8). The interaction of an individual antibody with most Fc receptors is weak. Only when an opsonized target is encountered is this Fc receptor-antibody binding amplified to the point where the myeloid cell remains attached and becomes activated. Dependent

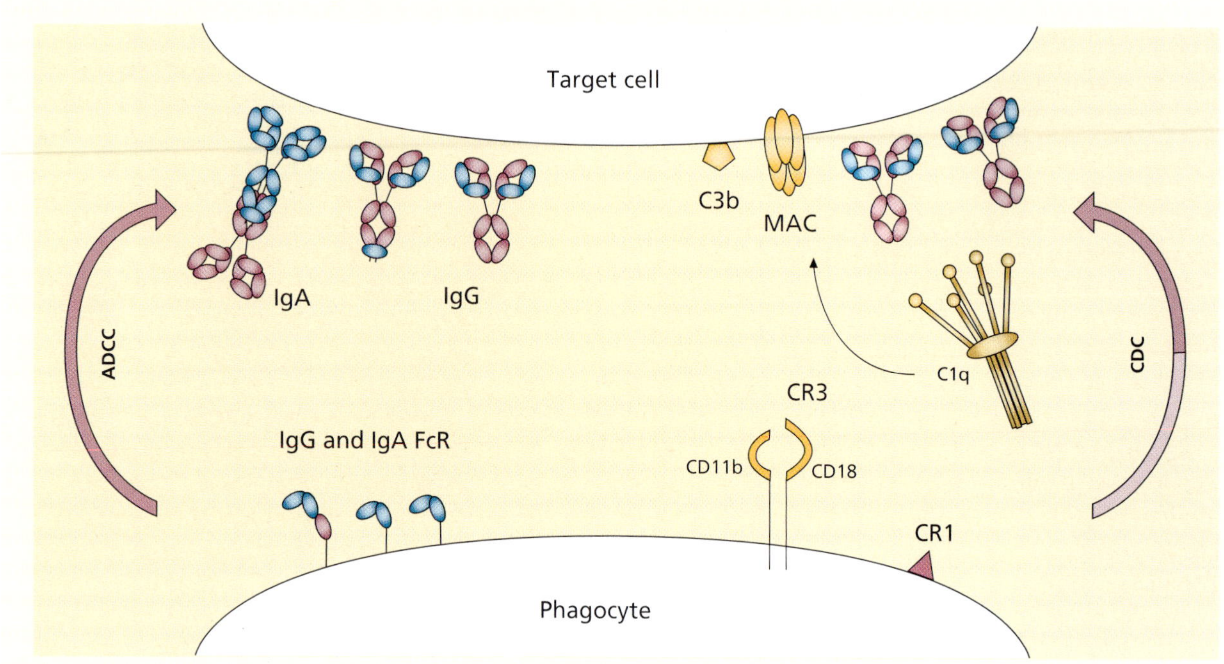

Figure 13.6. **Antibody effector functions.** In the presence of specific antibodies, target cells (such as infectious agents, tumor cells) become opsonized. Surface-bound IgG and IgM antibodies can interact with the C1q component of the classical complement pathway and efficiently activate the lytic complement pathway (CDL), the end result of which is the formation of the membrane attack complex (MAC, C5–C9). Furthermore, complement factors (C1q, C3b, C4b) can stimulate phagocytes via complement receptors CR1 and CR3 (CD11b and CD18), while MAC can lead to death of the target cell by lysis. IgG and IgA can interact directly with specific receptors on phagocytes (FcR) that potently stimulate antibody-dependent cell-mediated cytotoxicity (ADCC) and phagocytosis.

on the type of myeloid cell, this activation can lead to the engulfment (phagocytosis) of the opsonized target, or it can lead to the release of toxic substances, such as reactive oxygen intermediates, nitric oxide, hydrolytic enzymes, and specific cytokines (such as tumor necrosis factor α). The end result is the destruction of the opsonized target.

Development of Monoclonal Antibodies as Therapeutics

All functions together make the antibody a formidable weapon, which can be employed for therapeutic purposes. The first therapeutic monoclonal antibody to be registered was OKT3, a murine antibody used in the prevention of renal transplant rejection (Table 13.1). Since 1986, eight additional therapeutic monoclonal antibody-based products have been registered. In addition to products already on the market, some 59 monoclonal antibody-based products are currently in clinical trials. The major indication (31 products) is cancer. Additional indications include transplantation and respiratory, skin, and neurological disorders, as well as autoimmune conditions.

For biotechnological applications perhaps the most important property is antigen recognition. Antibodies can be isolated that recognize a near infinite variety of antigenic molecules. In addition, antibodies can be isolated which have desired affinity for any chosen antigen. IgG antibodies are favored in the development of therapeutics. As shown in Table 13.2, IgG antibodies have a long biological half-life (about 21 days), and are capable of effectively triggering ADCC and CDC. All of these properties together make IgG the molecule of choice for developing antibody therapy for cancer.

Murine Antibodies

Several types of human tumors express molecules on their cell surface which distinguish tumor cells from normal cells. This expression makes tumors potential targets for antibodies that recognize tumor-specific surface molecules. The first monoclonal antibodies used for therapy were derived from mouse hybridomas. While effective in some cases, repeated treatment with mouse antibodies caused severe immune reactions in human cancer patients. This problem derives from the fact that although antibody genes from mice and humans are highly conserved, there are many differences between rodent immunoglobulins and human immunoglobulins. The injection of mouse monoclonal antibodies into a human patient usually results in an immune response, which leads to the development of human anti-mouse antibodies (HAMA). In most cases, HAMA are detectable at about 8–12 days after injection, and reach a peak at about 25–30 days. This immune response can cause severe allergic reactions and usually precludes treatment beyond ten days. Importantly, it also precludes re-treatment of the same patient with a different rodent antibody. In view of the increasing number of antibody-based therapeutics appearing on the market this is not an ideal situation.

A solution to the immunogenicity of rodent monoclonal antibodies in human therapy would be to use human monoclonal antibodies. Generation of hybridomas from human B-cells producing human antibodies of desired specificity has not met with great success. Most therapeutic targets are 'self' proteins, and B-cells producing antibodies recognizing self-proteins are generally eliminated before they reach maturity. However, several approaches have been developed to enable the production of monoclonal antibodies which are largely humanized, or even completely human. These are schematically depicted in Figure 13.7 and will be described below.

Chimeric Antibodies

Genes encoding functional heavy and light chains of a desired mouse monoclonal antibody can be isolated from a hybridoma. Functional genes encoding heavy and light chain genes can also be isolated from human B-cells. By exchanging the variable regions (Fv) of the human antibody heavy and light chain genes for those derived from the mouse genes, one creates chimeric genes. When re-introduced into eukaryotic cells (usually CHO: Chinese hamster ovary cells), these genes express a chimeric antibody. These antibodies are approximately 75% human. The antigen specificity is in most cases identical to that of parental mouse antibodies, but the *in vivo* half-life and effector functions are human. Although less immunogenic than the original mouse antibodies, chimeric antibodies can still trigger significant antibody responses (HACA: human anti-chimeric antibody). Several chimeric antibodies have now successfully reached the market and are used to treat cancer, rheumatoid arthritis, myocardial infarction, and transplant rejection (see Table 13.1 and appendix B and C for details on basiliximab/Simulect, abciximab/Reopro).

Humanized Antibodies

As described above, the amino-acid residues that make actual contact with the epitope on an antigen are largely located in the complementarity determining regions (Figure 13.4). It is possible to engraft mouse CDRs onto a human framework region and thereby recapitulate the antigen-binding characteristics of the original mouse antibody. The resulting humanized antibody is >90% human. This 'CDR-grafting' is by no means a straightforward procedure. It can lead to a drop in affinity and is not guaranteed to work for every mouse antibody. However, several remarkable successes have been obtained and three humanized antibodies have recently reached the market (see Table 13.1 and appendix for further details on trastuzumab/Herceptin and basiliximab/Zenapax). Although very few cases have been reported, there is not enough data at this moment to fully assess the immunogenicity of these humanized antibodies

Human Antibodies

The ultimate goal for immunotherapeutics should be to achieve full biocompatibility. For antibodies, this means they should ideally consist of completely human polypeptides. Two approaches that achieve this goal are described below.

Human Antibodies Derived through Phage Display

As depicted in Figure 13.3, antibody variable regions are derived from several different gene segments. The human heavy chain variable region is formed by combining one (out of a possible 65) Vh segment with one (out of a possible 27) Diversity segments and one (out of six) Joining segments. This combination yields approximately 10,000 different heavy chain variable regions using just germ line segments. The human κ light chain locus contains approximately 40 functional Vκ-gene segments. The κ light chain variable region consists of one of these 40 Vκ segments combined with one (out of five) joining segments. These individual segments can be isolated and cloned into an expression vector. In an antibody, Vh and Vκ are part of different polypeptide chains. It has proven possible to express heavy and light chain variable regions as part of the same polypeptide chain and create functional antigen-binding proteins. These mini-antibodies are called single-chain variable fragments (ScFv, Figure 13.10). The Vκ and Vh segments are joined by a linker that facilitates orientation of the CDRs towards the antigen in a similar fashion as occurs in natural antibodies. This Vκ–linker-Vh segment is attached to a segment of one of the constituent proteins of the phage outer coat (i.e. M13 coat protein III, gP3). Then ScFv are expressed on the outside of a

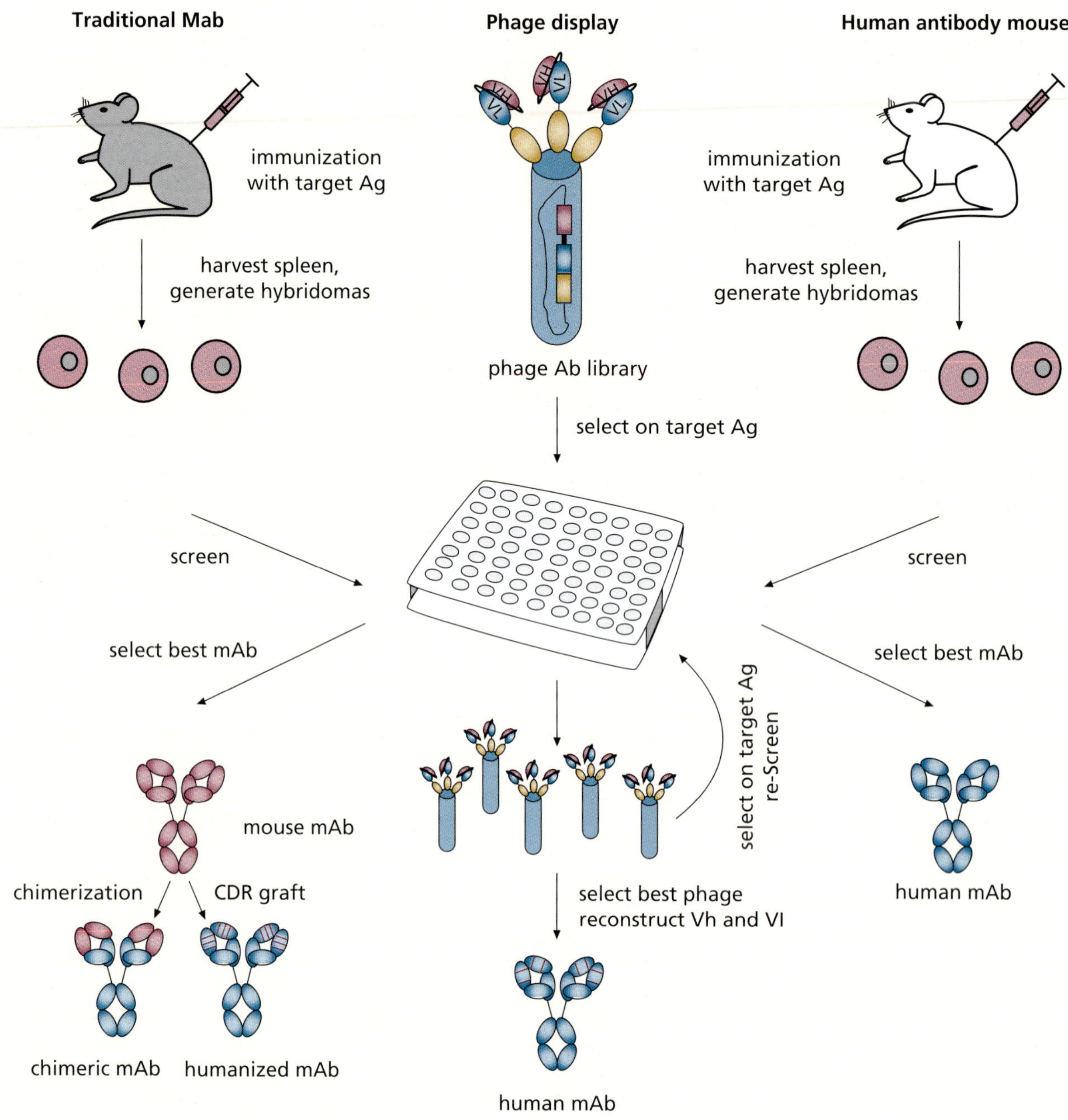

Figure 13.7. **Generation of human monoclonal antibodies.** Depicted are three ways of obtaining therapeutic antibodies with reduced/absent immunogenicity. On the left the procedure for obtaining mouse, chimeric and humanized antibodies is shown. The middle part shows a procedure for obtaining human antibodies through phage display. The right part depicts the procedure of obtaining human antibodies with the aid of genetically engineerd "human antibody" mice.

bacteriophage. The recombinant ScFv-gP3 gene is cloned into a plasmid, which allows for bacterial expression and replication (cf. Chapter 1). By allowing these bacteriophages to replicate in a bacterial cell culture containing the ScFv-g3p library, the entire array of possible ScFv proteins will be expressed as part of the bacteriophage outer protein coat. The construction of a ScFv-phage library is illustrated in Figure 13.8

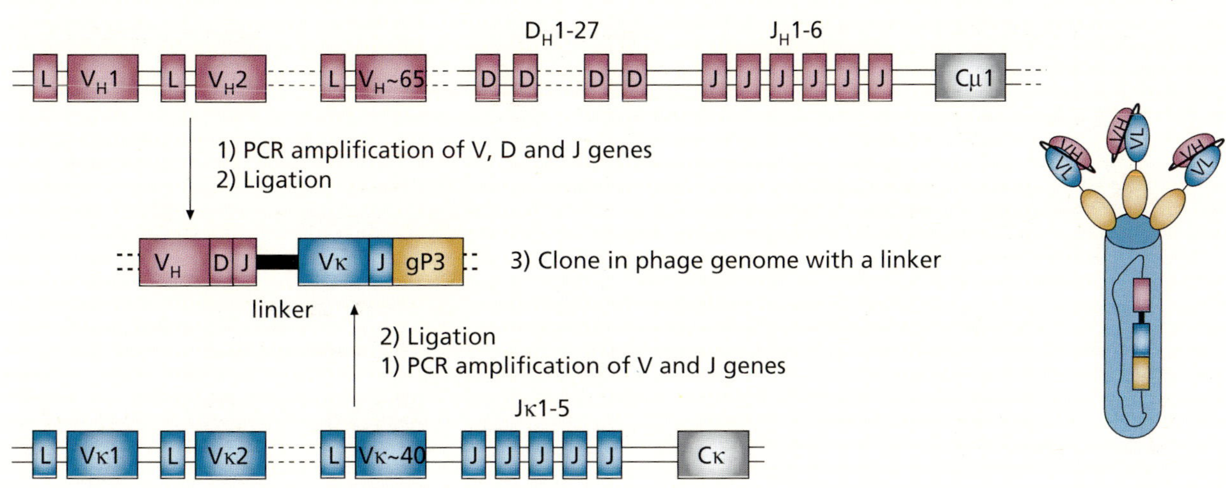

Figure 13.8. **Phage display.** In phage display methods, the antibody repertoire, or the V (D) and J genes are amplified, and joined randomly together. Subsequently, assembled V-genes from both heavy and light chains are cloned upstream of a gene encoding part of a surface-exposed protein (i.e. gP3) with a predetermined linker between them. The pool of randomly assembled ScFv-gP3-encoding plasmids is used to transform *E.coli*. When bacteriophages are allowed to replicate in these transformed *E.Coli* the resulting library phages express ScFv fragments that are capable binding a wide variety of antigens.

If a library was created that contained every possible combination of germ-line heavy and light chain variable regions it would yield a total of approximately two million different molecules. While impressive, this number is still far less than the capacity of the human B-cell system to generate antibody diversity, as encountered in humans. In addition to the combination of germ-line segments, B-cells use two other mechanisms. The imperfect joining and insertion of random nucleotides between V, D and J segments can lead to the usage of alternative reading frames (see Chapter 1). Furthermore, the process of somatic mutation introduces random mutations into the CDRs and to a lesser extent in framework regions. Together, these processes augment the primary diversity of two million by an estimated ten thousand- to hundred thousand-fold. To be able to isolate antibodies with high affinity to every conceivable antigen, a library must be generated which approaches the complexity of the human B-cell system. There are currently several libraries that approximate this complexity. By exposing such a library of bacteriophages to immobilized antigen, one can selectively isolate the correct ScFv-containing phage from the library. Using large repertoires of naive and semi-synthetic libraries, it was shown that ScFv antibodies can be isolated that recognize foreign as well as self antigens, comparable in affinity to those of a late immune response.

When a high affinity ScFv has been isolated, the Vκ and Vh regions can be isolated and used to reconstruct a complete antibody, similar to the process of making a chimeric antibody. The difference is that the resulting antibody is human. Phage display of ScFv, followed by genetic reconstruction of intact antibodies is a way of reproducing the amazingly efficient process of antibody formation in living organisms in vitro. It offers the possibility of selecting ScFv antibodies directed against self proteins, which is difficult in living organisms. However, most human protein targets are sufficiently different from their rodent counterparts to avoid generating self antibodies and allow for the successful generation of therapeutically useful monoclonal antibodies by conventional hybridoma technology.

HUMAN ANTIBODIES FROM GENETICALLY ENGINEERED MICE

An elegant way of producing completely human monoclonal antibodies is to make use of genetically engineered mice. As described in Chapter 6, techniques have been developed which make it possible to introduce new genes into mice, or functionally disable the mouse's own genes. These techniques have been used to create mice in which the gene clusters encoding the heavy and κ light chain genes are disabled (knocked out). These mice cannot produce antibodies and do not have mature B-cells. Subsequently, these mice are supplied with DNA segments containing large parts of the human heavy and κ light chain gene

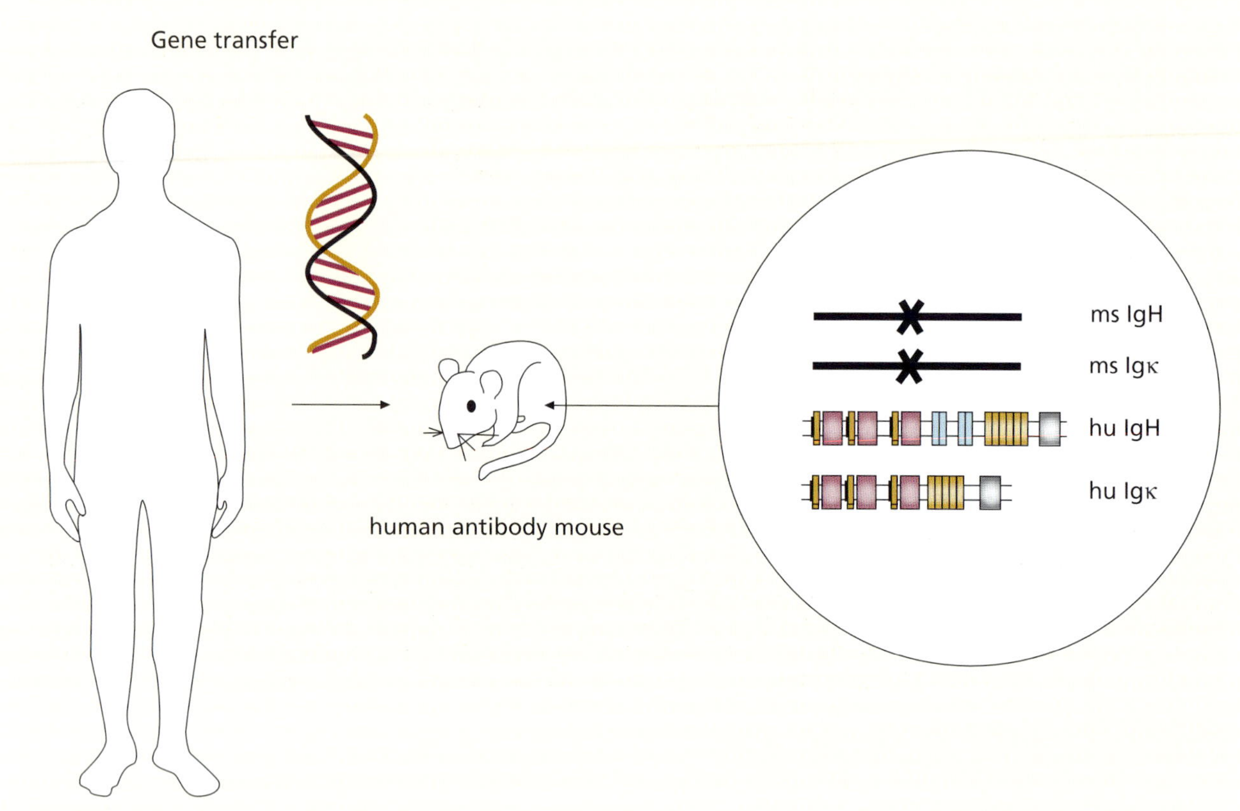

Figure 13.9. **Human antibody mouse.** To obtain a mouse capable of producing a wide array of fully human antibodies, the mouse heavy and kappa light chain genes are inactivated first. Subsequently, large human heavy and light gene fragments are incorporated into the mouse genome by gene transfer. The resulting mouse can be immunized with target antigens to generate human monoclonal antibodies (see Figure 13.7).

clusters. The human antibody mouse is schematically depicted in Figure 13.9. The human DNA segments are fully functional in these mice. These human antibody mice (appropriately called "HuMab mice" by one company) can be immunized with antigens and produce high affinity antibodies in a very similar fashion to normal mice. When the spleens of these immunized HuMab mice are fused with myeloma cells, the resulting hybridomas will produce fully human monoclonal antibodies. This process is schematically depicted in Figure 13.7.

A recent major achievement in genetic engineering is represented by trans-chromosomic mice. In addition to their normal contingent of 21 chromosome pairs, these mice carry human mini-chromosomes in every cell. These mini-chromosomes are derived from human chromosomes 14 and 2 and contain the complete germ-line gene clusters for immunoglobulin heavy and κ light chain, respectively. These mice reproduce the human immunoglobulin gene environment nearly completely, and should provide a full recapitulation of the human antibody response in mice. Several human antibodies from genetically engineered mice are currently in clinical trials.

ANTIBODY DERIVATIVES

Antibodies contain two functionally and molecularly separable modules: a module for antigen recognition (Fv or Fab) and one for triggering effector functions (Fc). The combination of these properties and the concomitant long half-life gave researchers the idea of using monoclonal antibodies for cancer treatment. Not all therapeutic applications require the presence of both the antigen binding and the immune triggering modules. For many applications the ability to recognize a target antigen is sufficient, or alternative effector mechanisms are required. Several alternatives to the use of whole antibodies are discussed below.

Antigen recognition can directly influence the function of the antigen: in the case where the antigen is an enzyme, antibodies can be isolated that will bind closely to the enzyme's active site and prevent access of the enzyme substrate, thereby functionally inhibiting the enzyme. In the case that the antigen is a receptor protein expressed on the surface of a cell, an inactivating antibody can be isolated that prevents ligand binding. Alternatively, activating antibodies can be isolated that mimic ligand binding

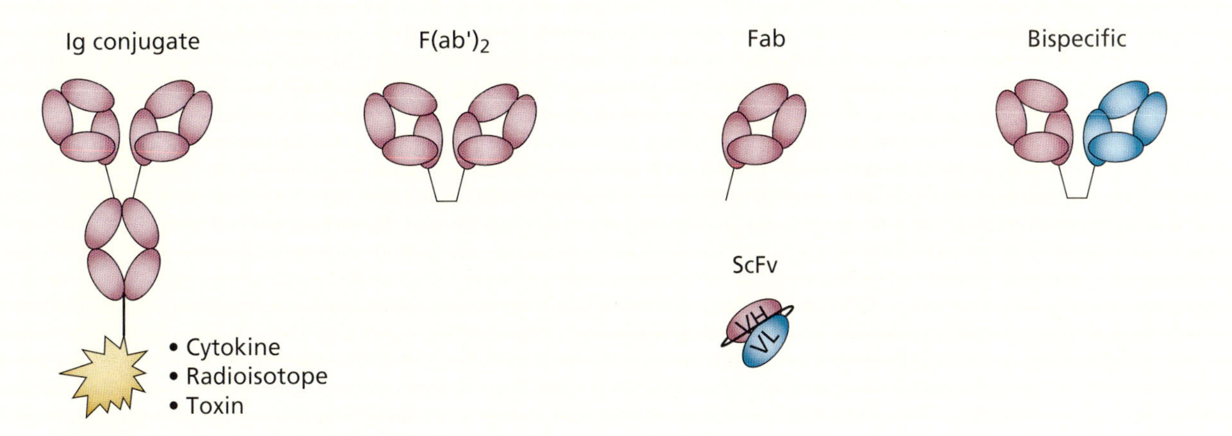

Figure 13.10. **Ways to modify functional properties of antibody molecules.** Alternative effector modules (e.g. radioisotopes, toxins, cytokines) can be connected to antibodies by genetic or chemical means to add or change functional properties. To eliminate Fc effector functions and change antibody valency, whole antibodies can be cleaved with proteolytic enzymes to generate or F(ab'). An alternative is generation of recombinant single-chain mini-antibodies (ScFv), which only harbor the V-regions from both heavy and light chains (no CH1, Cκ or Cλ), attached with a linker. Two Fab fragments derived from antibodies with different antigen specificity can also be joined together to generate F(ab')2 molecules with dual specificity (bispecific antibodies).

in a way that activates the receptor. In the reverse situation, antibodies can be developed that neutralize receptor ligands like hormones or cytokines, or toxins such as snake venom. For these applications it is not necessary to have the Fc portion present. In the case of receptor blockade or activation it may, however, still be useful to have the Fc portion present for increasing the biological half-life of the antibody. However, care must be taken to use an isotype or modified isotype that does not trigger ADCC or CDC, otherwise receptor-bearing cells are not merely activated or inhibited, but actually destroyed.

For antibodies that are meant to be used for inactivation of hormones or toxins a smaller size is beneficial, as it allows more rapid clearance of the undesired substance via the kidney.

ALTERNATIVE EFFECTOR FUNCTIONS (CF. CHAPTER 4 FOR MORE DETAILED INFORMATION)

The antigen recognition module can also be envisioned as a homing device; in the case of a whole antibody it delivers the effector part to the site where the antigen is found. It can also be used to deliver various alternative effectors to the site where antigens are located. Many different antigen-binding/effector combinations have been designed. Figure 13.10 depicts some of the most frequently used derivatives. Several of these approaches are currently being evaluated in clinical trials.

Alternative effectors can be attached to any antibody derivative by chemical means or by genetic engineering. Examples of alternative effectors are:

Toxins

Toxins can be used to kill cells by attaching them to an antibody that binds to a surface molecule and induces uptake of the surface molecule-mAb toxin complex. Once inside the target cell the toxin detaches from the antibody and enters the cytoplasm, where it inactivates the protein synthesis machinery of the cell. Ricin-A and calichaemicin are frequently used for this purpose.

Radioisotopes

Depending on the nature and dose of the radioisotopes they can be used for radioactive imaging or treatment of tumors (low dose, γ emitters or high dose, α or β emitters with limited penetration). Several radiodiagnostic antibodies are currently on the market. They are being used for the detection of tumor masses and micrometastases that are difficult to find by other diagnostic strategies. Radioisotopes are coupled to antibodies by chemical means. Several antibody derivatives can be used for this purpose, depending on the pharmacokinetic profiles required (Fab, F(ab')$_2$, ScFv). Smaller molecules give better tumor penetration and are more rapidly cleared. This rapid clearance reduces toxicity to other non-tumor tissues. This is beneficial when used for tumor treatment, and also for imaging, as it reduces background signals caused by binding to Fc receptors on normal cells.

Cytokines

Cytokines modulate functions of the immune system. By attaching cytokines to an antibody(-derivative) and directing them to tumor antigens, it is theoretically possible to increase the local concentration of such cytokine in the tumor to the point where the immune system is triggered and starts destroying tumors. Several approaches have been tested successfully in animal models, and are currently under clinical investigation. Tumor necrosis factor α and interleukin-2 represent two of the most frequently used cytokines in this respect.

Bispecific Antibodies

This term is used to indicate a molecule containing two distinct antigen recognition modules (see Figure 13.10). Traditionally, bispecific antibodies consist of Fab molecules isolated by proteolytic cleavage from two different parent antibodies and coupled by chemical cross-linking. Alternatively, genetic engineering allows for the generation of bispecific fusion proteins, bypassing the need for cleavage and chemical conjugation. Bispecific antibodies are predominantly designed to bring cells of the immune system into close contact with tumor cells. For this purpose, one Fab specifically binds to a surface molecule expressed on tumor cells and the other Fab binds to a molecule present on specific effector cells, such as cytotoxic T-cells, granulocytes or neutrophils. Ideally, the bispecific antibody should not only bring the effector cell into close contact with tumor cells; it should also activate effector cells. This activation can be achieved by mimicking the function of the natural ligand for a receptor expressed on immune cells. Examples of receptor molecules used for this purpose are CD64, CD89 and CD3, but there are many more examples. Bispecific molecules of which one part is directed against CD64 have been extensively tested in clinical trials and are currently in Phase III.

Production

All antibodies that are currently on the market are produced from mammalian cell cultures. Traditional murine antibodies can be produced directly from the original hybridoma. Chimeric, humanized and phage display-derived mAbs are produced from recombinant genes which need to be reintroduced into mammalian cells to enable proper folding and glycosylation. Like traditional murine monoclonal antibodies, human antibodies from genetically engineered mice can also be produced directly from the original hybridoma. Production of biologically active whole antibody from non-mammalian cell culture systems such as yeast or bacteria has not met with great success, due to problems in achieving proper folding and glycosylation. However, production in plants shows some promise (cf. Chapter 6).

Production of mAb in mammalian cell culture is expensive. To be economically acceptable, a cell culture system must be able to produce >100 micrograms of antibody per mL. Typically, treatment of, for instance, cancer patients requires repeated administrations of doses of several hundreds of milligrams at a time (see appendix for details on Herceptin). Although effective, it makes the cost of treatment high. Development of transgenic animals like goats or cows, which are able to produce monoclonal antibodies in their milk may offer more economical alternatives in the long run (cf. Chapters 3 and 6). ■

Further Reading

- Immunology Today, Vol 21 issue 8 (August 2000).
  This issue is dedicated solely to antibodies and contains a wealth of information and web-links relevant to the field of antibody-based therapeutics.
- Using Antibodies: A Laboratory Manual (1999). Ed Harlow and David Lane. Cold Spring Harbor Laboratory press. Immunology. IM Roitt, J Brostoff and DK Male, London, Mosby, 1998, 5th edition.

References

- **Clynes RA, Towers TL, Presta LG, Ravetch JV**: *Inhibitory Fc receptors modulate in vivo cytoxicity against tumor targets. Nat Med* 2000, **6**:443–446.
- **Miller RA, Maloney DG, Warnke R, Levy R**: *Treatment of B-cell lymphoma with monoclonal anti-idiotype antibody. N Engl J Med* 1982, **306**:517–522.
- **Fisher RG, Johnson JE, Dillon SB, Parker RA, Graham BS**: *Prophylaxis with respiratory syncytial virus F-specific humanized monoclonal antibody delays and moderately suppresses the native antibody response but does not impair immunity to late rechallenge. J Infect Dis* 1999, **180**:708–713.
- **Carter P, Presta L, Gorman CM, Ridgway JB, Henner D, Wong WL, Rowland AM, Kotts C, Carver ME, Shepard HM**: *Humanization of an anti-p185HER2 antibody for human cancer therapy. Proc Natl Acad Sci U S A* 1992, **89**:4285–4289.
- **Hakimi J, Chizzonite R, Luke DR, Familletti PC, Bailon P, Kondas JA, Pilson RS, Lin P, Weber DV, Spence C, *et al.***: *Reduced immunogenicity and improved pharmacokinetics of humanized anti- Tac in cynomolgus monkeys. J Immunol* 1991, **147**:1352–1359.
- **Hoogenboom HR, Henderikx P, de Haard H**: *Creating and engineering human antibodies for immunotherapy. Adv Drug Deliv Rev* 1998, **31**:5–31.
- **Vaughan TJ, Osbourn JK, Tempest PR**: *Human antibodies by design. Nat Biotechnol* 1998, **16**:535–539.
- **Bruggemann M, Taussig MJ**: *Production of human antibody repertoires in transgenic mice. Curr Opin Biotechnol* 1997, **8**:455–458.
- **Fishwild DM, O'Donnell SL, Bengoechea T, Hudson DV, Harding F, Bernhard SL, Jones D, Kay RM, Higgins KM, Schramm SR, *et al.***: *High-avidity human IgG kappa monoclonal antibodies from a novel strain of minilocus transgenic mice. Nat Biotechnol* 1996, **14**:845–851.
- **Harding FA, Lonberg N**: *Class switching in human immunoglobulin transgenic mice. Ann N Y Acad Sci* 1995, **764**:536–546.
- **Lonberg N, Huszar D**: *Human antibodies from transgenic mice. Int Rev Immunol* 1995, **13**:65–93.
- **Tomizuka K, Shinohara T, Yoshida H, Uejima H, Ohguma A, Tanaka S, Sato K, Oshimura M, Ishida I**: *Double trans-chromosomic mice: maintenance of two individual human chromosome fragments containing Ig heavy and kappa loci and expression of fully human antibodies. Proc Natl Acad Sci U S A* 2000, **97**:722–727.
- **Kuroiwa Y, Tomizuka K, Shinohara T, Kazuki Y, Yoshida H, Ohguma A, Yamamoto T, Tanaka S, Oshimura M, Ishida I**: *Manipulation of human minichromosomes to carry greater than megabase- sized chromosome inserts. Nat Biotechnol* 2000, **18**:1086–1090.
- **Fischer R, Hoffmann K, Schillberg S, Emans N**: *Antibody production by molecular farming in plants. J Biol Regul Homeost Agents* 2000, **14**:83–92.
- **Larrick JW, Yu L, Chen J, Jaiswal S, Wycoff K**: *Production of antibodies in transgenic plants. Res Immunol* 1998, **149**:603–608.
- **Russell DA**: *Feasibility of antibody production in plants for human therapeutic use. Curr Top Microbiol Immunol* 1999, **240**:119–138.
- **Pollock DP, Kutzko JP, Birck-Wilson E, Williams JL, Echelard Y, Meade HM**: *Transgenic milk as a method for the production of recombinant antibodies. J Immunol Methods* 1999, **231**:147–157.

Self-Assessment Questions

Question 1: *Which isotype or derivative would be appropriate for the development of a therapeutic antibody intended to functionally block a membrane-expressed hormone receptor, but not kill the receptor-expressing cell?*

Question 2: *What are the limitations for therapeutic use of traditional murine monoclonal antibodies?*

Question 3: *By which means can partially or completely human therapeutic antibodies be developed?*

Question 4: *What type of molecules can be used as targets for therapeutic antibodies?*

Answers

Answer 1: It depends on the desired effect and pharmacokinetics. IgG4 is a good choice if a long half-life is needed, without activation of ADCC or complement. F(ab) is a good choice when shorter circulation times are needed or more direct control of circulating antibody levels.

Answer 2: They are regarded as foreign proteins, and as such will elicit vigorous immune responses in humans. This immune response will neutralize the therapeutic effect, and in addition will cause severe allergic reactions upon re-exposure. A second reason murine antibodies are of limited use is that they are not efficient in activating human effector functions (ADCC and CDC). This inefficiency particularly limits their use as cancer therapeutics.

Answer 3: Chimerization or humanization of murine antibodies, and expressing the resultant recombinant antibody in (mammalian) cells.

Panning human-Vh/Vl derived phage display library, followed by genetic re-modeling of the isolated human ScFv into an intact human antibody and expressing the resultant recombinant antibody in (mammalian) cells.

Immunization of human heavy/light-chain transgenic or transchromosomic mice followed by conventional hybridoma development.

Answer 4: Antibodies do not enter into cells by themselves. The primary targets are therefore extracellular molecules, such as cytokines, chemokines and transmembrane proteins.

Nomenclature

The nonproprietary (or generic) names of small molecule drug products provide a suffix and/or prefix clue to the molecule's chemical class and therapeutic class. The nonproprietary names of monoclonal antibodies provide similar clues. The US Adopted Name (USAN) Council has been involved in creating generally accepted names for the various biological pharmaceutical products just as they have for small molecule pharmaceuticals. For instance, the nonproprietary name of the monoclonal antibody product distributed as ReoPro is "abciximab." This name tells us that the molecule is a chimeric monoclonal antibody that targets the cardiovascular system.

USAN Council has developed the following guidelines for naming monoclonal antibodies ():

1) The suffix *–mab* is used for monoclonal antibodies and fragments.
2) The source of the antibody is designated within the name. The animal source is an important safety factor when considering the potential for development of antibodies to the therapeutic monoclonal antibody in patients. The following are approved identifiers:

   a = rat
   e = hamster
   i = primate
   o = mouse
   u = human
   xi = chimera
   zu = humanized

   Thus, <u>xi</u>mab indicates a <u>chimeric</u> monoclonal antibody.
3) The general disease state subclass is included in the nonproprietary name by inclusion of a code syllable approved by the USAN Council.

   viral = *-vir-*
   bacterial = *-bac-*
   immunomodulator = *-lim-*
   infectious lesions = *-les-*
   tumors-colon = *-col-*
   tumors-melanoma = *-mel-*
   tumors-mammary = *-mar-*
   tumors-testis = *-got-*
   tumors-ovary = *-gov-*
   tumors-prostate = *-pr(o)-*
   tumors-miscellaneous = *-tum-*
   cardiovascular = *-cir-*

   A distinct, compatible syllable is selected as the beginning prefix in order to create a unique name.
5) The order for combining the various key elements is as follows: unique prefix followed by disease state/target followed by source of antibody followed by "mab".
6) If the product is conjugated to another chemical or is radiolabeled, recognition is made by the addition of a second word.

Source: USP Dictionary of USAN and International Drug Names, 2000 Ed., U.S. Pharmacopeia, Rockville, MD, 2000, p. 1096.

Diagnostic Monoclonal Antibodies

A selection of U.S. Food and Drug Approved Diagnostic Mabs.

Mab	Trade Name	Detection/Indication
Technetium-99m-arcitumomab	CEA-Scan	metastatic colorectal cancer
Imiciromab pentetate	MyoScint	myocardial infarction
Satumomab pendetide	OncoScint CR/OV	colorectal and ovarian cancer
Capromab	ProstaScint	prostate adenocarcinoma
Nofetumomab	Verluma	small-cell lung cancer

13A Appendix A to Monoclonal Antibody-Based Pharmaceuticals

Trastuzumab/Herceptin®

Daniel L. Combs

Introduction

Herceptin® (trastuzumab) is a recombinant humanized monoclonal antibody that binds with high affinity to the extracellular domain of the HER2 receptor on cells over-expressing the HER2 gene. The antibody was engineered by inserting the complementary determining region amino acid residues of the murine parent (muMAb 4D5) into the framework of a consensus human IgG1 (Carter *et al.*, 1992). It has a molecular mass of 148 kDa and is glycosylated. Trastuzumab binds with somewhat greater affinity than does muMAb 4D5. Furthermore, unlike muMAb 4D5, it induces antibody-dependent cellular cytoxicity (ADCC) against HER2 overexpressing human tumor cell lines in the presence of human peripheral blood mononuclear cells. Trastuzumab is produced in a suspension culture of the mammalian Chinese Hamster Ovary (CHO) cell line. The formulation approved for clinical use is referred to as Herceptin® and the actual monoclonal antibody has the generic name trastuzumab.

Herceptin® is approved in the United States for the treatment of metastatic breast cancer in patients whose tumors overexpress the HER2 receptor (Herceptin® Package Insert, September 2000). Overexpression is scored on a scale of 0, 1+, 2+, or 3+ as determined by immunohistochemical assay of tumor biopsy samples. Herceptin® as a single agent is indicated for the treatment of those patients who have received one or more chemotherapy regimens for their metastatic disease. Herceptin®, in combination with the taxane drug paclitaxel, is indicated for the treatment of those patients who have not received chemotherapy for their metastatic disease.

Background

The HER2 proto-oncogene, commonly referred to as HER2, is a member of the epidermal growth factor receptor (EGFR) family by virtue of its structural homology to EGFR (HER1) (Slamon *et al.*, 1987 and 1989; Hynes, 1993). Approximately one-quarter of women with breast cancer overexpress HER2. Overexpression is primarily due to gene amplification (Kraus *et al.*, 1987) and has been shown to correlate with poor clinical prognosis, shorter disease free interval and overall survival, and a more aggressive disease in general (Hynes and Stern, 1994).

The epidermal growth factor family of receptors are tyrosine kinase mediators of cell growth, differentiation, and survival (Groenen *et al.*, 1994; Lemke, 1996). The family is comprised of four distinct members: HER1 (ErbB1 or epidermal growth factor receptor), HER2 (ErbB2), HER3 (ErbB3), and HER4 (ErbB4) (Carraway and Cantley, 1994; Earp *et al.*, 1995; Pinkas-Kramarski *et al.*, 1997; Burden and Yarden, 1997; Riese *et al.*, 1995; Pinkas-Kramarski *et al.*, 1996). HER2 is the only member of this family without a known ligand. Inclusion of HER2 in receptor complexes results in enhanced signaling. Hence, overexpression of HER2 is theorized to lead to an increased signal for unchecked cell proliferation resulting in cancer (Sliwkowski *et al.*, 1994; Karunagaran *et al.*, 1996). The extracellular domain of the HER2 receptor, referred to here as shed antigen, can be released from the cell surface by endogenous proteolytic activity and is detectable in the serum of some patients.

Pharmacology

Mechanism of Action

Trastuzumab has demonstrated both cytostatic and cytotoxic activity *in vitro* and *in vivo* against a number of HER2-overexpressing cell lines. The precise molecular mechanisms behind these activities are unclear. Cytostatic activity is likely due to a trastuzumab blockade of the HER2 receptor, resulting in the forced formation of HER2 homodimers. This result prevents the enhancement of growth-signaling that results from the association of HER2 with other EGFR family members. Growth factor signaling may also be reduced as a result of down modulation and internalization of HER2 (Baulida, 1996; Sarup *et al.*, 1991; De Santes *et al.*, 1992) (Table 13.A1),

The cytotoxic activity of trastuzumab is due to antibody-dependent cell-mediated cytotoxicity (ADCC) (Lewis *et al.*, 1993; Pegram *et al.*, 1997; Hotaling *et al.*, 1996). The FcγRIII receptor on natural killer (NK) cells, and on monocytes and T-cells, binds to the Fc region of trastuzumab on opsonized tumor cells (Figure 13.A1). The efficacy of these cell types in mediating ADCC has been characterized by a quantitative *in vitro* assay which measures

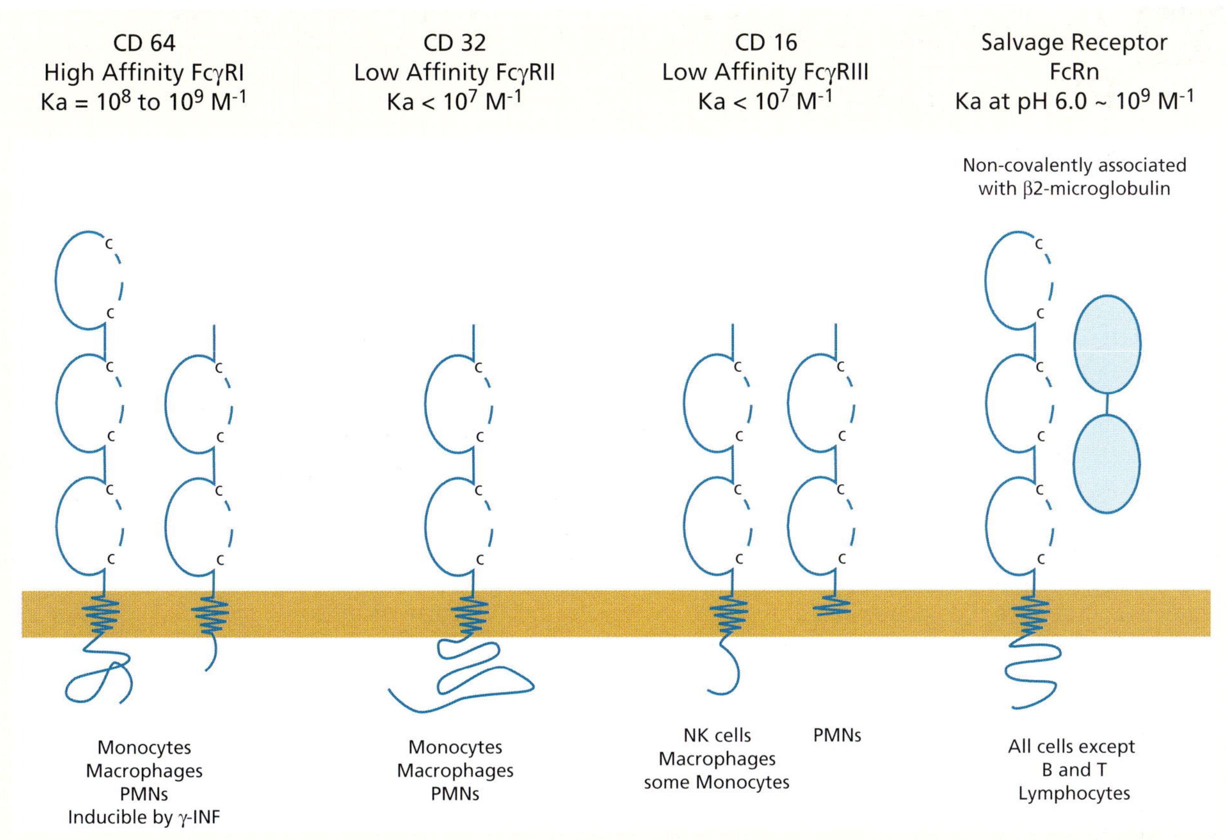

Figure 13A.1. Diagrammatic representation of the Fcγ receptors. These receptors are believed to mediate the ADCC activity of trastuzumab as well as the disposition processes accounting for trastuzumab pharmacokinetics.

Cell Line	HER2 Expression	Immuno-Histochemistry Score	Relative HER2 Expression after Exposure to Trastuzumab	
			1 Day	5 Days
MCF7	normal	0	49%	-
SK-BR-3	high	3^+	76%	43%

Table 13A.1. Trastuzumab-mediated downregulation of HER2.

the potentiating effect of a drug on an effector lymphocyte cell population that has cytotoxic activity against a target tumor cell-line. The target cell-lines are SKBR3, MCF-7, or BT-474, which are breast cancer cell-lines that express various levels of the HER2 gene. An example of the concentration-response curve of trastuzumab in this assay is shown in Figure 13.A2. These studies showed that monocytes and NK cells are extremely potent in killing trastuzumab-coated target cells (Figure 13.A3). When antibodies that block various lymphocyte receptors were added to this assay, CD16 (low affinity Fcγ RIII) was identified as necessary in mediating the activity of trastuzumab (Figure 13.A4).

Because some tumor cells overexpress the HER2 receptor in high density, there is an avidity component to trastuzumab induced ADCC as demonstrated by differential sensitivity of HER2 overexpressing cells to ADCC. This avidity enhancement is a consequence of high levels of Fcγ receptor-bearing cells binding to tumor cells opsonized by trastuzumab. Thus, trastuzumab activity is preferentially targeted to HER2-expressing cells with 2+ and 3+ level of overexpression rather than 1+ and non-expressing cells.

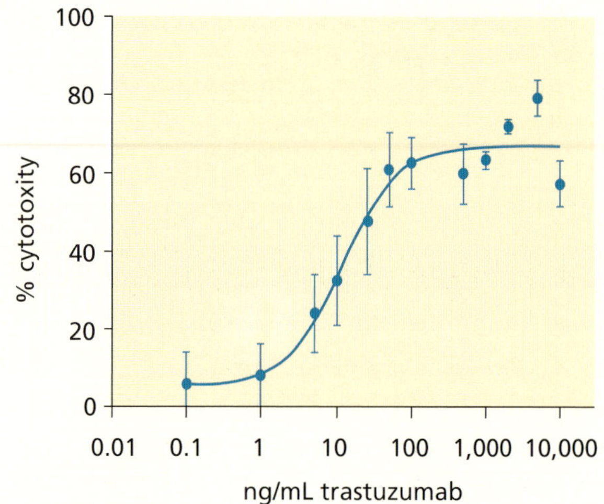

Figure 13A.2. ADCC assay showing cytotoxic activity of trastuzumab at various concentrations. The effector cell population was pooled lymphocytes from 3 human donors. In this example, the effector to target cell-ratio was held constant and the optimum trastuzumab concentration was selected for further study.

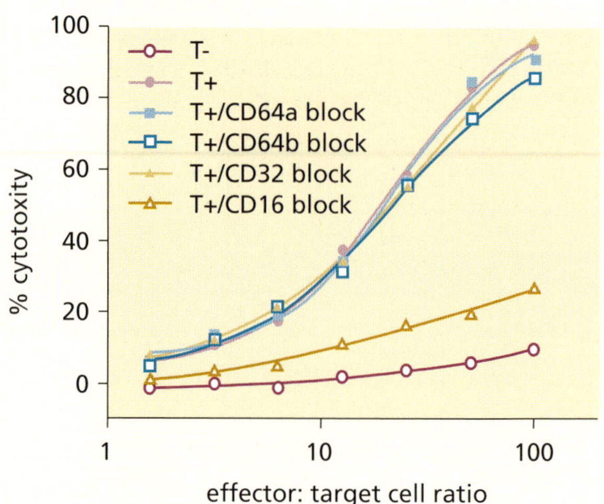

Figure 13A.4. In vitro assay of ADCC showing that the CD16 Fcγ receptors are necessary for mediating the cytotoxic activity of trastuzumab. The effector cells were NK cells. In this example, the optimum trastuzumab was maintained and the effector to target cell-ratio was varied from 1 to 100.

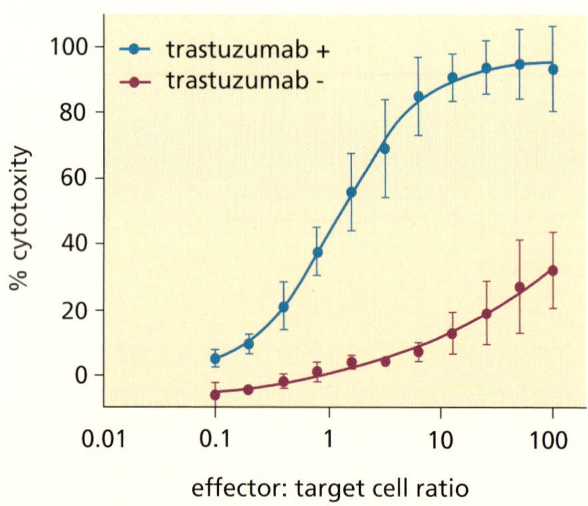

Figure 13A.3. In vitro assay of ADCC showing significant cytotoxic activity of trastuzumab at increasing ratios of effector to target cells. The effector cells were NK cells. In this example, the optimum trastuzumab concentration was maintained and the effector to target cell-ratio was varied from 0.1 to 100.

This preferential targeting contributes to the safety profile of trastuzumab in that normal cells show less susceptibility to ADCC.

Although trastuzumab contains a human IgG1 Fc region, *in vitro* studies indicated that it is not capable of fully activating complement to mediate complement dependent cytotoxicity, presumably because of inhibitory molecules present on the tumor cell surface.

In Vitro / In Vivo Efficacy Models

In vitro studies of tumor cell lines grown in culture have shown that monoclonal antibodies can block the HER2 receptor and inhibit cell growth (Baselga and Mendelson, 1994; Drebin *et al.*, 1985; Hancock *et al.*, 1991; Kasprzyk *et al.*, 1992; Stancovski *et al.*, 1991; Harwerth *et al.*, 1992). The maximum inhibitory effect was seen at an antibody concentration between 1 – 10 μg/mL (Hudziak *et al.*, 1989). Similarly, xenograft studies in nude mice transfected with human tumor cells overexpressing the HER2 gene demonstrated inhibition of tumor growth using a panel of antibodies directed against the HER2 receptor.

The most effective monoclonal antibody identified early in this work was muMAb 4D5, the murine parent of Trastuzumab. muMAb 4D5 was found to be active in the inhibition of tumor growth when moderately high HER2-overexpressing Paxton ovarian tumors and Murray breast tumors were transplanted into nude mice.

Unfortunately, the clinical utility of muMAb 4D5 was limited by immunogenicity. Therefore, it was humanized to create trastuzumab (Carter *et al.*, 1992). The murine complementary determining region amino acid residues associated with HER2 binding were inserted into a framework of a generic IgG1 human antibody. The resulting humanized antibody, trastuzumab, is highly homologous to human immunoglobulin and, unlike the murine parent antibody, has ADCC activity.

The efficacy of trastuzumab was determined relative to muMAb 4D5 in a nude mouse xenograft model using MCF7-HER2, a breast cancer cell-line that had been engineered to overexpress HER2. Dose related response in inhibition of tumor growth was observed and trastuzumab was significantly superior to muMAb 4D5. Trastuzumab was similarly evaluated in a xenograft model with another breast tumor cell line, BT-474 (Figure 13.A5), which naturally overexpresses HER2 and is therefore a better model for the human cancer. Dose dependent growth inhibition was observed and antitumor activity plateaued at doses above 1 mg/kg.

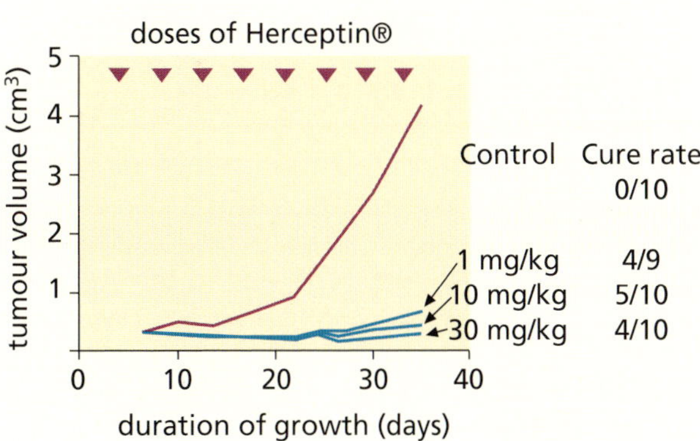

Figure 13A.5. Trastuzumab as a single agent in a murine xenograft model of tumor growth inhibition. The breast tumor cell-line used (human BT-474) naturally overexpress HER2 receptor.

Models in Combination with Cytotoxic Chemotherapeutic Agents

Trastuzumab was found to have additive and synergistic effects with certain commonly used cancer chemotherapeutic drugs. Combination studies of cisplatin and trastuzumab, muMAb 4D5 and other anti-HER2 monoclonal antibodies revealed potentiation of cytotoxicity by decreasing DNA repair following cisplatin-induced DNA damage (Pietras *et al.*, 1994; Arteaga *et al.*, 1994). *In vitro* studies in SK-BR3 HER2-overexpressing cells led to *in vivo* mouse xenograft studies using both MCF7 and the naturally overexpressing breast cancer cell-line BT-474 (Pegram *et al.*, 1999). The panel of chemotherapeutic drugs included drugs from several different classes: doxorubicin, paclitaxel, etoposide, methotrexate, cisplatin, vinblastine, thiotepa, cyclophosphamide, 5-flurouracil. In the mouse xenograft model using BT-474 cells, treatment with doxorubicin or paclitaxel resulted in greater inhibition of tumor growth than was observed with any agent alone (Baselga *et al.*, 1998) (Figure 13.A6). These studies demonstrated that trastuzumab augments the tumor killing capability of chemotherapy.

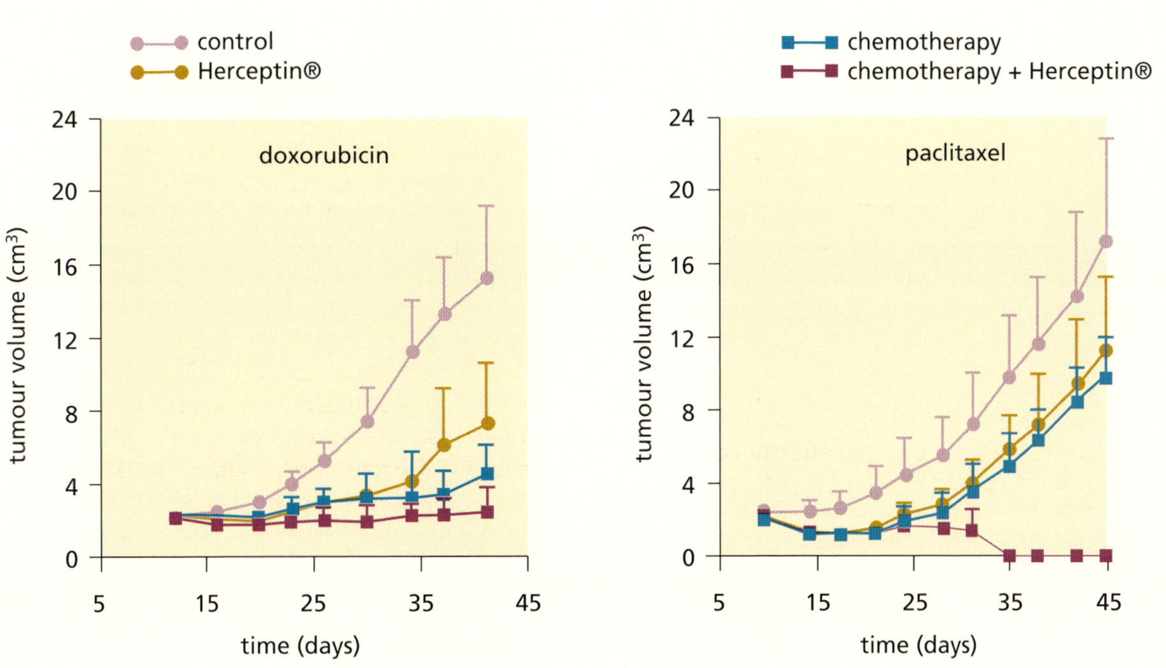

Figure 13A.6. Chemotherapy, trastuzumab as a single agent, and trastuzumab plus chemotherapy in a murine xenograft model of tumor growth inhibition using the BT-474 human breast tumor cell line (reproduced with permission from Baselga J, *et al.*, 1998).

Disposition

Biological Disposition Pathways

All full-length monoclonal antibodies constructed upon the human IgG consensus framework theoretically share the same generic disposition pathways. Differences in disposition kinetics should differ only in those pathways related to antigen-specific binding processes related to the complementary determining regions. However, unexplained differences in disposition exist between similar IgG1 antibodies when examined in animal models where only non-specific binding occurs. Apparently, other factors still remain to be discovered in order to explain these observed disposition differences.

Nevertheless, trastuzumab disposition kinetics can be roughly categorized into generic and antigen-specific pathways. Because trastuzumab is constructed upon a human IgG consensus framework, it is theoretically susceptible to the same binding and internalization through low and high-affinity Fcγ receptors (see Figure 13.A1) of the mononuclear phagocyte system (MPS) that eliminates endogenous antibodies (Mariani and Strober, 1990). Elimination through the MPS consists of intracellular trafficking to lysozomes followed by protein degradation. The long half-life of trastuzumab and endogenous antibodies is likely due to recycling through the FcRn salvage receptor, which protects the antibody from degradation during internalization, intracellular transit, return to the cellular membrane and release back into the extracellular space. It has been demonstrated that engineered gene knockout mice lacking the FcRn salvage receptor have abnormally short IgG half-lives (Ghetie *et al.*, 1996).

The specific disposition of trastuzumab is due to either antigen-specific binding to the HER2 receptor on the cell surface or to the shedding of HER2 extracellular domain circulating in the bloodstream (cf. Chapter 4). Total body tumor burden may or may not correlate with the extent of trastuzumab disposition depending upon whether first-order or zero-order kinetics apply, which in turn depends upon the ratio of antibody to antigen.

In this overview of trastuzumab disposition, reversible binding processes are considered to contribute to distribution volume, whereas irreversible binding processes leading to protein degradation contribute to clearance.

Pharmacokinetics

The pharmacokinetics of trastuzumab were studied in metastatic breast cancer patients. Short duration intravenous infusions of 10 to 500 mg given as single doses demonstrated dose-dependent pharmacokinetics (Figure 13.A7). When administered as weekly infusions, these same dose-levels also showed dose-dependent kinetics. Mean half-life

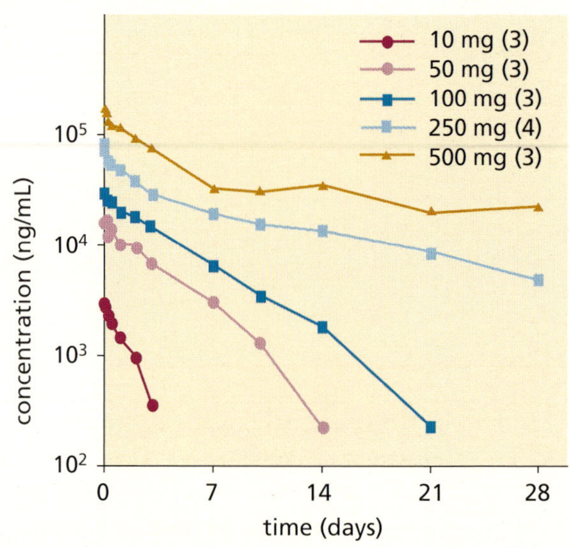

Figure 13A.7. Phase I mean serum concentrations of trastuzumab in metastatic breast cancer patients following single fixed-doses of 10, 50, 100, and 500 mg. N = 3 for all groups except the 250 group, where N = 4 patients.

increased and clearance decreased with increasing dose level. The half-life averaged 1.7 days at the 10 mg dose and 12 days at the 500 mg dose. Volume of distribution was approximately that of serum volume (44 mL/kg). At the highest weekly dose studied (500 mg), mean peak serum concentrations were 377 μg/mL.

Herceptin® is approved in the United States for administration on a body-weight basis as a 4 mg/kg loading dose followed by weekly maintenance doses of 2 mg/kg (Herceptin® Package Insert, September 2000). Phase III studies of this regimen resulted in a mean half-life of 5.8 days (range = 1 to 32 days). Trastuzumab reached an apparent steady-state level following 16 to 32 weeks of administration with mean trough and peak concentrations of approximately 79 μg/mL and 123 μg/mL, respectively (Table 13.A2 and Figure 13.A8). It should be noted that the half-life of trastuzumab was determined by fitting a one-compartment model to a peak and trough sampling schedule, which underestimated the true half-life and therefore could not account for the observed steady-state concentrations. The observed steady state suggested a longer half-life for trastuzumab, more consistent with that of other IgG1 monoclonal antibodies. Further clinical trials, in-progress or planned, will provide a better estimate of half-life.

Detectable concentrations of shed antigen were found in 62% to 71% of patients at pretreatment baseline measurement and tended to be higher in those patients with greater HER2 overexpression (3+ compared to 2+ overexpressers).

Phase/Dose (n)	Half-life (days)	Clearance (mL/day/kg)	Volume (mL/kg)	Css (µg/mL)
Phase I Studies (alone):				
10 mg (n = 6)	1.7 ± 0.2	21 ± 8	52 ± 23	NA[b]
50 mg (n = 6)	5.1 ± 2.5	9.0 ± 5.1	51 ± 6	NA
100 mg (n = 6)	8.0 ± 2.0	5.2 ± 2.0	56 ± 7	NA
250 mg (n = 6)	8.6 ± 4.9	5.5 ± 4.6	53 ± 30	NA
500 mg (n = 8)	12 ± 5.5	6.0 ± 5.3	77 ± 31	NA
Phase II Studies (alone or in combination with cisplatin):				
250 mg LD[c] 100 MD[c] (n = 82)	9 ± 10	6.3 ± 7.4	51 ± 23	51 ± 23
Phase III Studies (alone or in combination with AC or Paclitaxel)[d]:				
4.0 mg/kg LD[c] 2.0 mg/kg MD[c] (n = 159)	5.8 ± 4.3	5.1 ± 2.5	36 ± 17	56 ± 18

Table 13A.2. Cross-Study summary of mean (±SD) pharmacokinetic parameters following once weekly IV administration of trastuzumab[a].

[a] For Phase I and II Studies: Pharmacokinetic parameters were computed out to the last sampling time, which varied for each patient. For Phase III Studies: Pharmacokinetic parameters were computed for the first 8 weeks of treatment only after which the first tumor response evaluation was performed.

[b] NA = Not Available, since Css was not computed in Phase I studies.

[c] LD = loading dose, MD = maintenance dose.

[d] n = 109 for Herceptin® in combination with chemotherapy, and n = 50 for Herceptin® as a single agent.

Complexes of shed antigen and trastuzumab have been found to have intermediate clearances between those of free trastuzumab and shed antigen. Thus, high levels of shed antigen in patients can add to the overall clearance of trastuzumab. The median shed antigen concentration in patients was measured at approximately 11 ng/mL and in 6.3% to 15% of patients concentrations were greater than 500 ng/mL. The highest shed antigen concentration observed was 1880 ng/mL. Patients with higher levels of shed antigen at baseline were more likely to have lower trastuzumab serum concentrations (Figure 13.A9). However, with weekly dosing, most patients with elevated shed antigen levels had normal trastuzumab concentrations after six weekly doses. Thus, the clearance of drugs by shed antigen is not considered a barrier to effective treatment for the majority of patients and dosing for them does not need to be adjusted based upon shed antigen levels.

The influence of total HER2 antigen concentration (shed HER2 antigen and total body tumor burden of HER2) on trastuzumab clearance and volume of distribution, although consistent with its mechanism of action, is not currently ascertainable due to a lack of data on patient tumor burden. Likewise, the correlation between shed antigen level and clinical prognosis is unclear.

Pharmacokinetic/Pharmacodynamic Relationships

There are no known pharmacodynamic endpoints that are reliably predictive of clinical response to Herceptin® treatment or have proved useful in any pharmacokinetic/pharmacodynamic evaluation. Although high shed antigen is associated with lower serum trastuzumab concentration, there is no correlation between baseline shed antigen and clinical response.

In general, higher trastuzumab serum concentrations are associated with a trend towards better tumor response. After eight weeks of treatment, patients responding to

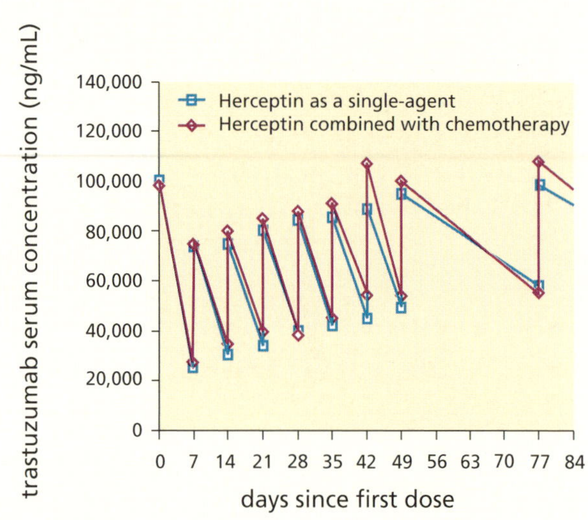

Figure 13A.8. Mean serum concentrations of trastuzumab in metastatic breast cancer patients following a loading-dose of 4 mg/kg and weekly maintenance doses of 2 mg/kg. Squares: Herceptin®administerd as a single-agent; Diamonds: Herceptin® administerd in combination with chemotherapy (AC or Paclitaxel).

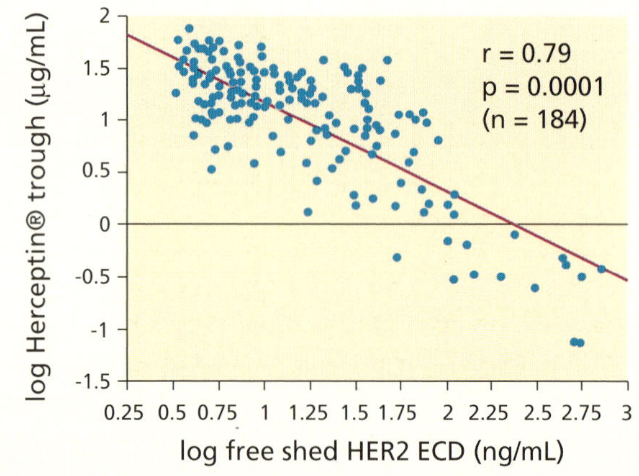

Figure 13A.9 Relationship between serum shed antigen (extracellular domain of the HER2 receptor) and trastuzumab trough serum concentration in metastatic breast cancer patients (reproduced with permission from Pegram M, *et al.* Journal of Clinical Oncology, 1998; 16:2659–71).

Herceptin® monotherapy displayed a significantly higher trastuzumab trough concentration (60 ± 20 µg/mL) compared to non-responders (33 ± 25 µg/mL). However, the clinical trials were not designed to determine a minimally effective or target concentration.

A higher maintenance dose of 4 mg/kg has been evaluated in approximately 100 patients across three different studies. Due to the small number of responses in this group, it was not possible to assess the possibility of an enhanced dose-response at this higher maintenance dose.

Clinical usage

Key Clinical Experience

The safety and efficacy of Herceptin® were studied in a randomized, controlled clinical trial in combination with chemotherapy (469 patients) and an open-label single agent trial (222 patients). Patients in both trials had metastatic breast cancer with tumors overexpressing the HER2 protein as assessed by immunohistochemical assay. Patients were eligible if their level of tumor overexpression was 2+ or 3+ on a scale from 0 to 3+.

In both trials Herceptin® was administered by IV-infusion with a 4 mg/kg loading dose (90 minutes) followed by weekly maintenance doses of 2 mg/kg weekly (30 minutes).

Herceptin® in Combination with Chemotherapy

In the combination trial Herceptin® was administered with either paclitaxel (175 mg/m^2) or with an anthracycline plus cyclophosphamide (AC). The anthracycline used was either doxorubicin (60 mg/m^2) or epirubicin (75 mg/m^2). Cyclophosphamide was administered at 600 mg/m^2. Chemotherapeutic regimens were given every 21 days for at least six cycles. Two other arms in this trial consisted of the paclitaxel or AC chemotherapeutic regimens in the absence of Herceptin®.

Compared with patients receiving chemotherapy alone, patients also receiving Herceptin® experienced a significantly longer median time to disease progression, a higher overall response rate, a longer median duration of response, and a higher one-year survival rate (79% alive for Herceptin® plus chemotherapy versus 68% for chemotherapy alone) (Table 13.A3). These treatment differences were observed both in patients receiving Herceptin® plus paclitaxel and in those receiving Herceptin® plus AC; however the magnitude of the treatment effects was greater in the paclitaxel subgroup.

Specifically, patients receiving Herceptin® had a median time to disease progression that was 2.7 months longer than patients receiving chemotherapy alone and an overall response rate of 45% compared to 29%. Addition of Herceptin® made the biggest improvement in treatment effect in the subgroup receiving paclitaxel, increasing time to progression by 4.2 months over paclitaxel alone.

	Combined results		Paclitaxel Subgroup		AC Subgroup	
	Herceptin® + All Chemotherapy (n = 235)	All Chemotherapy (n = 234)	Herceptin® + Paclitaxel (n = 92)	Paclitaxel (n = 96)	Herceptin® + AC[a] (n = 143)	AC (n = 138)
Primary Endpoint: Time to Progression[b,c]						
Median (months)	7.2	4.5	6.7	2.5	7.6	5.7
95% confidence interval	6.9–8.2	4.3–4.9	5.2–9.9	2.0–4.3	7.2–9.1	4.6–7.1
p-value (log rank)	< 0.0001		< 0.0001		0.002	
Secondary Endpoint: Overall Response Rate[b]						
Rate (percent)	45	29	38	15	50	38
95% confidence interval	39–51	23–35	28–48	8–22	42–58	30–46
p-value (χ2-test)	< 0.001		< 0.001		0.10	
1-Year Survival[c]						
Percent Alive	79	68	73	61	83	73
95% confidence interval	74–84	62–74	66–80	51–71	77–89	66–82
p-value (Z-test)	< 0.01		0.08		0.04	

Table 13A.3. Efficacy of Herceptin® when Combined with first-line chemotherapy.
[a] AC = anthracycline (doxorubicin or epirubicin) and cyclophosphamide.
[b] Assessed by an independent Response Evaluation Committee.
[c] Kaplan-Meier estimate.

Herceptin® as a Single Agent

In the single agent trial, Herceptin® was studied in HER2 overexpressing metastatic breast cancer patients who had relapsed following one or two prior chemotherapy regimens for metastatic disease. The overall response rate was 14% (complete + partial responders) with a 2% complete response rate and a 12% partial response rate. Complete responses were observed only in those patients with disease limited to skin and lymph nodes.

Treatment Effect and HER2 Overexpression

In both efficacy studies, the degree of HER2 overexpression was a predictor of treatment effect such that the beneficial treatment effects were largely limited to patients with the highest level of overexpression (3+).

Safety Concerns

Patients receiving anthracycline chemotherapy are at risk of cardiotoxicity, which is thought to be caused by excessive intracellular production of free radicals within the myocardium. This risk is increased when Herceptin® is added to anthracycline therapy or when patients previously treated with anthracycline are given Herceptin®. In spite of this cardiotoxicity, there was a survival benefit attributable to Herceptin® treatment in the clinical trials.

Cardiotoxicity takes the form of ventricular dysfunction and congestive heart failure. The exact mechanism by which Herceptin® appears to exacerbate anthracycline-induced cardiotoxicity is not known but may be related to the role of the HER family of receptors in development (Lemke, 1996). In clinical trials, class III–IV congestive heart failure (New York Heart Association) was observed in 5% of

	Herceptin® alone[a] (n = 213)	Herceptin® + Paclitaxel[b] (n = 91)	Paclitaxel[b] (n = 95)	Herceptin® + AC[b] (n = 143)	AC[b] (n = 135)
Any Cardiac Dysfunction	7%	11%	1%	28%	7%
Class III-IV[c]	5%	4%	1%	19%	3%

Table 13A.4. Incidence and severity of cardiac dysfunction.
[a] Open-label single-agent Phase III study (94% of patients received prior anthracyclines).
[b] Randomized Phase III study comparing chemotherapy plus Herceptin® to chemotherapy alone, where chemotherapy was either anthracycline/cyclophosphamide or paclitaxel.
[c] New York Heart Association.

patients receiving Herceptin® alone, 4% of patients receiving Herceptin® plus paclitaxel and 1% of patients receiving paclitaxel alone. The highest incidence of this class of congestive heart failure was found in patients receiving Herceptin® plus AC (19%) as compared to patients receiving AC alone (3%) (Table 13.A4).

Careful cardiac monitoring is recommended for any patient undergoing Herceptin® treatment and discontinuation of Herceptin® should be considered for patients who develop clinically significant congestive heart failure. In the clinical trials, most patients with cardiac dysfunction responded to appropriate medical therapy, often including the discontinuation of Herceptin®.

Infrequent severe hypersensitivity reactions including anaphylaxis have occurred and have been most commonly associated with the first infusion. Rare severe infusion reactions have also been observed to occur, again mostly associated with the first infusion. In some cases these reactions have been fatal. Some patients suffering severe reactions have been readministered Herceptin® following recovery. The majority were prophylactically treated with pre-medications including antihistamines and/or corticosteroids. Rare instances of severe pulmonary events leading to death have been reported with the use of Herceptin®. These include dyspnea, pulmonary infiltrates, pleural effusions, non-cardiogenic pulmonary edema, pulmonary insufficiency and hypoxia, and acute respiratory distress syndrome.

Pharmaceutical considerations

Formulation

Herceptin® is a sterile, white to pale-yellow, preservative-free lyophilized powder for intravenous administration. The nominal content of each vial is 440 mg trastuzumab, 9.9 mg L-histidine HCL, 6.4 mg L-histidine, 400 mg alfa,alfa-trehalose dihydrate, and 1.8 mg polysorbate 20, USP. Reconstitution with 20 mL bacteriostatic water for injection USP containing 1.1% benzyl alcohol preservative yields a multi-dose solution of 21 mg/mL trastuzumab at a pH of approximately 6. If intended for multiple use, this reconstituted solution should be stored at 2–8 °C (36–46 °F) which maintains sterility and stability for up to 28 days. If Herceptin® is reconstituted with unpreserved sterile water for injection, it should be used immediately and the unused portion discarded. For infusion the appropriate volume of 21 mg/mL solution should be computed for either a 4 mg/kg loading dose or a 2 mg/kg maintenance dose and added to an infusion bag containing 250 mL of 0.9% sodium chloride injection USP. This infusion solution may be stored at 2–8 °C (36–46 °F) for up to 24 hours prior to use. Dextrose solution (5%) should not be used in preparing infusion solutions.

Other Routes of Administration / Dosing Regimens

Herceptin® has not been studied clinically as a subcutaneously injectable drug, although such administration may be feasible for convenience to the patient and clinical staff. Maintenance doses of 4 mg/kg have been studied in fewer than 100 patients. Currently the clinical feasibility of a q3 week regimen of 8 mg/kg loading dose and 6 mg/kg maintenance dose is being evaluated in a small trial.

Acknowledgements

The author wishes to thank the following Genentech researchers for contributing material for this chapter: Judith Fox, Tim Hotaling and Mark Sliwkowski. ■

Further Reading

- **Aguilar Z, Akita RW, Finn RS, Ramos BL, Pegram MD, Kabbinavar FF, *et al.*** (1999). Biological effects of heregulin/neu differentiation factor on normal and malignant human breast and ovarian epithelian cells. *Oncogene*, 18, 6050–6062.
- **Baselga J, Tripathy D, Mendelsohn J, Baughman S, Benz CC, Dantis L, *et al.*** (1999). Phase II study of weekly intravenous trastuzumab (Herceptin) in patients with HER2/neu-overexpressing metastatic breast cancer. *Seminars in Oncology*, 26(4 Suppl 12):78–83.
- **Borden EC, Esserman L, Linder DJ, Campbell MJ and Fulton AM.** (1999). Biological therapies for breast carcinoma: concepts for improvement in survival [Review]. *Seminars in Oncology*, 26(4 Suppl 12):28–40.
- **Bridges AJ.** (1999). The rationale and strategy used to develop a series of highly potent, irreversible, inhibitors of the epidermal growth factor receptor family of tyrosine kinases [Review]. *Current Medicinal Chemistry*. 6(9):825–43.
- **Burden S, Yarden Yosef.** (1997). Neuregulins and their receptors: a versatile signaling module in organogenesis and oncogenesis. *Neuron*, 18:847–55.
- **Burris HA 3rd.** (2000). Docetaxel (Taxotere) in HER-2-positive patients and in combination with trastuzumab (Herceptin) [Review]. *Seminars in Oncology*, 27(2 Suppl 3):19–23.
- **Feldman AM, Lorell BH, Reis SE.** (2000). Trastuzumab in the treatment of metastatic breast cancer: anticancer therapy versus cardiotoxicity [Review]. *Circulation*, 102(3):272–4.
- **Hung MC, Lau YK.** (1999). Basic science of HER-2/neu: a review [Review]. *Seminars in Oncology*, 26(4 Suppl 12):51–9.
- **Kirschbaum MH, Yarden Y.** (2000). The ErbB/HER family of receptor tyrosine kinases: a potential target for chemoprevention of epithelial neoplasms. *J Cell Biochem*, Suppl 34:52–60.
- **Miller KD, Sledge GW Jr.** (1999). Toward checkmate: biology and breast cancer therapy for the new millennium [Review]. *Investigational New Drugs*, 17(4):417–27.
- **Norton L.** (1999). Kinetic concepts in the systemic drug therapy of breast cancer [Review]. *Seminars in Oncology*, 26(1 Suppl 2):11–20.
- **Perez EA.** (1999). Current management of metastatic breast cancer [Review]. *Seminars in Oncology*, 26(4 Suppl 12):1–10.
- **Ryu DD, Nam DH.** (2000). Recent progress in biomolecular engineering [Review]. *Biotechnology Progress*, 16(1):2–16.
- **Shak S.** (1999). Overview of the trastuzumab (Herceptin) anti-HER2 monoclonal antibody clinical program in HER2-overexpressing metastatic breast cancer. Herceptin Multinational Investigator Study Group. [Review]. *Seminars in Oncology*, 26(4 Suppl 12):71–7.
- **Sledge GW Jr, Miller K.** (1999). Breast cancer: challenges and opportunities[Review]. *Seminars in Oncology*, 26(6 Suppl 18):1–5.
- **Sliwkowski MX, Lofgren JA, Lewis GD, Hotaling TE, Fendly BM and Fox JA.** (1999). Nonclinical studies addressing the mechanism of action of trastuzumab (Herceptin) [Review]. Seminars in Oncology, 26(4 Suppl 12):60–70.
- **Sznol M, Holmlund J.** (1997). Antigen-specific agents in development [Review]. *Seminars in Oncology*, 24(2):173–86.
- **Weiner LM.** (1999). Monoclonal antibody therapy of cancer [Review]. *Seminars in Oncology*, 26(5 Suppl 14):43–51.
- **Yu D, Hung MC.** (2000). Role of erbB2 in breast cancer chemosensitivity [Review]. *Bioessays*, 22(7):673–80.

References

- **Arteaga CL, Winnier AR, Poirier MC, Lopez-Larraza DM, Shawver LK, Hurd SD, *et al.*** (1994). p185$^{c\text{-}erbB\text{-}2}$ signaling enhances cisplatin-induced cytotoxicity in human breast carcinoma cells: association between an oncogenic receptor tyrosine kinase and drug-induced DNA repair. *Cancer Res*, 54, 3758–65.
- **Baselga J, Mendelsohn J.** (1994). Receptor blockade with monoclonal antibodies as anti-cancer therapy. *Pharmacol Ther*, 64, 127–54.
- **Baselga J, Norton L, Albanell J, Kim Y-M and Mendelsohn J.** (1998). Recombinant humanized anti-HER2 antibody (Herceptin™) enhances the antitumor activity of paclitaxel and doxorubicin against HER2/neu overexpressing human breast cancer xenografts. *Cancer Res*, 58, 2825–31.
- **Baulida J, Kraus MH, Alimandi M, Di Fiore PP and Carpenter G.** (1996). All ErbB receptors other than the epidermal growth factor receptor are endocytosis impaired. *J Biol Chem*, 271, 5251–7.
- **Burden S and Yarden Y.** (1997). Neuregulins and their receptors: a versatile signaling module in organogenesis and oncogenesis. *Neuron*, 18, 847–55.
- **Carraway KL III and Cantley LC.** (1994). A neu acquaintance for erbB3 and erbB4: a role for receptor heterodimerization in growth signaling. *Cell*, 78, 5–8.
- **Carter P, Preta L, Gorman CM, Ridgway JB, Henner D, Wong WL, *et al.*** (1992). Humanization of an anti-p185^{HER2} antibody for human cancer treatment. *Proc Natl Acad Sci USA*, 89, 4285–9.
- **De Santes K, Slamon D, Anderson SK, Shepard M, Fendly B, Maneval D, *et al.*** (1992). Radiolabeled antibody targeting of the HER-2/neu oncoprotein. *Cancer Res*, 52, 1916–23.
- **Drebin JA, Link VC, Stern DF, Weinberg RA and Greene MI.** (1985). Down-modulation of an oncogene protein product and reversion of the transformed phenotype by monoclonal antibodies. *Cell*, 41, 697–706.

- **Earp HS, Dawson TL, Li X and Yu H.** (1995). Heterodimerization and functional interaction between EGF receptor family members: a new signaling paradigm with implications for breast cancer research. *Breast Cancer Res Treat*, 35, 115–32.
- **Ghetie V, Hubbard JG, Kim J-K, Tsen M-F, Lee Y and Ward ES.** (1996). Abnormally short serum half-lives of IgG in β2-microglobulin-deficient mice. *Eur J Immunol*, 26, 690–696.
- **Groenen LC, Nice EC and Burgess AW.** (1994). Structure-function relationships for the EGF/TGF-α family of mitogens. *Growth Factors*, 11, 235–57.
- **Hancock MC, Langton BC, Chan T, Toy P, Monahan JJ, Mischak RR, *et al.*** (1991). A monoclonal antibody against the c-erbB-2 protein enhances the cytotoxicity of cis-diamminedichloroplatinum against human breast and ovarian tumor cell lines. *Cancer Res*, 51, 4575–80.
- **Harwerth I-M, Wels W, Marte BM and Hunes NE.** (1992). Monoclonal antibodies against the extracellular domain of the erbB-2 receptor function as partial ligand agonists. *J Biol Chem*, 267, 15160–7.
- **Herceptin®** (Trastuzumab) Package Insert, September 2000. Genentech, Inc. 1 DNA Way, South San Francisco, CA 94080-4990, www.gene.com
- **Hotaling TE, Reitz B, Wofgang-Kimball D, Bauer K and Fox JA.** (1996). The humanized anti-HER2 antibody rhuMAb HER2 mediates antibody dependent cell-mediated cytotoxictiy via FcγR III [abstract]. *Proc Annu Meet Am Assoc Cancer Res*, 37, 471.
- **Hudziak RM, Lewis GD, Winget M, Fendly BM, Shepard HM and Ulrich A.** (1989). p185^{HER2} monoclonal antibody has antiproliferative effects in vitro and sensitizes human breast tumor cells to tumor necrosis factor. *Mol Cell Biol*, 9, 1165–72.
- **Hynes NE and Stern DF.** (1994). The biology of erbB-2/neu/HER-2 and its role in cancer. *Biochim Biophys Acta*, 1198, 165–84.
- **Hynes NE.** (1993). Amplification and overexpression of the erbB-2 gene in human tumors: its involvement in tumor development, significance as a prognostic factor, and potential as a target for cancer therapy. *Sem Cancer Biol*, 4, 19–26.
- **Karunagaran D, Tzahar E, Beerli RR, Chen X, Graus-Porta D, Ratzkin BJ, *et al.*** (1996). ErbB-2 is a common auxiliary subunit of NDF and EGF receptors: implications for breast cancer. *EMBO J*, 15, 254–64.
- **Kasprzyk PG, Song SU, Di Fiore PP, King CR.** (1992). Therapy of an animal model of human gastric cancer using a combination of anti-erbB-2 monoclonal antibodies. *Cancer Res*, 52, 2771–6.
- **Kraus MH, Popescu NC, Amsbaugh SC and King CR.** (1987). Overexpression of the EGF receptor-related proto-oncolgene erbB-2 in human mammary tumor cell lines by different molecular mechanisms. *EMBO J*, 6, 605–10.
- **Lemke G.** (1996). Neuregulins in development. *Mol Cell Neurosci*, 7, 247–62.
- **Lewis GD, Figari I, Fendly B, Wong WL, Carter P. Gorman C, *et al.*** (1993). Differential responses of human tumor cell lines to anti-p185HER2 monoclonal antibodies. *Cancer Immunol Immunother*, 37, 255–63.
- **Mariani G and Strober W.** (1990). Immunoglobulin metabolism In: Metzger H (editor). Fc receptors and the action of antibodies. *Am Soc for Microbiol*, 94–177.
- **Pegram M, Hsu S, Lewis G, Pietras R, Beryt M, Sliwkowski M, *et al.*** (1999). Inhibitory effects of combinations of HER2/neu antibody and chemotherapeutic agents for treatment of human breast cancers. *Oncogene*, 18, 2241–51.
- **Pegram MD, Baly D, Wirth C, Gilkerson E, Slamon DJ, Sliwkowski MX, *et al.*** (1997). Antibody dependent cell-mediated cytotoxicity in breast cancer patients in Phase III clinical trials of a humanized anti-HER2 antibody [abstract], *Proc Am Assoc Cancer Res*, 38, 602.
- **Pietras RJ, Fendly BM, Chazin VR, Pegram MD, Howell SB and Slamon DJ.** (1994). Antibody to HER-2/neu receptor blocks DNA repair after cisplatin in human breast and ovarian cancer cells. *Oncogene*, 9, 1829–38.
- **Pinkas-Kramarski R, Alroy I and Yarden Y.** (1997). ErbB receptors and EGF-like ligands: cell lineage determination and oncogenesis through combinatorial signaling. *J Mammary Gland Biology and Neoplasia*, 2, 97–107.
- **Pinkas-Kramarski R, Soussan L, Waterman H, Levkowitz G, Alroy I, Klapper L, *et al.*** (1996). Diversification of Neu differentiation factor and epidermal growth factor signaling by combinatorial receptor interactions. *EMBO J*, 15, 2452–67.
- **Riese DJ II, van Raaij TM, Plowman GD, Andrews GC and Stern DF.** (1995). The cellular response to neuregulins is governed by complex interactions of the erbB receptor family. *Mol Cell Biol*, 15, 5770–6.
- **Sarup JC, Johnson RM, King KL, Fendly BM, Lipari MT, Napier MA, *et al.*** (1991). Characterization of an anti-p185HER2 monoclonal antibody that stimulates receptor function and inhibits tumor cell growth. *Growth Regul*, 1, 72–82.
- **Slamon DJ, Clark GM, Wong SG, Levin WJ, Ullrich A and McGuire WL.** (1987). Human breast cancer: correlation of relapse and survival with amplification of the HER-2/neu oncogene. *Science*, 235, 177–82.
- **Slamon DJ, Godolphin W, Jones LA, Holt JA, Wong SG, Keith DE, *et al.*** (1989). Studies of the HER-2/neu proto-ongogene in human breast and ovarian cancer. *Science*, 244, 707–12.
- **Sliwkowski MX, Schaefer G, Akita RW, Lofgren JA, Fitzpatrick VD, Nuijens A, *et al.*** (1994). Coexpression of erbB2 and erbB3 proteins reconstitutes a high affinity receptor for heregulin. *J Biol Chem*, 269, 14661–5.
- **Stancovski I, Hurwitz E, Leitner O, Ullrich A, Yarden Y and Sela M.** (1991). Mechanistic aspects of the opposing effects of monoclonal antibodies to the ERBB2 receptor on tumor growth. *Proc Natl Acad Sci USA*, 88, 8691–5.

Self-Assessment Questions

Question 1: *Given the high binding affinity (low KD) and pharmacokinetic characteristics of trastuzumab (Herceptin), the receptor occupancy should be quite high (> 90% based upon the law of mass-balance). Why then do tumor response rates not approach 100%?*

Question 2: *Trastuzumab (Herceptin) can form a complex with circulating shed extracellular domain (ECD) of the HER2 receptor (shed ECD). Given that the relative magnitude of clearance is: free ECD > complex > free trastuzumab, will the profile of total ECD concentrations rise or fall with repeated dosing? What about total trastuzumab concentrations? (Total ECD is measured by an assay that measures free ECD and ECD in the complex, whereas the total trastuzumab assay is specific for free trastuzumab and trastuzumab in the complex.)*

Question 3: *What are the major elimination pathways for Herceptin in patients? Would one expect the same pathways to be present in healthy cynomolgus and rhesus monkeys that were used in Herceptin toxicology studies? The rat is a useful animal model to study the cardiotoxicity sometimes observed in patients receiving Herceptin plus anthracycline chemotherapeutics. However, the rat version of the HER2 receptor does not bind trastuzumab. Knowing this, what clearance pathways would the rat have in common with patients?*

Question 4: *Given that normal healthy tissue also contains cells expressing the HER2 receptor, why does trastuzumab treatment not result in the general destruction of healthy tissues along with cancerous tissues?*

Question 5: *It would be considerably more convenient for the patient and medical staff if Herceptin could be delivered via subcutaneous injection as opposed to the 30 to 90 minute intravenous infusion now given each week. If the maximum dose volume acceptable for subcutaneous injection were 4 mL and the bioavailability by this route of administration were 35%, what would be the concentration required for the reconstituted vial? (Note: monoclonal antibodies, including Herceptin, generally have considerably higher subcutaneous bioavailability than the low value of 35% used in this example.)*

Answers

Answer 1: Estimates of receptor occupancy based upon KD and pharmacokinetics are valid only for the biological compartment where the pharmacokinetics are measured. This is usually the serum or plasma. Except for hematological malignancies, most tumors are not located in the blood. Consequently, without knowledge of drug levels at the surface or interior of the tumor, receptor occupancy cannot be determined where it is most meaningful. A target that is mostly or entirely located in the blood compartment is a better candidate for using receptor occupancy as a tool in choosing dosage regimens. It should also be kept in mind that tumor cells are heterogeneous and often develop biological strategies to overcome the activity of a chemotherapeutic drug, regardless of the efficiency of receptor blockade. Many other factors (e.g. organ function, global health status, immune function) contribute to the ability of patients to respond to chemotherapy.

Answer 2: With repeated dosing more and more of total ECD is comprised of ECD bound up in the complex. As a consequence of the slower clearance of the complex relative to free ECD, over time the serum profile of total ECD shows an accumulation to a higher level. For total trastuzumab however, the complex of trastuzumab and ECD clears more quickly than free trastuzumab. Nevertheless, with repeated dosing at the prescribed dose, less and less of total trastuzumab is comprised of the complex; most of total drug is due to free trastuzumab. Thus, serum profiles of trastuzumab following dosing at steady state should show a lower clearance compared to single-dose profiles. It should be kept in mind that in a small minority of patients shed ECD is consistently maintained at high levels. In these patients, enough trastuzumab is bound up in the more highly cleared complex to result in reduced trastuzumab serum concentrations leading to a failure to attain therapeutic drug levels.

Answer 3: Trastuzumab is eliminated in patients by specific biological processes related to the Fab binding regions of the antibody that target the HER2 receptor on both normal and tumor cell surfaces, as well as circulating ECD. Trastuzumab is also eliminated by non-specific biological processes in common with endogenous IgG antibodies, including elimination by Fcγ receptors of the mononuclear phagocyte system (MPS). Also, FcRn receptors constitute a common antibody salvage pathway, resulting in a prolonged half-life in the body. Because trastuzumab is cross-reactive with the monkey HER2 receptor, the same clearance processes are present with the exception that monkeys do not have tumors. Therefore, this component of trastuzumab clearance, present in patients, is missing in the monkey model. Rats similarly do not have HER2 overexpressing tumors; moreover since trastuzumab is not cross-reactive in rats, specific elimination via binding to the HER2 receptor is absent. As a consequence of this lack of receptor homology, standard rat models used to study the impact of chronic blockade of the HER2 receptor must be performed with a substitute (surrogate) monoclonal antibody specific to the rat version of the HER2 receptor.

Answer 4: There is an avidity component to trastuzumab's cytotoxic effect, which results in greater killing of tumor cells compared to healthy cells. Cells overexpressing HER2 at the 2+ and 3+ level are usually tumor cells, while healthy cells expressing HER2 generally express at the 1+ level. Therefore, trastuzumab bound to tumor cells heavily opsonizes the cell surface. Immune cells mediating antibody dependent cellular cytotoxicity (ADCC) express Fcγ receptors that bind to the Fc portion of cell-bound Herceptin. Since the extent of opsonization of the tumor cell is high, this leads to a high density of bound immune cells, or avidity (often described as the velcro effect). Thus, ADCC-mediating immune cells bind with much higher density to 2+ and 3+ overexpressing tumor cells than to 1+ normal cells. Hence, this difference in avidity acts to preferentially target tumor cells and spares normal cells from destruction.

Answer 5: The current regimen requires administration of a maintenance dose of 2 mg/kg. For a 60 kg patient, this would be 120 mg of Herceptin delivered in 4 mL maximum injection volume. Thus, the concentration would need to be 30 mg/mL in the reconstituted vial. If the bioavailability were only 35%, maintaining the same average serum concentration would require $100/35 \times 2$ mg/kg = 5.71 mg/kg dosed or $100/35 \times 30$ mg/mL = 85.7 mg/mL in the reconstituted vial. On the other hand, the infusion administration calls for reconstitution of a 440 mg vial with 20 mL bacteriostatic water for injection, resulting in a reconstituted vial of 21 mg/mL (final volume is actually 20.95 mL). The appropriate volume of this solution is then added to an infusion bag of 250 mL. Given the assumptions of this example, the manufacturing feasibility of a subcutaneous formulation of Herceptin requires that it be possible to maintain in solution a vial reconstituted to 85.7 mg/mL. This is in comparison to 21 mg/mL for the infusion route of administration.

13B Appendix B to Monoclonal Antibody-Based Pharmaceuticals

Abciximab/Reopro®

Robert E. Jordan, Lawrence I. Deckelbaum and Marian T. Nakada

Introduction

Abciximab is the Fab fragment of the human/murine chimeric monoclonal antibody 7E3 (Knight, *et al.*, 1995). Abciximab binds and blocks platelet GPIIb/IIIa (α_{IIb}/β_3) and the related integrin receptor, $\alpha_v\beta_3$. The parent molecule of abciximab is the murine 7E3 monoclonal antibody that was originally characterized by Coller (Coller, 1985). Antibody 7E3 also interacts with the integrin receptor $\alpha_M\beta_2$ (Mac-1) present on white blood cells (Altieri and Edgington, 1988). Abciximab is a potent inhibitor of platelet aggregation and is indicated as an adjunct to percutaneous coronary intervention (PCI) for the prevention of cardiac ischemic complications in patients undergoing procedures such as balloon angioplasty and stent implantation and in patients with unstable angina not responding to conventional medical therapy when PCI is planned within 24 hours.

Molecular structure

Abciximab is produced from the human-murine chimeric monoclonal antibody, chimeric 7E3 IgG. Chimeric 7E3 IgG is a recombinant protein containing murine variable regions and human constant domains (Figure 13B.1). The chimeric 7E3 antibody is produced by continuous perfusion in mammalian cell culture. Abciximab is produced by the papain digestion of purified chimeric 7E3 IgG which yields the Fab fragments and the Fc domain. The 47.6 kDa Fab fragment is purified by a series of steps involving specific viral inactivation and removal procedures, and column chromatography. The final abciximab product contains 439 amino acids and consists of 50% murine and 50% human sequences. Abciximab possesses no detectable carbohydrate groups and has an isoelectric point (pI) of approximately 8.3.

Pharmacology

Mechanism of Action

Abciximab binds to the platelet GPIIb/IIIa receptor, a member of the integrin family of adhesion molecules, and the major platelet surface receptor for a variety of ligands involved in platelet aggregation (Plow and Ginsberg, 1989). Abciximab inhibits platelet aggregation by preventing the binding of fibrinogen, the von Willebrand factor, and other

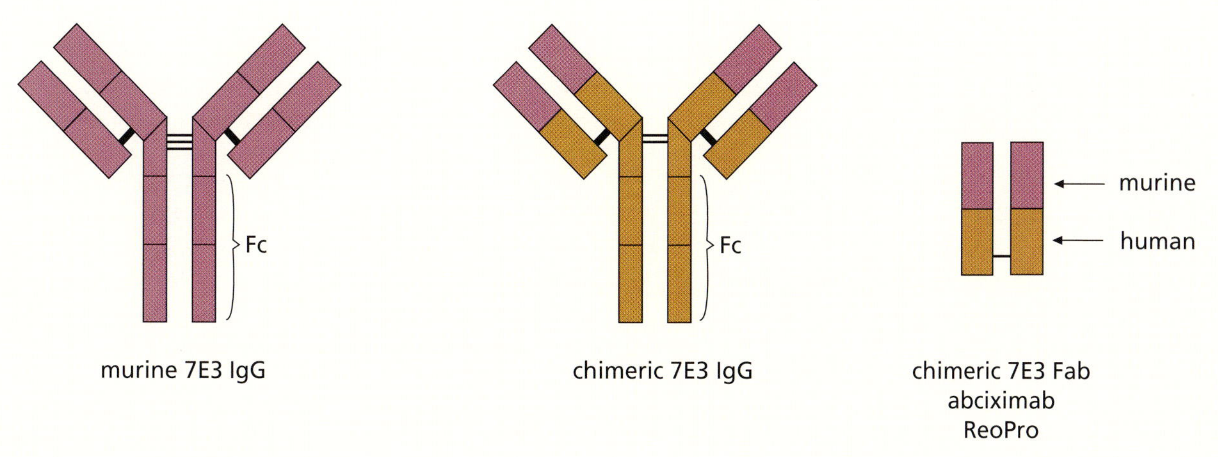

Figure 13B.1. Schematic depiction of murine 7E3 IgG (left), chimeric 7E3 IgG (center) in which human constant domains have replaced the original murine domains, and chimeric 7E3 Fab produced by proteolytic digestion of chimeric 7E3 IgG with papain.

adhesive molecules that bind to GPIIb/IIIa on activated platelets (Coller *et al.*, 1991). The mechanism of action of abciximab involves steric hindrance and/or conformational effects within GPIIb/IIIa to block access of large adhesive molecules to the receptor. The binding of platelet GPIIb/IIIa by abciximab blocks the ability of platelets to aggregate in response to a wide variety of stimuli, including collagen, adenosine diphosphate (ADP), thrombin, and others. The acute *in vivo* antithrombotic activity of abciximab in blocking platelet thrombus formation in coronary arteries is correlated directly to its binding to the platelet GPIIb/IIIa receptor. In addition to binding to the GPIIb/IIIa receptor, abciximab binds to the vitronectin ($\alpha_v\beta_3$) receptor, which mediates the procoagulant properties of platelets (Reverter *et al.*, 1996) and the proliferative properties of vascular endothelial and smooth muscle cells (Coller, 1999). *In vitro* studies showed that abciximab blocked $\alpha_v\beta_3$-mediated effects, including cell adhesion, and more effectively blocked the burst of thrombin generation that followed platelet activation than did agents inhibiting GPIIb/IIIa alone. The relation of these data to clinical efficacy is uncertain.

Abciximab also reacts with the integrin receptor $\alpha_M\beta_2$ (Mac-1). Mac-1 is present on granulocytes, monocytes, and leukocytes and is an important mediator of inflammation. The importance of this cross-reactivity is uncertain (Coller, 1999).

Preclinical Experience

Near maximal inhibition of platelet aggregation was observed when at least 80% of surface GPIIb/IIIa receptors were blocked by abciximab. In non-human primates, abciximab bolus doses of 0.25 mg/kg generally achieved a blockade of at least 80% of platelet receptors (Jordan *et al.*, 1996). Inhibition of platelet function was temporary following a bolus dose, but receptor blockade could be sustained at ≥ 80% by continuous intravenous infusion. The inhibitory effects of abciximab were substantially reversed by the transfusion of platelets in monkeys (Lemmer, 2000).

Pharmacodynamics

Intravenous administration in humans of single bolus doses of abciximab of 0.15, 0.20, 0.25 and 0.30 mg/kg produced dose-dependent inhibition of platelet function as measured by *ex vivo* platelet aggregation in response to ADP or by prolongation of bleeding time (Jordan *et al.*, 1992; Jakubowski *et al.*, 1999). At the two highest doses (0.25 and 0.30 mg/kg) at two hours post injection, over 80% of the GPIIb/IIIa receptors were blocked and platelet aggregation in response to 20 μM ADP was almost completely abolished. The median bleeding time increased to over 30 minutes at both doses compared to a baseline value of approximately five minutes. Importantly, the inhibition of platelets occurs rapidly as shown by the full inhibition of platelet function by the Ultegra Rapid Platelet Function assay within ten minutes following the 0.25 mg/kg bolus (Kereiakes *et al.*, 1999).

Intravenous administration in humans of a single bolus dose of 0.25 mg/kg, followed by a continuous infusion of 10 μg/min for periods of 12 hours, produced sustained high-grade GPIIb/IIIa receptor blockade (≥ 80%) and inhibition of platelet function (*ex vivo* platelet aggregation in response to 5 μM or 20 μM ADP less than 20% of baseline and bleeding time greater than 30 minutes) (Mascelli *et al.*, 1998). Similar results were obtained when a weight-adjusted infusion dose (0.125 μg/kg/min to a maximum of 10 μg/min) was used in patients weighing up to 80 kg. In a separate study, 28 of 30 subjects receiving the 0.125 μg/kg/min infusion for 48 hours achieved > 80% receptor blockade for the duration of the infusion (Freedman *et al.*, 1999).

Low levels of GPIIb/IIIa receptor blockade are present for up to 15 days following cessation of the infusion (Mascelli *et al.*, 1998). After discontinuation of abciximab infusion, platelet function returns gradually to normal. Bleeding time returned to ≤ 12 minutes within 12 hours following the end of infusion in 15 of 20 patients (75%) and within 24 hours in 18 of 20 patients (90%). *Ex vivo* platelet aggregation in response to 5 μM ADP returned to ≥ 50% of baseline within 24 hours following the end of infusion in 11 of 32 patients (34%) and within 48 hours in 23 of 32 patients (72%). In response to 20 μM ADP, *ex vivo* platelet aggregation returned to ≥ 50% of baseline within 24 hours in 20 of 32 patients (62%) and within 48 hours in 28 of 32 patients (88%).

The gradual recovery from receptor blockade results from the redistribution of abciximab among all of the platelets in circulation, and is not due to the effect of new uninhibited platelets that have entered circulation after cessation of abciximab treatment. Figure 13B.2 shows a series of flow cytograms of platelets from an individual who received a bolus plus 12-hour infusion of abciximab. The platelets obtained prior to abciximab treatment (upper panel) are non-fluorescent and indicate the FACS profile of platelets without bound abciximab. At 30 minutes after treatment, all circulating platelets are highly coated with abciximab, as indicated by the substantial right-shifted position of the histogram. Also indicated is the number of abciximab molecules per platelet quantified by an independent receptor blockade assay (102,000 per platelet at 30 minutes). At 24 hours after the bolus (12 hours post-cessation of the 12-hour infusion), a single unimodal histogram is still evident although less fluorescent than at the earlier 30-minute determination. The unimodal nature of the histogram indicates that all platelets contain bound

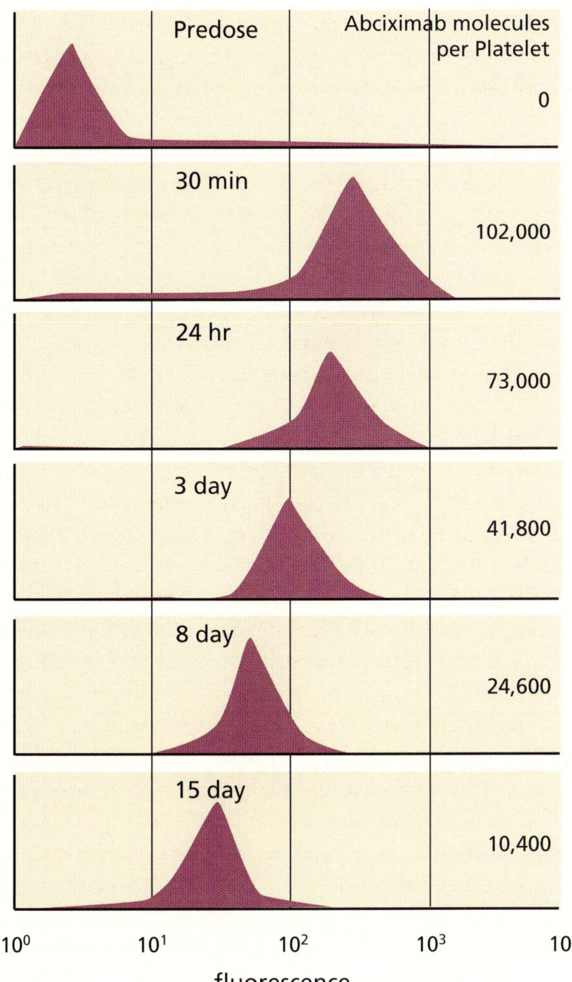

Figure 13B.2. Flow cytometric histograms of platelet samples obtained from a patient who received a 0.25 mg/kg bolus plus a 12-hour infusion of 10 μg/min of abciximab. Platelet samples were treated with a fluorescein-conjugated rabbit anti-abciximab antibody preparation and then fixed with 1% formalin. Samples were evaluated on a Becton-Dickinson FACScan flow cytometer. The predose sample exhibits a non-fluorescent peak of platelets corresponding to the absence of abciximab. Post-treatment samples demonstrate a single, unimodal fluorescent platelet peak without evidence of a second population of platelet without abciximab (Mascelli, *et al.*, 1998).

abciximab and that there are no uncoated platelets equivalent to those at pretreatment. Unimodal platelet histograms were also found at 3 days, 8 days and 15 days post-treatment. Although the average fluorescence of the platelet peaks decline progressively during this period, at no point was a second peak of uncoated platelets detected.

The average circulating lifetime of a platelet is seven to nine days which means that at 15 days post-therapy, all of the originally-circulating platelets were replaced by new platelets entering circulation. As indicated in the figure, approximately 10,000 molecules of abciximab were present per platelet at 15 days (Mascelli *et al.*, 1998). The persistence of platelet-bound abciximab at prolonged times suggests that abciximab continuously redistributes among circulating platelets, including those newly entered into the system. A continuous re-equilibration of abciximab among platelets was shown *in vitro* (Jordan *et al.*, 1996) and is the likely explanation for the results in the patient shown in Figure 13B.2 and for similar published examples (Christopoulos *et al.*, 1993). A corollary to this pharmacodynamic profile is that platelets have equivalent numbers of bound abciximab throughout the prolonged recovery period and that the gradually diminishing receptor blockade is a property of all of the platelets in circulation.

Despite the binding of specific quantities of abciximab to platelet GPIIb/IIIa receptors, little additional free plasma abciximab is detectable during and after treatment. This is due, in part, to the rapid receptor binding with close correspondence of the abciximab dose to the amount of platelet surface GPIIb/IIIa receptors. For most individuals, a 0.25 mg/kg dose of abciximab is typically less than twofold in excess of the total number of molecules needed to bind all GPIIb/IIIa receptors on circulating and splenic platelets (Coller *et al.*, 1991). Thus, the rapid disappearance of free plasma abciximab can be largely attributed to the rapid binding to platelets.

In contrast to the rapid decline of free plasma abciximab following the bolus dose, the bolus plus infusion regimen maintained a plasma concentration of abciximab (~200 ng/mL) in these patients for the duration of the infusion. Following the cessation of the 12-hour infusion, abciximab disappeared rapidly from the plasma.

The importance of the continuous infusion for the efficacy of abciximab is well established. The infusion provides a source of abciximab to prevent the gradual decline of receptor blockade. The clinical validity of this concept was illustrated by the marked and continued inhibition of ischemic events by the EPIC bolus plus infusion regimen but not by the bolus dose alone (see study description below). The progressive and uniform decline of receptor blockade on circulating platelets can be attributed to the continuous redistribution of abciximab among platelets, including to those newly synthesized platelets that may possess little or no receptor blockade. Abciximab that has dissociated from platelets likely undergoes rapid clearance in the kidney as is typical for immunoglobulin Fab fragments.

The pharmacodynamic and pharmacokinetic profiles of abciximab therapy provide a means to reverse the therapeutic effects. In a preclinical model, the transfusion of donor platelets after abciximab treatment resulted in an immediate, partial normalization of platelet function (Lemmer, 2000). Reversal occurs immediately because of the low concentration of free plasma abciximab that is insufficient to inhibit the function of the newly transfused platelets. Redistribution of bound Abciximab to these newly transfused platelets results in a decrease in mean platelet receptor blockade. Platelet transfusion to reverse abciximab has also been successfully performed in patients requiring emergency coronary bypass surgery (Kereiakes, 1998; Tcheng *et al.*, 1994).

Clinical usage

Key Clinical Experience

Four large, randomized, placebo-controlled phase III clinical trials with more than 8500 enrolled patients have provided definitive evidence that the potent and sustained GPIIb/IIIa receptor blockade by abciximab prevents cardiac ischemic complications associated with percutaneous coronary interventions (PCI). Three of these trials evaluated abciximab as adjunctive therapy at the time of PCI (EPIC, EPILOG, EPISTENT). The fourth trial (CAPTURE) was designed to evaluate the use of abciximab in unstable angina patients not responding to conventional medical therapy and for whom PCI was planned within 24 hours.

The EPIC Trial

The first phase III trial of abciximab was EPIC (Evaluation of c7E3 to Prevent Ischemic Complications). EPIC was carried out in 2099 patients who were at high risk of ischemic complications during or after percutaneous transluminal coronary angioplasty (PTCA) or directional coronary atherectomy (The EPIC Investigators, 1994). In a double-blind study design, patients were randomly assigned to one of three treatment arms. Patients in the placebo arm received a placebo bolus plus placebo infusion for 12 hours. Patients in the bolus arm received a 0.25 mg/kg bolus of abciximab plus placebo infusion for 12 hours. Patients in the bolus plus infusion arm received a 0.25 mg/kg bolus plus a 10 μg/min abciximab infusion for 12 hours. The primary composite end point of the trial was the occurrence by 30 days of death from any cause, MI, or need for urgent coronary intervention. Patients were subsequently evaluated in a blinded fashion at six months, one year and three years.

An intent-to-treat analysis showed that the primary endpoint event rates in the bolus plus infusion treatment group were significantly reduced in the first 48 hours (placebo 9.9%; abciximab, 6.6%; relative reduction, 33%; P = 0.025). At 30 days the formal primary composite end point was sustained with a 35% relative reduction (P = 0.008) in the bolus plus infusion treatment group, compared with the placebo group (Figure 13B3).

Blinded evaluations of patients were continued through six months and three years. At the six-month follow-up visit, there was a relative reduction of 23% in the composite end point of death, MI, or repeat revasularization (PCI or CABG) intervention (P = 0.001). At three years, for the composite of death, MI, or urgent intervention there was a 20% relative reduction (P = 0.027). When both urgent and nonurgent interventions were included, there was a 13% relative reduction (P = 0.009). Using standard doses of heparin, the incidence of bleeding was increased in patients treated with abciximab.

The EPILOG Trial

The EPILOG (Evaluation of PTCA to Improve Longterm Outcome by c7E3 GPIIB/IIa receptor blockade) trial was a prospective, multicenter, randomized, double-blind, placebo-controlled trial in which abciximab was evaluated in a broad population of patients undergoing PCI. EPILOG was designed to test the hypothesis that abciximab in conjunction with a low-dose, weight-adjusted heparin regimen, early sheath removal, improved access-site and patient management, and weight adjustment of the abciximab infusion dose could significantly lower the bleeding rate yet maintain the efficacy seen in the EPIC trial. EPILOG was a three-treatment arm trial of abciximab plus standard-dose, weight-adjusted heparin (target activated clotting time (ACT) ≥ 300 seconds); abciximab plus low-dose, weight-adjusted heparin (target ACT ≥ 200 seconds); and placebo plus standard-dose, weight-adjusted heparin. For those receiving abciximab, a bolus of 0.25 mg/kg of body weight was administered 10 to 60 minutes before the procedure and was followed by an infusion of 0.125 μg/kg/min (to a maximum of 10 μg/min) for 12 hours. Based on positive interim findings, an independent Safety and Efficacy Monitoring Committee recommended that EPILOG be stopped after an analysis at 1500 patients, with a final enrollment of 2792 of the planned 4800 patients (Ferguson, 1996).

Compared to the placebo group in EPILOG, there was a relative reduction in the primary composite end point of death or MI of 59% at 48 hours and a 59% relative reduction at 30 days in the group receiving abciximab plus low-dose, weight-adjusted heparin. The composite secondary end point of death, MI, or urgent intervention at 48 hours demonstrated a 57% relative reduction and at 30 days demonstrated a 56% relative reduction (EPILOG Investigators, 1997).

At six months, there was a 48% relative reduction (P = 0.001) in the incidence of death or MI, a 43% relative reduction (P < 0.001) in the composite of death, MI, or urgent intervention and a 12% relative reduction

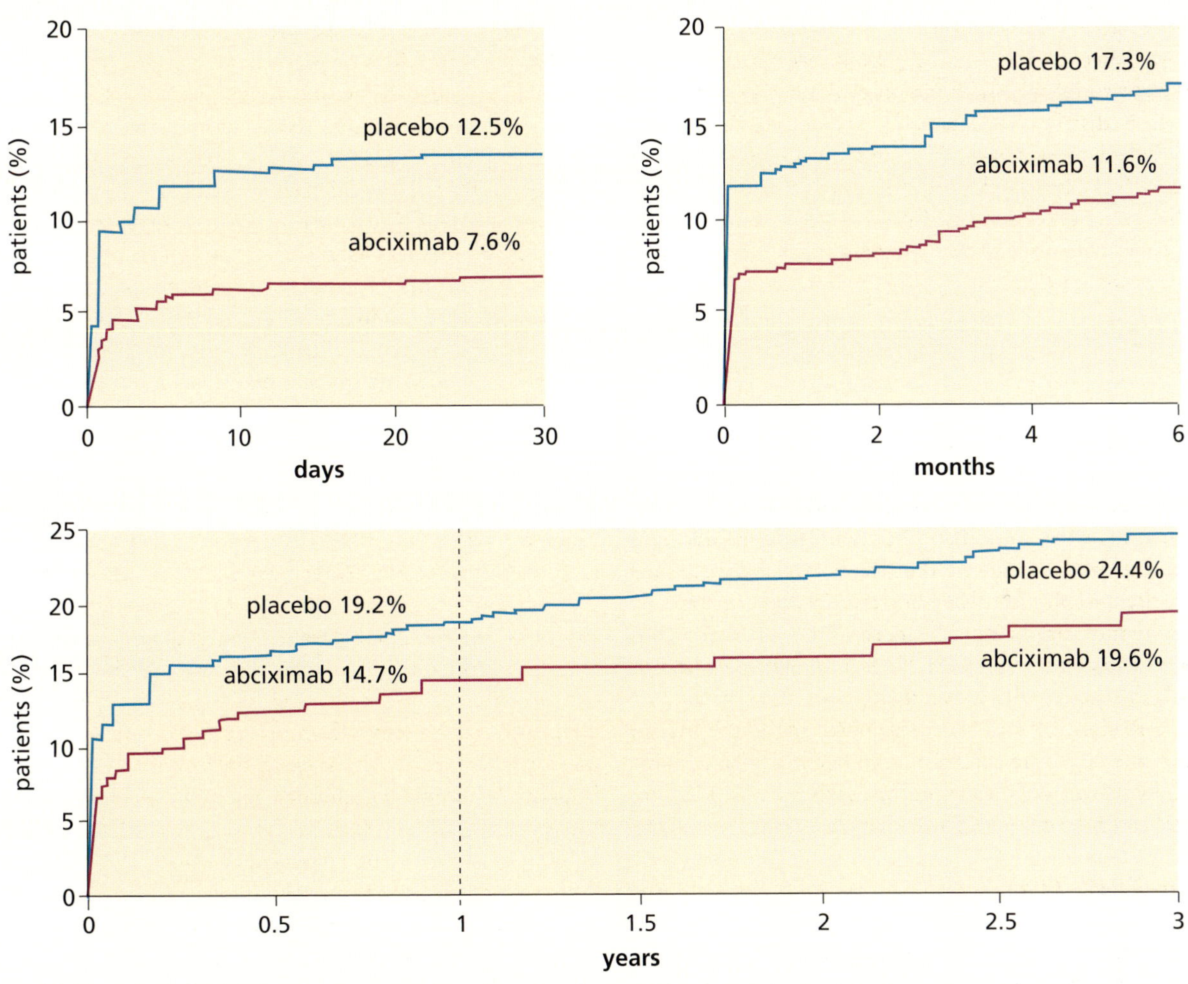

Figure 13B.3. A comparison of the composite endpoint of death, myocardial infarction and urgent intervention in patients who received standard therapy (placebo) and in patients who received the bolus plus 12-hour infusion of abciximab. Results are shown for the initial 30-day period, for 0 to 6 months and for extended follow-up through 1 and 3 years in the EPIC trial.

(P = 0.034) in the composite of death, MI, or any repeat intervention (urgent or nonurgent) in the group receiving abciximab plus low-dose heparin, compared with the placebo group (Lincoff *et al.*, 1999). Follow-up at one year demonstrated a 49% relative reduction (P < 0.001) in the composite of death and MI; a 41% relative reduction (P < 0.001) in the composite end point of death, MI, or urgent intervention; and a 9% relative reduction in the composite of death, MI, or any repeat intervention (urgent or nonurgent). The results of the EPILOG trial confirmed the efficacy of abciximab bolus plus 12-hour infusion in a broad population of patients undergoing PCI. Bleeding rates were reduced in the EPILOG trial by use of modified heparin dosing regimens (Table 13B.1) and specific patient management techniques.

The EPISTENT Trial

The EPISTENT (Evaluation of Platelet Inhibition in Stenting) study was a multicenter, randomized placebo-controlled trial that enrolled patients suitable for either primary stent implantation or conventional angioplasty/atherectomy. Patients were randomly assigned to one of three treatment arms: abciximab plus low-dose, weight-adjusted heparin and conventional angioplasty/atherectomy (abciximab plus PTCA); primary stent implantation with abciximab plus low-dose, weight-adjusted heparin (abciximab plus stent); or primary stent with placebo plus standard-dose, weight-adjusted heparin (placebo plus stent).

Data for all 2399 randomized patients were included in the primary end-point analysis of death, MI, or urgent

	Placebo (n = 939)	Abciximab + Standard Dose Heparin (n = 918)	Abciximab + Low-dose Heparin (n = 935)
Major	10 (1.1)	17 (1.9)	10 (1.1)
Minor	32 (3.4)	70 (7.6)	37 (4.0)
Requiring Transfusion*)	10 (1.1)	7 (0.8)	6 (0.6)

Table 13B.1. Non-CABG bleeding in the EPILOG trial. Number of patients with bleeding events (%).
*) Packed red blood cells or whole blood.

intervention at 30 days (EPISTENT Investigators, 1998). There was a significant relative reduction of 51% (P < 0.001) in the abciximab plus stent group and a 36% (P = 0.007) relative reduction in the abciximab plus PTCA group, compared with the placebo plus stent group. At the six-month follow-up, the event rates of death, MI, or urgent intervention were lower in both abciximab groups, compared with the placebo plus stent group. At the one-year follow-up, the event rates of death, MI, or target vessel intervention were significantly lower in the abciximab-plus-stent group, compared with the placebo-plus-stent group (P = 0.039) (Topol *et al.*, 1999). The mortality benefit of abciximab plus stent is shown as a Kaplan-Meier plot in Figure 13B.4. After one year the combined treatment resulted in a lower mortality rate than with placebo plus stent or abciximab plus PTCA. At one year, the mortality rate was 2.4% in the placebo plus stent group, compared with 1.0% in the abciximab plus stent group, a statistically significant 57% relative reduction (P = 0.037).

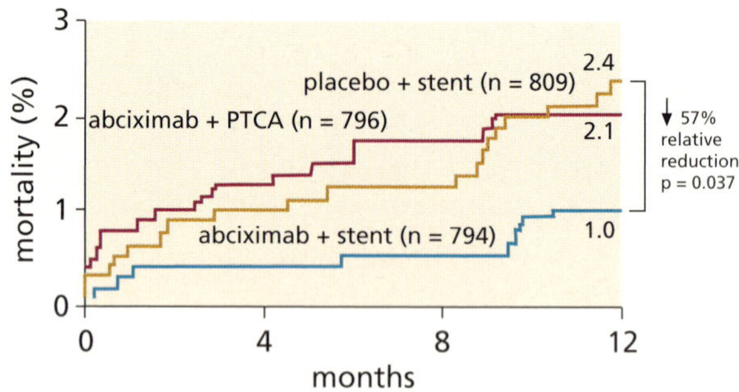

Figure 13B.4. The EPISTENT mortality results through 1 year for patients receiving 3 different treatment regiments; 1) placebo plus stent, 2) abciximab plus PTCA and 3) abciximab plus stent.

The CAPTURE Trial

The CAPTURE (Chimeric c7E3 Fab Antiplatelet Therapy in Unstable Refractory angina) trial was a randomized, double-blind, multicenter, placebo-controlled trial in unstable angina patients not responding to conventional medical therapy and for whom PCI was planned but not immediately performed (CAPTURE Investigators, 1997). The objective was to determine whether abciximab could improve outcomes by reducing ischemic complications before, during, and after PCI. The abciximab dose was a 0.25 mg/kg bolus administered 18 to 24 hours prior to PCI that was followed by a continuous infusion at a rate of 10 μg/min until one hour after completion of the intervention.

The CAPTURE trial was halted on the advice of the independent Safety and Efficacy Monitoring Committee based on positive efficacy results at an interim analysis. Total enrollment was 1265 of the planned 1400 patients. An intent-to-treat analysis showed that the primary endpoint of death, MI, or urgent intervention at 30 days was reduced by 29% in the abciximab-treated patients, compared with those receiving placebo. There was a 47% relative reduction (P = 0.003) in the event rate of death or MI in the abciximab-treated group, compared with the placebo group.

Blinded evaluations of patients were continued until six months after randomization. There was a 17% relative reduction in the event rates over time for the composite end point of death or MI (P = 0.19). The event rates for the composite end point of death, MI, or any repeat intervention (urgent or nonurgent) were not different between the abciximab group (31%) and the placebo group (31%). This lack of sustained benefit contrasts with the results from EPIC, EPILOG, and EPISTENT trials, where an abciximab 12-hour infusion following the intervention was given. However, these results are similar to the results from the abciximab bolusonly arm in the EPIC trial, in which the early benefit of abciximab was not sustained at six months.

Safety Concerns

Abciximab has the potential to increase the risk of bleeding, particularly in the presence of anticoagulants, e.g. heparin or thrombolytics, but this risk can be decreased by the use of low-dose heparin. The total incidence of intracranial hemorrhage and non-hemorrhagic stroke in clinical trials was not significantly different for placebo patients and for abciximab treated patients. Patients treated with abciximab are more likely than patients treated with placebo to experience decreases in platelet counts. In EPILOG, the incidence of a decrease in platelet count went to less than 50,000/μL and was 0.4% for placebo patients and 0.6% for abciximab treated patients. Additional details are available in the full prescribing information for abciximab.

Pharmaceutical Considerations

Formulation

The recommended dosage of abciximab in adults is an intravenous bolus of 0.25 mg/kg administered 10–60 minutes before the start of PTCA, followed by a continuous infusion of 0.125 μg/kg/min (to a maximum of 10 μg/min) for 12 hours.

Abciximab (2 mg/mL) is supplied in 5 mL vials containing 10 mg. Abciximab is a clear, colorless, non-pyrogenic solution for intravenous (IV) use. Abciximab is formulated in a buffered solution (pH 7.2) of 0.01 M sodium phosphate, 0.15 M sodium chloride and 0.001% polysorbate 80 in Water for Injection. No preservatives are added. Vials should be stored at 2 to 8 °C. (36 to 46 °F). Do not shake. Do not use beyond the expiration date. Discard any unused portion left in the vial. Under correct storage conditions, abciximab has been shown to be stable for three years. Insert information can be found at www.reopro.com. ■

References

- **Altieri DC, Edgington TS**. A monoclonal antibody reaction with distinct adhesion molecules defines a transition in the functional state of the receptor CD11b/CD18 (Mac-1). J Immunol. 1988;141:2656–2660.
- **CAPTURE Investigators**. Randomised placebo-controlled trial of abciximab before and during coronary intervention in refractory unstable angina: the CAPTURE study. *Lancet.* 1997;349:1429–1435.
- **Christopoulos C, Mackie I, Lahiri A, Machin S**. Flow cytometric observations on the *in vivo* use of Fab fragments of a chimaeric monoclonal antibody to platelet glycoprotein IIb-IIIa. *Blood Coagulation and Fibrinolysis.* 1993;4:729–737.
- **Coller BS**. Blockade of platelet GPIIb/IIIa receptors as an antithrombotic strategy. *Circulation.* 1995;92:273–2380.
- **Coller BS, Scudder LE, Beer J, Gold HK, Folts JD, Cavagnaro J, Jordan R, Wagner C, Iuliucci J, Knight D, Ghrayeb J, Smith C, Weisman HF, Berger H**. Monoclonal antibodies to platelet glycoprotein IIb/III as antithrombotic agents. *Ann NY Acad Sci.* 1991;614:193–213.
- **Coller BS**. Binding of abciximab to αvβ3 and activated αMβ2 receptors: with a review of platelet leukocyte interactions. *Thrombosis Haemost.* 1999;82(2):326–336.
- **EPILOG Investigators**. Platelet glycoprotein IIb/IIIa receptor blockade and low dose heparin during percutaneous coronary revascularization. *N Engl J Med.* 1997;336:1689–1696.
- **EPISTENT Investigators**. Randomised placebo-controlled and balloon-angioplasty-controlled trial to assess safety of coronary stenting with use of platelet glycoprotein-IIb/IIIa blockade. *Lancet.* 1998;352:87–92.
- **Freedman JE, Pezzullo JC, Abernethy DR**. Acute coronary syndromes: from pathophysiology to clinical outcomes. Circulation. 1999;100(18, Suppl):I-431.
- **Ferguson III, JJ**. EPILOG and CAPTURE trials halted because of positive interim results. *Circulation.* 1996;93:637.
- **Jakubowski JA, Jordan RE, Weisman HF**. Current antiplatelet therapy. In *Handbook of Experimental Pharmacology, Antithrombotics.* 1999;132:176–207.
- **Jordan RE, Wagner CL, Mascelli MA, Treacy G, Nedelman MA, Woody JN, Weisman HF, Coller BS**. Preclinical development of c7E3 Fab; a mouse/human chimeric monoclonal antibody fragment that inhibits platelet function by blockade of GPIIb/IIIa receptors with observations on the immunogenicity of c7E3 Fab in humans. *In Adhesion Receptors as Therapeutic Targets,* edited by MA Horton. London: CRC, 1996;81–305.
- **Jordan RE, Mascelli MA, Nakada MT, Weisman HF**. Pharmacology and clinical development of abciximab (c7E3 Fab, ReoPro): A monoclonal antibody inhibitor of GPIIb/IIIa and $\alpha_v\beta_3$. In New Therapeutic Agents in *Thrombosis and Thrombolysis,* edited by AA Sasahara. New York:Marcel Dekker, 1997;291–313.
- **Kereiakes DJ**. Prophylactic platelet transfusion in abciximab-treated patients requiring emergency coronary bypass surgery. *Am J Cardiol.* 1998;81:373.
- **Kereiakes DJ, Broderick TM, Roth EM, *et al.*** Time course, magnitude, and consistency of platelet inhibition of abciximab, tirofiban or eptifibatide in patients with unstable angina pectoris undergoing percutaneous coronary intervention. *Am J Cardiol.* 1999;84:391–395.
- **Knight DM, Wagner C, Jordan R, McAleer MF, DeRita R, Fass DN, Coller BS, Weisman HF, Ghrayeb J**. The

immunogenicity of the 7E3 murine monoclonal Fab antibody fragment variable region is dramatically reduced in humans by substitution of human for murine constant regions. *Mol Immunol,* 1995;32:1271–1281.

- **Lemmer JH Jr**. Clinical experience in coronary bypass surgery for abciximab-treated patients, *Ann Thorac Surg.* 2000;70:533–537.
- **Lincoff AM, Tcheng JE, Califf RM, *et al.***, for the EPILOG Investigators. Sustained suppression of ischemic complications of coronary intervention by platelet GPIIb/IIIa blockade with abciximab: one-year outcome in the EPILOG trial. *Circulation.* 1999;99:1951–1958.
- **Plow EF, Ginsberg MH**. Cellular adhesion: GPIIb/IIIa as a prototypic adhesion receptor. *Prog Hemost Thromb.* 1989;9:117–156.
- **Reverter JC, Beguin S, Kessels H, Kumar R, Hemker HC, Coller BS**. Inhibition of platelet-mediated, tissue factor-induced thrombin generation by the mouse/human chimeric 7E3 antibody. *J Clin Invest.* 1996;98:863–874.
- **Tcheng JE, Ellis SG, George BS, Kereiakes DJ, Kleiman NS, Talley JD, Wang AL, Weisman HF, Califf RM, Topol EJ**. Pharmacodynamics of chimeric glycoprotein IIb/IIIa integrin antiplatelet antibody Fab 7E3 in high-risk coronary angioplasty. *Circulation.* 1994;90:1757–1764.
- **The EPIC Investigators.** (1994). Use of a monoclonal antibody directed against the platelet glycoprotein IIb/IIIa receptor in high-risk coronary angioplasty. *NEJM.* 1994;330:956–961.
- **Topol EJ, Califf RM, Weisman HF, Ellis SG, Tcheng JE, Worley S, Ivanhoe R, George BS, Fintel D, Weston M, Sigmon K, Anderson KM, Lee KL, Willerson JT** on behalf of the EPIC investigators. Randomised trial of coronary intervention with antibody against platelet IIb/IIIa integrin for reduction of clinical restenosis: results at six months. *Lancet.* 1994;343:881–886
- **Topol EJ, Plow EF**. Clinical trials of platelet receptor inhibitors. *Thromb Haemost.* 1993;70:94–98.
- **Topol EJ, Mark DB, Lincoff AM, *et al.*** Outcomes at 1 year and economic implications of platelet glycoprotein IIb/IIIa blockade in patients undergoing coronary stenting: results from a multicentre randomised trial. *Lancet.* 1999;354:2019–2024.
- **Weisman HF**. ReoPro clinical development: Future directions and therapeutic approaches. *J Invasive Cardiology,* 1996;8:51B–61B.
- **Weisman HF, Schaible TF, Jordan RE, Cabot CF, Anderson KM.** Anti-platelet monoclonal antibodies for the prevention of arterial thrombosis: experience with ReoPro, a monoclonal antibody directed against the platelet GPIIb/IIIa receptor. *Therapeutic Monoclonals.* 1995;23:1052–1057.

13C Appendix C to Monoclonal Antibody-Based Pharmaceuticals

Daclizumab/Zenapax® and Basiliximab/Simulect®

David S. Ziska

Introduction

Background

Daclizumab and basiliximab are humanized, murine monoclonal antibodies that bind to the α-subunit of the interleukin-2 (IL-2) receptor on activated T-cells (Zenapax® Package Insert, 1997; Simulect® Package Insert, 1998). This 55-kDa subunit, also designated Tac or CD25, plays a key role in the proliferation and differentiation of only activated T-cells. Both anti-Tac products possess highly selective pharmacological activity and thus, because of this specificity, have few adverse effects occurring with greater incidence than placebo (Vincenti *et al.*, 1998; Kahan *et al.*, 1999).

Molecular Characteristics of Chimeric Anti-CD25's Antibodies

To synthesize each of these murine/human glycoproteins, human and murine antibody genes are recombined (Queen *et al.*, 1989; Amlot *et al.*, 1995) (cf. Chapter 13). Molecular weights of both glycoproteins produced from this recombination are estimated to be about 144 kDa, although the murine antibody segments of each are unique. Daclizumab amino acid sequences are 90% human and 10% murine, whereas basiliximab sequences are less human and more murine (Zenapax® Package Insert, 1997; Simulect® Package Insert, 1998). These structural differences result from different recombination strategies. Daclizumab utilizes only those sequences from the murine hypervariable anti-Tac genes, whereas the basiliximab construct utilizes the sequences coding for the entire heavy and light chains of the variable region of murine monoclonal anti-Tac (Queen *et al.*, 1989; Amlot *et al.*, 1995). Human IgG_1 sequences code for the human portion of both heavy and light constant constructs. Although, as implied previously, daclizumab differs in that it includes human variable sequences utilizing only the complementarity-determining regions (also known as hypervariable regions) of the murine monoclonal anti-Tac.

Pharmacology

Pharmacokinetics

Given their numerous similarities, these monoclonal antibodies have surprisingly significant pharmacokinetic differences. The adult elimination half-life ($t^1/_2$) of daclizumab is reported to be about 20 days, which is very similar to that of human immunoglobulin G (IgG), yet basiliximab is reported to have an average adult elimination $t^1/_2$ of about 7.5 days (Vincenti *et al.*, 1998; Kovarik *et al.*, 1999). These significant differences in elimination do not directly impact dosing regimens. Mean steady state volume of distribution of daclizumab is about 5.5 L and for basiliximab it is around 8 L (Zenapax® Package Insert, 1997; Kovarik *et al.*, 1999). Exposure-response to these two products also differs significantly. For adequate saturation of the CD25 subunit in transplant recipients concentrations of daclizumab between 5 to 10 μg/mL are necessary, whereas for basiliximab concentrations of only 0.2 μg/mL or greater are sufficient (Zenapax® Package Insert, 1997; Kovarik *et al.*, 1999).

Clinical Usage

Indications

Currently each product has been FDA approved for the prophylaxis of acute organ rejection in adult renal transplant patients. Each antibody product must be combined with a cocktail of drugs for induction of immunosuppression containing at least cyclosporine and corticosteroids (Zenapax® Package Insert, 1997; Simulect® Package Insert, 1998). A number of transplant centers also combine these antibody products with mycophenolate mofetil or azathioprine as part of a quadruple induction regimen (Vincenti *et al.*, 1998; Oberholzer *et al.*, 2000; Wiseman *et al.*, 1999). Other indications being investigated for these agents include immunosuppression induction in liver, heart and pancreas/islet transplant, as well as use in the treatment of acute rejection in solid organ transplant and T-cell mediated uveitis (Beniaminovitz *et al.*, 2000; Nashan *et al.*, 1996; Nussenblatt *et al.*, 1999; Shapiro *et al.*, 2000).

Immunosuppression Induction in Renal Allograft – Daclizumab

Initial indication for both products is for the prevention of acute rejection in renal transplantation. Vincenti *et al.* (1998) describe clinic experience in this setting with daclizumab being added to cyclosporine, azathioprine and corticosteroids. One milligram (mg) per kilogram (kg) of daclizumab or placebo was administered intravenously less than 24 hours before transplantation. To complete the five-dose regimen, the other four doses were administered two, four, six and eight weeks after transplantation. The primary end point – incidence of biopsy-confirmed acute rejection within six months after transplantation – was significantly reduced from 35% to 22% in the placebo versus daclizumab group respectively, P = 0.03. Time to first rejection was increased versus placebo from 30 days to 73 days (P = 0.008). Also of note, three patients died of different fungal and bacterial infections in the placebo group and no patients died of infections in the daclizumab group, although one patient died of lymphoma.

Another study reports one-year experience with daclizumab as five-dose induction of immunosuppression combined with cyclosporine, corticosteroids and ± azathioprine (Ekberg *et al.*, 2000). Acute rejection was reduced from 43.3% to 27.7% (P = 0.0001), as was anti-lymphocyte therapy for acute rejection, 15.3% to 7.9%, for placebo and daclizumab, respectively. One-year graft survival, as well as patient survival, was also significantly increased with the use of daclizumab. This difference did not reach statistical significance in the Vincenti study (Vincenti *et al.*, 1998). The Ekberg study also confirmed that infectious disease did not increase with the addition of daclizumab. For example, cytomegalovirus infection occurred in 15% of the daclizumab and 17.5% of the placebo groups.

A minority renal transplant patient population receiving daclizumab immunosuppression induction with daclizumab or placebo and calcineurin inhibitor, mycophenolate mofetil and corticosteroid was analyzed by Meier-Kriesche *et al.* (2000). Minority transplant populations are an important group to study because their risk of acute rejection is historically higher than transplant recipients of Northern European heritage. In this study daclizumab induction reduced both total corticosteroid exposure as well as the incidence of early acute rejections. If confirmed in larger cohorts, this regimen could significantly reduce acute rejection rates in minority populations.

Immunosuppression Induction in Renal Allograft – Basiliximab

Kahan *et al.* (1999) reported the United States initial basiliximab clinical experience. Basiliximab or placebo was added to a cyclosporine microemulsion and corticosteroids for the induction of immunosuppression and the prevention of acute rejection in renal transplantation. Two 20 mg doses of basiliximab or placebo were administered as part of an immunosuppression induction regimen, with the first dose administered immediately before the transplantation and the second dose administered on day 4 after transplantation. One-year results documented a significant reduction in biopsy-confirmed acute rejection episodes similar to the daclizumab experience. Episodes were reduced from 49.1% in placebo to 35.3% in the basiliximab groups, respectively. Patient and graft survival rates were not significantly increased compared to placebo.

A combined European/Canadian experience reported similar results with basiliximab in this setting (Nashan *et al.*, 1997). Interestingly, Kahan *et al.* (1999) also analyzed the impact of basiliximab on various demographic factors. In this analysis males, those less than 50 years old and African-Americans all experienced fewer rejection episodes when basiliximab induction immunosuppression was compared to placebo (Kahan *et al.*, 1999).

Immunosuppression Induction in Other Solid Organs

As with other immunosuppression drugs initially FDA approved for use in one type of solid organ transplantation. Investigation into using these chimeric monoclonal products with other types of solid organ transplantation has been started. Already there are reports of using these products for the induction of liver, islet, islet/kidney and heart transplantation. The safety and potential for extending the efficacy of already successful induction of immunosuppression regimens are compelling reasons for pursuing research into the application of these products in numerous applications.

Acute Rejection Treatment

Research into using these products for the treatment of acute rejection is scant. Biologically it is plausible that there exists a potential for this indication with anti-Tac antibody products. One case study describes an experience of reversing a late acute rejection episode that had been treated with a rabbit antithymocyte product, then a murine anti-CD3 monoclonal product and finally with daclizumab every other week for ten weeks. Only after daclizumab therapy was pursued was an enduring remission realized in this recipient of a combined islet-kidney transplant (Oberholzer *et al.*, 2000).

Other Applications

Several autoimmune diseases are caused, at least in part if not primarily, by activated T-lymphocytes. Humanized anti-Tac mAb may one day prove an effective and safe addition to current therapies. In one of these non-infectious autoimmune disorders – intermediate and posterior uveitis – daclizumab appears to be effective in a long term, open-labeled trial (Nussenblatt *et al.*, 1999). The trial suggests that daclizumab may be an effective follow-up or replacement therapy for conventional immunosuppressants.

Safety Concerns

Of the commonly used antithymocyte products FDA approved in the United States, chimeric monoclonal antibody products are much safer than the murine monoclonal, muromonab-CD3 and rabbit antithymocyte globulin (Orthoclone® OKT3 Package Insert, 1995; Thymoglobulin® Package Insert, 1999). Several studies also establish that somatic and infectious adverse effects occur at about the same rate as placebo when a chimeric anti-Tac monoclonal antibody is combined with standard immunosuppression cocktails. Some of the most striking differences between the older antithymocyte products and the chimeric products are that the newer products do not induce cytokine release syndrome (CRS) (Vincenti *et al.*, 1998; Kahan *et al.*, 1999). Thus, meticulous application of pre- and post-administration CRS prevention protocols with corticosteroids and antihistamines is unnecessary. Even when these CRS prevention protocols are followed with the older products there still exists a significant risk of other morbidities. Life-threatening infections are one of the most common causes of morbidity associated with the older products (Orthoclone® OKT3 Package Insert, 1995; Thymoglobulin® Package Insert, 1999). Daclizumab and basiliximab represent a significant improvement in reducing adverse effects associated with induction immunosuppression. Initial studies indicated that herpetic infections could be reduced when an anti-Tac product was used for induction and CMV occurred less frequently (Kahan *et al.*, 1999). Furthermore, selecting one of the newer products might lead to reduced calcineurin inhibitor exposure during the induction phase (Golconda *et al.*, 2000).

Pharmaceutical considerations

Formulation

Zenapax™ is supplied as a sterile, clear, colorless concentrate for further dilution and intravenous administration. Each 25 mg/5mL preservative-free vial contains 5 mg of daclizumab, 3.6 mg sodium phosphate monobasic monohydrate, 11 mg sodium phosphate dibasic heptahydrate, 4.6 mg sodium chloride, 0.2 mg polysorbate 80 and may contain hydrochloric acid or sodium hydroxide to adjust the pH to 6.9. The concentrated contents of each vial must be diluted before injection. Reconstitution consists of diluting the calculated volume in 50 mL of sterile 0.9% sodium chloride solution before intravenous admixture. Mixing this solution by gentle inversion avoids foaming and ensures that the product maintains activity. Any unused portion should be discarded as each vial is intended for single use. Once prepared, Zenapax™ admixture should be administered within four hours if not refrigerated. It can also be stored between 2° to 8 °C for up to 24 hours. (Zenapax™ Package Insert, 1997).

Simulect™ is supplied as a sterile, colorless water soluble lyophilisate. Each 6 mL preservative-free vial contains 20 mg of basiliximab, 7.21 mg monobasic potassium phosphate, 0.99 mg disodium hydrogen phosphate (anhydrous), 1.61 mg sodium chloride, 20 mg sucrose, 80 mg mannitol and 40 mg glycine, to be reconstituted in 5 mL of Sterile Water for Injection, USP.

The lyophilized powder of each vial must be reconstituted before injection. Reconstitution consists of adding 5 mL of Sterile Water for Injection, USP, to the vial and gently agitating until the powder is dissolved. Mixing this solution by gentle inversion avoids foaming and ensures that the product maintains activity. The new solution should then be diluted to a volume of 50 mL with normal saline or dextrose 5% for infusion, and gently inverted to avoid foaming. Any unused portion should be discarded as each vial is intended for single use. Once prepared, Simulect™ admixture should be administered within four hours if not refrigerated. It can also be stored between 2° to 8 °C for up to 24 hours. (Simulect™ Package Insert, 1998).

Pediatric Dosing Regimen

Simulect™ has received FDA approval for use in children. In children from 2 through 15 years of age, two doses of 12 mg/m² each, up to a maximum of 20 mg/dose, are recommended. As with adults, the first dose should be given two hours prior to transplantation surgery and the second dose given four days after that surgery (Simulect™ Package Insert, 1998).

Summary

Daclizumab and basiliximab are remarkable new drugs from many perspectives. These highly specific, potent, and effective new immunosuppressants are associated with an unmatched safety profile. Given their favorable characteristics these products and ones like them come closest to approaching the 'magic bullet' drug ideal. Structurally and pharmacokinetically, these products differ significantly; although, from clinical experience it is apparent that these antibody products are similar in efficacy and safety. As experience grows with daclizumab and basiliximab many other indications and applications will happily emerge for these unique products. Because of this initial clinical success, the technology employed to construct and produce humanized monoclonal antibodies will likely be applied to numerous diseases and clinical applications. ■

References

- **Amlot PL, Rawlings E, Fernando ON, Griffin PJ, Heinrich G, Schreier MH, Castaigne JP, Moore R, Sweny P.** (1995). Prolonged action of a chimeric interleukin-2 receptor (CD25) monoclonal antibody used in cadaveric renal transplantation. Transplantation. Oct 15;60(7):748–56.
- **Beniaminovitz A, Itescu S, Lietz K, Donovan M, Burke EM, Groff BD, Edwards N, Mancini DM.** (2000). Prevention of rejection in cardiac transplantation by blockade of the interleukin-2 receptor with a monoclonal antibody. N Engl J Med. Mar 2;342(9):613–9.
- **Ekberg H, Backman L, Tufveson G, Tyden G, Nashan B, Vincenti F.** (2000). Daclizumab prevents acute rejection and improves patient survival post transplantation: 1 year pooled analysis. Transpl Int. 13(2):151–9.
- **Golconda MS, Rayhill SC, Hunsicker LG**. Daclizumab Permits delayed introduction of calcineurin inhibitors in renal transplant recipients at risk for delayed graft function. Abstract 175, Transplant 2000: The first joint Transplant Meeting of the AST and ASTS (2000).
- **Kahan BD, Rajagopalan PR, Hall M.** (1999). Reduction of the occurrence of acute cellular rejection among renal allograft recipients treated with basiliximab, a chimeric anti-interleukin-2-receptor monoclonal antibody. United States Simulect Renal Study Group. Transplantation. 67(2):276–84.
- **Kovarik JM, Kahan BD, Rajagopalan PR, Bennett W, Mulloy LL, Gerbeau C, Hall ML.** (1999). Population pharmacokinetics and exposure-response relationships for basiliximab in kidney transplantation. The U.S. Simulect Renal Transplant Study Group. Transplantation. 68(9):1288–94.
- **Meier-Kriesche HU, Palenkar SS, Friedman GS, Mulgaonkar SP, Goldblat MV, Kaplan B.** (2000). Efficacy of Daclizumab in an African-American and Hispanic renal transplant population. Transpl Int. 13(2):142–5, 2000.
- **Nashan B, Moore R, Amlot P, Schmidt AG, Abeywickrama K, Soulillou JP.** (1997). Randomised trial of basiliximab versus placebo for control of acute cellular rejection in renal allograft recipients. CHIB 201 International Study Group. Lancet 350(9086):1193–8.
- **Nashan B, Schlitt HJ, Schwinzer R, Ringe B, Kuse E, Tusch G, Wonigeit K, Pichlmayr R.** (1996). Immunoprophylaxis with a monoclonal anti-IL-2 receptor antibody in liver transplant patients. Transplantation. 61(4):546–54.
- **Nussenblatt RB, Fortin E, Schiffman R, Rizzo L, Smith J, Van Veldhuisen P, Sran P, Yaffe A, Goldman CK, Waldmann TA, Whitcup SM.** (1999). Treatment of noninfectious intermediate and posterior uveitis with the humanized anti-Tac mAb: a phase I/II clinical trial. Proc Natl Acad Sci U S A. 96(13):7462–6.
- **Oberholzer J, Triponez F, Martin PY, Williamson C, Morel P.** (2000). Daclizumab as escape therapy for late acute kidney rejection in the presence of FK506 nephrotoxicity. Transpl Int. 13(2):169–71.
- Orthoclone OKT®3 (muromonab-CD3) Sterile Solution For Intravenous Use Only. (June 1995). Ortho Biotech Inc. Package Insert, Raritan, NJ 08869.
- **Queen C, Schneider WP, Selick HE, Payne PW, Landolfi NF, Duncan JF, Avdalovic NM, Levitt M, Junghans RP, Waldmann TA.** (1989). A humanized antibody that binds to the interleukin 2 receptor. Proc Natl Acad Sci U S A. 86(24):10029–33.
- Simulect® (basiliximab) For Injection. Novartis Pharmaceuticals Corporation. (May 1998). Package Insert. East Hanover, NJ 07936.
- Thymoglobulin® (rabbit antithymoglobulin) SangStat Medical Corporation. (January 1999). Package Insert. Menlo Park, CA 94025.
- **Vincenti F, Kirkman R, Light S, Bumgardner G, Pescovitz M, Halloran P, Neylan J, Wilkinson A, Ekberg H, Gaston R, Backman L, Burdick J.** (1998). Interleukin-2-receptor blockade with daclizumab to prevent acute rejection in renal transplantation. Daclizumab Triple Therapy Study Group. N Engl J Med. 338(3):161–5.
- **Wiseman LR, Faulds D.** (1999). Daclizumab: a review of its use in the prevention of acute rejection in renal transplant recipients. Drugs. 58(6):1029–42.

Zenapax® (daclizumab) Sterile Concentrate For Injection. Roche Pharmaceuticals Inc. (December 1997). Package Insert. Nutley, NJ 07110.

Self-Assessment Questions

Question 1: *Why are the humanized anti-Tac monoclonal products so much safer than the murine anti-CD3 monoclonal product?*

Question 2: *Which anti-Tac product contains greater portions of murine amino acid sequences?*

Answers

Answer 1: The anti-Tac products do not induce a cytokine release syndrome (CRS). CRS is the most life-threatening short-term risk with murine anti-CD3. Some infectious diseases also occur less frequently with the anti-Tac products. This phenomenon is probably related to less intense induction of immunosuppression necessary with anti-Tac based induction cocktails.

Answer 2: Daclizumab amino acid sequences are 90% human and 10% murine, whereas basiliximab sequences are less human and more murine. Given that basiliximab contains more murine amino acid sequences there might be theoretical concerns about safety or HAMA production. At this time there is no clinical evidence to suggest that one product is clinically safer than the other.

14 Recombinant Thrombolytic Agents

Nishit B. Modi

Introduction

Coagulation and fibrinogenolysis exist in a mutually compensatory or balanced state. Endogenous regulatory mechanisms ensure that the process of hemostasis and blood coagulation at a site of injury, and the subsequent fibrinolysis of the blood clot, is localized and well controlled. This localization and control ensures a rapid and efficient hemostatic response at a site of injury while simultaneously avoiding thrombogenic events at sites distant from the site of injury. Such control also prevents the hemostatic response from persisting beyond its physiologic need. This chapter will focus on the therapeutic aspects of tissue-type plasminogen activator and second-generation thrombolytic agents that are now available through recombinant technology.

Tissue-type Plasminogen Activator

Deposition of fibrin and platelets in the vasculature leads to thromboembolic diseases that are responsible for considerable mortality and morbidity. Early thrombolytic therapy can decrease mortality and improve coronary artery patency in patients with acute myocardial infarction (AMI). During fibrinolysis, the inactive zymogen plasminogen is enzymatically converted to the active moiety, plasmin, by various physiologic plasminogen activators, such as tissue-type plasminogen activator (t-PA) and single-chain urokinase-type plasminogen activator (scu-PA). Plasmin subsequently digests the insoluble fibrin matrix of a thrombus to yield soluble fibrin degradation products (Figure 14.1). Tissue-type plasminogen activator exhibits fibrin-specific plasminogen activation, with minimal systemic fibrinogenolysis. The relative absence of systemic fibrinogenolysis with t-PA means that there are fewer systemic side-effects compared to other plasminogen activators. Furthermore, t-PA is not associated with the allergic and hypotensive effects reported for the non-endogenous plasminogen activators, streptokinase and acylated plasminogen-streptokinase activator complex (APSAC).

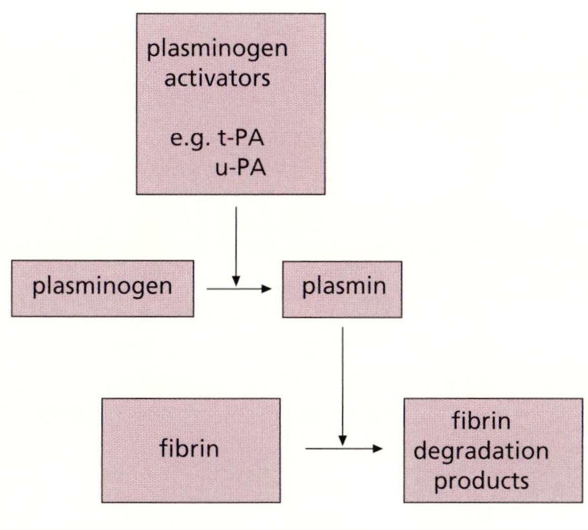

Figure 14.1. Schematic representation of the fibrinolytic pathway.

Structure

Native tissue-type plasminogen activator (t-PA) is a serine protease synthesized by vascular endothelial cells as a single-chain polypeptide of 527 amino acids with a molecular mass of 64 kDa (Pennica *et al.*, 1983). Approximately 6–8% of the molecular mass consists of carbohydrate. A schematic of the primary structure of human t-PA is shown in Figure 14.2. There are 17 disulfide bridges and four putative N-linked glycosylation sites recognized by the consensus sequence Asn-X-Ser/Thr at residues 117, 184, 218, and 448 (Pennica *et al.*, 1983). In addition, the presence of a fucose attached to Thr61 via an O-glycosidic linkage has been reported (Harris *et al.*, 1991). Two forms of t-PA that differ by the absence or presence of a carbohydrate moiety at Asp184 have also been characterized (Bennett, 1983): Type I t-PA is glycosylated at asparagine 117, 184, and 448, whereas Type II t-PA lacks a glycosylation at asparagine 184. The asparagine at amino acid 218 is normally not occupied in either form of t-PA (Vehar *et al.*, 1984a). Asparagine 117 contains a high-mannose oligosaccharide whereas Asn184 and Asn448 are

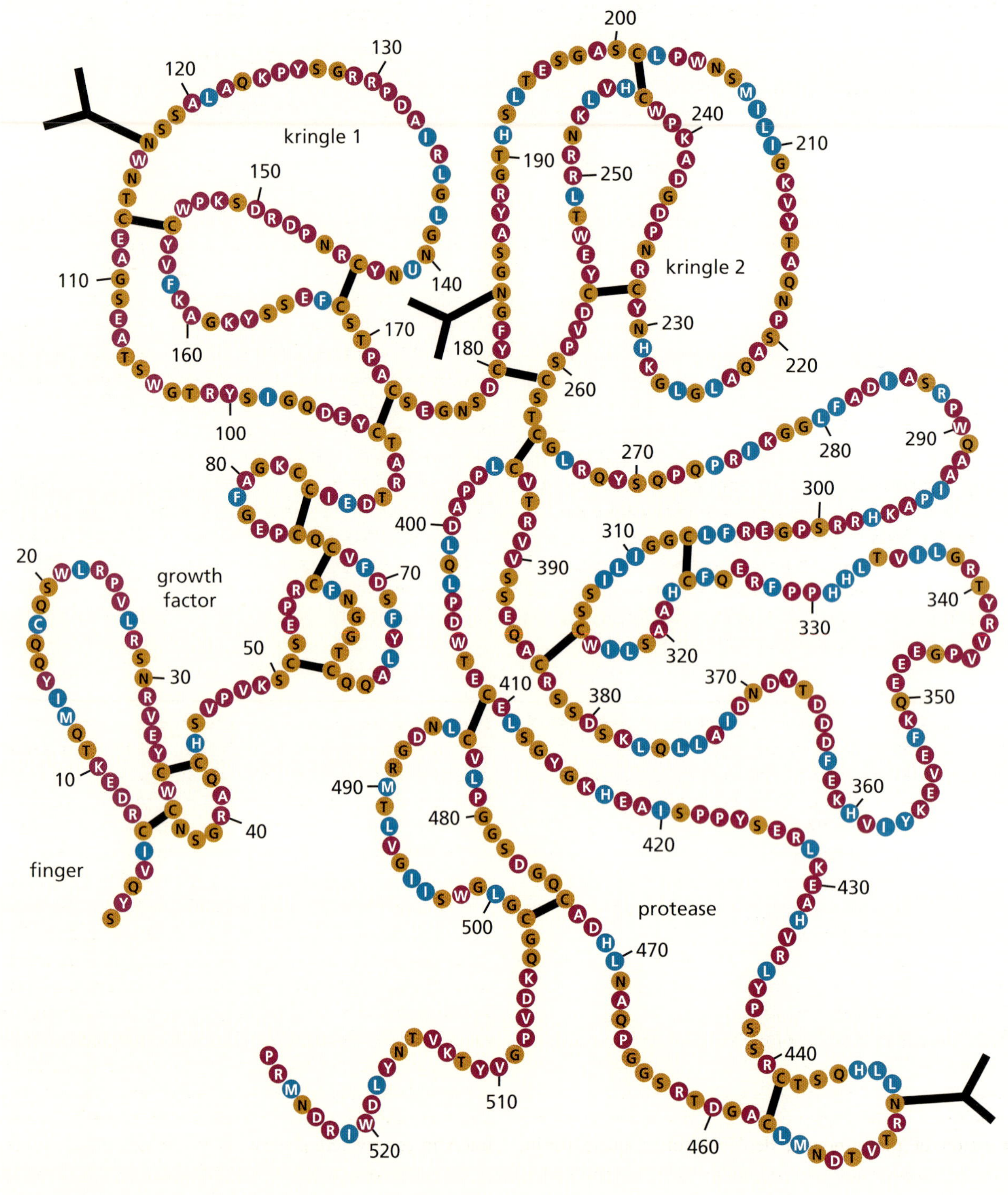

Figure 14.2. Primary structure of tissue-plasminogen activator.

of the complex carbohydrate type (Spellman *et al.*, 1989). Complex N-linked glycan structures contain a disaccharide Galβ(1,4)GlcNac and terminate in sialic acid residues, while an oligomannose (high mannose)-type glycan contains only mannose in the outer arms (see "Further Reading" for more details on protein glycosylation). Type II t-PA has a slightly higher specific activity *in vitro* compared with Type I t-PA (Einarsson *et al.*, 1985).

During fibrinolysis, the single-chain t-PA polypeptide is cleaved between Arg275 and Ile276 by plasmin to yield two-chain t-PA. Two-chain t-PA consists of a heavy chain (A-chain) derived from the amino terminus and a light chain (B-chain) linked by a single disulfide bridge between Cys264 and Cys395. The A-chain consists of the finger, growth factor, and two kringle domains. The finger domain and the second kringle are responsible for t-PA binding to fibrin and for the activation of plasminogen. The function of the first kringle is not known. The B-chain contains the serine protease domain consisting of the His-Asp-Ser triad that cleaves plasminogen (Pennica *et al.*, 1983).

Pharmacology

During fibrinolysis the inactive zymogen plasminogen is converted to the active enzyme plasmin by hydrolysis of the Arg560–Val561 peptide bond by the action of plasminogen activators. Plasmin then degrades the insoluble fibrin clot into soluble degradation products. Tissue plasminogen activator has a high affinity for fibrin and is a strong activator of plasminogen. In the absence of fibrin, t-PA is a poor enzyme, but in the presence of fibrin, t-PA enhances the activation of plasminogen by more than 600-fold (Hoylaerts *et al.*, 1982). Plasminogen activators are inhibited by the action of plasminogen activator inhibitors 1 and 2 (PAI-1 and PAI-2), which normally circulate at a concentration of 5–20 μg/L in the plasma (Collen and Lijnen, 1994). Mean t-PA antigen concentrations at rest in humans are approximately 5 μg/mL and can increase 1.5–2-fold in venous occlusion (Holvoet *et al.*, 1987). Circulating plasmin is rapidly inactivated by α_2-antiplasmin, whereas plasmin formed on the fibrin clot surface is only slowly inactivated. This slow inactivation allows for efficient plasminogen activation at the target site (the fibrin clot) with less systemic activation and fewer systemic side-effects compared with thrombolytic agents that are less fibrin-specific. If the amount of fibrin produced is sufficient to deplete the available α_2-antiplasmin, a systemic fibrinolytic state can occur, which is characterized by the activation of plasminogen, depletion of α_2-antiplasmin, decreased fibrinogen levels and increased fibrinogen degradation products. This degradation can subsequently lead to hemorrhagic complications. Decreases in plasma levels of fibrinogen (to 54–61% of baseline), plasminogen (to 54–70% of baseline), and α_2-antiplasmin (to 20–35% of baseline) have been reported following 100 mg rt-PA (recombinant t-PA) administered over 1.5–3.0 hours (Seifried *et al.*, 1989; Tanswell *et al.*, 1992). These effects reverted to 70–88% of baseline values by 24 hours after treatment.

First Generation Recombinant Thrombolytic Agents

Recombinant t-PA (rt-PA)

Recombinant t-PA (rt-PA) (alteplase) is identical to endogenous human t-PA. Like melanoma-derived t-PA, rt-PA lacks glycosylation at Asn218 and exists in two forms that differ by the absence or presence of a carbohydrate at residue Asn184 (Vehar *et al.*, 1986). Initially, rt-PA was produced as a two-chain form in Chinese Hamster Ovary (CHO) cells using a roller bottle (RB) process. Most of the initial pharmacokinetic and clinical studies were conducted using rt-PA derived from this process. Subsequently, a large-scale suspension culture (SC) process that produced primarily (80%) single-chain rt-PA was developed for commercialization. A pharmacokinetic comparison of rt-PA derived from the RB and SC processes showed that SC-derived rt-PA was cleared from the circulation approximately 30% faster than RB-derived rt-PA (Data on file, Genentech, Inc.). However, when used at doses that give similar concentrations, both RB- and SC-derived rt-PA had similar pharmacodynamic and therapeutic properties.

Pharmacokinetics of t-PA

The pharmacokinetics of rt-PA have been studied in mice, rats, rabbits, primates, and humans. After intravenous administration, plasma concentrations decline rapidly with an initial dominant half-life of less than five minutes in all species. Plasma clearance ranges from 27 mL/min in rabbits (Hotchkiss *et al.*, 1988), to 29 mL/min in monkeys (Baughman, 1987), and to 620 mL/min in humans (Tanswell *et al.*, 1989). Recombinant t-PA exhibits nonlinear (Michaelis-Menten) pharmacokinetics at high plasma concentrations (Tanswell *et al.*, 1990). The estimated Km (Michaelis-Menten constant) and Vmax (maximum elimination rate or catabolic capacity) values estimated by simultaneously fitting multiple plasma concentration-time curves following several doses were 12- to 15 μg/mL and 3.7 μg/mL/hr, respectively, with little species variation in these parameters. The pharmacokinetics are essentially linear in cases where plasma concentrations do not exceed 10% to 20% of Km (i.e. 1.5–3 μg/mL). Table 14.1 presents a pharmacokinetic summary of alteplase following intravenous administration in humans. These data show that recombinant t-PA has an initial volume of distribution approximating plasma volume and a rapid plasma clearance. The initial half-life was less than five minutes. There was no difference in the pharmacokinetics following the different infusion regimens. A lower plasma clearance was noted following intravenous bolus injection, possibly suggesting saturation of clearance mechanisms.

Administration regimen	Health status	Cmax (μg/mL)	CL (L/min)	V_1 (L)	V_{ss} (L)	$t_{1/2\alpha}$ (min)	$t_{1/2\beta}$ (min)	$t_{1/2\gamma}$ (h)	Reference
0.25 mg/kg/30 min 0.5 mg/kg/30 min	Healthy Healthy	0.96±0.18 1.8±0.3	0.64±0.05	4.6±0.3	8.1±0.8	4.4±0.2	39±3	–	Tanswell *et al.*, 1989
100 mg/2.5 h	AMI	3.3±1.0	0.38±0.07	2.8±0.9	9.3±5.0	3.6±0.9	16±5	3.7±1.4	Seifried *et al.*, 1989
100 mg/1.5 h	AMI	4±1	0.57±0.10	3.4±1.5	8.4±5.0	3.4±1.4	72±68	–	Tanswell *et al.*, 1992
100 mg/1.5 h	AMI	–	0.45±0.17	7.2±4.0	29±22	–	144±100	–	Modi *et al.*, 2000
Bolus	AMI	9.8±3.6	0.48±0.15	4.5±1.3	31±18	4.8±1.0	17±6	9.1±3.1	Tebbe *et al.*, 1989

Table 14.1. Pharmacokinetic parameters (mean±SD) for alteplase antigen following intravenous administration in healthy volunteers and patients with AMI. Cmax = maximum plasma concentration; CL = plasma clearance; V_1 = initial volume of distribution; V_{ss} = steady-state volume of distribution; $t_{1/2}$ = half-life.

The primary route of alteplase clearance is via receptor-mediated clearance mechanisms in the liver. Three cell types in the liver are responsible for the clearance of t-PA: parenchymal cells, endothelial cells, and Kupffer cells. Kupffer cells and endothelial cells mediate t-PA clearance via the mannose receptor. Parenchymal cells clear t-PA via a carbohydrate-independent, receptor-mediated mechanism. Data suggest that this carbohydrate-independent clearance is mediated by the low-density lipoprotein receptor-related protein (LRP) (Bu *et al.*, 1993).

Several reports have shown a correlation between change in hepatic blood flow and plasma concentrations of thrombolytic agents in healthy volunteers (De Boer *et al.*, 1992, van Griensven *et al.*, 1996). The therapeutic implications of pharmacokinetic and pharmacodynamic drug interactions with thrombolytic agents have been reviewed (De Boer and van Griensven, 1995). Clinical data correlating hepatic blood flow with rt-PA plasma concentrations in patients with AMI are currently lacking, and it is unclear if dose adjustments of thrombolytic agents are therapeutically necessary in patients receiving drugs that might affect hepatic blood flow.

Clinical Usage

Recombinant human t-PA (alteplase t-PA) is indicated for use in the management of acute myocardial infarction (AMI) and acute massive pulmonary embolism in adults. It is also indicated for the management of acute ischemic stroke if therapy is initiated within three hours after the onset of stroke symptoms and after exclusion of intracranial hemorrhage by cranial computerized tomography scan.

Two dose regimens, the 90-minute accelerated regimen and the three-hour regimen, have been studied in patients experiencing AMI; controlled studies comparing the clinical outcome of the two regimens have not been conducted. For the accelerated regimen, the recommended dose is based on patient weight, not to exceed 100 mg alteplase. For patients weighing more than 67 kg, the recommended dose regimen is 100 mg as a 15-mg intravenous bolus injection, followed by 50 mg infused over 30 minutes, and then 35 mg infused over the next 60 minutes. For patients weighing no more than 67 kg, the recommended dose regimen is a 15-mg intravenous bolus injection, followed by 0.75 mg/kg infused over 30 minutes not to exceed 50 mg, and then 0.5 mg/kg over the next 60 minutes and not to exceed 35 mg.

For the three-hour regimen, the recommended dose is 100 mg administered as 60 mg in the first hour (6–10 mg as a bolus), 20-mg over each of the second and third hours. For patients weighing less than 65 kg, the dose is 1.25 mg/kg over three hours. Infarct artery-related patency rates of 70–77% are achieved at 90 minutes with this three-hour regimen (Vestraete *et al.*, 1985). Patency grades of blood flow in the infarct-related artery are defined by the Thrombolysis in Myocardial Infarction (TIMI) scale and are assessed angiographically with TIMI grade 0 representing no flow; grade 1, minimal flow; grade 2, sluggish flow; and grade 3, complete or full, brisk flow.

The efficacy of the accelerated 90-minute regimen was demonstrated in an international, multicenter trial (GUSTO) that enrolled approximately 41,000 patients (The GUSTO Investigators, 1993a,b). The GUSTO trial demonstrated a higher infarct-related artery patency rate at 90-minutes in the group treated with rt-PA with heparin compared with streptokinase with either intravenous or subcutaneous heparin. The patency in the alteplase group was 81.3% compared with 53.5–59.0% in the streptokinase groups. In addition, the alteplase group had a reduced mortality (an additional ten lives saved per 10,000 patients treated). The intracranial hemorrhage rate was approximately 1%.

In a multicenter, open-label study in 461 patients with AMI randomized to receive 100 mg alteplase over 90 minutes or two 50-mg bolus doses 30 minutes apart, the 90-minute angiographic patency rate was 74.5% for the double bolus group and 81.4% in the infusion group (p = 0.08). The 30-day mortality rates were 4.5% in the bolus group and 1.7% in the infusion group (not significantly different) (Bleich *et al.*, 1998). Similarly, the Continuous Infusion Versus Double-Bolus Administration of Alteplase (COBALT) trial in 7,169 patients with AMI showed a higher incidence of 30-day mortality in the double bolus alteplase group (7.98%) compared with the accelerated-infusion group (7.53%). There was also a slightly higher incidence of intracranial hemorrhage in the double bolus group (COBALT Investigators, 1997).

For acute ischemic stroke, the recommended dose is 0.9 mg/kg not to exceed 90 mg infused over 60 minutes, with 10% of the total dose administered as an initial intravenous bolus over one minute. The safety and efficacy of this regimen with concomitant use of heparin and aspirin during the first 24 hours has not been investigated.

The recommended dose for treatment of pulmonary embolism is 100 mg administered by intravenous infusion over two hours. Heparin therapy should be instituted or reinstituted near the end of or immediately following alteplase infusion when the partial thromboplastin time or thrombin time returns to twice normal or less.

Safety Concerns

Since thrombolytic therapy increases the risk of bleeding, alteplase is contraindicated in patients with a history of cerebrovascular accidents, or patients who have any kind of active internal bleeding, intracranial neoplasm, arteriovenous malformation, or aneurism, or who have had recent intracranial, intraspinal surgery, or trauma.

Pharmaceutical Considerations

Recombinant human t-PA (Alteplase; Activase®, Genentech, Inc; Actilyse®, Boehringer Ingelheim) is supplied as a sterile, white to off-white lyophilized powder. Recombinant t-PA is practically insoluble in water, so arginine is included in the formulation to increase aqueous solubility (cf. Chapter 4). Phosphoric acid and/or sodium hydroxide may be used to adjust the pH. The sterile lyophilized powder should be stored at controlled room temperatures not to exceed 30 °C, or refrigerated at 2–8 °C, and protected from excessive light.

The powder is reconstituted by adding the accompanying Sterile Water for Injection, USP to the vial, resulting in a colorless to pale yellow transparent solution containing 1 mg/mL rt-PA, with a pH of approximately 7.3 and an osmolality of approximately 215 mOs/kg. Recombinant t-PA is stable in solution over a pH range of 5–7.5. Since the reconstituted solution does not contain any preservatives, it should be used within eight hours of preparation and should be refrigerated prior to use. The solution is incompatible with bacteriostatic water for injection. Other solutions, such as Sterile Water for Injection or preservative-containing solutions, should not be used for further dilution. The 1-mg/mL solution can be diluted further with an equal volume of 0.9% Sodium Chloride for Injection, USP, or 5% Dextrose Injection, USP, to yield a solution with a concentration of 0.5 mg/mL. This solution is compatible with glass bottles and polyvinyl chloride bags.

Second-Generation Recombinant Thrombolytic Agents

The rapid clearance of rt-PA from the circulation by the liver necessitates administration as an intravenous infusion. Although alteplase provides more rapid thrombolysis and superior patency compared with streptokinase and urokinase, at therapeutic doses there is some fibrinogenolysis and the administration scheme is relatively complicated. Thus, there is room for further improvements in efficacy and safety. Considerable nonclinical and clinical research has been underway to identify rt-PA variants that are fibrin specific and that have a simpler administration regimen compared with alteplase. Several reviews (e.g. Higgins and Bennett, 1990) have outlined the progress of efforts to develop second-generation thrombolytic agents. Strategies that have been used to develop t-PA variants have included domain deletions, glycosylation changes, and site-directed amino acid substitutions. A number of these second-generation thrombolytic agents are currently in late-stage clinical trials, or have been approved for marketing.

Reteplase

Reteplase is a 355 amino acid deletion variant of t-PA, consisting of the protease and kringle 2 domains of human t-PA. It is expressed in *Escherichia coli* cells as a single-chain, non-glycosylated, 39.6 kDa peptide.

Pharmacology

Like alteplase, reteplase is a fibrin-specific activator of plasminogen. *In vitro*, the plasminogenolytic activity of reteplase is 2–3.8-fold lower than alteplase on a molar basis (Kohnert *et al.*, 1993), which may be attributed to the absence of the finger domain in reteplase. Reteplase had a similar *in vitro* maximal efficacy (Emax) compared with alteplase, however, the molar concentration required to produce 50% clot lysis (EC_{50}) was 6.4-fold higher for

Dose (U)	n	Cmax (ng/mL)	CL (L/h)	$t_{1/2\alpha}$ (min)	$t_{1/2\beta}$ (h)	Reference
10	4	4620	6.24	19.2	6.3	Sefried *et al.*, 1992
15	9	5060	8.34	18.8	6.3	Sefried *et al.*, 1992
15	9	5170	8.70	21.4	5.0	Grünewald *et al.*, 1997
10 + 5	7	3610	9.12	16.3	5.4	Grünewald *et al.*, 1997
10 + 10	8	3370	6.90	17.0	5.5	Grünewald *et al.*, 1997

Table 14.2. Pharmacokinetic parameters for reteplase antigen from Phase II studies in patients with acute myocardial infarction.

reteplase than for alteplase (Martin *et al.*, 1993). The data also suggested that *in vitro* reteplase has a lower thrombolytic potency in lysing aged and platelet-rich clots compared with alteplase.

Table 14.2 presents a summary of the pharmacokinetics of reteplase in humans.

CLINICAL USAGE

Reteplase (Retavase®, Centocor) is indicated for use in the management of acute myocardial infarction in adults for the improvement of ventricular function following AMI, the reduction of the incidence of congestive heart failure, and the reduction of mortality associated with AMI.

The potency of reteplase is expressed in units using a reference standard that is specific for reteplase and not comparable with units used for other thrombolytic agents. Reteplase is administered as a double bolus injection regimen consisting of 10 U each. Each bolus is administered as an intravenous bolus injection of two minutes via an intravenous line in which no other medications are being administered simultaneously. The second bolus injection is given 30 minutes after the first. Heparin and reteplase are incompatible when combined in solution, and should not be administered simultaneously through the same intravenous line. If reteplase is administered through an intravenous line containing heparin, normal saline or 5% Dextrose solution should be flushed through the intravenous line prior to and following reteplase.

The INJECT trial evaluated the effects of reteplase (10 + 10 U) and streptokinase (1.6 million units over 60 minutes) on 35-day mortality in 6010 AMI patients in a double-blind randomized fashion. The 35-day mortality was 9.0% for patients treated with reteplase and 9.5% for those treated with streptokinase with no difference between the two groups. The incidence of stroke was also similar between the groups; however, more patients treated with reteplase experienced hemorrhagic strokes.

Two open-label angiographic studies (RAPID 1 and RAPID 2) have compared reteplase with alteplase. In RAPID 1 patients were treated with reteplase (10 + 10 U, 15 U, or 10 + 5 U) or the standard alteplase regimen (100 mg over three hours) within six hours of symptoms. Figure 14.3 shows the 90-minute TIMI 3 grade flow and 30-day mortality rates for the treatment groups. Ninety minute TIMI grade 3 flow was seen in 63% of patients in the 10 + 10 U reteplase group and 49% of the patients in the standard regimen alteplase group.

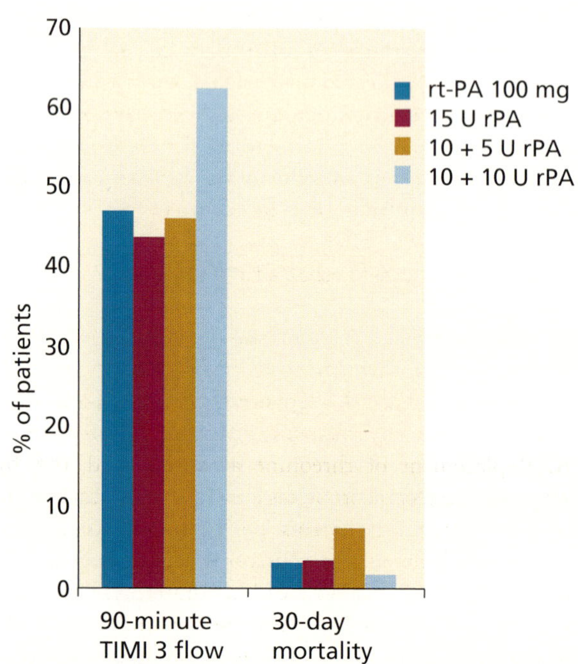

Figure 14.3. Correlation between TIMI flow and mortality demonstrating a decrease in mortality with improvement in TIMI flow.

RAPID 2 was an open-label, randomized trial in 320 patients comparing 10 + 10 U reteplase and accelerated alteplase within 12 hours of symptom onset. Percentages of patients with TIMI grade 3 flow at 90 minutes were 59.9% in the reteplase group and 45.2% in the alteplase group. There was no significant difference in the 35-day mortality between the two groups. Neither trial was powered to compare the efficacy or safety with respect to mortality or incidence of stroke.

The more favorable results for reteplase compared with alteplase noted in smaller trials were not replicated in a large, randomized, double-blind trial. In the GUSTO-III trial, 15,059 patients were randomized in a 2:1 fashion to receive reteplase in two bolus doses of 10 U 30 minutes apart or up to 100 mg alteplase infused over 90 minutes. The 30-day mortality rates were 7.47% for reteplase and 7.24% for alteplase (The Global Use of Strategies to Open Occluded Coronary Arteries (GUSTO III) Investigators, 1997). The stroke rate was 1.64% for reteplase and 1.79% for alteplase (p=0.50). Reteplase, while easier to administer than accelerated alteplase, did not demonstrate any survival advantage.

Safety Concerns

As with other thrombolytic agents, reteplase is contraindicated in cases of active internal bleeding, history of cerebrovascular accident, recent intracranial or intraspinal surgery or trauma, intracranial neoplasm, arteriovenous malformation, or aneurism, in cases of known bleeding diathesis, or in severe uncontrolled hypertension.

Pharmaceutical Considerations

Reteplase is supplied as a sterile, white, lyophilized powder for intravenous injection after reconstitution with Sterile Water for Injection, USP, supplied as part of the kit. Following reconstitution, the pH of the solution is 6.0.

Tenecteplase

Tenecteplase (TNKase™, Genentech, Inc) is a t-PA variant that has amino acid substitutions in three regions of t-PA. Replacement of threonine at amino acid 103 by asparagine (T103N) incorporates a complex oligosaccharide carbohydrate structure at this position. Replacement of arginine at position 117 by glutamine (N117Q) results in removal of the high mannose carbohydrate present at this site. A tetra-alanine substitution at positions 496–499 (KHRR496–499AAAA) contributes to increased fibrin-specificity. These three design modifications result in a thrombolytic that, compared to the parent t-PA molecule, is approximately 10- to 14-fold more fibrin-specific, is 80-fold more resistant to local inactivation, and has an 8-fold slower clearance in rabbits (Keyt *et al.*, 1994). Allometric scaling of pharmacokinetic data in animals predicted that tenecteplase would have a five-fold slower plasma clearance compared with alteplase (McCluskey *et al.*, 1997).

Pharmacology

In an *in vitro* clot lysis model, tenecteplase had 80% of the plasma clot lysis activity as t-PA (Keyt *et al.*, 1994). The plasma clearance of tenecteplase in rabbits was 1.9 mL/min/kg compared with 16 mL/min/kg for alteplase. A dose-ranging study in rats indicated no decrease in clearance over a range of 0.3 to 50 mg/kg, whereas in dogs the clearance decreased from 17 mL/min/kg at 0.3 mg/kg to 3.5 mL/min/kg at 30 mg/kg. Tissue distribution studies in rats indicate that the liver is the major organ of clearance (McCluskey *et al.*, 1997).

Like alteplase, tenecteplase has Type I and Type II glycoforms. Type I has three carbohydrate structures at asparagine 103, 184, and 448 and Type II lacks the carbohydrate at asparagine 184. Carbohydrate structures on tenecteplase are all of the complex oligosaccharide type with no high mannose structures. For this reason, the rapid mannose receptor-mediated clearance observed for alteplase does not occur with tenecteplase. Rather, tenecteplase is thought to be cleared by galactose receptors present in liver sinusoidal cells.

Enzymatic removal of terminal sialic acid from tenecteplase has been shown to increase the clearance in rabbits and is likely due to increased exposure of underlying galactose sugars. This de-sialylation effect is more profound with tenecteplase than with alteplase and is probably due to the predominant mannose-receptor mediated clearance for alteplase. A second possible clearance pathway for tenecteplase is a non-carbohydrate mediated mechanism via the low density lipoprotein-receptor related protein (LRP) that is also a clearance pathway for alteplase (Camani *et al.*, 1998).

The thrombolytic effects of tenecteplase have been demonstrated in a rabbit model of coronary artery thrombosis (Benedict *et al.*, 1995) and in an embolic stroke model (Thomas *et al.*, 1994). In these studies the thrombolytic potency of tenecteplase was five to ten-fold greater than alteplase. The slower clearance of tenecteplase results in a longer exposure of the clot to the thrombolytic agent, which likely offsets the slightly lower activity. The higher fibrin specificity of tenecteplase results in lower systemic activation of plasminogen and an observed conservation of fibrinogen.

Clinical Usage

Tenecteplase is indicated for the reduction of mortality associated with acute myocardial infarction. The recommended total dose of tenecteplase should not exceed 50 mg and is based on patient weight according to the following weight-adjusted dosing table:

Patient Weight (kg)	Tenecteplase Dose (mg)
<60	30
≥60 to <70	35
≥70 to <80	40
≥80 to <90	45
≥90	50

Treatment should be initiated as soon as possible after the onset of AMI symptoms. Tenecteplase is contraindicated in patients with known bleeding diathesis or active internal bleeding, history of cerebrovascular accident, recent intracranial, intraspinal surgery or trauma, intracranial neoplasm, arteriovenous malformation, aneurysm, or severe uncontrolled hypertension due to an increased risk of bleeding.

Two studies (TIMI 10A and TIMI 10B) have examined the clinical pharmacokinetics of tenecteplase. TIMI 10A was a Phase I pilot safety study in patients with AMI. Pharmacokinetic data were obtained in 82 patients following intravenous bolus doses of 5 to 50 mg. Tenecteplase plasma concentrations decreased in a biphasic manner with an initial half-life of 11 to 20 minutes and a terminal half-life of 41 to 138 minutes. Mean plasma clearance of tenecteplase ranged from 125 to 216 mL/min and decreased with increasing dose (Modi *et al.*, 1998).

TIMI 10B was a dose-finding Phase II efficacy study comparing 30, 40 and 50 mg doses of bolus tenecteplase to 100 mg alteplase administered via the accelerated infusion regimen. Table 14.3 summarizes the pharmacokinetic data from TIMI 10B. Tenecteplase plasma clearance was approximately 100 mL/min compared to 453 mL/min for accelerated alteplase. In contrast to TIMI 10A, no dose-dependent decrease in plasma clearance was noted in TIMI 10B, probably a result of the narrower dose range examined. Additionally, the plasma clearance noted in TIMI 10B was slightly lower than that noted in TIMI 10A at comparable doses (Modi *et al.*, 2000). The 30, 40 and 50mg doses in TIMI 10B produced TIMI grade 3 flow in 54.3%, 62.8%, and 65.8% of the patients, respectively. TIMI grade 3 flow was seen in 62.7% of patients in the accelerated alteplase group, not significantly different from that in the 40 mg tenecteplase group. An additional finding of this dose-finding efficacy trial was that dose-adjusted dosing was important in achieving optimal reperfusion (Cannon *et al.*, 1998). In addition, tenecteplase resulted in a lower change from baseline in systemic coagulation factors compared with alteplase.

The safety and efficacy of tenecteplase were studied in a large double-blind, randomized trial (ASSENT-2). This trial in 16,949 AMI patients showed that the 30-day mortality rates for single bolus tenecteplase and accelerated alteplase were almost identical (6.18% for tenecteplase and 6.15% for alteplase) (Assessment of the Safety and Efficacy of a New Thrombolytic [ASSENT-2] Investigators, 1999). Intracranial hemorrhage rates were similar in both groups (0.9%), but fewer non-cerebral hemorrhages and a lower need for blood transfusion was noted in the tenecteplase group. In conclusion, tenecteplase and 90-minute alteplase are equivalent in terms of mortality and rates of intracranial hemorrhage. The single-bolus regimen for tenecteplase may facilitate thrombolytic therapy.

PHARMACEUTICAL CONSIDERATIONS

Tenecteplase is supplied as a sterile, white to off-white, lyophilized powder in a 50 mg vial under a partial vacuum. It should be stored at controlled room temperature not to exceed 30 °C (86 °F) or it should be stored refrigerated at 2 to 8 °C (36–46 °F). Tenecteplase is intended for intravenous bolus injection following reconstitution with Sterile Water for Injection. Each vial nominally contains 52.5 mg tenecteplase (comprising a 5% overfill), 0.55 g L-arginine, 0.17 g phosphoric acid, and 4.3 mg polysorbate 20. Biological potency of tenecteplase is determined by an *in vitro* clot lysis assay and is expressed in tenecteplase-specific activity units. The specific activity of tenecteplase has been defined as 200 units/mg protein.

Dose (mg)	n	Cmax (µg/mL)	CL (L/h)	$t_{1/2\alpha}$ (min)	$t_{1/2\beta}$ (min)
30	48	10.0	98.5	21.5	116
40	31	10.9	119	23.8	129
50	20	15.2	99.9	20.1	90.4

Table 14.3. Pharmacokinetic parameters for tenecteplase antigen from a Phase II study in patients with acute myocardial infarction (Modi *et al.*, 2000).

Lanoteplase

Lanoteplase is currently in development and published information is limited at this time. Lanoteplase is a t-PA variant in which the fibronectin fingerlike and epidermal growth factor domains have been removed (Collen *et al.*, 1988). In addition, an asparagine to glutamine substitution at amino acid 117 provides reduced clearance (Hansen *et al.*, 1988). Lanoteplase is produced in CHO cells. Lanoteplase has enhanced fibrinolytic activity in the presence of fibrin-related plasminogen and it is more fibrin-specific compared with streptokinase and urokinase. Preliminary pharmacokinetic data in humans showed a half-life of ~37±11 minutes, indicating that lanoteplase can be administered as an intravenous bolus over two to four minutes (Liao *et al.*, 1997).

The Intravenous nPA for Treatment of Infarcting Myocardium Early (InTIME) study was a multicenter, double-blind, randomized, double placebo, dose-ranging study in 613 patients comparing four doses of lanoteplase with accelerated alteplase. Patients were randomized to receive intravenous bolus doses of 15, 30, 60, or 120 kU/kg (not to exceed 12,000 kU) of lanoteplase or accelerated alteplase (den Heijer *et al.*, 1998). A statistically significant increase in the proportion of patients with TIMI grade 3 flow at 60 minutes was noted with increasing lanoteplase dose ($p < 0.001$). Patients given the highest lanoteplase dose appeared to have a higher rate of TIMI grade 3 flow at 90-minutes compared with alteplase (57% versus 46%), although this may be a result of the unusually low TIMI grade 3 flow in the alteplase arm of this small study. There was no difference in the 30-day composite endpoint of death, heart failure, major bleeding, or nonfatal infarction (Ross, 1999).

A larger randomized, multicenter equivalence trial (InTime II) in 15,078 patients compared the safety and efficacy of 120 kU/kg lanoteplase with that of accelerated alteplase (Ferguson, 1999). Patients were randomized in a 2:1 fashion to the lanoteplase arm or the alteplase arm. The primary endpoint of the study was 30-day mortality with an incidence of 6.7% for lanoteplase and 6.6% for alteplase. The difference in the incidence of stroke was not statistically significantly different between the treatment groups (1.89% for lanoteplase and 1.52% for alteplase). Intracranial hemorrhage was significantly more frequent in the lanoteplase arm than in the alteplase arm (1.13% versus 0.62%).

Conclusions

Recombinant technology has brought about significant advances in the availability of thrombolytic agents. Several thrombolytic agents with varying fibrin specificity and ease of administration have received regulatory approval. However, improvements in the patency of the infarct-related artery have generally been incremental. Research continues to better understand the role of glycosylation in clearance mechanisms and to look at alternative delivery modalities. ■

Further reading

- **Furukawa K and Kobata A.** (1992) Protein glycosylation. Curr Opinion Biotech, 3, 554–559.
- **Froehlich J and Stump DL.** (1995) Recombinant Tissue Plasminogen Activator in Thrombolytic Therapy for Peripheral Vascular Disease. Comerota AJ (Ed). J. B. Lippincot Company.
- **Lis H and Sharon N.** (1993) Protein glycosylation. Structural and functional aspects. Eur J Biochem, 218, 1–27.

References

- **Assessment of the Safety and Efficacy of a New Thrombolytic (ASSENT-2) Investigators.** (1999). Single-bolus tenecteplase compared with front-loaded alteplase in acute myocardial infarction: the ASSENT-2 double-blind randomized trial. Lancet, 354, 716–722.
- **Baughman RA.** (1987). Pharmacokinetics of tissue plasminogen activator. In Tissue Plasminogen Activator in Thrombolytic Therapy, edited by B Sobel, D Collen and E Grossbard. New York: Markel Dekker, pp. 41–53.
- **Bennett WF.** (1983). Two forms of tissue-type plasminogen activator (tPA) differ at a single specific glycosylation site. Thromb Haemost, 50, 106.
- **Benedict CR, Refino CJ, Keyt BA, Pakala R, Paoni NF, Thomas GR, Bennett WF.** (1995). New variant of human tissue plasminogen activator (tPA) with enhanced efficacy and lower incidence of bleeding compared with recombinant human tPA. Circulation, 92, 3032–3040.
- **Bleich SD, Adgey AAJ, McMechan SR, Love TW.** (1998). An angiographic assessment of alteplase: Double-bolus and front-loaded infusion regimens in myocardial infraction. Am Heart J 136, 74–78.
- **Bu G, Maksymovitch EA, Schwartz AL.** (1993). Receptor-mediated endocytosis of tissue-type plasminogen activator by low density lipoprotein receptor-related protein on human hepatoma HepG2 cells. J Biol Chem 268, 13002–13009.

- **Camani C, Gavin O, Bertossa C, Samatani E, Kruithof EK.** (1998). Studies on the effect of fucosylated and non-fucosylated finger/growth factor constructs on the clearance of tissue type plasminogen activator mediated by the low-density lipoprotein-receptor related protein. Eur J Biochem 251, 804–11.
- **Cannon CP, Gibson CM, McCabe CH, Adgey AAJ, Schwiger MJ, Sequeira RF, Grollier G, Giugliani RP, Frey M, Mueller HS, Steingart RM, Weaver WD, Van de Werf F, Braunwald E.** (1998). TNK-tissue plasminogen activator compared with front-loaded alteplase in acute myocardial infarction. Circulation, 98, 2805–2814.
- **Collen D, Stassen JM, Larsen GR.** (1988). Pharmacokinetics and thrombolytic properties of deletion mutants of human tissue-type plasminogen activator in rabbits. Blood, 71, 216–219.
- **Collen D, Lijnen HR.** (1994). Fibrinolysis and the control of hemostasis. In The Molecular Basis of Blood Diseases, edited by G Stamatoyannopoulos, AW Nienhuis, PW Majerus and H Varmus. Philadelphia: WB Saunders Company, pp. 725–752.
- **De Boer A, Kluft C, Kroon JM, Kasper FJ, Shoemaker HC, Pruis J, Breimer DD, Soons PA, Emeis JJ, Cohen AF.** (1992). Liver blood flow as a major determinant of the clearance of recombinant human tissue-type plasminogen activator. Thromb Haemost, 67, 83–87.
- **De Boer A, van Greisven JMT.** (1995). Drug interactions with thrombolytic agents. Current perspectives. Clin Pharmacokinet, 28, 315–326.
- **Einarsson M, Brandt J, Kaplan L.** (1985). Large-scale purification of human tissue-type plasminogen activator using monoclonal antibodies. Biochim Biophys Acta, 830, 1–10.
- **Ferguson JJ.** (1999). Meeting highlights. Highlights of the 48th scientific sessions of the American College of Cardiology. Circulation, 100, 570–575.
- **The Global Use of Strategies to Open Occluded Coronary Arteries (GUSTO) Investigators** (1993a). An international randomized trial comparing four thrombolytic strategies for acute myocardial infarction. N Engl J Med, 329, 673–682.
- **The Global Use of Strategies to Open Occluded Coronary Arteries (GUSTO) Investigators** (1993b). The effects of tissue plasminogen activator, streptokinase, or both on coronary-artery patency, ventricular function, and survival after acute myocardial infarction. N Eng J Med, 329, 1615–1622.
- **The Global Use of Strategies to Open Occluded Coronary Arteries (GUSTO III) Investigators** (1997). A comparison of reteplase with alteplase for acute myocardial infarction. N Engl J Med 337, 1118–1123.
- **Grünewald M, Müller M, Ellbrück D, Osterhues H, Mnohren M, Schirmer G, Ziesche S, Güloglu A, Bock R, Seifried E.** (1997). Double- versus single-bolus thrombolysis with reteplase for acute myocardial infarction: a pharmacokinetic and pharmacodynamic study. Fibrinolysis & Proteolysis, 11, 137–145.
- **Hansen L, Blue Y, Barone K, Collen D, Larsen GR.** (1988). Functional effects of asparagine-linked oligosaccharide on natural and variant human tissue-type plasminogen activator. J Biol Chem, 263, 15713–15719.
- **Harris RJ, Leonard CK, Guzzetta AW, Spellman MW.** (1991). Tissue plasminogen activator has an O-linked fucose attached to Threonine-61 in the epidermal growth factor domain. Biochemistry, 30, 2311–2314.
- **Higgins DL, Bennett WF.** (1990). Tissue plasminogen activator: The biochemistry and pharmacology of variants produced by mutagenesis. Annu Rev Pharmacol Toxicol, 30, 91–121.
- **Holvoet P, Boes J, Collen D.** (1987). Measurement of free, one-chain tissue-type plasminogen activator in human plasma with an enzyme-linked immunosorbent assay based on an active site-specific murine monoclonal antibody. Blood, 69, 284–289.
- **Hotchkiss A, Refino CJ, Leonard CK, O'Connor JV, Crowley C, McCabe J, Tate K, Nakamura G, Powers D, Levinson A, Mohler M, Spellman MW.** (1988). The influence of carbohydrate structure on the clearance of recombinant tissue-type plasminogen activator. Thromb Haemost, 60, 255–261.
- **Keyt BA, Paoni NF, Refino CJ, Berleau L, Nguyen H, Chow A, Lai J, Pena L, Pater C, Ogez J, Etcheverry T, Botstein D, Bennett WF.** (1994). A faster-acting and more potent form of tissue plasminogen activator. Proc Natl Acad Sci (USA), 91: 3670–3674.
- **Kohnert U, Horsch B, Fischer S.** (1993). A variant of tissue plasminogen activator (t-PA) comprised of the kringle 2 and the protease domain shows a significant difference in the in vitro rate of plasmin formation as compared to the recombinant human t-PA from transformed Chinese hamster ovary cells. Fibrinolysis, 7, 365–372.
- **Liao W-C, Beierle FA, Stouffer BC, Dockens RA, Abbud ZA, Tay LK, Knaus DM, Raymond RH, Chew PH, Kostis JB.** (1997). Single bolus regimen of lanoteplase (nPA) in acute myocardial infarction: pharmacokinetic evaluation from InTime-I study. Circulation 96(Suppl 1), I-260–I-261.
- **Martin U, Sponer G, Strein K.** (1993). Differential fibrinolytic properties of the recombinant plasminogen activator BM 06.022 in human plasma and blood clot systems in vitro. Blood Coag Fibrinolysis, 4, 235–242.
- **McCluskey ER, Keyt BA, Refino CJ, Modi NB, Zioncheck TF, Bussiere JL, Love TW.** (1997). Biochemistry, pharmacology, and initial clinical experience with TNK-tPA in New therapeutic agents. in Thrombosis and Thrombolysis. Sasahara AA and Loscalzo (Eds). Marcel Dekker, Inc. New York. pp. 475–593.
- **Modi NB, Eppler S, Breed J, Cannon CP, Braunwald E, Love T.** (1998). Pharmacokinetics of a slower clearing tissue plasminogen activator variant, TNK-tPA, in patients with acute myocardial infarction. Thromb Haemost 79, 134–139.
- **Modi NB, Fox NL, Clow F-W, Tanswell P, Cannon CP, Van de Werf F, Braunwald E.** (2000). Pharmacokinetics and pharmacodynamics of tenecteplase: Results from a Phase II study in patients with acute myocardial infarction. J Clin Pharmacol, 40, 508–515.
- **Pennica D, Holmes WE, Kohr WJ, Harkins RN, Vehar GA, Ward CA, Bennett WF, Yelverton E, Seeburg PH, Heyneker HL, Goeddel DV, Collen D.** (1983). Cloning and expression of

human tissue-type plasminogen activator cDNA in E. coli. Science, 301, 214–221.

- **Ross AM.** (1999). New plasminogen activators: A clinical review. Clin Cardiol, 22, 165–171.
- **Seifried E, Tanswell P, Ellbrück D, Haerer W, Schmidt A.** (1989). Pharmacokinetics and haemostatic status during consecutive infusions of recombinant tissue-type plasminogen activator in patients with acute myocardial infarction. Thromb Haemost, 61, 497–501.
- **Spellman MW, Basa LJ, Leonard CK, Chakel JV, O'Connor JV, Wilson S, Van Halbeck H.** (1989). Carbohydrate structures of human tissue plasminogen activator expressed in Chinese Hamster Ovary cells. J Biol Chem 264, 14100–14111.
- **Tanswell P, Seifried E, SU PCAF, Feuerer W, Rijken DC.** (1989). Pharmacokinetics and systemic effects of tissue-type plasminogen activator in normal subjects. Clin Pharmacol Ther, 46, 155–162.
- **Tanswell P, Heinzel G, Greischel A, Krause J.** (1990). Nonlinear pharmacokinetics of tissue-type plasminogen activator in three animal species and isolated perfused rat liver. J Pharmacol Exp Ther, 255, 318–324.
- **Tanswell P, Tebbe U, Neuhaus K-L, Gläsle-Schwarz L, Wojcik J, Seifried E.** (1992). Pharmacokinetics and fibrin specificity of alteplase during accelerated infusions in acute myocardial infarction. J Am Coll Cardiol, 19, 1071–1075.
- **Tebbe U, Tanswell P, Seifried E, Feuerer W, Scholz K-H, Herrmann KS.** (1989). Single-bolus injection of recombinant tissue-type plasminogen activator in acute myocardial infarction. Am J Cardiol, 64, 448–453.
- **The Continuous Infusion Versus Double-Bolus Administration of Alteplase (COBALT) Investigators.** (1997). A comparison of continuous infusion and alteplase with double-bolus administration for acute myocardial infarction. New Engl J Med, 337, 1124–1130.
- **Thomas GR, Thibodeaux H, Errett CJ, Badillo JM, Keyt BA, Refino CJ, Zivin JA, Bennett WF.** (1994). A long-half-life and fibrin-specific form of tissue plasminogen activator in rabbit models of embolic stroke and peripheral bleeding. Stroke, 25, 2072–8.
- **van Griensven JMT, Huisman LGM, Stuurman T, Dooijewaard G, Kroon R, Schoemaker RC, Kluft K, Cohen AF.** (1996). Effects of increased liver blood flow on the kinetics and dynamics of recombinant tissue-type plasminogen activator. Clin Pharmacol Ther, 60, 504–511.
- **Vehar GA, Kohr WJ, Bennett WF, Pennica D, Ward CA, Harkins RN, Collen D.** (1984). Characterization studies on human melanoma cell tissue plasminogen activator. Bio/Tech, 2, 1051–1057.
- **Vehar GA, Spellman MW, Keyt BA, Ferguson CK, Keck RG, Chloupek RC, Harris R, Bennett WF, Builder SE, Hancock WS.** (1986). Characterization studies of human tissue-type plasminogen activator produced using recombinant DNA technology. Cold Spring Harbor Symp Quant Biol, 51, 551–562.
- **Verstraete M, Bernard R, Bory M, Brower RW, Collen D *et al.*** (1985). Randomized trial of intravenous streptokinase in acute myocardial infarction. Report from the European Cooperative Study Group for recombinant tissue-type plasminogen activator. Lancet, 1, 842–847.

Self-Assessment Question

Question 1: *A number of second-generation thrombolytic agents have either been approved or are in late stages of development. Discuss some of the limitations that the second-generation thrombolytic agents are designed to address.*

Answer

Answer 1 Although alteplase demonstrated an increased patency rate in the infarct-related artery and a decrease in mortality, several areas were identified where further improvements could be made in the treatment of acute myocardial infarction. Second-generation thrombolytic agents are designed to address some of these shortcomings.

(i) Due to the rapid clearance of rt-PA from the circulation by the liver, the current administration is via intravenous infusion over 90-minutes or three hours. Second-generation thrombolytic agents have a slower plasma clearance allowing administration as a single or double bolus regimen (see Tables 14.1–3).

(ii) Although alteplase is more fibrin-selective compared to streptokinase and urokinase, there is still a 30%- to 50% fall in systemic fibrinogen levels. Second-generation thrombolytic agents are more fibrin-specific and could result in further reduction in systemic fibrinogenolysis.

15 Recombinant Coagulation Factors

Nishit B Modi

Introduction

Blood coagulation may be initiated by the exposure of blood to tissue factor (extrinsic pathway) or by the activation of plasma factors (intrinsic pathway). The two pathways converge into a common pathway leading to the generation of thrombin. A schematic of the two pathways is presented in Figure 15.1. Normally hemostasis is a highly efficient and tightly regulated process for ensuring that generation of thrombin occurs quickly and is localized. Abnormalities that result in a delay in blood coagulation are associated with a bleeding tendency termed hemophilia. Hemophilia is an X-linked recessive disorder. The incidence of hemophilia is estimated at five to six people per 100,000 males. Hemophilia A (classical hemophilia) patients have decreased, defective or absent production of Factor VIII, whereas patients with Hemophilia B lack Factor IX. The availability of recombinant coagulation factors has been a major advance in the area of hemophilia, providing patients improved safety and reducing the risk of infections transmitted by transfusion (Roddie and Ludlam, 1997).

Factor VIII

Factor VIII (antihemophilia factor) is a plasma protein that functions as a cofactor by increasing the Vmax in the activation of Factor X by Factor IXa in the presence of calcium ions and negatively charged phospholipid (Jackson and Nemerson, 1980). The congenital absence of Factor VIII is

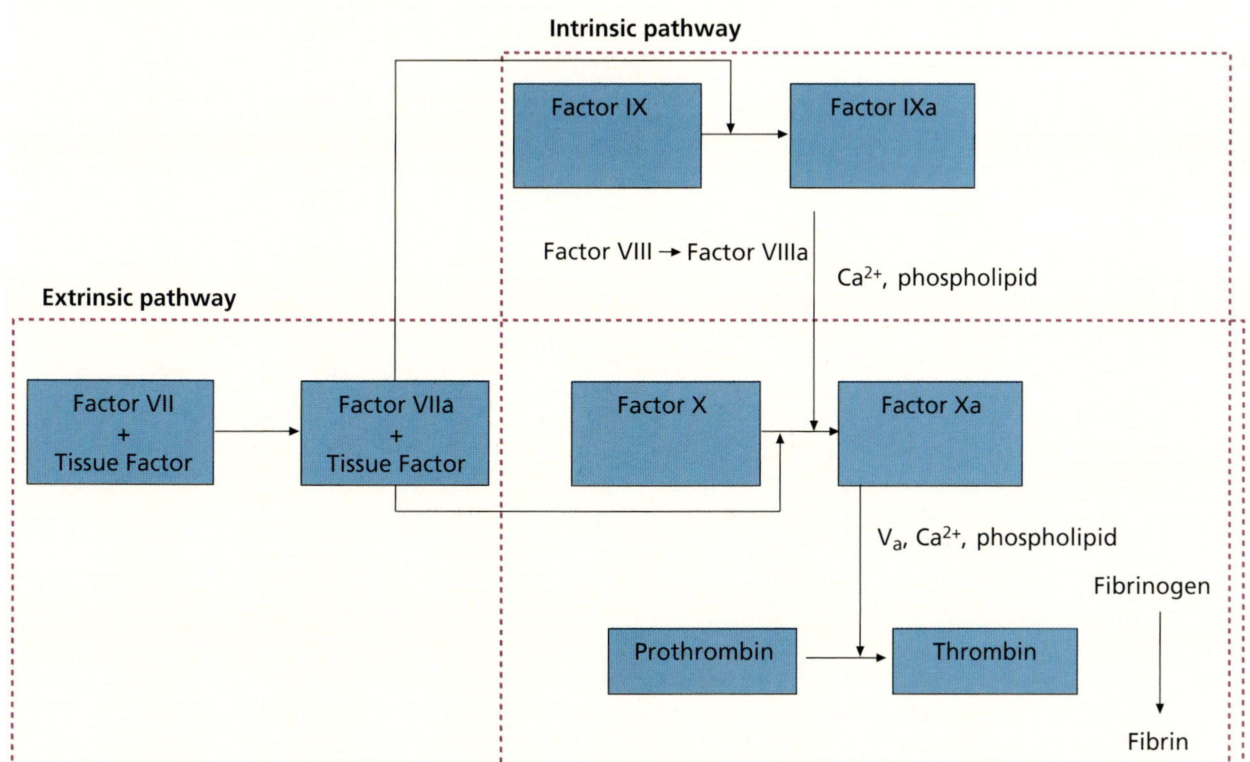

Figure 15.1. Simplified scheme showing the role of Factor VIII in the coagulation pathway.

termed Hemophilia A and afflicts approximately one in 10,000 males (Antonarakis *et al.*, 1987). The introduction of Factor VIII concentrates derived from plasma increased the quality of life and the life expectancy of individuals with hemophilia A, however, reliance on plasma as a source for Factor VIII also exposed patients to alloantigens and to risks associated with transfusion-associated viral diseases. The availability of Factor VIII derived from recombinant technology has the potential to eliminate many of the shortcomings of plasma-derived antihemophilia factor and to be available in an unlimited supply.

Structure

Factor VIII is synthesized as a single-chain polypeptide of 2332 amino acids (Eaton *et al.*, 1987). Shortly after synthesis, cleavage occurs and most plasma Factor VIII circulates as an 80 kDa light chain associated with a series of 210 kDa heavy chains in a metal ion-dependent complex. There are 25 potential N-linked glycosylation sites and 22 cysteines (Vehar *et al.*, 1984). The heterogeneity of the heavy chain is due to proteolytic cleavage, which reduces the molecular size of the heavy chain from 210 kDa to 90 kDa via a number of intermediates. The 90 kDa species lacks the amino acid residues 741–1648 (the B-domain), which are dispensable for Factor VIII activity (Eaton *et al.*, 1986).

Pharmacology

The concentration of Factor VIII in plasma is about 200 ng/mL (Hoyer, 1981). It is not known where Factor VIII is synthesized. There is evidence that several different tissues, including the spleen, liver, and kidney, may play a role. Factor VIII is normally covalently associated with a 50-fold excess of von Willebrand factor. Von Willebrand factor protects Factor VIII from proteolytic cleavage and allows concentration at sites of hemostasis. Circulating von Willebrand factor is bound by exposed subendothelium and activated platelets at sites of injury allowing localization of von Willebrand factor and Factor VIII.

Factor VIII circulates in the body as a large precursor polypeptide devoid of coagulant activity. Cleavage by thrombin at Arg372-Ser373, Arg740-Ser741, and Arg1689-Ser1690 results in procoagulant function (Vehar *et al.*, 1984). While cleavage at Arg740 is not essential for coagulant activity, cleavage at the other two sites is necessary. Although Factor VIII is synthesized as a single-chain polypeptide, shortly after synthesis, the single-chain polypeptide is cleaved and most of the Factor VIII in plasma exists as an 80 kDa light chain and a series of heavy chains. Factor VIII circulates as a heterodimer of the 80 kDa light chain and a variable (90–210 kDa) heavy chain in a metal ion-dependent complex.

Recombinant Factor VIII

Recombinant Factor VIII is available from three sources: Baxter Healthcare, Bayer Corporation, and Genetics Institute/American Home Products. Recombinant Factor VIII from Baxter Healthcare (Recombinate®) and Genetics Institute (Refacto®) is produced using transfected CHO cells, whereas that from Bayer Inc (Kogenate®) is produced using transfected Baby Hamster Kidney cells. A major difference between recombinant Factor VIII from Bayer and Baxter Healthcare is the presence of a Galα1–>3Gal carbohydrate moiety in the Baxter product (Hironaka *et al.*, 1992). The recombinant product from Baxter and Bayer comprises full-length Factor VIII which, like plasma-derived Factor VIII, consists of a dimer of the 80 kDa light chain and a heterogeneous heavy chain of 90–210 kDa (Schwartz *et al.*, 1990). The Genetics Institute product differs from the other two in that it is a deletion mutant in which the heavy chain lacks nearly the entire B-domain (Roddie and Ludlam, 1997).

Disposition of Recombinant Factor VIII

Several studies have evaluated the clinical pharmacokinetics of recombinant Factor VIII. The pharmacokinetic profile is summarized in Table 15.1. Following administration, the increase in Factor VIII concentration is dose-proportional and the disposition is similar following single and chronic dosing. The terminal half-life is 14–16 hours and the initial volume of distribution approximates plasma volume.

Pharmaceutical Considerations

Recombinant Factor VIII (Kogenate®, Bayer; Recombinate®, Baxter; Refacto®, Genetics Institute) is supplied as sterile, single-dose vials containing 250 to 1000 IU of Factor VIII activity. The preparation is lyophilized and stabilized with human albumin (Kogenate® and Recombinate®) or polysorbate 80 (Refacto®). Recently a reformulated product, Kogenate® FS (Bayer), has become available. This product is similar to its predecessor Kogenate Antihemophilic Factor (Recombinant) but incorporates a revised purification and formulation process that eliminates the addition of human albumin as a stabilizer, using histidine instead. The products contain no preservatives and should be stored at 2–8 °C. The lyophilized powder may be stored at room temperature (up to 25 °C) for up to three months without loss of biological activity. Freezing should be avoided. Factor VIII should be reconstituted with the diluent provided. The reconstituted product must be administered intravenously by direct syringe injection or drip infusion within three hours of reconstitution.

Administration regimen	CL (mL/h/kg)	V (mLkg)	$t_{1/2}$ (h)	MRT (h)	Reference
50 U/kg Recombinate®	3.1±1.2	62±18[a]	14.5±4.3	NR[b]	Morfini *et al.*, 1992
50 IU/kg Kogenate®[c]	2.5±0.8	51±13[d]	15.8±3.9	21.2±5.3	Schwartz *et al.*, 1990
	2.6±0.9	48±12	13.9±3.2	19.1±4.5	
	2.2±0.7	49±18	16.6±3.0	22.6±4.1	
50 U/kg Kogenate®	2.4±0.7	51±13	16.5±4.9	22.2±4.9	Harrison *et al.*, 1991

Table 15.1. Clinical pharmacokinetic profile of recombinant Factor VIII following intravenous administration in patients with hemophilia A. [a] $V_{d\ area}$; [b] Not reported; [c] Data reported for weeks 1, 13 and 25; [d] V_{dss}.

Clinical Usage

Recombinant Factor VIII (Kogenate® and Kogenate® FS, Bayer Corporation) is indicated for the treatment of classical hemophilia (hemophilia A) in which there is a demonstrated deficiency of activity of Factor VIII. Recombinant Factor VIII provides a means of temporarily replacing the missing coagulation factor in order to correct or prevent bleeding episodes, or in order to perform emergency or elective surgery in hemophiliacs. Recombinant Factor VIII can also be used for the treatment of hemophilia A in certain patients with inhibitors to Factor VIII. The dosage may be different in the presence of inhibitors.

Schwartz *et al.* (1990) investigated the pharmacokinetics, safety and efficacy of recombinant Factor VIII (Kogenate®) in patients with hemophilia A. In this study, the mean residence time and elimination half-life of recombinant Factor VIII were equal to or exceeded that for plasma-derived Factor VIII, whereas the clearance and steady-state volumes of distribution for recombinant Factor VIII were slightly smaller than that for plasma-derived Factor VIII. In the safety and efficacy portion of the study, the mean incremental recovery of Factor VIII following 50 IU/kg of recombinant Factor VIII given at weeks 1, 5, 9, 13, and 25 was 2.49–2.92% per IU administered per kilogram and was not statistically dependent on multiple dosing.

The pharmacokinetics of Kogenate® FS was similar to Kogenate®. The mean biological half-life was 13 hours, similar to that noted for Kogenate® and for plasma derived antihemophilic factor. The recovery and half-life data were unchanged after 24 weeks of treatment indicating continued efficacy and the absence of antibodies against Factor VIII that interfered with its pharmacokinetic profile.

The incidence of inhibitors to recombinant Factor VIII (Kogenate®) in previously untreated patients is approximately 20% (Lusher *et al.*, 1993). This incidence rate is similar to that for plasma derived Factor VIII, where approximately 10–15% of patients treated develop antibodies that neutralize Factor VIII and result in resistance to treatment (McMillan *et al.*, 1988). A direct comparison of incidence rates is difficult since studies investigating the incidence of inhibitor development to recombinant Factor VIII used previously untreated patients, whereas those investigating plasma derived Factor VIII were conducted in previously treated patients, a group that may be at lower risk for inhibitor development (Lusher *et al.*, 1993) The study by Lusher *et al.* (1993) showed that the risk of developing antibodies to recombinant Factor VIII correlated with the severity of disease and the intensity of exposure to Factor VIII. Inhibitors were detected 1 to 15 months after the initial exposure to Factor VIII. In several of the patients in whom inhibitors were detected, they disappeared completely or remained at a low level (≤ 10 Bethesda units) despite continued treatment with Factor VIII.

Dosage of recombinant Factor VIII (in International Units, IU) must be individualized to the needs of the patient, the severity of the deficiency and of the hemorrhage, the presence of inhibitors, and to the desired increase in Factor VIII activity (in IU/dL, or percentage of normal). Appropriate assays for Factor VIII levels should follow therapy with Factor VIII. As a guide, the *in vivo* percent elevation in Factor VIII level may be estimated using the following equation (Abildgaard *et al.*, 1966):

Dosage Required (IU) = Body Wt (kg) × Desired Increase in Factor VIII (%) × 0.5 IU/kg %

Safety Concerns

Since trace amounts of mouse or hamster protein may be present in recombinant Factor VIII as contaminants from the expression system, caution should be exercised when administering recombinant Factor VIII to individuals with known hypersensitivity to plasma-derived antihemophilic factor or with hypersensitivity to biological preparations with trace amounts of murine or hamster proteins.

Factor VIIa

Development of recombinant Factor VIIa was motivated by the fact that a small fraction of patients with hemophilia (15–20% of patients with hemophilia A and 2–5% of patients with hemophilia B) develop antibodies (inhibitors) to Factor VIII or Factor IX. For these patients the high titers of inhibitors make it impossible to give sufficient coagulation factor to overcome the inhibitor and therapy is ineffective or is associated with unacceptable side effects. Sometimes porcine Factor VIII or (partially activated) prothrombin complex concentrate (aPCC) may be used. However, porcine Factor VIII can produce thrombocytopenia and allergic reactions and aPCC is effective in only 62% of treatment episodes (Lusher *et al.*, 1980) and can result in myocardial infarction or disseminated intravascular coagulation. Intensive plasmapheresis, which has sometimes been used in combination with immune adsorption to reduce inhibitor titers, is time consuming and an anamnestic response may make it difficult to keep inhibitor levels low enough.

Factor VIIa can be valuable in these instances since in the absence of tissue factor it has very low proteolytic activity despite it being in an activated form. Tissue factor is normally only expressed by damaged endothelium, thus localizing the effects of Factor VIIa to sites of tissue injury. Initially Factor VIIa was derived from plasma purification, however, the very low concentration (0.5 μg/mL) in plasma made large scale purification difficult.

Structure

Factor VII is a vitamin K-dependent glycosylated serine protease proenzyme. Synthesis of Factor VII occurs in hepatocytes. Factor VII has 406 amino acids and the molecular weight is ~ 50kDa. The protein is not functionally active unless it is γ-carboxylated. There are two sites of N-linked glycosylation on Factor VII. There are three distinct domains: the Gla-domain that interacts with cell surface tissue factor, two tandem EGF-domains, and the serine-protease domain. Factor VII is synthesized as a proenzyme that becomes activated and cleaved upon hydrolysis of Arg-152 and Ile-153.

Recombinant Factor VIIa

Recombinant Coagulation Factor VIIa is produced in Baby Hamster Kidney cells using recombinant DNA technology. Recombinant Factor VII is expressed in a single-chain form and is spontaneously activated to Factor VIIa during purification. Characterization of the protein indicates that it is very similar to plasma-derived Factor VIIa with regard to amino acid sequence, carbohydrate composition, and γ-carboxylation (Thim *et al.*, 1988).

Pharmacokinetics and Pharmacodynamics

The single-dose pharmacokinetics of recombinant Factor VIIa were investigated in 15 patients with hemophilia with severe Factor VIII or Factor IX deficiency (Lindley *et al.*, 1994). Table 15.2 summarizes the pharmacokinetics from this study. Following an intravenous dose of 17.5, 35, and 70 μg/kg, the plasma clearance was 30.3, 32.4, and 36.1 mL/h/kg, respectively. The pharmacokinetics were linear and no difference in clearance was noted between non-bleeding and bleeding episodes. Median clearance was 31.0 mL/h in non-bleeding episodes and 32.6 mL/h in bleeding episodes. The median half-life was 2.9 h in non-bleeding episodes and 2.3 h in bleeding episodes. There was considerable interindividual variability whereas intraindividual variability appeared to be lower.

Based on preclinical studies in dogs, a concentration of > 8 U/mL should result in immediate hemostasis, whereas a concentration of 4 U/mL seems to be below the hemostatic level (Hedner, 1996). Based on the results of several pharmacokinetic/pharmacodynamics studies, it is necessary

	Dose (μg/kg)		
	17.5	35	70
Cmax (U/ml)	4.92	10.8	19.6
Cl (ml/h/kg)	30.3	32.5	36.1
$t_{1/2}$ (h)	2.6	2.7	2.8
MRT (h)	3.3	3.3	3.4
Vss (ml/kg)	98.1	110	120
Recovery (%)	50.1	49.0	42.6

Table 15.2. Clinical pharmacokinetic profile of recombinant Factor VIIa (Lindley *et al.*, 1994). Cmax values are presented in IU/ml based on a specific activity of 21–25 IU/μg.

to maintain plasma levels above 5–6 U/mL for adequate hemostasis. This plasma level maintenance may be accomplished by administering sufficiently high initial concentrations or by maintaining a strict two-hour dosing interval following doses of 70–90 μg/kg (Hedner, 1996).

Pharmaceutical Considerations

Novoseven® (Novo Nordisk) is formulated with sodium chloride, calcium chloride dihydrate, glycylglycine, polysorbate 80 and mannitol. The pH is adjusted to 5.3–6.3. The product does not contain any stabilizing protein. Prior to reconstitution, NovoSeven should be stored refrigerated (2–8 °C), avoiding exposure to direct sunlight.

NovoSeven® should be reconstituted with Sterile Water for Injection, USP (2.2 mL for the 1.2 mg vial and 8.5 mL for the 4.8 mg vial). After reconstitution with the appropriate volume of diluent, each vial contains approximately 0.6 mg/mL. Following reconstitution, NovoSeven® may be stored at refrigerated or at room temperature for up to three hours. NovoSeven® should not be mixed with infusion solutions until further clinical data are available to justify this.

Clinical Usage

Recombinant Factor VIIa (NovoSeven®) is indicated for the treatment of bleeding episodes in patients with hemophilia A or B with the presence of inhibitors to Factor VIII or Factor IX. The recommended dose of recombinant factor VIIa for patients with hemophilia A or B with inhibitors is 90 μg/kg every two hours until hemostasis is achieved or until treatment is judged to be inadequate. In order to achieve hemostasis, Factor VII:coagulation activity (FVII:C) levels should be maintained above 6 U/mL (Hedner, 1996; Lusher *et al.*, 1998).

Clinical trials with recombinant Factor VIIa have included a single dose comparative study of 35 and 70 μg/kg in joint, muscle, and mucocutaneous bleeds (Macik *et al.*, 1993), a comparative study in surgery (Cooper *et al.*, 1997), and a home treatment study (Key, 1997).

The study by Copper *et al.* (1997) was a double-blind, randomized, multicenter trial evaluating Novoseven® doses of 35 μg/kg and 90 μg/kg in patients hospitalized for preplanned surgical treatment. Doses were administered intravenously in a blinded fashion just prior to surgery and every two hours for 48 hours beginning at wound closure. Blinded dosing continued every two to six hours for an additional three days. The 35 μg/kg dose provided hemostasis through Day 5 in 70–100% of patients undergoing minor surgery and 40% of patients undergoing major surgery. The 90 mg/kg dose was effective in 83–100% of patients undergoing minor or major surgery. In the home treatment study, 88% of bleeds were effectively treated and there was no evidence of decreased efficacy with multiple use (Key, 1997).

Although specific drug interaction studies have not been conducted, to date there have been more than 50 episodes of concomitant use of antifibrinolytic agents (e.g. tranexamic acid, epsilon-aminocaproic acid) and recombinant Factor VIIa.

Based on the clinical safety database of 1989 bleeding episodes in 298 patients with hemophilia A or B with inhibitors, adverse events reported at rates of more than 2% of patients treated include fever, hemorrhage, decreased fibrinogen, hemarthrosis, and hypertension.

Safety Concerns

Recombinant Factor VIIa (NovoSeven®) should not be administered to patients with known hypersensitivity to recombinant Factor VIIa or any of the components of recombinant Factor VIIa. Recombinant Factor VIIa is contraindicated in patients with known hypersensitivity to mouse, hamster, or bovine proteins.

Factor IX

Factor IX is activated by Factor VII/tissue factor complex in the extrinsic pathway and by Factor XIa in the intrinsic pathway (Figure 15.1). Activated Factor IX, in combination with activated factor VIII, activates Factor X, resulting in the conversion of prothrombin to thrombin. Thrombin then converts fibrinogen to fibrin forming a blood clot at a site of hemorrhage.

Recombinant Coagulation Factor IX

Recombinant Coagulation Factor IX (BeneFix®, Genetics Institute) is produced in a CHO cell line. The transfected cell line secretes recombinant Factor IX in the culture medium from which the protein is purified via several chromatographic steps. Recombinant Factor IX is a glycoprotein with a Mr of ~ 55 kDa consisting of 415 amino acids in a single-chain.

While plasma-derived Factor IX carries a Thr/Ala dimorphism at position 148, the primary amino acid sequence of recombinant Factor IX is identical to the Ala148 allelic form. As a result of post-translational modifications, recombinant and plasma-derived Factor IX differ in a number of respects (White *et al.*, 1997). First, plasma-derived Factor IX carries 12 gamma-carboxyglutamic acid (Gla) residues in its amino-terminal Gla-domain, whereas 40%

of recombinant Factor IX is undercarboxylated, lacking gamma-carboxylation at Glu40. Crossover studies in dogs have suggested that these two isoforms have similar pharmacokinetics and pharmacodynamics (McCarthy *et al.*, 1997). Other differences between recombinant and plasma-derived Factor IX are in the activation peptide region (residues 146–180), which is cleaved off upon Factor IX activation. These include the lack of sulfation at Tyr155, and of phosphorylation at Ser158, as well as different N-linked glycosylation patterns at Asn157 and Asn167. While these structural differences have no apparent impact on the biological activity of recombinant Factor IX, they may contribute to the observed difference in pharmacokinetics (see section Clinical Usage).

The potency of recombinant Factor IX is determined in International Units using an *in vitro* clotting assay. One IU is the amount of Factor IX activity present in a milliliter of pooled normal human plasma. The specific activity of BeneFix® is greater than or equal to 200 IU/mg protein.

Pharmacology

Non-clinical studies have been conducted in mice, rats, and dogs. Comparison of recombinant Factor IX and monoclonal-purified plasma derived Factor IX in a hemophilia B dog model showed that both products corrected both whole blood clotting time and partial thromboplastin time (Schaub *et al.*, 1998). Treatment with recombinant Factor IX or plasma derived Factor IX decreased partial thromboplastin time (PTT) from 135 to >150 seconds to 46–96 seconds or 59–62 seconds, respectively (Brinkhous *et al.*, 1996).

Preclinical studies have indicated that recombinant Factor IX has low thrombogenic potential (Schaub *et al.*, 1998). Studies in a modified Wessler stasis model showed that none of the rabbits treated with 50, 500, or 1000 IU/kg developed thrombosis. At 150 IU/kg one of six rabbits developed thrombosis (Ferranti *et al.*, 1995). Toxicology studies in mice, rats, and dogs showed that recombinant Factor IX was well tolerated, with the only toxicology noted in mice (activation of coagulation), a fact which has also been noted with plasma derived products. In beagle dogs, administration of recombinant Factor IX once daily for 14 days at doses of 50, 100, or 200 IU/kg in beagles showed a dose-proportional increase in Cmax and AUC. The elimination half-life ranged between 10.9 and 15.8 hours and was independent of dose (McCarthy *et al.*, 1995). In addition, the pharmacokinetics were similar between Day 1 and Day 7. Pharmacokinetic and pharmacodynamic studies have indicated that increases in recombinant Factor IX plasma concentrations are correlated ($r = 0.86$) with Factor IX activity as measured by a clotting assay (Schaub *et al.*, 1998). Comparison of recombinant Factor IX and plasma-derived Factor IX in a dog model of hemophilia B indicated that while plasma-derived Factor IX had a higher AUC and Cmax compared with recombinant Factor IX, the efficacy of the two products was similar (Keith *et al.*, 1995).

Pharmaceutical Considerations

Recombinant Factor IX (BeneFix®) is supplied as a sterile, lyophilized powder in single use vials containing nominally 250, 500, or 1000 IU per vial intended for IV injection. Recombinant Factor IX should be stored refrigerated (2–8 °C). It may also be stored at room temperature (25 °C) for up to six months. Freezing should be avoided to prevent damage to the diluent vial.

Recombinant Factor IX should be reconstituted with Sterile Water for Injection (diluent), which is provided. After reconstitution, BeneFix® should be injected intravenously over several minutes. The product does not contain a preservative and should be used within three hours of reconstitution.

Clinical Usage

BeneFix® is indicated for the control and prevention of hemorrhagic episodes in patients with hemophilia B, including the control and prevention of bleeding in surgical settings.

Following an IV dose of 50 IU/kg over ten minutes in 36 patients, the mean increase in Factor IX activity was 0.8±0.2 IU/dl per IU/kg infused. The mean biological half-life was 19.4±5.4 h. The *in vivo* recovery using BeneFix® was 28% less than the recovery using highly purified plasma-derived Factor IX, whereas there was no difference in the biological half-life (White *et al.*, 1998). Factor IX clotting activity are highly correlated ($r = 0.97$) with plasma concentrations of recombinant Factor IX (White *et al.*, 1998).

The dosage and duration of treatment with BeneFix® depends on the severity of Factor IX deficiency, the location and extent of bleeding, the clinical condition, patient age and the desired recovery in Factor IX. A guide to the dose of BeneFix® is provided by the following empirical finding that one International Unit (IU) of Factor IX is expected, on average, to increase the circulating level of Factor IX by 0.8±0.2 IU/dL (range 0.4–1.4) per IU/kg infused:

Factor IX Dosage Required (IU) = Body Wt (kg) × Desired Increase in Factor IX (%) × 1.2 IU/kg %. The amount of Factor IX to be infused, as well as the frequency of infusion, will vary with each patient. Close monitoring of plasma Factor IX activity should be performed, as should the calculation of recovery and half-life, as clinically indicated, in order to adjust doses as appropriate. Higher doses of Factor IX may be necessary in patients with inhibitors. If the expected levels of Factor IX are not attained, or if bleeding is not controlled, biological testing may be merited to determine if Factor IX inhibitors are present.

SAFETY CONCERNS

Since BeneFix® is produced in a CHO cell line, it may be contraindicated in patients with known history of hypersensitivity to hamster protein and other constituents in the preparation. ■

Further Reading

- **Lynch TJ**. (2000) Biotechnology: alternatives to human plasma-derived therapeutic proteins Baillieres Best Pract Res Clin Haematol 13:669–688.
- **Shord SS, Lindley CM.** (2000) Coagulation products and their uses. Am J Health Syst Pharm 57:1403–1417.

References

- **Abildgaard CF, Simone JV, Corrigan JJ, Seeler RA, Edelstein G, Vanderheiden J, Schulman I.** (1966). Treatment of hemophilia with glycine-precipitated Factor VIII. N Eng J Med, 275, 471–475.
- **Antorakis SE, Youssoufian H, Kazazian HH Jr.** (1987). Molecular genetics of hemophilia A in man (Factor VIII deficiency). Mol Biol Med, 4, 81–94.
- **Brinkhous KM, Sigman JL, Read MS, Stewart PF, McCarthy KP, Timony GA, Leppanen SD, Rup BJ, Keith JC, Garzone PD, Schaub RG.** (1996). Recombinant human factor IX: Replacement therapy, prophylaxis, and pharmacokinetics in canine hemophilia B. Blood 88, 2603–2610.
- **Cooper HA, Hoots WK, Shapiro A.** (1997). Comparison of two doses of recombinant factor VIIa (rFVIIa) for producing hemostasis during and after surgery in patients (PTS) with hemophilia A or B and inhibitors and PTS with acquired inhibitors. Thromb Haemostas, (Suppl), 167.
- **Eaton D, Rodriguez H, Vehar GA.** (1986). Proteolytic processing of human factor VIII. Correlation of specific cleavages by thrombin, factor Xa, and activated protein C with activation and inactivation of factor VIII coagulant activity. Biochemistry, 25, 505–512.
- **Eaton DL, Hass PE, Riddle L, Mather J, Weibe M, Gregory T, Vehar GA** (1987). Characterization of recombinant human Factor VIII. J Biol Chem, 262, 3285–3290.
- **Ferranti TJ, Misra BR, Schaub RG *et al.*** (1995). Recombinant human factor IX has low thrombogenicity in the Wessler stasis mode. Thromb Haemost 73, 1014.
- **Harrison JF, Bloom AL, Abildgaard CF.** (1991). The pharmacokinetics of recombinant Factor VIII. The rFactor VII Clinical Trial Group. Semin Hematol, 28 (suppl 1), 29–35.
- **Hedner U** (1996). Dosing and monitoring NovoSeven® treatment. Haemostasis 216(suppl 1), 102–108.
- **Hironaka T, Furukawa K, Esmon PC, Fournel MA, Sawada S, Kato M, Minaga T, Kobata A.** (1992). Comparative study of the sugar chains of factor VIII purified from human plasma and from the culture media of recombinant baby hamster kidney cells. J Biol Chem, 267, 8012–8020.
- **Hoyer LW.** (1981). The Factor VIII complex: Structure and function. Blood, 58, 1–13.
- **Jackson CM, Nemerson Y.** (1980). Blood coagulation. Ann Rev Biochem, 49, 767–811.
- **Keith JC, Ferranti, Misra B, Fredrick T, Rup B, McCarthy K, Faulkner R, Bush I, Schaub RG.** (1995). Evaluation of recombinant human factor IX: pharmacokinetic studies in the rat and dog. Thromb Haemost, 73, 101–105.
- **Key NS** (1997). Efficacy of recombinant factor VIIa (rFVIIa) when administered in the home to control joint muscle and mucocutaneous bleeds in hemophiliacs with inhibitors. Thromb Haemostas, (Suppl), 51.
- **Lindley CM, Sawyer WT, Macik G, Lusher JM, Harrison JF, Baird-Cox K, Birch K, Glazer S, Roberts HR.** (1994). Pharmacokinetics and pharmacodynamics of recombinant factor VIIa. Clin Pharmacol Ther 55, 638–648.
- **Lusher JM, Shapiro SS, Palascak JE, Rao AV, Levine PH, Blatt PM.** (1980). Efficacy of prothrombin-complex concentrates in hemophiliacs with antibodies to factor VIII. N Engl J Med.303, 421–425.
- **Lusher JM, Arkin S, Abildgaard CF, Schwartz RS, and the Kogenate previously untreated patient study group.** (1993). Recombinant Factor VIII for the treatment of previously untreated patients with hemophilia A. N Eng J Med, 328, 453–459.
- **Lusher J, Ingerslev J, Roberts H, Hedner U.** (1998). Clinical experience with recombinant factor VIIa. Blood Coag Fibrinolysis, 9, 119–128.
- **Macik BG, Lindley CM, Lusher J *et al.*** (1993). Safety and initial clinical efficacy of three dose levels of recombinant activated factor VII (rFVIIa): results of a Phase I study. Transfusion, 33, 878.
- **McCarthy KP, Timony GA, DeCoste MT, *et al.*** (1995). Pharmacokinetics of recombinant factor IX in beagle dogs. Thromb Haemost 73, 1016.
- **McCarthy KP, Brinkhous KM, Stewart PF, *et al.*** (1997). The pharmacokinetics of fully µ-carboxylated factor IX and factor IX lacking µ-carboxylation at Glu-40 are similar in the hemophilia

beagle dog. XVI Congress of the International Society of Thrombosis and Haemostasis. June 8–10, Florence, Italy.

- **McMillan CW, Shapiro SS, Whitehurst D, Hoyer LW, Rao AV, Lazerson J.** (1988). The natural history of factor VIII:C inhibitors in patients with hemophilia A: a natural cooperative study. II. Observations on the initial development of factor VIII:C inhibitor. Blood, 71, 344–348.
- **Morfini M, Longo G, Messori A, Lee M, White G, Mannucci P, and the Recombinate Study Group.** (1992). Pharmacokinetic properties of recombinant factor VIII compared with a monoclonally purified concentrate (Hemofil® M). Thromb Haemostas, 68, 433–435.
- **Roddie PH, Ludlam CA** (1997). Recombinant coagulation factors. Blood Reviews 11, 169–177.
- **Schaub R, Garzone P, Bouchard P, Rup B, Keith J, Brinkhous K, Larsen G.** (1998). Preclinical studies of recombinant factor IX. Semin Hematol, 2 (suppl 2), 28–32.
- **Schwartz RS, Abildgaard CF, Aledort LM, *et al.*** (1990). Human recombinant DNA-derived antihemophilic factor (Factor VIII) in the treatment of hemophilia A. N Engl J Med, 323, 1800–1805.
- **Thim L, Bjoern S, Christensen M, *et al.*** (1988). Amino acid sequence and posttranslational modifications of human factor VIIa from plasma and transfected baby hamster kidney cells. Biochemistry 27:7785–7793.
- **Vehar GA, Keyt BA, Eaton D, Rodrigues H, O'Brien DP, Rotblat F, Opperman H, Keck RG, Wood WI, Harkins RN, Tuddenham EGD, Lawn RM, Capon DJ.** (1984). Structure of human Factor VIII. Nature, 312, 337–342.
- **White G, Shapiro A, Ragni M, Garzone P, Goodfellow J, Tubridy K, Courter S.** (1998). Clinical evaluation of recombinant factor IX. Semin Hematol, 2 (suppl 2), 33–38.
- **White G, Beeb A, Nielsen B** (1997). Recombinant Factor IX. Thromb. Haemostasis 78, 261–265.

Self-Assessment Questions

Question 1: *Design a therapeutic regimen for a 30 kg patient with a laceration. Assume that the desired plasma concentration of Factor VIII is 30 IU/dL*

Question 2: *What criteria should Factor VIII dosage be based on?*

Answers

Answer 1: Dose = 30 IU/dL × 50 mL/kg (volume of distribution) × 30 kg = 450 IU.

Answer 2: Dosage should be individualized based on the needs of the patient, severity of deficiency, presence of inhibitors, and the desired increase in Factor VIII.

16 Recombinant Human Deoxyribonuclease

Melinda Marian and Dominick Sinicropi

Introduction

Deoxyribonuclease I (DNase) is a human endonuclease, normally present in saliva, urine, pancreatic secretions and blood, which catalyzes the hydrolysis of extracellular DNA into oligonucleotides. Aerosolized recombinant human DNase (rhDNase) has been developed for inhalation to assist in the treatment of pulmonary disease in patients with cystic fibrosis (CF).

Cystic fibrosis (CF) is the most common autosomal recessive, lethal disease in Caucasians and is caused by mutations of a gene that regulates the synthesis of a chloride ion transfer protein (Riordan *et al.*, 1989). Clinical manifestations of the disease include obstruction of the airways and pancreatic ducts. The abnormal ion transport has been implicated in the formation of the dehydrated, viscous mucus found in the airway secretions of CF patients. Retention of viscous purulent mucus in the airways contributes both to reduced pulmonary function and to exacerbations of infection (Boat *et al.*, 1988; Collins, 1992). A cycle of pulmonary obstruction and infection leads to progressive lung destruction and eventual death before the age of thirty for most CF patients.

Macromolecules that contribute to the physical properties of lung secretions are mucus glycoproteins, filamentous actin and DNA. Experiments in the 1950s and 1960s revealed that DNA is present in very large concentrations (3–14 mg/mL) in infected – but not in uninfected – lung secretions (Matthews *et al.*, 1963). Degenerating neutrophils that accumulate in response to infection release the high levels of extracellular DNA (Potter *et al.*, 1969). Such high concentrations of DNA make the secretions very viscous. The DNA-rich secretions also bind aminoglycoside antibiotics commonly used for treatment of pulmonary infections and may reduce their efficacy (Bataillon *et al.*, 1992).

Early *in vitro* studies in which lung secretions were incubated for several hours with partially purified bovine pancreatic DNase I showed a large reduction in viscosity (Armstrong and White, 1950). Based on these observations, bovine pancreatic DNase I (Dornavac or Pancreatic Dornase) was approved in the United States for human use in 1958. Numerous uncontrolled clinical studies in patients with pneumonia and one study in patients with cystic fibrosis suggested that bovine pancreatic DNase I was effective in reducing the viscosity of lung secretions (Lieberman, 1968). However, severe adverse reactions did occasionally occur, perhaps as a consequence of allergic reactions to a foreign protein or 'irritation' due to contaminating proteases, as up to 2% trypsin and chymotrypsin were present in the final product (Lieberman, 1962). Both bovine DNase I products were eventually withdrawn from the market.

Recombinant human deoxyribonuclease I (rhDNase) was cloned, sequenced and expressed (Shak *et al.*, 1990) to re-evaluate the potential of DNase I as a therapeutic for cystic fibrosis. *In vitro* incubation with catalytic concentrations of rhDNase reduced the viscoelasticity of purulent sputum from CF patients (Shak *et al.*, 1990). The reduction in viscoelasticity was directly related to both rhDNase concentration and to reduction in the size of the DNA in the samples. Therefore, reduction of high molecular weight DNA into smaller fragments by treatment with aerosolized rhDNase was proposed as a mechanism to reduce the mucus viscosity and improve mucus clearability from obstructed airways in patients. It was hoped that improved clearance of the purulent mucus would enhance pulmonary function and reduce recurrent exacerbations of respiratory symptoms requiring parenteral antibiotics.

Protein Chemistry and Structure

The protein chemistry of human DNases including DNase I, has been recently reviewed (Lazarus, 2002). Recombinant human DNase I is a monomeric, 260-amino acid glycoprotein produced in Chinese hamster ovary (CHO) cells (Shak *et al.*, 1990). The molecule has four cysteines and two potential N-linked glycosylation sites. The molecule has an approximate molecular weight from polyacrylamide gel electrophoresis (PAGE) of 37 kDa. The predicted molecular mass from the amino acid sequence is 29.3 kDa. The higher molecular weight and the broad band observed on PAGE gels are due to glycosylation. The primary amino acid structure (Figure 16.1) is identical to that of the native human enzyme purified from urine. DNase I is an endonuclease that cleaves double-stranded DNA, or to a much lesser degree single-stranded DNA,

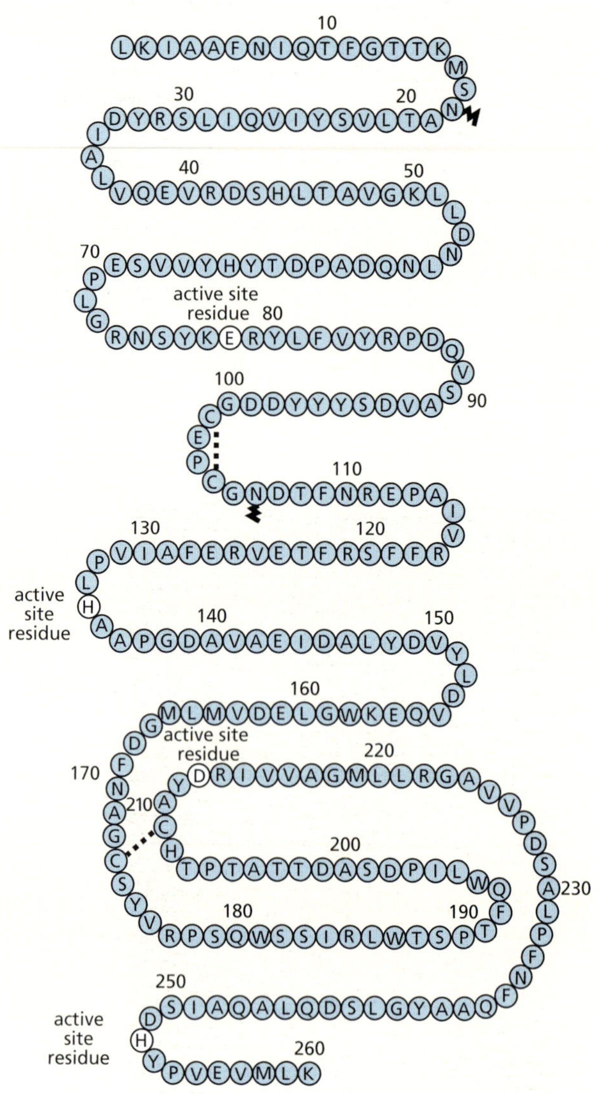

Figure 16.1. Primary amino acid sequence of rhDNase.

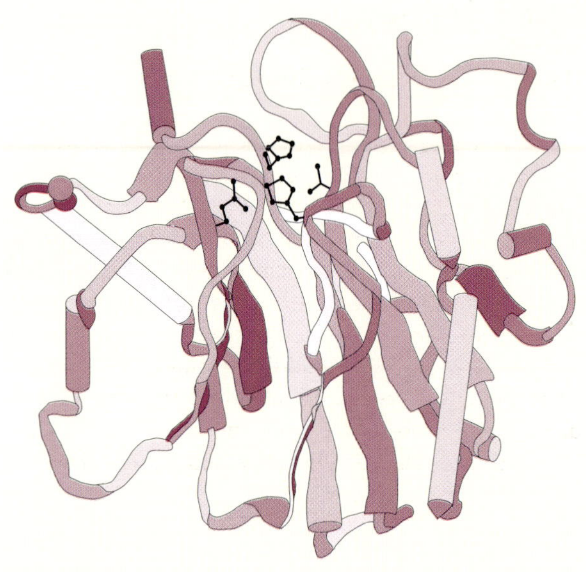

Figure 16.2 Ribbon diagram of rhDNase. The active site residues are shown in black.

into 5′-phosphate-terminated oligonucleotides. Optimal DNase enzymatic activity depends upon the presence of calcium and magnesium ions. DNase is inactivated by heat, is specifically inhibited by actin or EDTA, and shows optimal activity at neutral (5.5–7.5) pH. The active site includes two histidine residues (residues 134 and 252) and their hydrogen bond pairs (residues Glu78 and Asp 212) which are involved in the catalysis of phosphodiester bonds. These and other residues involved in the binding of structural Ca^{2+}, the coordination of divalent metal ion binding at the active site and DNA contact residues have been identified by mutational analysis (Pan *et al.*, 1998).

The X-ray crystal structure of rhDNase has been solved at 2.2 Å (Wolf *et al.*, 1995). Only minor deviations were observed between the crystal structure of rhDNase and bovine pancreatic DNase, which share a sequence identity of 78%. A ribbon diagram of rhDNase based on the crystal structure coordinates reveals a core of beta sheets surrounded by eight alpha-helices and several loops (Figure 16.2).

Several variants of rhDNase with desired properties have been engineered by site-directed mutagenesis. The methods for production of the variants and the assays to characterize them were reviewed recently (Pan *et al.*, 2001; Sinicropi and Lazarus, 2001). Actin-resistant variants were made that retain full catalytic activity but are not inhibited by monomeric actin (Ulmer *et al.*, 1996). These actin-resistant rhDNase variants were approximately 50-fold more potent than wild-type rhDNase in reducing sputum viscoelasticity and degradation of DNA in cystic fibrosis sputum. In addition, introducing positively charged residues at the DNA binding interface has altered the catalytic mechanism of rhDNase. These so-called 'hyperactive' rhDNase variants are as much as 10,000-fold more active than wild-type rhDNase and are not inhibited by physiological saline. The greater catalytic activity of the hyperactive variants appears to be due to a change in the catalytic mechanism from a "single strand nicking" activity in the case of wild-type rhDNase to a "processive nicking" activity in the hyperactive rhDNase variants (Pan and Lazarus, 1997), resulting in a higher frequency of double strand cleavages.

Pharmacology

In vitro Actions on Sputum

In vitro, rhDNase hydrolyzes the DNA in sputum of CF patients and reduces sputum viscoelasticity (Figure 16.3a, Shak *et al.*, 1990). Effects of rhDNase were initially examined using a "pourability" assay. Pourability was assessed qualitatively by inverting the tubes and observing the movement of sputum after a tap on the side of the tube. Catalytic amounts (50 μg/mL) greatly reduced the viscosity of the sputum, rapidly transforming it from a viscous gel to a flowing liquid. More than 50% of the sputum moved down the tube within 15 minutes of incubation, and all the sputum moved freely down the tube within 30 minutes. The qualitative results of the pourability assay were confirmed by quantitative measurement of viscosity using a Brookfield Cone-Plate viscometer. The reduction of viscosity by rhDNase is rhDNase concentration-dependent (Figure 16.3a) and is associated with reduction in size of sputum DNA as measured by agarose gel electrophoresis (Figure 16.3b).

An alternative mechanism for the reduction of CF sputum viscoelasticity by rhDNase was proposed by Vasconcellos *et al.* (1994). They demonstrated that filamentous actin (F-actin) contributes to the viscoelastic properties of CF

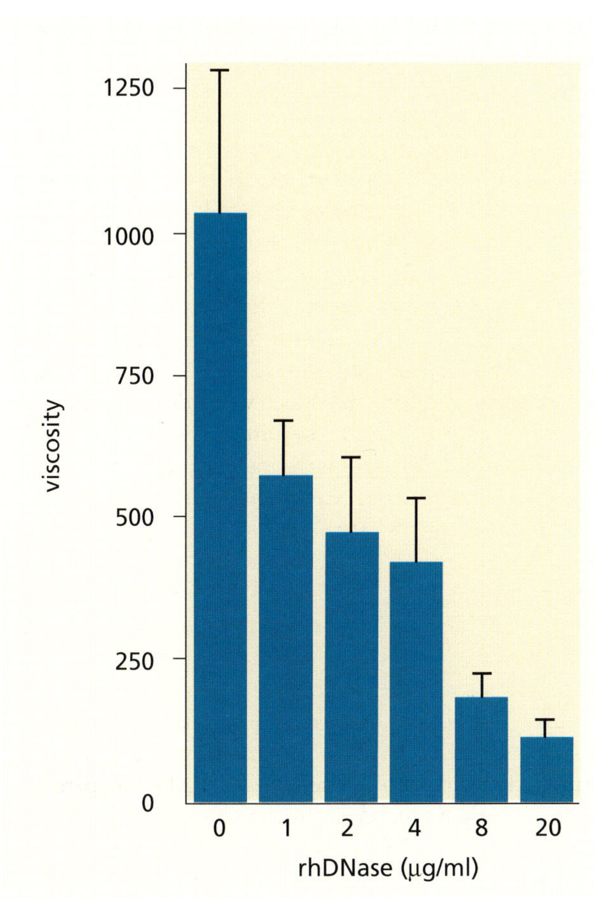

Figure 16.3a. In vitro reduction in viscosity in $10^3.kg.m^{-1}.s^{-1}$ of cystic fibrosis sputum by cone-plate viscometry. Cystic fibrosis sputum was incubated with various concentrations of rhDNase for 15 minutes at 37° C.

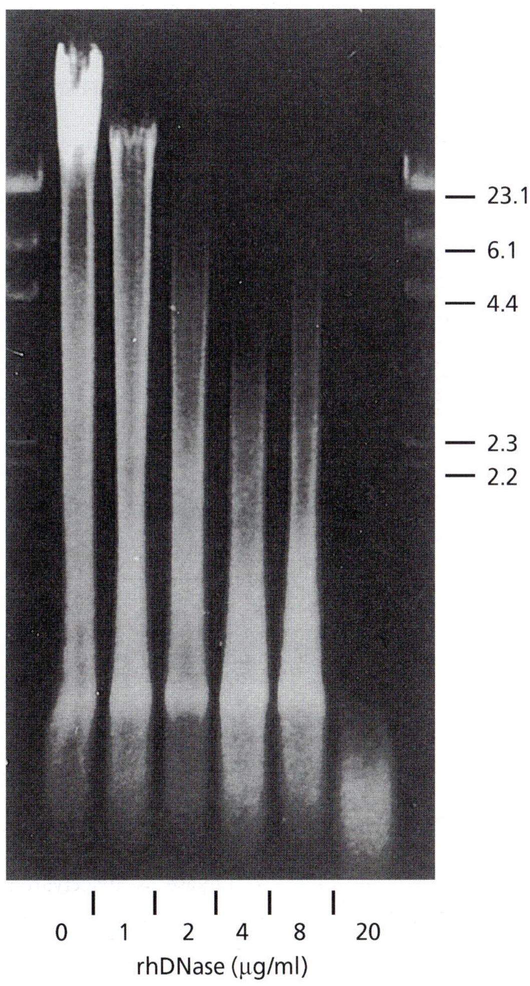

Figure 16.3b *In vitro* reduction in sputum DNA size as measured by agarose gel electrophoresis. Cystic fibrosis sputum was incubated with increasing concentrations (0–20 μg/mL) of rhDNase for 150 minutes at 37°C. Outside lanes are molecular weight standards for DNA in Kilodaltons.

sputum and that an actin-depolymerizing protein, gelsolin, can reduce sputum viscoelasticity similarly to rhDNase. F-actin is in equilibrium with its monomeric form (G-actin) which binds to rhDNase with high affinity and is a potent inhibitor of rhDNase activity. rhDNase is known to depolymerize F-actin by binding to G-actin with high affinity, shifting the equilibrium in favor of rhDNase/G-actin complexes. Vasconcellos and coworkers proposed that rhDNase might work by a gelsolin-like mechanism; that is, by depolymerization of F-actin in sputum rather than by degradation of DNA. To elucidate the mechanism by which rhDNase reduces sputum viscoelasticity, the activity of two types of rhDNase variants were compared in CF sputum (Ulmer *et al.*, 1996). Active site variants were engineered that were unable to catalyze the hydrolysis of DNA but retained the ability to bind to G-actin. Actin-resistant variants that were unable to bind to G-actin but still catalyze DNA hydrolysis were also made. The active site variants did not degrade DNA in CF sputum and did not decrease sputum viscoelasticity. Since the active site variants retained the ability to bind G-actin these results argue against depolymerization of F-actin as the mechanism by which rhDNase reduces sputum viscoelasticity. In contrast, the actin-resistant variants were more potent than wild-type rhDNase in their ability to degrade DNA and reduce sputum viscoelasticity. The increased potency of the actin-resistant variants indicated that G-actin was a significant inhibitor of wild-type rhDNase in CF sputum and confirmed that hydrolysis of DNA was the mechanism by which rhDNase decreases sputum viscoelasticity. Additional *in vitro* studies characterizing the relative potency of actin-resistant and hyperactive rhDNase variants in serum and CF sputum have been reported by Pan *et al.*, 1998b.

In vivo Actions of rhDNase on Sputum

In vivo confirmation of the proposed mechanism of action for rhDNase has been obtained from direct characterization of apparent DNA size (Figure 16.4) and measurements of enzymatic and immunoreactive (ELISA) activity of rhDNase (Figure 16.5) in sputum from cystic fibrosis patients (Sinicropi *et al.*, 1994a). Sputum samples were obtained one to six hours postdose from adult cystic fibrosis patients after inhalation of 5 to 20 mg of rhDNase. rhDNase therapy produced a sustained reduction in DNA size in recovered sputum (Figure 16.4).

Inhalation of the therapeutic dose of rhDNase produced sputum levels of rhDNase which have been shown to be effective *in vitro* (Figure 16.5) (Shak, 1995). The recovered rhDNase was also enzymatically active. Enzymatic activity was directly correlated with rhDNase concentrations in the sputum. Viscoelasticity was reduced in the recovered sputum, as well.

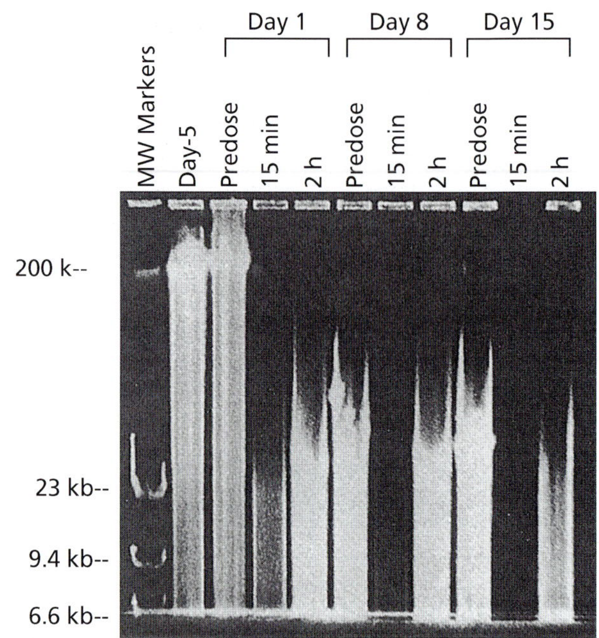

Figure 16.4 Sustained reduction in DNA length in sputum recovered from a CF patient treated with 2.5 mg rhDNase BID for up to 15 days. Samples analysed by pulsed field agarose field gel electrophoresis,

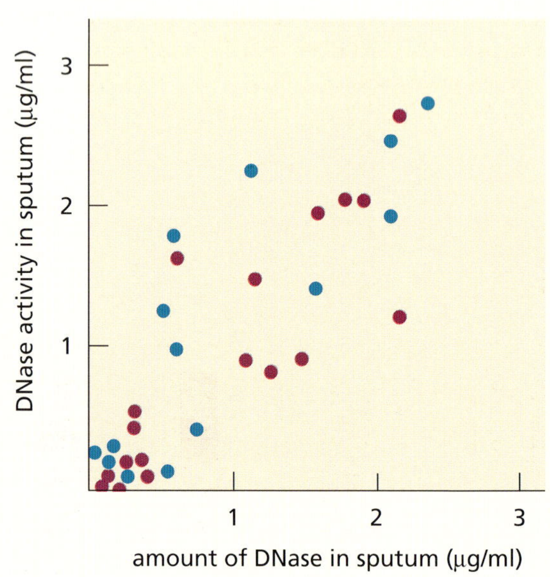

Figure 16.5. Immunoreactive concentrations and enzymatic activity of DNase in sputum following aerosol administration of either 10 mg (●) or 20 mg (●) rhDNase to patients with cystic fibrosis. Each data point is a separate sample measured in duplicate.

Pharmacokinetics and Metabolism

Non-clinical ADME data in rats and monkeys suggest minimal systemic absorption of rhDNase following aerosol inhalation of clinically-equivalent doses. rhDNase is cleared from the systemic circulation without any accumulation in tissues following acute exposure (Green, 1994). Additionally, non-clinical metabolism studies suggest that the low rhDNase concentrations present in serum following inhalation will be bound to binding proteins (Mohler *et al.*, 1993; Green, 1994). The low concentrations of endogenous DNase normally present in serum and the low concentrations of rhDNase in serum following inhalation are inactive due to the ionic composition and presence of binding proteins in serum (Prince *et al.*, 1998).

When 2.5 mg of rhDNase was administered twice daily by inhalation to 18 CF patients, mean sputum concentrations of 2 µg/mL DNase were measurable within 15 minutes after the first dose on Day 1 (Figure 16.6). Mean sputum concentrations declined to an average of 0.6 µg/mL two hours following inhalation. The peak rhDNase concentration measured two hours after inhalation on Days 8 and 15 increased to 3.0 and 3.6 µg/mL, respectively. Sputum rhDNase concentrations measured six hours after inhalation on Days 8 and 15 were similar to Day 1. Predose trough concentrations of 0.3–0.4 µg/mL rhDNase measured on Day 8 and Day 15 (sample taken approximately 12 hours after the previous dose) were, however, higher than Day 1, suggesting possible modest accumulation of rhDNase with repeated dosing. Inhalation of up to 10 mg three times daily of rhDNase by four CF patients for six consecutive days did not result in significant elevation of serum concentrations of DNase above normal endogenous levels (Aitken *et al.*, 1992; Hubbard *et al.*, 1992; Sinicropi *et al.*, 1992). After administration of up to 2.5 mg of rhDNase twice daily for six months to 321 CF patients, no accumulation of serum DNase was noted (assay limit of detection = approximately 0.5 ng DNase/mL serum).

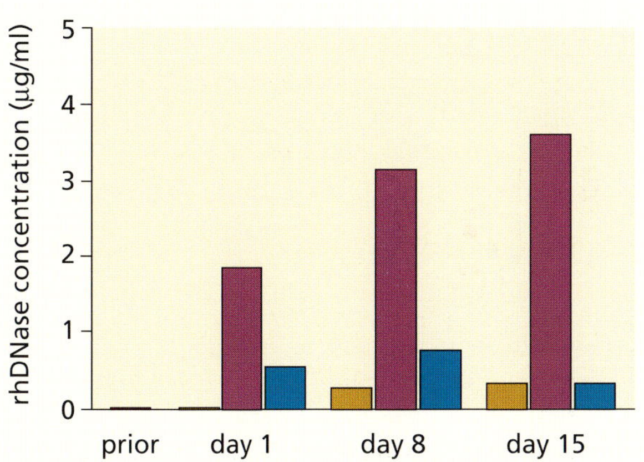

Figure 16.6. rhDNase concentration in sputum following administration of 2.5 mg of rhDNase twice daily by inhalation to CF patients. Mean ±SD. N = 18.

Protein Manufacture and Formulation

Genentech's approved rhDNase product (Pulmozyme® [dornase alpha]) is a sterile, clear, colorless aqueous solution containing 1.0 mg/mL dornase alpha, 0.15 mg/mL calcium chloride dihydrate and 8.77 mg/mL sodium chloride. The solution contains no preservative and has a nominal pH of 6.3. Pulmozyme® is administered by the inhalation of an aerosol mist produced by a compressed air-driven nebulizer system. Pulmozyme® is supplied as single-use ampoules, which deliver 2.5 mL of solution to the nebulizer.

The choice of formulation components was determined by a need to provide one to two years of stability and to meet additional requirements unique to aerosol delivery. A simple colorimetric assay for rhDNase activity was used to evaluate the stability of rhDNase in various formulations (Sinicropi *et al.*, 1994b). In order to avoid adverse pulmonary reactions, such as cough or bronchoconstriction, aerosols for local pulmonary delivery should be formulated as isotonic solutions with minimal or no buffer components and should maintain pH >5.0. rhDNase has an additional requirement for calcium to be present for optimal enzymatic activity. Limiting formulation components raised concerns about pH control, since protein stability and solubility can be highly pH-dependent. Fortunately, the protein itself provided sufficient buffering capacity at 1 mg/mL to maintain pH stability over the storage life of the product.

The droplet or particle size of an aerosol is also important in defining the site of deposition of the drug in the patient's airways (Gonda, 1990). A distribution of particle or droplet size of 1–6 µm was determined to be optimal for the uniform deposition of rhDNase in the airways (Cipolla *et al.*, 1994). Jet nebulizers were used since they are the simplest method of producing aerosols in the desired respirable range. However, recirculation of protein solutions under high shear rates in the nebulizer bowl presented risks to the integrity of the protein molecule. rhDNase survived recirculation and high shear rates during the nebulization process with no apparent degradation in protein quality or enzymatic activity (Cippola *et al.*, 1994).

Approved nebulizer systems for the administration of rhDNase include the Hudson T and Marquest Acorn II used with a PulmoAide air compressor. These nebulizers produce aerosol droplets in the respirable range (1–6 µm) with a mass median aerodynamic diameter (MMAD) of 4–6 μm. Recently, Geller *et al.* (1998) postulated that the delivery of rhDNase with a device that produces smaller droplets leads to more peripheral deposition in the smaller airways and thereby improve efficacy. Results obtained in 749 CF patients with mild disease confirmed that patients randomized to the Sidestream nebulizer powered by the MobilAire Compressor (MMAD = 2.1 μm) tended to have greater improvement in pulmonary function than patients using the Hudson T nebulizer with PulmoAide Compressor (MMAD = 4.9 μm). These results indicate that the efficacy of rhDNase is dependent, in part, on the physical properties of the aerosol produced by the delivery system.

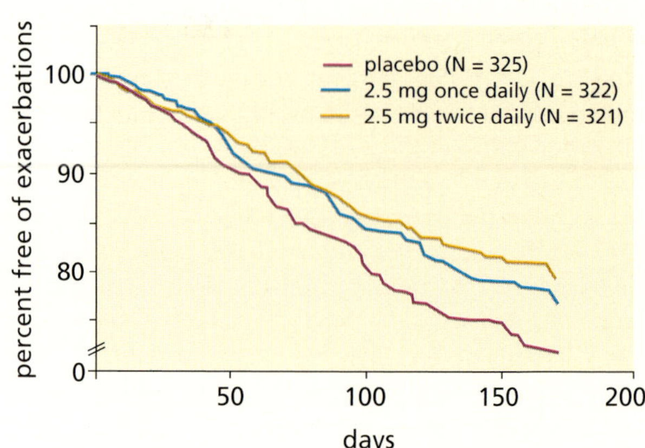

Figure 16.7. Proportion of patients free of exacerbations of respiratory symptoms requiring parenteral antibiotic therapy from a 24-week study.

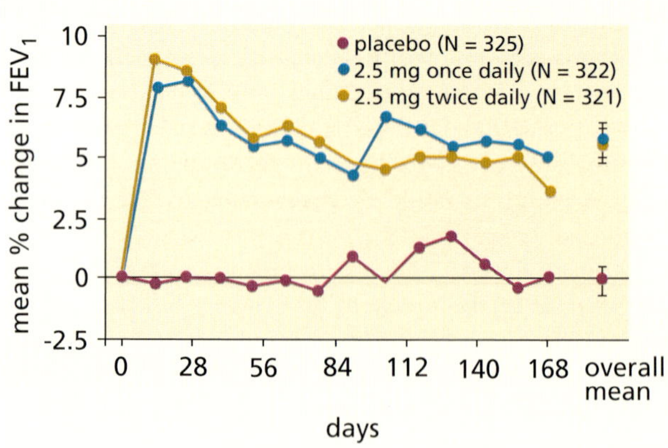

Figure 16.8. Mean percent change in FEV1 from baseline through a 24-week study.

Clinical Usage

Indication and Clinical Dosage

rhDNase (Pulmozyme®) is currently approved for use in cystic fibrosis patients, in conjunction with standard therapies, to reduce the frequency of respiratory infections requiring parenteral antibiotics and to improve pulmonary function. The recommended dose for use in most cystic fibrosis patients is one 2.5 mg dose inhaled daily using a tested, recommended nebulizer.

Clinical Experience

Clinical usage and therapeutic potential of rhDNase is summarized in reviews by Fuchs *et al.* (1994) and Shak (1995).

CYSTIC FIBROSIS

rhDNase has been evaluated in a large, randomized, placebo-controlled trial of clinically stable CF patients, 5 years of age or older, with baseline forced vital capacity (FVC) greater than or equal to 40% of predicted (Fuchs *et al.*, 1994). All patients were receiving additional standard therapies for CF. Patients were treated with placebo, 2.5 mg of rhDNase once or twice a day for six months. When compared to placebo, both once daily and twice daily doses of rhDNase resulted in a 28–37% reduction in respiratory tract infections requiring use of parenteral antibiotics (Figure 16.7). Within eight days of the start of treatment with rhDNase, mean forced expiratory volume in one second (FEV_1) increased 7.9% in patients treated once a day and 9.0% in those treated twice a day compared to the baseline values. The mean FEV_1 observed during long-term therapy increased 5.8% from baseline at the 2.5 mg daily dose level and 5.6% from baseline at the 2.5 mg twice daily dose level (Figure 16.8). The risk of respiratory tract infection was reduced even in patients whose pulmonary function (FEV_1) was not improved. This finding is thought to result from improved clearance of mucus from the small airways in the lung which may have little effect on FEV_1 or FVC, but may significantly reduce the risk of exacerbations of infection (Shak, 1995). The administration of rhDNase also lessened shortness of breath, increased the general perception of well-being, and reduced the severity of other cystic fibrosis-related symptoms.

OTHER STUDIES

rhDNase did not produce a pulmonary function benefit in short-term usage in the most severely ill CF patients (FVC less than 40% of predicted) (Shah *et al.*, 1995). These patients with end-stage lung disease represent approximately 7% of the CF population. Many are being prepared for lung transplantation but die while still awaiting an organ due to the shortage of donors. Studies are in progress to assess the impact of chronic usage on pulmonary function and infection risk in this population.

RhDNase therapy may provide clinical benefit for young CF patients with mild disease by slowing progression of the disease. Therefore, a study was done to investigate the safety and deposition of rhDNase in the airways of CF patients < 5 years old (3 months – 5 years) compared with patients 5–10 years of age (Wagener *et al.*, 1998). After two weeks of daily administration of 2.5 mg rhDNase, comparable levels of rhDNase were deposited in the lower airways of both age groups. Moreover, rhDNase was well-tolerated in the younger age group with an adverse event frequency similar to that in the older age group.

Clinical trials have indicated that rhDNase therapy can be continued or initiated during an acute respiratory exacerbation (Wilmott *et al.*, 1993). Short-term dose ranging studies demonstrated that doses in excess of 2.5 mg twice daily did not provide further improvement in FEV_1 (Hubbard *et al.*, 1992; Aiken *et al.*, 1992; Ramsey *et al.*, 1993). Patients who have received drug on a cyclical regimen (i.e. administration of rhDNase 10 mg twice daily for 14 days, followed by a 14-day washout period) showed rapid improvement in FEV_1 with the initiation of each cycle and a return to baseline with each rhDNase withdrawal (Eisenberg *et al.*, 1997).

Other agents for CF therapy, such as N-acetylcysteine which acts on mucus glycoproteins, amiloride which blocks sodium absorption in airway epithelial cells, anti-*Pseudomonas* antibodies, anti-proteases, gelsolin, ibuprofen and gene therapy are under active investigation (Rosenstein, 1994). Further clinical studies are necessary to determine whether use of these agents in combination with rhDNase and/or other standard CF therapies will result in significant improvements in the management of CF. Recently, the intermittent administration of aerosolized tobramycin was approved for use in CF patients with or without concomitant use of rhDNase (Ramsey *et al.*, 1999). Aerosolized tobramycin was well tolerated, improved pulmonary function and decreased the density of *P. aeruginosa* in sputum. In combination with rhDNase, a larger treatment effect was noted but did not reach statistical significance. No differences in safety profile were observed following aerosolized tobramycin in patients that did or did not use rhDNase.

SYSTEMIC LUPUS ERYTHEMATOSUS

Complexes of DNA with antibodies to DNA have been implicated as a causative factor underlying the clinical pathogenesis of systemic lupus erythematosus (SLE) (Koffler *et al.*, 1973; Lefkowith *et al.*, 1996). The observation that DNase-deficient mice develop a lupus-like syndrome supports the hypothesis that a reduction in serum DNase may be a factor in the initiation of SLE (Napirei *et al.*, 2000). Therefore, systemic administration of rhDNase may be effective in the treatment of SLE (Lachmann, 1996; Macanovic *et al.*, 1996). Degradation of extracellular DNA or the DNA component of DNA/anti-DNA immune complexes may be of clinical benefit in SLE by decreasing inflammation in tissues or by reducing the antigen load leading to a decrease in production of antibodies to DNA. A recent clinical study demonstrated that that systemic administration of rhDNase was well tolerated and did not induce the production of antibodies to rhDNase (Davis *et al.*, 1999). However, serum concentrations of rhDNase were insufficient for catalytic activity of rhDNase in serum (Prince *et al.*, 1998). Therefore, additional studies utilizing higher doses or more potent rhDNase variants are needed to determine whether systemic administration of rhDNase may have a clinical benefit in SLE.

Safety Concerns

The administration of rhDNase has not been associated with an increase in major adverse events. Most adverse events were not more common with rhDNase than with placebo treatment and probably reflect complications related to the underlying lung disease. Most events associated with dosing were mild, transient in nature, and did not require alterations in dosing. Observed symptoms included hoarseness, pharyngitis, laryngitis, rash, chest pain, and conjunctivitis. Within all the studies a small percentage (average 2–4%) of patients treated with rhDNase developed serum antibodies to rhDNase. None of these patients developed anaphylaxis, and the clinical significance of serum antibodies to rhDNase in unknown.

Summary

DNase, a human enzyme responsible for the digestion of extracellular DNA, has been developed as a safe and effective adjunctive agent in the treatment of pulmonary disease in cystic fibrosis patients. rhDNase reduced the viscoelasticity and improved the transport properties of viscous mucus both *in vitro* and *in vivo*. Inhalation of aerosols of rhDNase reduced the risk of infections requiring antibiotics, improved pulmonary function and improved the well-being of CF patients with mild to moderate disease. Continuing studies will assess the usefulness of rhDNase in early-stage CF pulmonary disease and other disease states.

Acknowledgments

This review benefited greatly from the contributions and comments of DNase project team members at Genentech, notably Robert A Lazarus, and Robert Fick. Charles Eigenbrot is thanked for the ribbon diagram of rhDNase. ■

Further Reading

- **Boat TF.** (1988). Cystic fibrosis. In *Textbook of respiratory medicine 1*, edited by J.F. Murray and J.A. Nadel, pp. 1126–1152. WB Saunders: Philadelphia.
- **Cipolla DC, Gonda I, Meserve KC, Weck S and Shire SJ.** (1994). Formulation and aerosol delivery of recombinant deoxyribonucleic acid derived human deoxyribonuclease I. In *Formulation and Delivery of Protein and Peptides*, ACS Symposium Series 567, edited by J.L. Cleland and R. Langer, pp. 322–342. American Chemical Society: Washington, DC.
- **Collins FS.** (1992). Cystic fibrosis: molecular biology and therapeutic implications. *Science*, 256, 774–779.
- **Fuchs HJ, Borowitz DS, Christiansen DH, Morris EM, Nash ML, Ramsey BW, *et al*.** (1994). Effect of aerosolized recombinant human DNase on exacerbations of respiratory symptoms and on pulmonary function in patients with cystic fibrosis. *New Engl. J. Med.*, 331, 637–642.
- **Lazarus RA.** (2002). Human Deoxyribonucleases. In *Wiley Encyclopedia of Molecular Medicine*, edited by T.E. Creighton, pp. 1025–1028. New York: John Wiley and Sons.
- **Rosenstein BJ**. (1994). Cystic fibrosis in the year 2000. *Semin. Respir.Crit. Care Med.*, 15, 446–451.
- **Shak S**. (1995). Aerosolized recombinant human DNase I for the treatment of cystic fibrosis. *Chest*, 107(suppl), 65s–70s.
- **Shak S, Capon DJ, Helmiss R, Marsters SA and Baker CL.** (1990). Recombinant human DNase I reduces the viscosity of cystic fibrosis sputum. *Proc. Natl. Acad. Sci. USA*, 87, 9188–9192.

References

- **Aiken ML, Burke W, McDonald G, Shak S, Montgomery AB and Smith A**. (1992). Recombinant human DNase inhalation in normal subjects and patients with cystic fibrosis. *J. Am. Med. Assoc.*, 267(14), 1947–1951.
- **Armstrong JB and White JC**. (1950). Liquifaction of viscous purulent exudates by deoxyribonuclease. *Lancet*, 2, 739–742.
- **Bataillon V, Lhermitte M, Lafitte J-J, Pommery J and Roussel P.** (1992). The binding of amikacin to macromolecules from the sputum of patients suffering from respiratory diseases. *J. Antimicrob. Chemother.*, 29, 499–508.
- **Davis JC Jr, Manzi S, Yarboro C, Rairie J, Mcinnes I, Averthelyi D *et al*.** (1999). Recombinant human DNase I (rhDNase) in patients with lupus nephritis. *Lupus*, 8, 68–76.
- **Eisenberg JD, Aitken ML, Dorkin HL, Harwood IR, Ramsey BW, Schidlow DV, *et al*.** (1997). Safety of repeated intermittent courses of aerosolized recombinant human deoxyribonuclease in patients with cystic fibrosis. J Ped, 131, 118–124.
- **Geller DE, Eigen H, Fiel SB, Clark A, Lamarre AP, Johnson CA, *et al*.** (1998). Effect of smaller droplet size of Dornase Alfa on lung function in mild cystic fibrosis. *Ped Pulmonol*, 25, 83–87.
- **Gonda I**. (1990). A semi-empirical model of aerosol deposition in the human respiratory tract. *J. Pharm. Pharmacol.*, 33, 692–696.
- **Green JD.** (1994). Pharmaco-toxicological expert report, Pulmozyme™, rhDNase, Genentech, Inc., *Human & Expt. Tox.*, 13, Suppl 1, S1–S42.
- **Hubbard RC, McElvaney NG, Birrer P, Shak S, Robinson WW, Jolley C, *et al*.** (1992). A preliminary study of aerosolized recombinant human deoxyribonuclease I in the treatment of cystic fibrosis. *New Engl. J. Med.*, 326, 812–815.
- **Koffler D, Agnello V and Kunkel HG.** (1973). Polynucleotide immune complexes in serum and glomeruli of patients with systemic lupus erythematosus. *Am J Pathol*, 74, 109–124.
- **Lachmann PJ.** (1996). The in vivo destruction of antigen – a tool for probing and modulating an autoimmune response. *Clin Exp Immunol*,106, 187–189.
- **Lefkowith JB and Gilkeson GS.** (1996). Nephritogenic autoantibodies in lupus: current concepts and continuing controversies. *Arthritis Rheum*, 39, 894–903.
- **Lieberman J.** (1968). Dornase aerosol effect on sputum viscosity in cases of cystic fibrosis. *J. Am. Med. Assoc.*, 205, 312–313.
- **Lieberman J.** (1962). Enzymatic dissolution of pulmonary secretions. *Am. J. Dis. Child*, 104, 3342–348.
- **Macanovic M, Sinicropi D, Shak S, Baughman S, Thiru S and Lachmann PJ.** (1996). The treatment of systemic lupus erythematosus (SLE) in NZB/W F1 hybrid mice; studies with recombinant murine DNase and with dexamethasone. *Clin Exp Immunol*, 106, 243–252.
- **Matthews LW, Spector S, Lemm J and Potter JL.** (1963). The over-all chemical composition of pulmonary secretions from patients with cystic fibrosis, bronchiectatis and laryngectomy. *Am. Rev. Respir. Dis.*, 88, 119–204.
- **Mohler M, Cook J, Lewis D, Moore J, Sinicropi D, Championsmith A *et al*.** (1993). Altered pharmacokinetics of recombinant human deoxyribonuclease in rats due to the presence of a binding protein. *Drug Met. Disp.*, 21, 71–75.
- **Napirei M, Karsunky H, Zevnik B, Stephan H, Mannherz HG and Moroy T.** (2000). Features of systemic lupus erythematosus in DNase 1-deficient mice. *Nature Gen*, 25, 177–181.

- **Pan CQ and Lazarus RA.** (1997). Engineering hyperactive variants of human deoxyribonuclease I by altering its functional mechanism. *Biochem*, 36, 6624–6632.
- **Pan CQ, Ulme JS, Herzka A and Lazarus RA.** (1998a). Mutational analysis of human DNase I at the DNA binding interface: Implications for DNA recognition, catalysis and metal ion dependence. *Prot Sci*, 7, 628–636.
- **Pan CQ, Dodge TH, Baker DL, Prince WS, Sinicropi DV and Lazarus RA.** (1998b) Improved potency of hyperactive and actin-resistant human DNase I variants for treatment of cystic fibrosis and systemic lupus erythematosus. *J Biol Chem*, 273, 18374–18381.
- **Pan CQ, Sinicropi DV and Lazarus RA.** (2001) Engineered properties and assays for human DNase I mutants. In *Nuclease Methods and Protocols, Methods in Molecular Biology Vol. 160*, edited by C.H. Schein, pp. 309–32. Humana Press: Totowa.
- **Potter JL, Spector S, Matthews LW and Lemm J.** (1969). Studies on pulmonary secretions. 3. The nucleic acids in whole pulmonary secretions from patients with cystic fibrosis bronchiectasis and laryngectomy. *Am. Rev. Resp. Dis.*, 99, 909–915.
- **Prince WS, Baker DL, Dodge AH, Ahmed AE, Chestnut RW and Sinicropi DV.** (1998). Pharmacodynamics of recombinant human DNase I in serum. *Clin Exp Immunol*, 113, 289–296.
- **Ramsey BW, Astley SJ, Aitken ML, Burke W, Colin AA, Dorkin HL, *et al.*** (1993). Efficacy and safety of short-term administration of aerosolized recombinant human deoxyribonuclease in patients with cystic fibrosis. *Am. Rev. Resp. Dis.*, 148, 145–151.
- **Ramsey BW, Pepe MS, Quan JM, Otto KL, Montgomery AB and Williams-Warren J *et al.*** (1999). Intermittent administration of inhaled tobramycin in patients with cystic fibrosis. *N Eng J Med*, 340, 23–30.
- **Riordan JR, Rommens JM, Kerem B, Alon N, Rozmahel R, Grzelczak Z, *et al.*** (1989). Identification of the cystic fibrosis gene: genetic analysis. *Science*, 245, 1073–1080.
- **Shah PL, Bush A, Canny GJ, Colin AA, Fuchs HJ, Geddes DM *et al.*** (1995). Recombinant human DNase I in cystic fibrosis patients with severe pulmonary disease: a short-term, double-blind study followed by six months of open-label treatment. *Eur. Respir. J.*, 8, 954–958.
- **Sinicropi D, Williams R, Baker D, Fuchs H and Shak S.** (1992). Endogenous serum DNase levels in normal and cystic fibrosis subjects determined by a sensitive fluorimetric ELISA. *Pediatr. Pulmonol.*, Suppl 8, 302.
- **Sinicropi DV, Williams M, Prince WS, Lofgren JA, Lucas M, DeVault A *et al.*** (1994a). Sputum pharmacodynamics and pharmacokinetics of recombinant human DNase I in cystic fibrosis. *Am. J. Respir. Crit. Care Med.*, 149, suppl 4, A671.
- **Sinicropi D, Baker DL, Prince WS, Shiffer K and Shak S**. (1994b). Colorimetric determination of DNase I activity with a DNA-methyl green substrate. *Anal Biochem*, 222, 351–358.
- **Sinicropi DV and Lazarus RA**. (2001) Assays for human DNase I activity in biological matrices. In *Nuclease Methods and Protocols, Methods in Molecular Biology Vol. 160*, edited by C.H. Schein, pp. 323–333. Humana Press: Totowa.
- **Ulmer JS, Herzka A, Toy KJ, Baker DL, Dodge AH, Sinicropi D *et al.*** (1996). Engineering actin-resistant human DNase I for treatment of cystic fibrosis. *Proc Natl Acad Sci USA*, 93, 8225–8229.
- **Vasconcellos CA, Allen PG, Wohl ME, Drazen JM, Janmey PA and Stossel TP.** (1994). Reduction in viscosity of cystic fibrosis sputum in vitro by gelsolin. *Science*, 263, 969–971.
- **Wagener JS, Rock MJ, McCubbin MM, Hamilton SD, Johnson CA and Ahrens RC.** (1998). Aerosol delivery and safety of recombinant human deoxyribonuclease in young children with cystic fibrosis: A bronchoscopic study. *J Pediatr*, 133, 486–491.
- **Wilmott R, Amin RS, Collin A. *et al.*** (1993). A phase II, double-blind, multicenter study of the safety and efficacy of aerosolized recombinant human DNase I (rhDNase) in hospitalized patients with CF experiencing acute pulmonary exacerbations. *Pediatr. Pulmonol.*, Suppl 9, 154.
- **Wolf E, Frenz J and Suck D.** (1995). Structure of human pancreatic DNase I at 2.2 Å resolution. *Protein Eng.*, 8 (Suppl), 79.

Self-Assessment Questions

Question 1: *Why would reduction in the apparent size of DNA molecules in mucus improve pulmonary function and/or reduce the risk of infections?*

Question 2: *What factors must be considered when choosing formulation components for an aerosolized protein?*

Answers

Answer 1: Reduction in DNA size reduces the viscoelasticity of mucus and improves the clearability of the mucus from the airways. Clearance of the DNA-rich mucus from the airways may also improve the efficacy of antibiotics typically administered for chronic lung infections since the aminoglycoside antibiotics commonly used have been shown to bind to DNA.

Answer 2: The formulation should be isotonic, have minimal additives (buffer agents, surfactants, etc) and maintain a pH >5.0. Stability of the protein and development of possible protein aggregates should be carefully monitored if using minimal buffering agents and surfactants.

17 Follicle-Stimulating Hormone

Tom Sam and Marjo Peters

Introduction

About 15% of all couples experience infertility at some time during their reproductive lives. Increasingly, infertility can be treated by the use of assisted reproductive technologies, such as *in vitro* fertilization (IVF), gamete intra-fallopian transfer (GIFT) and intracytoplasmic sperm injection (ICSI). Gonadotropin treatment to increase the number of oocytes is a common element of these programs. A major cause for female infertility is chronic anovulation. Patients suffering from this condition are also treated with gonadotropins with the aim to achieve monofollicular development.

Gonadotropin preparations for infertility treatment are traditionally derived from postmenopausal urine. The urinary preparations contain Follicle-Stimulating Hormone (FSH), but are typically less than 5% pure. The preparations also contain Luteinizing Hormone (LH) as a contaminant. Recombinant DNA technology allows the reproducible manufacturing of FSH preparations of high purity and specific activity, devoid of urinary contaminants. Recombinant FSH is produced using a Chinese Hamster Ovary (CHO) cell line, transfected with the genes encoding for the two human FSH subunits (van Wezenbeek, 1990; Howles, 1996). The isolation procedures render a product of high purity (at least 97%), devoid of LH activity and very similar to natural FSH.

Currently, there are two clinically approved recombinant FSH-containing drug products on the market. These are Gonal-F®, manufactured by Serono/S.A., and Puregon®, with the brand name of Follistim® in the USA, manufactured by NV Organon. Regulatory authorities have issued two distinct International Non-proprietary Names for the two corresponding recombinant FSH drug substances, i.e. follitropin α (Gonal-F®) and follitropin β (Puregon®/Follistim®). Thus, the two products should be considered similar, but not identical preparations containing distinct active ingredients.

Biological Role

The primary function of the glycoprotein hormone FSH in the female is the regulation of follicle growth. FSH is produced and secreted by the anterior lobe of the pituitary, a gland at the base of the brain. Its target is the FSH receptor at the surface of the granulosa cells that surround the oocyte. FSH acts synergistically with oestrogens and LH to stimulate proliferation of these granulosa cells, which leads to follicular growth. This process explains why deficient endogenous production of FSH may cause infertility.

Chemical Description

Follicle-stimulating hormone belongs to a family of structurally related glycoproteins which includes luteinizing hormone (LH), chorionic gonadotropin (CG) and thyroid-stimulating hormone (TSH). Each hormone is a dimeric protein consisting of two non-covalently associated glycoprotein subunits, denoted α and β. The α-subunit is identical for all these gonadotropins, and it is the β-subunit that provides each hormone with its specific biological function.

The glycoprotein subunits of FSH consist of two polypeptide backbones with carbohydrate side-chains attached to the two asparagine (Asn) amino acid residues on each subunit. The oligosaccharides are attached to Asn-52 and Asn-78 on the α-subunit (92 amino acids), and to Asn-7 and Asn-24 on the β-subunit (111 amino acids). The glycoprotein FSH has a molecular mass of approximately 35 kDa. For the FSH preparation to be biologically active, the two subunits must be correctly assembled into their 3-dimensional dimeric protein structure and post-translationally modified (Figure 17.1).

Assembly and glycosylation are intracellular processes that take place in the endoplasmatic reticulum and in the Golgi apparatus. This glycosylation process leads to the formation of a population of hormone isoforms differing in their carbohydrate side-chain composition. The carbohydrate side-chains of FSH are essential for its biological activity since they 1) influence FSH receptor binding, 2) play an important role in the signal transduction into the FSH target cell and 3) affect the plasma residence time of the hormone.

Recombinant FSH contains approximately 36% carbohydrate on a mass per mass basis. The carbohydrate side-chains are composed of mannose, fucose, N-acetyl-glucosamine,

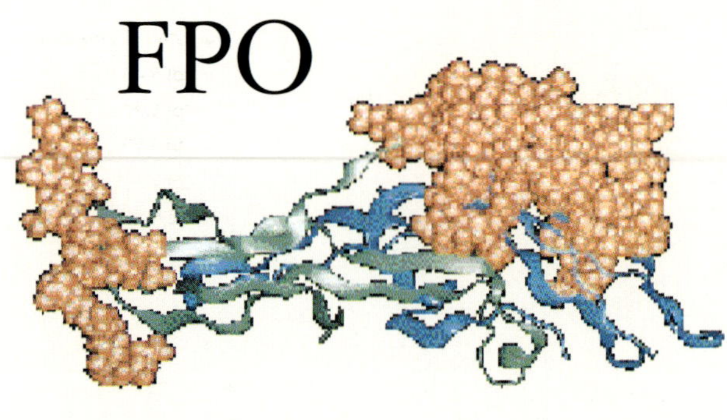

Figure 17.1. A 3-dimensional model of FSH. The ribbons represent the polypeptide backbones of the α-subunit (green ribbon) and the β-subunit (blue ribbon). The carbohydrate side chains (yellow and pink space filled globules) cover large areas of the surface of the polypeptide subunits. The sialic acid carbohydrates are depicted in pink.

galactose and sialic acid. Structure analysis by ^{1}H-NMR spectroscopy on oligosaccharides enzymatically cleaved from follitropin β, reveals minor differences with natural FSH. For instance, the bisecting GlcNAc residues are lacking in the recombinant molecule, simply because the FSH-producing CHO cells do not possess the enzymes to incorporate these residues. Furthermore, the carbohydrate side-chains of recombinant FSH exclusively contain α2-3 linked sialic acid, whereas in the natural hormone α1-6 linked sialic acid occurs, as well. All carbohydrate side-chains identified in recombinant FSH are, however, moieties normally found in other natural human glycoproteins.

Production of Recombinant FSH

The genes coding for the human FSH α-subunit and β-subunit were inserted in cloning vectors (plasmids) to enable efficient transfer into recipient cells. These vectors also contained promoters that could direct transcription of foreign genes in recipient cells. CHO cells were selected as recipient cells since they were easily transfected with foreign DNA, and are capable of synthesizing glycoproteins. Furthermore they could be grown in cell cultures on a large scale. To construct a FSH-producing cell line NV Organon, the manufacturer of Puregon®/Follistim®, used one single vector containing the coding sequences for both subunit genes (Olijve, 1996). Ares-Serono, the manufacturer of Gonal-F®, used two separate vectors, one for each subunit gene (Howles, 1996). Following transfection, a genetically stable transformant producing biologically active recombinant FSH was isolated. For the CHO cell line used for the manufacture of Puregon®/Follistim® it was shown that approximately 150–450 gene copies were present.

In order to establish a master cell bank (MCB) identical cell preparations of the selected clone are stored in individual vials and cryopreserved until needed. Subsequently a working cell bank (WCB) is established by the expansion of cells derived from a single vial of the MCB and aliquots are put in vials and cryopreserved, as well. Each time a production run is started cells from one or more vials of the WCB are cultured.

Both recombinant FSH products are isolated from cell culture supernatant. This supenatant is collected from a perfusion-type of bioreactor containing recombinant FSH-producing CHO cells grown on microcarriers. This is because CHO cells are anchorage-dependent cells, which implies that a proper surface must be provided for cell growth. The reactor is perfused with growth-promoting medium during a period that may continue for up to three months (cf. Chapter 3). The down-stream purification processes for the isolation of the two recombinant FSH products are different. For Puregon®/Follistim® a series of chromatographic steps, including anion and cation exchange chromatography, hydrophobic chromatography and size-exclusion chromatography is used. Recombinant FSH in Gonal-F® is obtained by a similar process of five chromatographic steps, but also includes an immunoaffinity step using a murine FSH-specific monoclonal antibody. In both production processes, each purification step is rigorously controlled in order to ensure the batch-to-batch consistency of the purified product.

Isohormones

Structural characteristics

As explained above, FSH exists in many distinct molecular forms (isohormones), with identical polypeptide backbones but differing in oligosaccharide structure, in particular in the degree of terminal sialylation. These isohormones can be separated by chromatofocusing or isoelectric focusing on the basis of their different isoelectric points (pI), as has been demonstrated for follotropin β (de Leeuw *et al.*, 1996, Figure 17.2). The typical pattern for FSH indicates an isohormone distribution between pI values of 6 and 4. To obtain structural information at the subunit level, the two subunits were separated by RP-HPLC and treated to release the N-linked carbohydrate side-chains. Fractions with low pI values (acidic fractions) displayed a high content of tri- and tetrasialooligosaccharides and a low content of neutral and monosialo oligosaccharides. For fractions with a high pI (basic fractions) value the reverse was found. The β-subunit carbohydrate side-chains appeared to be more heavily sialylated and branched than the α-subunit

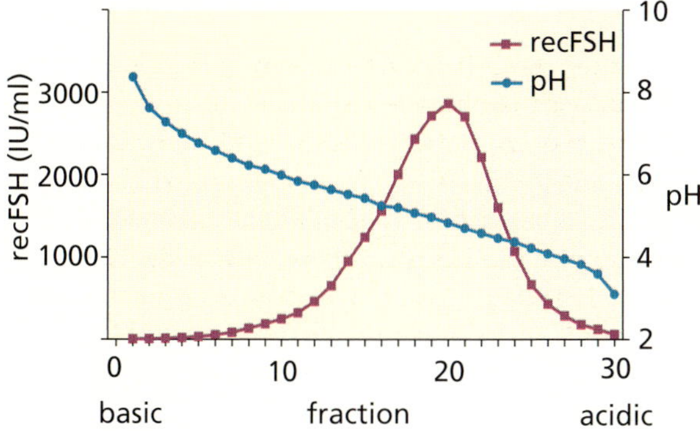

Figure 17.2. Isohormone profile of recombinant follicle stimulating hormone (follitropin beta) after preparative free flow focussing (De Leeuw et al., 1996). The FSH concentration was determined by a two-site immunoassay that is capable of quantifying the various isohormones equally well.

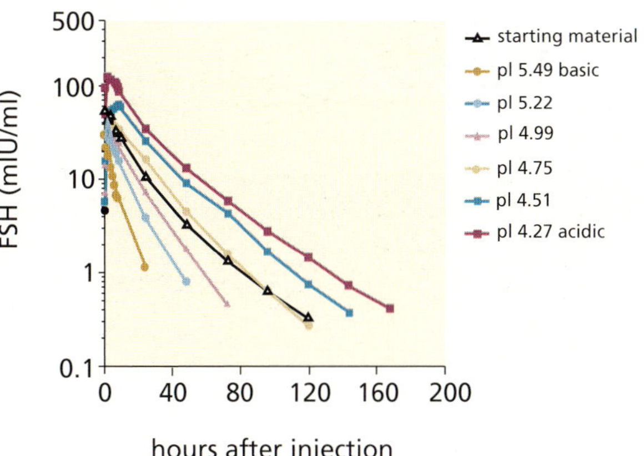

Figure 17.3. Kinetic behavior of FSH isoforms after a single intramuscular injection (20 IU/kg) in Beagle dogs.

carbohydrate side-chains. The low pI value isohormones of follitropin β have a high sialic acid/galactose ratio and are rich in tri- and tetra-antennary N-linked carbohydrate side-chains, as compared with the side-chains of the high pI value isohormones.

Biological properties of recombinant FSH isohormones

A FSH preparation can be characterized with four essentially different assays, each having its own specific merits. The immunoassay (1) determines FSH-specific structural features and provides a relative measure for the quantity of FSH. The receptor binding assay (2) provides information on the proper conformation for interaction with the FSH receptor. Receptor binding studies with calf testis membranes have shown that FSH isoform activity in follitropin β decreases when going from high to low pI isoforms. The *in vitro* bioassay (3) measures the capability of FSH to transduce signals into target cells (the intrinsic bioactivity). The *in vitro* bioactivity, assessed in the rat Sertoli cell bioassay, also decreases when going from high to low pI isoforms. The *in vivo* bioassay (4) provides the overall bioactivity of a FSH preparation. It is determined by the number of molecules, the plasma residence time, the receptor binding activity and the signal transduction. Surprisingly, in contrast to the receptor binding and *in vitro* bioassays, the *in vivo* biological activity determined in rats shows an approximate 20-fold increase between isoforms with a pI value of 5.49, as compared to those with a pI of 4.27. These results indicate that the basic isohormones exhibit the highest receptor binding and signal transduction activity, whereas the acidic isohormones are the more active forms under *in vivo* conditions.

Pharmacokinetic behavior of recombinant FSH isohormones

The pharmacokinetic behavior of follitropin β and its isohormones was investigated in Beagle dogs that were given an intramuscular bolus injection of a number of FSH isohormone fractions, each with a specific pI value. With a decrease in pI value from 5.49 (basic) to 4.27 (acidic), the AUC increased and the clearance rate decreased, each more than ten-fold (Figure 17.3). A more than two-fold difference in elimination half-life between the most acidic and the most basic FSH isohormone fraction was calculated. The absorption rate of the two most acidic isoforms was higher than the absorption rates of all other isoforms. The AUC and the clearance rate for the follitropin β preparation, being a mixture of all isohormone fractions, corresponded with the centre of the isohormone profile (Figure 17.3). In contrast, the elimination of the follitropin β preparation occurred at a rate similar to that of the most acidic fractions, indicating that the elimination rate is largely determined by the removal of the most acidic isoforms from the plasma.

Thus, for follitropin β isohormone fractions, a clear correlation exists between pI value and pharmacokinetic behavior. Increasing acidity leads to an increase in the extent of absorption and elimination half-life and to a decrease in clearance rates.

Pharmaceutical Formulations

Recombinant FSH preparations distinguish themselves by their high purity (at least 97%) e.g. from urinary FSH preparations, typically having a purity of less than 5%.

Market preparation	Freeze-dried presentation	Container	
Gonal-F® (follitropin alpha) Sereno/S.A.	powder powder powder	ampoule, vial ampoule multidose vial	75 and 150 IU 37.5 600 IU and 1200 IU
Puregon®/Follistim (follitropin beta) NV Organon	lyosphere cake solution for injection solution for injection	ampoule vial vial cartridge	50, 100 and 150 IU 75 and 150 IU 50, 75, 100, 150, 200, 225, 250 and 300 IU 300 and 600 IU

Table 17.1. The presentation forms of recombinant FSH products.

Pure proteins are, however, relatively unstable and are therefore usually lyophilized, unless some specific stabilizing measures can be taken. FSH preparations are available in different strengths and presentation forms, both as freeze-dried products (powder, cake, lyosphere) and as solutions for injection (see Table 17.1). Lyospheres are frozen drops of aqueous solution, which are freeze-dried in bulk and subsequently put in ampoules. Compared to the traditional freeze-dried cake formulation, lyospheres have the advantage of high dose uniformity, less adsorption to the glass walls of the ampoule, instantaneous dissolution, and in case of FSH, improved stability. Freeze-dried follitropin α is formulated with sucrose (bulking agent, lyoprotectant), sodium dihydrogen phosphate/disodium hydrogen phosphate, phosphoric acid and sodium hydroxide (for pH adjustment). Freeze-dried follitropin β is formulated with sucrose, sodium citrate (stabilizer), polysorbate 20 (lyoprotectant and agent to prevent adsorption losses), and hydrochloride/sodium hydroxide (for pH adjustment). The lyophilized preparations are to be reconstituted before use to obtain a ready-for-use solution for injection. In addition to the freeze-dried presentation form, a solution for injection with several strengths of follitropin β could be developed. To stabilize the solutions 0.25 mg of L-methionine had to be added. Furthermore, the solution in the cartridge contains benzyl alcohol as preservative.

The lyophilized formulations are registered in strengths from 37.5 to 1200 IU. The dosage is not fixed, but is individually titrated based on ovarian response. For the convenience of both patient and health care worker a solution presentation has been developed. The Puregon®/Follistim® solution for injection is available in vials and is very suitable for titration because of the large range of 50 to 300 IU of available strengths. A pen injector has been developed with multidose cartridges containing solution for injection, giving the patient optimal convenience.

The shelf-life of the freeze-dried recombinant FSH products is two years when stored in the containers in which they are supplied, at temperatures below 30 °C, not frozen and protected from light. The solutions for injection should be stored in the refrigerator for a maximum of three years with the container kept in the outer carton to protect the solution from light. The patient can keep the solutions at room temperature for a maximum of three months.

Clinical Aspects

Both recombinant FSH products on the market have been approved for two female indications. The first indication is anovulation (including polycystic ovarian disease) in women who are unresponsive to clomiphene citrate. The second indication is controlled ovarian hyperstimulation to induce the development of multiple follicles in medically assisted reproduction programs, such as IVF and embryo transfer. In addition, recombinant FSH may be used in men with congenital or required hypogonadotropic hypogonadism to stimulate spermatogenesis.

In anovulatory infertility in females, FSH treatment aims for the development of a single follicle, whereas IVF FSH treatment is aimed at multifollicular development. For the treatment of anovulatory patients it is recommended to start Puregon®/Follistim® treatment with 50 IU per day for 7 to 14 days and gradually increase dosing with steps of 50 IU if no sufficient response is seen. This gradual dose-increasing schedule is followed in order to prevent multifollicular development and the induction of ovarian hyperstimulation syndrome (a serious condition of unwanted hyperstimulation).

In the most commonly applied treatment regimens in IVF, endogenous gonadotropin levels are suppressed by a GnRH agonist or by the more recently approved GnRH antagonists (Cetrotide® and Orgalutran®/Antagon®). It is recommended to start Puregon® treatment with 100 – 200 IU of recombinant FSH followed by maintenance doses of 50 – 350 IU. The availability of a surplus of collected oocytes allows the replacement of two to three embryos. Similar treatment regimens are recommended for Gonal-F®.

Serum levels of FSH do not correlate with pharmacological responses, such as the production of oestradiol, inhibin response or follicular development. Moreover, there is a large variability found in the individual pharmacological response to a fixed dose of recombinant FSH. This variability emphasizes the importance of a patient individualized dosing and treatment regimen when using recombinant FSH.

Follitropin β has an elimination half-life of approximately 40 hours. Steady-state levels of follitropin β are therefore reached after four daily doses. At that time, the concentrations of circulating immunoreactive FSH are about a factor of 1.5–2.5 higher than after a single dose. This increase is relevant in attaining therapeutically effective plasma concentrations of FSH. Follitropin β can be administered via the intramuscular, as well as via the subcutaneous route, because the absence of impurities results in an improved local tolerance. Bioavailability via both routes is approximately 77%. Injections of the highly pure follitropin β preparations do not require medical personnel, but can be given by the patient herself or her partner. In a large number of patients treated with follitropin β, no formation of antibodies against recombinant FSH or CHO-cell derived proteins was observed.

Differences with Urinary FSH Preparations

In IVF, follitropin β treatment was found to be more effective and efficient than treatment with urinary FSH, since more follicles, oocytes, embryos and pregnancies are obtained with a lower total dose of recombinant FSH in a shorter treatment period. In a recent meta-analysis the occurrence of higher pregnancy rates with recombinant FSH versus urinary FSH was confirmed (Daya, 1999). Treatment of patients with anovulatory infertility with either follitropin β or urinary FSH was equally effective, but follitropin β treatment was more efficient (a lower total dose was needed in a shorter duration of treatment). ■

Further Reading

- **Damm, J.B.L.** (1995) Application of Glycobiology in the Biotechnological Production of Pharmaceuticals. Pharm. Tech. Europe, 9, 28–34.
- **Groves, M.J.** (1996) Pharmaceutical Biotechnology: Drugs for the Future, In: Sam, A.P., Fokkens, J.G., Innovations in drug delivery: impact on pharmacotherapy. 2nd Edition. Anselmus Society, Houten, the Netherlands, pp. 146–156.
- **Sam, A.P., Metsers, F.A.A.J.** (1997) Chemistry and Pharmacy Aspects of Applications for Marketing Authorisations for Peptide and Protein Medicines. In: Minutes 8th Intern. Pharm. Techn. Symp. "Recent Advances in Peptide and Protein Delivery", Ed. A.A. Hincal, Editions de Santé, Paris.

References

- **Daya, S., Gunby, J.** (1999) Recombinant versus urinary follicle stimulating hormone for ovarian stimulation in assisted reproduction. Human Reprod., 14, 2207–2215.
- **De Boer, W., Mannaerts, B.** (1990) Recombinant follicle stimulating hormone. II. Biochemical and biological characteristics. In: Crommelin, D.J.A., Schellekens, H. (Eds.), *From clone to clinic, Developments in Biotherapy.* Vol. 1. Kluwer Academic Publishers, Dordrecht, pp. 253–259.
- **De Leeuw, R., Mulders, J., Voortman, G., Rombout, F., Damm. J., Kloosterboer, L.** (1996) Structure-function relationship of recombinant follicle stimulating hormone (Puregon®). Mol. Human Reproduction, **2**, 361–369.
- **European Public Assessment Report Gonal-F** (Follitropin alpha), CPMP/415/95, revison 4, 6 December 2001 corrected. European Agency for the Evaluation of Medicinal Products.
- **European Public Assessment Report Puregon** (Follitropin beta), CPMP/003/96, revison 4, 15 January 2002. European Agency for the Evaluation of Medicinal Products.
- **Geurts, T.B.P., Peters, M.J.H., Bruggen, J.G.C. van, Boer, W. de, Out, H.J.** (1996) Puregon® (Org 32489) – Recombinant human follicle-stimulating hormone. Drugs of Today, 32, 239–258.
- **Howles, C.M.** (1996) Genetic engineering of human FSH (Gonal-F®) Human Reproduction Update, **2**, 172–191.
- **Olijve, W., de Boer, W., Mulders, J.W.M., van Wezenbeek, P.M.G.F.** (1996) Molecular biology and biochemistry of human recombinant follicle stimulating hormone (Puregon[R]). Mol. Human Reproduction, **2**, 371–382.
- **Out, H.J., Mannaerts, B.M.J.L., Driessen, S.G.A.J., Coelingh Bennink, H.J.T.** (1996) Recombinant follicle stimulating hormone (rFSH; Puregon) in assisted reproduction: More oocytes, more pregnancies. Results from five comparative studies. Human Reprod. Update, **2**, 162–171.
- **Voortman, G., Post, J. van de, Schoemaker, R.C., Gerwen, J. van.** (1999) Bioequivalence of subcutaneous injections of recombinant human follicle stimulating hormone (Puregon®) by Pen-injector and syringe. Human Reprod., 14, 1698–1702.

Self-Assessment Questions

Question 1: *What makes the formulation process of recombinant FSH difficult?*

Question 2: *What makes the profile of glycoprotein hormone preparations so complex?*

Answers

Answer 1: Recombinant proteins are highly purified preparations, not stabilised by the presence of other (contaminating) proteins. Urinary FSH preparations contain, for instance, more than 95% of proteins of largely undetermined origin. Recombinant protein formulations can be protected against the destabilizing effect of the freeze-drying process and against the effect of adsorption losses by the addition of albumin or gelatin in their formulations. However, this addition is not desirable, since it unnecessarily contaminates the highly purified protein, and may lead to immunological and/or local tolerance problems. Formulations based on low molecular weight compounds allow for more simple and reliable quality control. This formulation however requires optimisation of the formulation and the freeze-drying process.

Answer 2: FSH is a glycoprotein existing of a large array of isohormones, differing in the composition of their four carbohydrate side-chains. The fate of such an isohormone in an organism is a function of its intrinsic activity and its pharmacokinetics. It has been demonstrated that for recombinant FSH isohormone fractions, a clear correlation exists between their pI value and their receptor binding activity on the one hand and their pharmacokinetic behavior on the other. The relatively basic isoforms display high receptor binding and high intrinsic bioactivity with a short plasma residence time. Relatively acidic isohormones that are more heavily sialylated, combine low receptor binding and low intrinsic bioactivity with a long plasma residence time. Increasing acidity of the isohormone leads to an increase in absorption rate and elimination half-life, and to a decrease in clearance rate. The longer blood residence times of the acidic isohormones counterbalance their relatively lower intrinsic activities.

18 Dispensing Biotechnology Products: Handling, Professional Education and Product Information

Peggy Piascik and Gary H. Smith

Introduction

Pharmacists have traditionally been responsible for the preparation and/or dispensing of pharmaceuticals. Up until now most products for parenteral use have been available in ready to use containers or required dilution with water or saline prior to use without any special handling requirements. In hospitals, pharmacists have been involved with the preparation and dispensing of parenteral products for individual patients for many years. Biotechnology products are proteins subject to denaturation and thus require special handling techniques. While (hospital) pharmacists are skilled in handling parenteral products, biotechnology products may provide additional challenges which will be explained in more detail in this chapter.

Pharmacist Reluctance

Practicing pharmacists may be reluctant to provide pharmaceutical care services to patients who require therapy with biotechnology drugs for a variety of reasons including (1) lack of knowledge about the tools of biotechnology; (2) lack of understanding of the therapeutic aspects of recombinant protein products; (3) unfamiliarity of the side effects and patient counseling information; (4) unfamiliarity with the storage, handling and reconstitution of proteins; and (5) difficulty of handling reimbursement issues.

Some pharmacists may incorrectly view these drugs as quite different from traditional drug products which are normally dispensed as familiar oral dosage forms. However, in most respects the services offered by pharmacists when dispensing biotechnology products are basically the same as those provided for traditional tablets, or injectable products. In addition, pharmacists have dispensed insulin and a variety of other proteins routinely for years. As more of these novel protein products come to market and the indications for existing agents are expanded for ambulatory patients, pharmacists will be increasingly required to deal with protein pharmaceuticals. While the first protein/peptide recombinant products were used primarily in hospital sethings, many of those agents have become commonplace in ambulatory settings such as home health pharmacies and home infusion services. Even the traditional community pharmacy is now likely to be dispensing products like colony stimulating factors, growth hormone, and interferons to name a few.

Types of Information Needed by Pharmacists

What types of information do pharmacists require to be confident dispensers of biotech drugs? For pharmacists who have been out of school for more than five to ten years, a basic understanding of (or updated information regarding) the immune system, diseases related to immunosuppression and autoimmune mechanisms, and ways in which drugs may modify the immune system is essential. Several appropriate books that can provide a basic background in immunology are listed in Table 18.1. Additionally, practitioners may enroll in organized courses of continuing education programs which can provide up-to-date information in the area of immunology. Most current pharmacy students will be sufficiently trained in basic immunology as part of their professional curriculum.

Many pharmacists and pharmacy students upon hearing the word biotechnology imagine a discipline too technical or complicated to be understood by the typical practitioner. Pharmacists merely need to learn that biotechnology refers to a set of tools that has allowed great strides to be made in basic research, the understanding of disease and development of new therapeutic agents. All pharmacists should have a basic understanding of recombinant DNA technology and monoclonal antibody technology. It is not necessary that pharmacy practitioners know how to use these tools in the laboratory but rather how the use of these tools provides us with new products and a greater understanding of disease processes.

Pharmacists may also need to review or learn anew about protein chemistry and those characteristics that affect therapeutic activity, product storage and routes of administration of these drugs. Apart from this textbook, several publications, videotapes and continuing professional education programs from industry and academic institutions are available to pharmacists for learning about the technical aspects of product storage and handling. Pharmacists need to become familiar with the drug delivery systems currently in use for biotech drugs as well as those which are likely to be used in the next few years (cf. Chapter 4).

Cellular and Molecular Immunology. 4th ed.
Abbas AK, Lichtman AH, Pober JS.
Philadelphia: W.B. Saunders Company, 2000: 553 pp. *Softbound book providing basic immunology concepts and clinical issues.*

Immunology: a short course. 4th ed.
Benjamin E, Coico R, Sunshine G.
New York: Wiley-Liss, 2000: 528 pp.
Softbound elementary text with review questions for each chapter.

Concepts in Immunology and Immunotherapeutics. 3rd ed.
Koeller J, Tami J, eds. Bethesda, MD: American Society of Hospital Pharmacists, 1997: 537 pp.
Review of basic immunology including therapeutic applications.

Medical Immunology for Students.
Playfair JHL, Lydyard PM.
New York: Churchill Livingstone, 1995: 112 pp.
Softbound, simple overview of basic immunology, immunopathology and clinical immunology.

Immunology: clinical, fundamental and therapeutic aspects.
Ram BP, Harris MC, Tyle, P, eds.
New York: VCH, 1990: 364 pp.
Review of basic immunology, immunobiology, clinical immunology and related drugs; a scientific viewpoint.

Essential immunology. 9th ed.
Roitt IM.
Oxford; Boston: Blackwell Scientific Publications, 1997: 494 pp.
Softbound basic immunology textbook.

Table 18.1. Selected texts to enhance immunology knowledge.

Sources of Information for Pharmacists

Many pharmacists do not know where to obtain the information that will allow them to be good providers of products of biotechnology. This textbook provides much of the essential background information in one source.

A number of continuing education programs and journal articles in the past have focused on biotechnology methods describing recombinant DNA technology and how monoclonal antibodies are made. Many manufacturer-sponsored programs are now on the market describing biotech products that are currently available and those likely to come to market in the near future. An excellent source of information on biotechnology in general and specific products in particular is the biotech drug industry. Manufacturers are prepared to help pharmacists in the most effective provision of products and services to patients, both hospital-based and ambulatory (Table 18.2). However, many pharmacists are unaware of these services and how to obtain them.

A variety of manufacturer-sponsored programs and services are available to both health professionals and patients. The information provided by manufacturers can help pharmacists confidently provide biotechnology products to their patients. The services provided generally fall into three categories: reimbursement information, customer/medical services and support, and educational materials.

The Pharmacist and Handling of Biotech Drugs

For biotech based pharmaceuticals, it is logical for the pharmacist to be responsible for their storage, preparation and dispensing as well as patient education. However it will require, in many cases, that additional education be obtained by the pharmacist in order to be prepared for this role. This is especially true for pharmacists who practice primarily in the ambulatory care setting since many of these products will be administered by the patient him or herself in the home. The hospital as well as the community pharmacy of the future will handle different kinds of materials than they do today. The future community pharmacy will stock pumps, patches, timed-release tablets, liposomes, implants, and vials of tailored monoclonal antibodies. With gene therapy and gene splicing on the horizon it is not inconceivable that the pharmacist may well be involved with related products. A list of currently available and future products is presented in Chapters 8–17 and 20 (Check, 1984; Koeller *et al.*, 1991; Stewart *et al.*, 1989).

This chapter will discuss the general principles that pharmacists will need to know about storage, handling, preparation, administration of biotech products and issues related to outpatient/home care. Specific examples will be discussed for illustrative purposes. Most available products can be found in Table 18.3, which lists the products along with specific handling requirements. For more current information you may need to contact the manufacturer. A list of manufacturers and their telephone numbers can be found in Table 18.2.

Storage

Biotech products have special storage requirements which in most cases differ from the majority of products pharmacists

Manufacturer	Product	Professional services	Reimbursement hotline/ indigent patient programs
Amgen Inc.	Neupogen Epogen Infergen	1-800-772-6436[1]	1-800-272-9376[2]
Aventis	Lantus Refludan	1-800-633-1610	1-800-221-4025
Aventis-Behring	Helixate FS	1-800-504-5434	1-800-676-4266
Baxter Healthcare	Recombinate	1-800-423-2090	1-800-548-4448
Bayer Biological	KoGENate KoGENate FS	1-800-468-0894	1-800-288-8370
Bedford	GlucaGen	1-800--521-5169 1-800-562-4797	1-800-562-4797
Berlex	Betaseron	1-888-BERLEX-4 (1-888-237-5394)	1-888-237-5394
Biogen	Avonex	1-800-456-2255[3]	1-800-456-2255
Centocor	Retavase	1-800-457-6399	1-800-331-5773
Chiron	Proleukin	1-800-244-7668	1-800-775-7533
Genentech	Activase Protropin Pulmozyme Nutropin TNKase	1-800-821-8590	1-800-530-3083
Genetics	Neumega Benefix Refacto	1-888-638-6342	1-888-638-6342
Genzyme	Cerezyme Thyrogen	1-800-745-4447	1-800-745-4447
Glaxo-SmithKline (formerly SmithKline-Beecham and Glaxo Welcome)	Engerix-B LYMErix	1-888-825-5249	1-800-745-2967
Immunex	Leukine Enbrel	1-800-466-8639	Leukine-1-800-321-4669 Enbrel-1-800-282-7704
Intermune	Actimmune	1-888-696-8036[4]	1-800-577-9112
Ligand	Ontak	1-800-964-5836	1-877-654-4263

1. For Infergen. 1-888-508-8808.
2. In Washington, DC metropolitan area, phone 1-202-637-6698.
3. Also for general MS information and patient help via MS Active Source.
4. For clinical information on Actimmune, phone 1-510-923-9576.

Table 18.2. Toll-free assistance numbers for selected biopharmaceuticals in USA and Canada. With thanks to Richard Beasley for help updating this table.

Manufacturer	Product	Professional services	Reimbursement hotline/ indigent patient programs
Lilly	Humatrope ReoPro Glucagon Humulin Humulog (and Mix)	1-800-545-5979	1-800-545-5979
Merck	Comvax Recombivax HB	1-800-672-6372	1-800-672-6372[5]
Novo Nordisk	Novolin Novolog Norditropin	1-800-727-6500	1-800-727-6500
Organon	Follistim	1-800-631-1253	1-800-241-8812
Ortho Biotech	Procrit	1-800-325-7504	1-800-553-3851
Ortho-McNeil	Regranex	1-800-682-6532	1-800-899-4325
Pharmacia-UpJohn	Genotropin	1-888-768-5501	1-800-242-7014
Roche	Roferon A	1-800-526-6367	1-800-443-6676
Schering	Intron A Rebetron	1-800-222-7579	1-800-521-7157
Serono	Gonal-F Saizen	1-888-275-7376	1-800-283-8088[6]
Wyeth-Ayerst	Enbrel	1-800-934-5556 1-800-466-8639	1-800-282-7704 1-800-282-7704

5. Merck does not offer reimbursement information or options for their vaccines, this is a number for other Merck products.

6. Serono does not offer reimbursement information or options for Gonal-F or Saizen, this number is for other Serono products.

Table 18.2b. continued.

normally dispense. The shelf life of these products is often considerably shorter than for traditional compounds. E.g., interferon α 2a (McEvoy, 1995; Roche, 1992) is only stable in a refrigerator in the ready-to-use solution for 12 months. Since most of these products need to be kept at refrigerated temperatures some facilities may need to increase cold storage space in order to accommodate the storage needs.

Temperature Requirements

Since biotech products are primarily proteins, they are subject to denaturation when exposed to extreme temperatures. In general, most biotech products are shipped by the manufacturer in gel ice containers and need to be stored at 2–8 °C (Banga *et al.*, 1994). Once reconstituted, they should be kept stored under refrigeration until just prior to use. There are, of course, exceptions to this rule as exemplified by alteplase (tissue plasminogen activator). Alteplase is stable at room temperature for several years (Genentech, 1994). For individual product requirements for temperature requirements, the product brochure or the manufacturer should be contacted. Table 18.3 also lists temperature requirements for most of the available products. The variability between products with respect to temperature is exemplified by granulocyte-colony stimulating factor (G-CSF; filgrastim) (Amgen, 1992) and erythropoietin (Amgen, 1993) which are stable in ready-to-use form at

Product Name	Storage Temperature	Stability		Reconstitution sol	Stability after reconstitution, dilution	
		RT	Ref		RT	Ref
Aldesleukin	2–8 °C	48 h	18 m	SWFI	48 h	48 h
Alteplase	2–8 °C	24 m	24 m	dil (SWFI)	8 h	8 h
Baceplermin	2–8 °C	NA	ex da	NA	NA	NA
Denileukin diftitox	< −10 °C	6 h	ex da	NS	6 h	NA
Dornase alpha	2–8 °C	24 h	ex da	RTU	NA	NA
Erythropoetin alpha	2–8 °C	NA	ex da	RTU	NA	NA
Etanercept	2–8 °C	NA	ex da	dil (SBWFI)	6 h	6 h
Filgrastim	2–8 °C	24 h	ex da; syringes are sterile for 7 days	RTU	NA	NA
Follitropin alfa	2–25 °C	ex da	ex da	SWFI	NA	NA
Follitropin beta	2–25 °C	ex da	ex da	SWFI, 1/2NS	NA	NA
Glucagon	2–25 °C	12 m	ex da	SWFI	NA	NA
Hepatitis B vaccine	2–8 °C	NA	ex da	RTU	NA	NA
Imiglucerase	2–8 °C	NA	ex da	SWFI	12 h	12–24 h
Insulin (human)	2–8 °C	7 d	ex da	RTU	NA	NA
Insulin (human) aspart	2–8 °C	28 d	ex da	RTU	NA	NA
Insulin (human) glargine	2–8 °C	14–28 d*	ex da, 28 d opened	RTU	NA	NA
Insulin (human) lispro	2–8 °C	28 d	ex da	RTU	14 d	28 d
Interferon alpha 2a	2–8 °C	NA	ex da	RTU	NA	30 d
Interferon alpha 2b	2–8 °C	2–14 d*	ex da	dil (SBWFI)	NA	30 d
Interferon alfacon-1	2–8 °C	NA	ex da	RTU	NA	NA
Interferon beta 1a	2–8 °C	30 d	ex da	SWFI	NA	6 h
Interferon beta 1b	2–8 °C	7 d	ex da	dil	NA	3 h
Interferon gamma 1b	2–8 °C	12 h	ex da	RTU	NA	NA

Table 18.3a Storage, stability and reconstitution of selected biotechnology products

Table key: d = day; dil = supplied diluent; DNF = do not freeze; DNR = do not refrigerate; D5W = dextrose 5% in water; ex da = see expiration date on package; h = hours; IA = intraarterial; IC = intracoronary; IL = intralesional, IM = intramuscular injection; IO = intraorbital; IP = intraperitoneal; IVB = intravenous bolus; IVIF = intravenous infusion; IVIN = intravenous injection; m = months; mfg = contact manufacturer; NA = not available/applicable; NS = normal saline; PP = polypropylene; PVC = polyvinyl chloride; pwd = powder; Ref = refrigerator; RT = room temperature; RTU = ready to use solution; SBWFI = sterile bacteriostatic water for injection; sol = solution; SC = subcutaneous injection; SCI = subcutaneous infusion; SWFI = sterile water for injection; SWFIR = sterile water for irrigation; y = years. * varies with package size or concentration, see package insert. With thanks to Richard Beasley for help updating this table.

Product Name	Storage Temperature	Stability		Reconstitution sol	Stability after reconstitution, dilution	
		RT	Ref		RT	Ref
Lepirudin	2–25 °C	ex da	ex da	SWFI, NS	24 h	24 h
Lyme disease vaccine	2–8 °C	ex da	ex da	RTU	NA	NA
Oprelvekin	2–8 °C	NA	ex da	SWFI	3 h	3 h
Recombinant Factor VIII	2–8 °C	3–6 m*	ex da	SWFI, dil	3 h	DNR, DNF
Recombinant Factor IX	2–8 °C	6 m	ex da	SWFI, dil	3 h	DNR, DNF
Retavase	2–25 °C	ex da	ex da	SWFI	4 h	4 h
Sargramostim	2–8 °C	ex da	ex da	SWFI, SBWFI	6 h	6 h in SWFI; 20 d in SBWFI
Somatrem	2–8 °C	7 d	ex da	SBWFI	NA	14 d
Somatropin	2–8 °C	NA	ex da	dil, SBWFI	NA	24 h–14 d*
Tenectaplase	2–25 °C	ex da	ex da	SWFI	NA	8 h
Thyrotropin alpha	2–8 °C	NA	ex da	SWFI	NA	24 h

Table 18.3acont. Storage, stability and reconstitution of selected biotechnology products

Table key: d = day; dil = supplied diluent; DNF = do not freeze; DNR = do not refrigerate; D5W = dextrose 5% in water; ex da = see expiration date on package; h = hours; IA = intraarterial; IC = intracoronary; IL = intralesional, IM = intramuscular injection; IO = intraorbital; IP = intraperitoneal; IVB = intravenous bolus; IVIF = intravenous infusion; IVIN = intravenous injection; m = months; mfg = contact manufacturer; NA = not available/applicable; NS = normal saline; PP = polypropylene; PVC = polyvinyl chloride; pwd = powder; Ref = refrigerator; RT = room temperature; RTU = ready to use solution; SBWFI = sterile bacteriostatic water for injection; sol = solution; SC = subcutaneous injection; SCI = subcutaneous infusion; SWFI = sterile water for injection; SWFIR = sterile water for irrigation; y = years. * varies with manefacturer, see package insert.

room temperature for 24 hours and 14 days, respectively. Granulocyte macrophage-colony stimulating factor (GM-CSF; sargramostim) (Immunex, 1992) on the other hand is packaged as a lyophilized powder but still requires refrigeration and once reconstituted is stable at room temperature for 30 days or refrigerator for 2 years. Aldesleukin (interleukin-2) is stable for 48 hours at room temperature or up to 18 months in a refrigerator (Chiron, 1994). Betaseron (interferon β-1b) must be stored in a refrigerator and should be used within three hours after reconstitution (Berlex, 1994). While most products require refrigeration to maintain stability due to denaturation by elevated temperatures, extreme cold such as freezing may be just as harmful to most products. The key is to avoid extremes in temperature be it heat or cold (Banga *et al.*, 1994).

Storage in Dosing and Administration Devices

Most biotech products may adhere to either plastic or glass containers such as syringes, polyvinyl chloride (PVC) intravenous bags, infusion equipment, and glass intravenous bottles. The effectiveness of the product may be reduced by three or four fold due to adherence. In order to decrease the amount of adherence, human serum albumin (HSA) is usually added to the solutions (cf. Chapter 4). The relative loss through adherence is usually concentration dependent, i.e., the more concentrated the final solution the less significant the adherence becomes. The amount of human serum albumin added varies with the product (Banga *et al.*, 1994; Koeller *et al.*, 1991). Those products requiring the addition of HSA include filgrastim, sargromostim, aldesleukin, erythropoietin and interferon α. In the case of filgrastim at a concentration of 5–15 mcg/mL the addition of 2 mg/mL of HSA to the final solution is required (Amgen, 1992). With sargramostim, 1 mg/mL of HSA is required for concentrations of <10 mcg/mL. (Immunex, 1992). For aldesleukin 0.1% HSA is required for all concentrations (Chiron, 1995). For erythropoietin 2.5 mg HSA is required per injection, and 1 mg/vial of HSA for interferon α.

For additional information or to check on the most current information on this topic the manufacturer should be contacted.

Product Name	Compatibility with equipment	Compatibility with solution	Approved admin/route	Non approved admin/route
Aldesleukin	glass, PVC (re-commended), PP	D5W	IVIF	IV, SC
Alteplase	glass, PVC	D5W, NS	IVIF	IVB, IC, IA, IO
Becaplermin	cotton swabs, tongue depressors, or other aids	NS	topical (external use only)	NA
Denileukin diftitox	plastic syringe, PVC	NS	IVIF	IVB
Dornase alpha	nebulizer, compressor	NA	nebulizer/inhaler	NA
Erythropoetin alpha	plastic syringe	bacteriostatic NS	IVB, IVIN, SC	IP
Etanercept	plastic syringe	NA	SC	NA
Filgrastim	glass, PVC, PP polyolefin	D5W, (never NS)	SC, SCI, IVIF	IVIF-4 h
Follitropin alfa	plastic syringe	NS	SC	IV, IM
Follitropin beta	plastic syringe	NS	SC, IM, IV	NA
Glucagon	plastic syringe	NS	SC, IM, IV	NA
Hepatitis B vaccine	plastic or glass syringe	NS, but dilution is not recommended	IM	SC
Imiglucerase	glass, PVC, plastic syringes	NS	IVIF	NA
Insulin (human)	plastic syringes	NA	SC	NA
Insulin (human) aspart	plastic syringes	NA	SC	NA
Insulin (human) glargine	plastic syringes	none	SC	IV
Insulin (human) lispro	plastic syringes	SWFI, NS	SC	IV
Interferon alpha 2a	glass, PVC, plastic	NS	IM, SC	IVIF
Interferon alpha 2b	glass, PVC, plastic syringes	NS	IVIN, IVIF, IM, SC, IL	NA
Interferon alfacon-1	glass or plastic syringes	NA	SC	NA

Table 18.3b Compatibility and administration information of selected biotechnology products

Table key: d = day; dil = supplied diluent; DNF = do not freeze; DNR = do not refrigerate; D5W = dextrose 5% in water; ex da = see expiration date on package; h = hours; IA = intraarterial; IC = intracoronary; IL = intralesional, IM = intramuscular injection; IO = intraorbital; IP = intraperitoneal; IVB = intravenous bolus; IVIF = intravenous infusion; IVIN = intravenous injection; m = months; mfg = contact manufacturer; NA = not available/applicable; NS = normal saline; PP = polypropylene; PVC = polyvinyl chloride; pwd = powder; Ref = refrigerator; RT = room temperature; RTU = ready to use solution; SBWFI = sterile bacteriostatic water for injection; sol = solution; SC = subcutaneous injection; SCI = subcutaneous infusion; SWFI = sterile water for injection; SWFIR = sterile water for irrigation; y = years. With thanks to Richard Beasley for help updating this table.

Product Name	Compatibility with equipment	Compatibility with solution	Approved admin/route	Non approved admin/route
Interferon beta 1a	glass or plastic syringes	NA	IM	NA
Interferon beta 1b	glass or plastic syringes	NA	SC	NA
Interferon gamma 1b	glass or plastic syringes	NA	SC	IVIF, IM
Lepirudin	glass, PVC, plastic syringes	NS, D5W	IVB, IVIF, IVIN	NA
Lyme disease vaccine	plastic syringes	NA	IM	NA
Oprelvekin	plastic syringes	NA	SC	NA
Recombinant Factor VIII	plastic syringe, PVC	NA	IVIN, IVIF	NA
Recombinant Factor IX	plastic syringe, PVC	NA	IVIN, IVIF	NA
Retavase	plastic syringe, PVC	NS, D5W	IVB, IVIN	IM
Sargramostim	plastic syringe, PVC	NS	SC, IVIF	NA
Somatrem	plastic syringes	NA	SC, IM	NA
Somatropin	plastic syringes	NA	SC	NA
Tenectaplase	plastic syringe, PVC	NS only	IVB, IVIN	NA
Thyrotropin alfa	plastic syringes	NA	IM, SC	IV

Table 18.3b cont. Compatibility and administration information of selected biotechnology products

Table key: d = day; dil = supplied diluent; DNF = do not freeze; DNR = do not refrigerate; D5W = dextrose 5% in water; ex da = see expiration date on package; h = hours; IA = intraarterial; IC = intracoronary; IL = intralesional, IM = intramuscular injection; IO = intraorbital; IP = intraperitoneal; IVB = intravenous bolus; IVIF = intravenous infusion; IVIN = intravenous injection; m = months; mfg = contact manufacturer; NA = not available/applicable; NS = normal saline; PP = polypropylene; PVC = polyvinyl chloride; pwd = powder; Ref = refrigerator; RT = room temperature; RTU = ready to use solution; SBWFI = sterile bacteriostatic water for injection; sol = solution; SC = subcutaneous injection; SCI = subcutaneous infusion; SWFI = sterile water for injection; SWFIR = sterile water for irrigation; y = years.

Storage in IV Solutions

Biotech products may have variable stability when stored in the various available containers or syringes. Some products are only stable in plastic syringes, e.g. somatropin and erythropoietin, while others are stable in glass, polyvinyl chloride and polypropylene, e.g. aldesleukin. See Table 18.3 for a listing of all products and their compatibility with storage equipment. It is important to make sure that the product you wish to provide pre-filled syringes for is stable in the type of syringe you wish to use. This may present a challenge to home health care programs. Batch prefilling of syringes is possible and G-CSF is stable in Becton Dickinson (B-D) disposable plastic syringes for up to 7 days (Amgen, 1992; Amgen, 1995) while erythropoietin is stable for up to 14 days (Amgen, 1993; Amgen, 1995). Aldesleukin by Chiron Therapeutics (Chiron, 1995) is stable when administered in glass, PVC, and polypropylene while GM-CSF and G-CSF can be administered in either PVC or polypropylene (Immunex, 1995). See Table 18.3 for information of the other available products.

Light Protection

Some products are sensitive to light. Dornase alpha is packaged in protective foil pouches by the manufacturer to protect it from light degradation. The product should be stored in these original light protective containers. For patients who travel, the manufacturer will provide special travel pouches on request (Berlex, 1994). Alteplase in the lyophilized form also needs to be protected from light, but is not light sensitive when in solution (Genentech, 1995). As new products become available there will undoubtedly be more that will have specific storage requirements with respect to light.

Handling

Mixing and Shaking

Since the biotech products are complex proteins, improper handling can lead to denaturation. Shaking and severe agitation of most of these products will result in degradation. Therefore special techniques must be observed in preparing biotech products for use. Biotech products should not be shaken when adding any diluent. Shaking may cause the product to break down. Therefore once the diluent is added to the container it should be swirled as has been the case with insulin over the years. Some shaking during transport may be unavoidable and proper inspection should occur to make sure the products have not been harmed. Usually when this happens one can observe physical separation or frothing within the vial of liquid products. For lyophilized products agitation is not harmful until they have been reconstituted. In distributing individual products to patient or ward areas, pneumatic tubes should be avoided.

Travel Requirements

During travel with these products certain precautions should also be observed. They should be stored in insulated, cool containers. This can be accomplished by using ice packs to keep the biotech drug at the proper temperature in warmer climates, whereas the insulated container in colder climates may be all that is required. In fact, when traveling in sub-freezing weather, the products should be protected from freezing. When ice is used, care should be taken to not place the product directly on the ice. Dry ice should be avoided since it has the potential for freezing the product. When traveling by air, biotech products should be taken onto the plane in insulated packages and not placed in a cargo container. Aeroplane cargo containers may be cold enough to cause freezing (Banga, 1994; Koeller *et al.*, 1991).

Preparation

When preparing biotech products, aseptic technique should be adhered to as it is with other parenteral products. The pharmaceutical should be prepared in a clean room designed for this purpose with laminar air flow hoods, etc. Most of the products require reconstitution with sterile water or bacteriostatic water for injection depending on stability data. The compatibility of individual products varies and limited data is available. As mentioned previously when adding diluent to these products, care should be taken not to shake them, but to swirl the container between the palms of your hands. In the case of lyophilized products, the introduction of the diluent should be directed down the side of the vial and not directly on the powder to avoid denaturing the protein. Table 18.3 provides specific compatibility data regarding individual products. It is important to mention here that stability does not mean sterility. Biotech products are not any different in this regard than any other parenteral product. The same precautions need to be adhered to and are worth mentioning to be complete. Sterility is a particularly important consideration when pre-filling and pre-mixing various doses for administration at home. Once the manufacturer's provided sterile packaging is entered, sterility can no longer be assured nor will the manufacturer be responsible for any subsequent related problems. Individual manufacturers have not addressed the issue of sterility and each institution or organization must determine its own policy on this issue. Approximately half of the currently available biotechnology-produced products are provided as single-dose vials and thus, should not be reused. This does not, however, prevent preparing batches ("batching") of unit-of-use doses in order to be more cost efficient. Most of the patients receiving these agents are likely to have suppressed immune systems and are vulnerable to infection. Therefore, a policy involving the maintenance of sterility of biotech products should be developed by each health care organization, especially home health care programs. For example, policy at the University of Arizona Medical Center is that all parenteral products that are reconstituted are routinely given a 72 hour expiration date in accordance with infection control policy of the hospital. When products are made in a sterile environment under aseptic procedures they should remain sterile until used and thus could be stored for as long as physical compatibility data dictates. However, most institutions have shorter expiration dates, which are generally 72 hours or less, on reconstituted products. These expiration dates have been arbitrarily set due to lack of good sterility data to the contrary. Sterility studies should be performed in order to determine if reconstituted products could be stored for a longer period of time and still maintain sterility. For products reconstituted for home use in the pharmacy sterile products area, however, a 7 day expiration date is used, provided the product is stable and can be stored in the refrigerator. The American Society of Health-System Pharmacists has published a technical assistance bulletin on sterile products which should be consulted for developing policy on storage of reconstituted parenteral products (American Society of Hospital Pharmacy, 1993). Patients need to be informed about specific storage requirement and expiration dates to assure sterility and stability.

Administration

Prior to administering these products, pharmacists will need to observe extra caution in reviewing dosage regimens. This is primarily because the units of measure for the various products may be radically different. Some products are dosed in micrograms/kilogram (mcg/kg), while others in milligrams/kilograms (mg/kg). Also in some cases, units of measure are used which may be unique to the product, e.g. Chiron or Roche units. Dosage calculations need to be carefully checked to avoid any potential errors.

Routes of Administration

Biotech products, with the exception of dornase alpha, are restricted to parenteral administration. Some products may be given by either the intravenous or subcutaneous route while others are restricted to the subcutaneous route only. Table 18.3 lists the approved and non-approved routes of administration for each product. In some cases, new information may be available and the manufacturer should always be consulted in order to obtain supporting evidence for a particular route that is not approved, but may be more convenient for the patient. For example, G-CSF should be administered by the subcutaneous or intravenous route only, while GM-CSF is given by intravenous infusion over a two hour period (McEvoy, 1995). Aldesleukin is approved for intravenous administration only. But, subcutaneous administration, while not approved, has been used by some (Chiron, 1992). Erythropoietin should only be administered by the intravenous or subcutaneous routes (Amgen, 1993), while alteplase is only approved for the intravenous route (Genentech, 1992; McEvoy, 1995). Alteplase has also been administered by the intracoronary, intraarterial, and intraorbital routes as well (McEvoy, 1995).

Filtration

Filtering biotech products is not generally recommended since most of these proteins will adhere to the filter. Some hospitals and home infusion companies routinely use in line filters for all intravenous solutions to minimize the introduction of particulate matter into the patient. In the case of biotech products, they should be infused below the filter to avoid any possible decrease in the amount of drug delivered to the patient (Banga, 1994; Koeller *et al.*, 1991).

Flushing Solutions

Pharmaceutical biotechnology products are usually flushed with either saline or dextrose 5% in water. The product literature should be consulted and care should be taken to assure that the proper solution is used with each agent. In general, these biotech drugs should not be administered with other fluids or drugs since, in most cases, data does not exist about such compatibilities.

Outpatient/Home Care Issues

The management of patients in the outpatient and home settings is a growing aspect of health care delivery. The use of biotech products outside the hospital is no exception to this trend. Home infusion services is one of the fastest growing sectors of the health care market and they have become involved with all forms of parenterally-administered drugs including biotech products. Just as we have been educating insulin-dependent diabetics on the proper administration techniques, storage, and handling of insulin over the last several decades, we must also do this for patients receiving these other protein biotech products. The main difference with most of these newer products is that, unlike insulin, the dose may need to be prepared in the patient's home.

Patient Assessment and Education

Before a patient can be a candidate for home therapy, an assessment of the patient's capabilities must occur. The patient, family member, or care giver will need to be able to inject the medication and comply with all of the storage, handling, and preparation requirements. If the patient is incapable, then a patient care giver, relative, spouse, or friend will need to be solicited. The patient will need to be educated as to all of the storage, handling, preparation, and administering aspects as previously described. The use of aseptic technique is usually new to most patients and in some cases may be frightening. The health care provider must be sure that the patient is competent and willing to follow these procedures. Self-instructional tapes on specific products may be available from the manufacturer, and if so, should be provided to the patient providing they have the proper equipment for tape reviewing.

Proper storage facilities will need to be available in the patient's home as well as a clean area for preparation and administration. Ideally, the patient will be able to prepare each dose immediately prior to the time of administration. If this is not possible, the pharmacy will have to prepare prefilled syringes and provide appropriate storage and handling requirements to the patient. The patient will also need to be educated as to the proper handling, needed supplies and materials such as needles, syringes, alcohol wipes, etc. The proper disposal of these hazardous wastes must also be reviewed. Specific issues related to patient teaching include rotating injection sites, product handling, drug storage also during transporting/traveling, expiration dates, refrigeration, cleansing the injection site with alcohol, disposal of needles and syringes, drug side effects, and expected therapeutic outcome.

Monitoring

Like other injectables used by patients in the home, it is important that close patient monitoring occurs. This will require frequent phone calls to the patient and periodic home visits. Monitoring parameters should include adverse events, progress to expected outcomes, assessment of administration technique, review of storage and handling procedures, and adherence to aseptic technique.

Reimbursement

Reimbursement issues include third party billing information and availability of forms, cost sharing programs which limit the annual cost of therapy, financial assistance programs for patients who would otherwise have difficulty paying for therapy, and reimbursement assurance programs which are designed to remove reimbursement barriers which may exist when reimbursement has been denied. Any detailed discussion of reimbursement issues is beyond the scope of this book and is subject to practice location. This discussion will deal only with the availability of information to pharmacists to appropriately handle reimbursements for products and services in the United States.

Pharmacists need to know current insurer payment policies such as whether insurance companies will disallow claims for uses other than the labeled indications or if the product is to be used in the home rather than administered in a hospital or physician's office. Prior authorization is required for many products, particularly insurers with managed care or prepaid plans. Some manufacturers will contact the carrier to verify coverage, provide sample prior-approval letters, and will follow up on claims to determine the claim's status and continue to follow up until resolution of the case.

Manufacturers can also provide information that may convince the third-party payer to reconsider a denied claim. Some companies will intervene with the third party payer to determine the case for denial, provide additional clinical documentation or coding information, and will follow the appeal to conclusion. Pharmacists can act as facilitators to get qualified patients enrolled in programs to provide free medication to those who have insufficient insurance coverage or are otherwise unable to purchase the therapy.

Educational Materials

Therapy with biotech drugs is a rapidly growing, ever changing area of therapeutics. Pharmacists need to keep informed of current information about existing agents such as new indications, management of side effects, results of studies describing drug interactions or changes in information regarding product stability and reconstitution. Pharmacists will also be interested in the status of new agents as they move through the FDA approval process. Some good periodical sources of practical information about products of biotechnology are listed in Table 18.4.

- **Biotechnology Medicines in Development,** Communications Division, Pharmaceutical Manufacturers Association, Washington, D.C., *202-835-3400, updated approximately every 18 months.* http://www.phrma.org/charts/b_cøø.html
- **FDC Reports, "The Pink Sheet,"** Chevy Chase, MD, *published weekly.* http://www.fdcreports.com/pinkout.shtml
- **Biotechnology Update,** *a monthly column in* **Journal of the American Pharmaceutical Association.**
- **BioWorld Today,** Atlanta: Bioworld Publishing Group, *newspaper, 5 issues per week; also available on Netscape; Tel. (404)-262-7436; Fax (404)-814-0759.* http://www.bioworld.com
- **Bio/Technology,** New York: Nature Publishing Co., *a monthly journal dealing with all aspects of biotechnology.* http://www.nature.com/nbt
- **Genetic Engineering News,** New York: GEN Publishing, *bimonthly publication, Tel. (914)-834-3100; Fax (914)-834-3771.* http://www.genwirl.com/
- **Biotechnology News,** New Jersey: CTB International Publishing, *Tel. (201)-379-7749; Fax (201)-379-1158.* http://www.ctbintl.com/bio.htm

Table 18.4. Information sources for current trends in biotechnology.

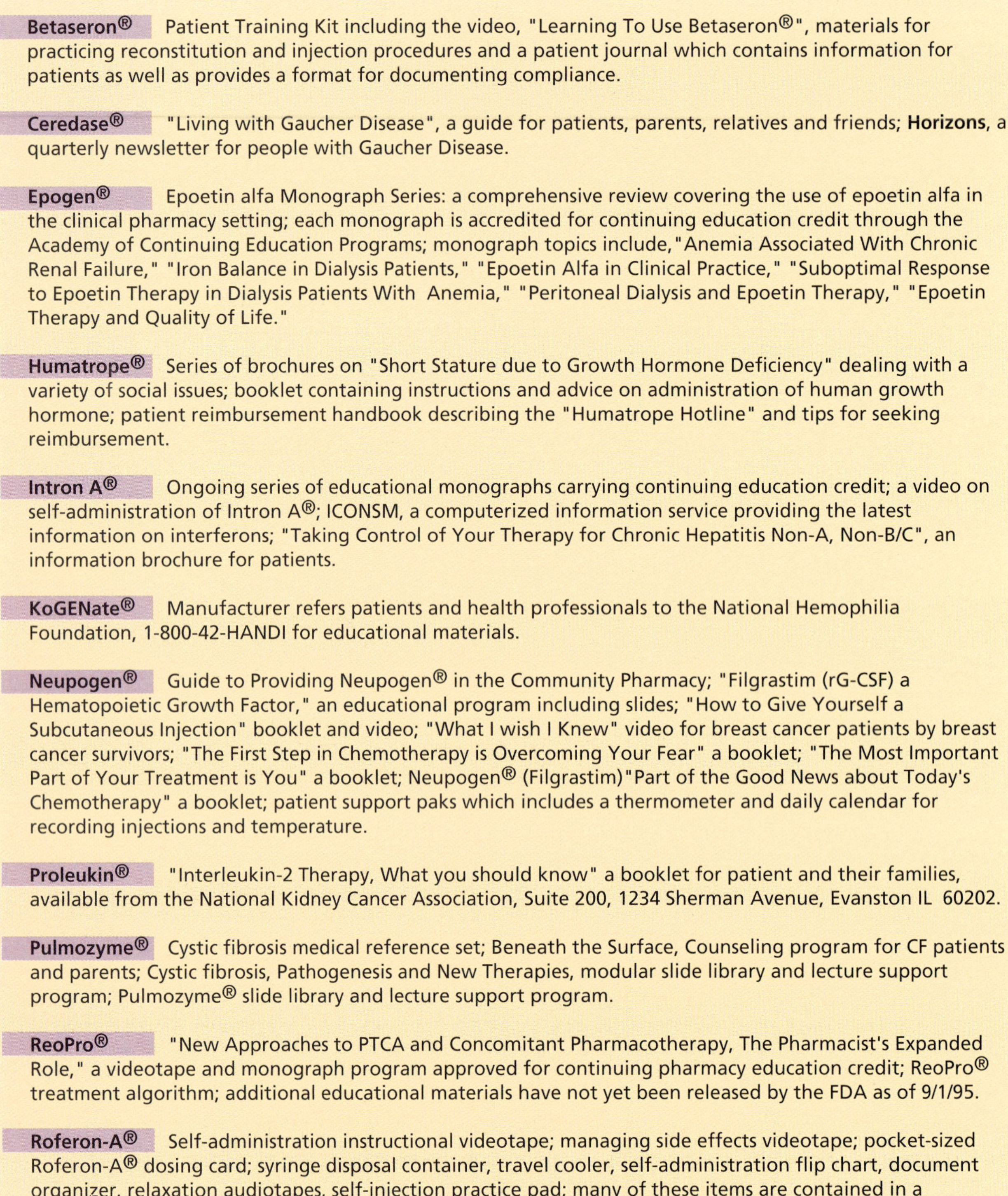

Betaseron® Patient Training Kit including the video, "Learning To Use Betaseron®", materials for practicing reconstitution and injection procedures and a patient journal which contains information for patients as well as provides a format for documenting compliance.

Ceredase® "Living with Gaucher Disease", a guide for patients, parents, relatives and friends; **Horizons**, a quarterly newsletter for people with Gaucher Disease.

Epogen® Epoetin alfa Monograph Series: a comprehensive review covering the use of epoetin alfa in the clinical pharmacy setting; each monograph is accredited for continuing education credit through the Academy of Continuing Education Programs; monograph topics include, "Anemia Associated With Chronic Renal Failure," "Iron Balance in Dialysis Patients," "Epoetin Alfa in Clinical Practice," "Suboptimal Response to Epoetin Therapy in Dialysis Patients With Anemia," "Peritoneal Dialysis and Epoetin Therapy," "Epoetin Therapy and Quality of Life."

Humatrope® Series of brochures on "Short Stature due to Growth Hormone Deficiency" dealing with a variety of social issues; booklet containing instructions and advice on administration of human growth hormone; patient reimbursement handbook describing the "Humatrope Hotline" and tips for seeking reimbursement.

Intron A® Ongoing series of educational monographs carrying continuing education credit; a video on self-administration of Intron A®; ICONSM, a computerized information service providing the latest information on interferons; "Taking Control of Your Therapy for Chronic Hepatitis Non-A, Non-B/C", an information brochure for patients.

KoGENate® Manufacturer refers patients and health professionals to the National Hemophilia Foundation, 1-800-42-HANDI for educational materials.

Neupogen® Guide to Providing Neupogen® in the Community Pharmacy; "Filgrastim (rG-CSF) a Hematopoietic Growth Factor," an educational program including slides; "How to Give Yourself a Subcutaneous Injection" booklet and video; "What I wish I Knew" video for breast cancer patients by breast cancer survivors; "The First Step in Chemotherapy is Overcoming Your Fear" a booklet; "The Most Important Part of Your Treatment is You" a booklet; Neupogen® (Filgrastim) "Part of the Good News about Today's Chemotherapy" a booklet; patient support paks which includes a thermometer and daily calendar for recording injections and temperature.

Proleukin® "Interleukin-2 Therapy, What you should know" a booklet for patient and their families, available from the National Kidney Cancer Association, Suite 200, 1234 Sherman Avenue, Evanston IL 60202.

Pulmozyme® Cystic fibrosis medical reference set; Beneath the Surface, Counseling program for CF patients and parents; Cystic fibrosis, Pathogenesis and New Therapies, modular slide library and lecture support program; Pulmozyme® slide library and lecture support program.

ReoPro® "New Approaches to PTCA and Concomitant Pharmacotherapy, The Pharmacist's Expanded Role," a videotape and monograph program approved for continuing pharmacy education credit; ReoPro® treatment algorithm; additional educational materials have not yet been released by the FDA as of 9/1/95.

Roferon-A® Self-administration instructional videotape; managing side effects videotape; pocket-sized Roferon-A® dosing card; syringe disposal container, travel cooler, self-administration flip chart, document organizer, relaxation audiotapes, self-injection practice pad; many of these items are contained in a "personal care kit."

Table 18.5. Examples of pharmacist/patient educational materials available from manufacturers.

Professional Services

Medical information services provided by manufacturers of biotech drugs are similar to the product, medical and patient management services provided by drug companies for traditional drug products. Information provided via this service generally includes appropriate indications, side effects, contraindications to use, results of clinical trials and investigational uses. Upon request, manufacturers can supply a product monograph and selected research articles that provide valuable information about each product.

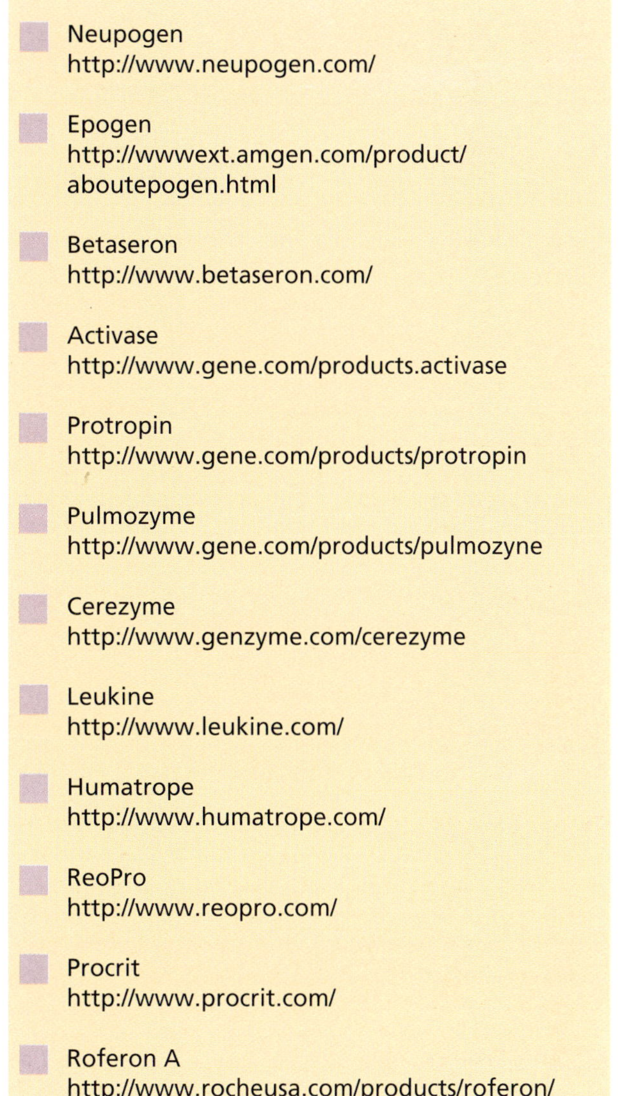

- Neupogen
  http://www.neupogen.com/
- Epogen
  http://wwwext.amgen.com/product/aboutepogen.html
- Betaseron
  http://www.betaseron.com/
- Activase
  http://www.gene.com/products.activase
- Protropin
  http://www.gene.com/products/protropin
- Pulmozyme
  http://www.gene.com/products/pulmozyne
- Cerezyme
  http://www.genzyme.com/cerezyme
- Leukine
  http://www.leukine.com/
- Humatrope
  http://www.humatrope.com/
- ReoPro
  http://www.reopro.com/
- Procrit
  http://www.procrit.com/
- Roferon A
  http://www.rocheusa.com/products/roferon/

Table 18.6. Individual product web-sites.

EDUCATIONAL MATERIALS FOR HEALTH PROFESSIONALS

Examples of pharmacist/patient educational materials provided by manufacturers are listed in Table 18.5. Numerous educational materials have been developed by manufacturers including continuing education programs for physicians, pharmacists and nurses; these programs sometimes include slides, videos and brochures. Since most biotechnology products are parenteral products, several manufacturers have produced videotapes which show the proper procedure for giving a subcutaneous injection. These instructional tapes are beneficial not just for patients but also for pharmacists who may not be skilled in injection techniques.

Amgen provides information on one of its products, Epogen®, through a monograph series which comprehensively reviews the use of the drug in the clinical pharmacy setting. Genentech supplies information on Pulmozyme® via a medical reference set, slide libraries and lecture support program. These and other materials are described in greater detail in Table 18.5.

EDUCATIONAL MATERIALS FOR PATIENTS

Examples of pharmacist/patient educational materials provided by manufacturers are listed in Table 18.5. Detailed patient information booklets exist for many of the products. Patient education materials can assist the patient and family members in learning more about his or her disease and how it will be treated. Education allows the patient to participate more actively in the therapy and to feel a greater level of control over the process. By contacting the manufacturer and acquiring patient educational materials, pharmacists can offer support to the patient in learning to use a new product. Many patients are already overwhelmed by dealing with a diagnosis of serious or chronic disease. Learning about a new therapy, especially if it involves the necessity of subcutaneous self-injection, can cause additional stress for the patient and family.

For example, both Genentech and Lilly have several booklets dealing with short stature, human growth hormone (Protropin®; Humatrope®) therapy and the "how to" of preparing and giving injections to children. A chart is included for recording of injections sites to insure that site rotation is maintained.

Berlex provides a patient training kit for multiple sclerosis patients to learn the reconstitution and injection procedures for Betaseron®. A journal is included for the patient to document compliance and record side effects which can be significant with this drug.

Some manufacturers also provide a referral to associations that can provide valuable information and services including a link to local chapters, meetings and support groups. For example, Bayer refers inquiries for patient information about KoGENate®, a recombinant clotting factor product (see Chapter 15), to the National Hemophilia

Internet Site	Type of Site	Web Address
A Doctor's Guide to the Internet	Biomedical news	www.docguide.com
BioOnline	Information library/catalog	www.bio.com
BioCentury	Biotechnology industry new	www.biocentury.com/
BioPharma	Database	www.biopharma.com/
Genetic Engineering News	On-line journal	www.genengnews.com
Nature Biotechnology	On-line journal	www. nature.com/nbt/
Pharmaceutical Research and Manufacturers of America	Professional organization	www.phrma.org/
Physicians Guide to the Internet	Biomedical news	www.webcom.com/pgi/
Reuter's Health Information Services, Inc.	Biomedical news	www.reutershealth.com/
The World Wide Web Virtual Library: Biotechnology	Information library/catalog	www.cato.com/biotech

Table 18.7. Sampling of some biotech-related Internet sites.

Foundation and Chiron Therapeutic, manufacturer of Proleukin®, refers families to the National Kidney Cancer Association.

Most commercially available biotech drugs now have individual web sites to provide updated information to patients. These sites usually contain the following types of information: disease background, reimbursement information, dosing information, references, referral to support groups and related organization web sites, frequently asked questions, administration and storage information, and information specifically for health professionals. A list of web sites for current products is provided in Table 18.6.

Toll-Free Access to Manufacturers' Services

Most manufacturers can be reached by toll-free numbers to request any of the types of information discussed above. Manufacturers of biotech products may have a separate number for reimbursement questions. Table 18.2 lists the manufacturers' toll-free assistance numbers for obtaining product and reimbursement information in North America. Vaccines and insulin products are not included in this table since these products were previously available in a non-recombinant form which was used in a similar manner. Moreover, the recombinant form is not significantly higher in price than the non-recombinant product.

The Internet and Biotech Information

The Internet has become a valuable site rich in up-to-date information concerning all aspects of pharmaceutical biotechnology. Sites including virtual libraries/catalogs, on-line journals (usually requiring a subscription), biomedical newsletters and biotechnology specific homepages abound on the Internet. Since the number of biotech-related sites are constantly increasing, only a small sampling of sites of interest could be provided in Table 18.7.

Concluding Remarks

Basically, the handling of biotechnology products requires similar skills and techniques as required for the preparation of other parenteral drugs, but there are often slightly difference nuances to the handling, preparation and administration of biotechnology-produced pharmaceuticals. The pharmacist can become an educator to others related to the pharmaceutical aspects of biotechnology products and can serve as a valuable resource to other health care professionals. In addition, biotech products give the pharmacist the opportunity to provide pharmaceutical care since patient education and monitoring is required. To play this role successfully, the pharmacist will need to keep abreast of new developments as new literature and products become available. ■

Further Reading

See Tables 18.1, 18.4 and 18.7 for lists of selected readings.

References

- **American Society of Health-System Pharmacists.** (1993). ASHP technical assistance bulletin on quality assurance for pharmacy-prepared sterile products. *Am J Hosp Pharm*, 50, 2386–2398.
- **Amgen Inc.** (1993). Epogen® package insert. Thousand Oaks, CA.
- **Amgen Inc.** (1992). Neupogen® package insert. Thousand Oaks, CA.
- **Amgen Inc.** (1995). Written information on storage, stability, compatibility, and administration. Thousand Oaks, CA.
- **Banga AK, Reddy IK.** (1994). Biotechnology drugs: pharmaceutical issues. *Pharmacy Times*, March, 68–76.
- **Bayer AG, Co.** (1993). Kogenate® package insert. Elkart, IN.
- **Baxter Health Care Corporation.** (1992). Recombinate® package insert. Glendale, CA.
- **Berlex Laboratories.** (1994). Betaseron® package insert. Richmond, CA.
- **Check WA.** (1984). New drug and drug-delivery systems in the year 2000. *Am J Hosp Pharm*, 41, 1536–15417.
- **Chiron Therapeutics.** (1994). Proleukin® package insert. Emeryville, CA.
- **Chiron Corporation.** (1995). Proleukin® written information on storage, reconstitution, compatibility, stability, and administration on file. Emeryville, CA.
- **Genentech, Inc.** (1990). Actimune® package insert. South San Francisco, CA.
- **Genentech, Inc.** (1991). Protropin® Package insert. South San Francisco, CA.
- **Genentech, Inc.** (1994). Activase® package insert. South San Francisco, CA.
- **Genentech, Inc.** (1994b). Pulmozyme® package insert. South San Francisco, CA.
- **Genentech, Inc.** (1995). Written information on storage, reconstitution, compatibility, stability, and administration on file. South San Francisco, CA.
- **Immunex Corporation.** (1992). Leukine® package insert. Seattle, WA.
- **Immunex Corporation.** (1995). Written information on storage, reconstitution, compatibility, stability, and administration on file. Seattle, WA.
- **Koeller J, Fields S.** (1991). The pharmacist's role with biotechnology products. Kalamazoo, MI: The Upjohn Company.
- **Lilly, Eli Company.** (1994). Humatrope® package insert. Indianapolis, IN.
- **Lilly, Eli Company.** (1995). Written information on storage, reconstitution, compatibility, stability, and administration on file. Indianapolis, IN.
- **McEvoy GK.** (1995). American Hospital Formulary Service Drug Information, American Society of Health-System Pharmacists. Bethesda, MD.
- **Roche Laboratories.** (1992). Referon® package insert. Nutley, NJ.
- **Schering Laboratories.** (1994). Intron® package insert. Kennilworth, NJ.
- **Schering Laboratories.** (1995). Written information on storage, reconstitution, compatibility, stability and administration on file. Kennilworth, NJ.
- **Stewart CF, Fleming RA.** (1989). Biotechnology products: new opportunities and responsibilities for the pharmacist. *Am J Hosp Pharm*, 46 (suppl 2) S4–S8.

Self-Assessment Questions

Question 1: *What are some of the causes of pharmacist reluctance to handling biotech products?*

Question 2: *In what areas of study do pharmacists and pharmacy students need to engage to be best prepared to provide pharmaceutical care services to patients receiving biotechnology therapeutic agents?*

Question 3: *What resources are available to pharmacy practitioners to learn more about biotechnology and the drug products of biotechnology?*

Question 4: *How do the storage requirements of biotech products differ from the majority of products pharmacists normally dispense?*

Question 5: *What is the most common temperature for the storage of biotech pharmaceuticals?*

Question 6: *Why is human serum albumin added to the solution of many biotech drugs?*

Question 7: *Why should biotech products not be shaken when adding any diluent?*

Question 8: *During travel, what precautions should also be observed with biotech products?*

Question 9: *Should biotech products be filtered prior to administration?*

Question 10: *What assessments must be done by the pharmacist before a patient can be considered a candidate for home therapy with a biotech product?*

Question 11: *What types of professional services information are provided by manufacturers of biotech drugs.*

Answers

Answer 1: Lack of understanding of the basics of biotechnology, lack of understanding of the therapeutics of recombinant protein products; unfamiliarity with the side effects and patient counseling information; lack of familiarity with the storage, handling and reconstitution of proteins; and the difficulty of handling reimbursement issues.

Answer 2: Basic biotechnology/immunological methods; protein chemistry; therapeutics of biotechnology agents; storage, handling, reconstitution and administration of biotechnology products.

Answer 3: Biotechnology/immunology texts, continuing education programs, manufacturers' information and toll-free assistance, biotechnology-oriented journals, the Internet (as described in Tables 18.1–18.6).

Answer 4: The shelf life of these products is often considerably shorter than has been the case with more traditional compounds. These products need to be kept at refrigerated temperatures. There are, of course, exceptions to this rule.

Answer 5: In general, most biotech products are shipped by the manufacturer in gel ice containers and need to be stored at 2–8 °C. Once reconstituted, they should be kept under refrigeration until just prior to use.

Answer 6: Most biotech products may adhere to either plastic or glass containers such as syringes and polyvinyl chloride (PVC) intravenous bags reducing effectiveness of the product. Human serum albumin is usually added to the solutions to prevent adherence.

Answer 7: Shaking may cause the product to break down (aggregation). Usually when this happens one can observe physical separation or frothing within the vial of liquid products.

Answer 8: They should be stored in insulated, cool containers. This can be accomplished by using ice packs to keep the biotech drug at the proper temperature in warmer climates, whereas the insulated container in colder climates may be all that is required. In fact, when traveling in sub-freezing weather, the products should be protected from freezing.

Answer 9: Filtering biotech products is not generally recommended since most of the proteins will adhere to the filter.

Answer 10: Before a patient can be a candidate for home therapy, an assessment of the patient's capabilities must occur. The patient, family member, or care giver will need to be able to inject the medication and comply with all of the storage, handling, and preparation requirements.

Answer 11: Medical information services provided by manufacturers of biotech drugs are similar to the product, medical and patient management services provided by drug companies for traditional drug products. Information provided via this service generally includes appropriate indications, side effects, contraindications to use, results of clinical trials and investigational uses. Upon request, manufacturers can supply a product monograph and selected research articles that provide valuable information about each product.

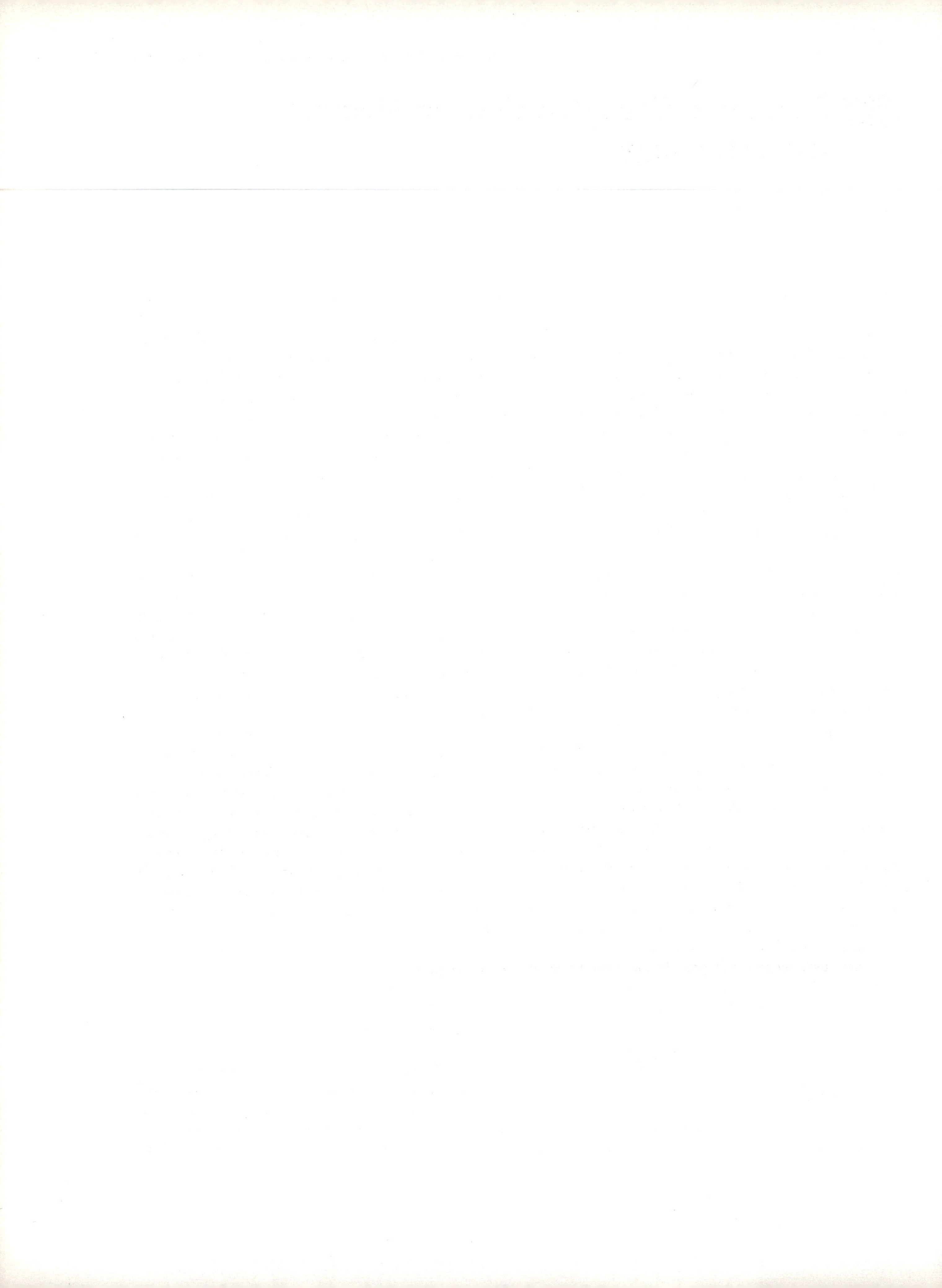

19 Economic Considerations in Medical Biotechnology

Eugene M. Kolassa

Introduction

The biotechnology revolution has coincided with another revolution in healthcare: the emergence of finance and economics as major issues in the use and success of new medical technologies. Healthcare finance has become a major social issue in nearly every nation, and the evaluation and scrutiny of the pricing and value of new treatments has become an industry unto itself. The most tangible effect of this change is the establishment of the so-called 'third hurdle' for new agents in many nations. Beyond the traditional requirements for demonstrating the efficacy and safety of new agents, some nations, and many private healthcare systems, now demand data on the economic costs and benefits of new medicines. Although currently required only in Canada (Blaker *et al.*, 1994) and Australia (Drummond, 1992), the governments of most developed nations are examining methods to extend similar prerequisites.

The licensing of new agents in most non-US nations has traditionally been accompanied by a parallel process of price and reimbursement approval, and the development of an economic dossier has emerged as a means to secure the highest possible rates of reimbursement. In recent years sets of economic guidelines have been developed and adopted by the regulatory authorities of several nations to help assist them in their decisions to reimburse new products. As many of the products of biotechnology are used to treat costly disorders, and the products themselves are often costly to discover and produce, these new agents have presented new problems to those charged with the financing of medical care delivery. The movement to require an economic rationale for the pricing of new agents brings new challenges to those developing such agents. These requirements also provide firms with new tools to help determine which new technologies will provide the most value to society, as well as contribute the greatest financial returns to those developing and marketing the products.

The Value of a New Medical Technology

The task of determining the value of a new agent should fall somewhere within the purview of the marketing function of a firm. Although some companies have established healthcare economic capabilities within the clinical research structure of their organizations, it is essential that the group that addresses the value of a new product does so from the perspective of the market and not of the company or the research team. This is important for two reasons. First, evaluating the product candidate from the perspective of the user, and not from the team that is developing it, can minimize the bias that is inherent in evaluating one's own creations. Second, and most importantly, a market focus will move the evaluation away from the technical and scientifically interesting aspects of the product under evaluation and toward the real utility the product might bring to the medical care marketplace. Although the scientific, or purely clinical, aspects of a new product should not be discounted, when it comes time to measure the economic contribution of a new agent those developing the new agent must move past these considerations. It is the tangible effects that a new treatment will have on the patient and healthcare system that determine its value, not the technology supporting it. The phrase to keep in mind is "value in use."

The importance of a marketing focus when evaluating the economic effects of a new agent, or product candidate, cannot be overstated. Failing to consider the product's value in use can result in overly optimistic expectations of sales performance and market acceptance. Marketing is often defined as the process of identifying and filling the needs of the market. If this is the case, the developers of new pharmaceutical technologies must ask "What does the market want?" Analysis of the pharmaceutical market in the first decade of the 21st Century will show that the market wants:

- lower costs
- controllable costs
- predictable cost
- improved outcomes

Note that this list does not include new therapeutic agents. From the perspective of many payers, authorities, and buyers a new agent, in and of itself, is a problem. The effort required to evaluate a new agent and prepare recommendations to adopt or reject it takes time away from other efforts. For many in the healthcare delivery system a new drug means more work. Not that they are opposed to innovation, but newness in and of itself, regardless of the technology behind it, has no intrinsic value. The value of new technologies is in their efficiency – their ability to render results that are not available through other methods or at costs significantly lower than other interventions. Documenting and understanding the economic effects of new technologies on the various healthcare systems helps the firm to allocate its resources more appropriately, accelerate the adoption of new technologies into the healthcare system, and reap the financial rewards of its innovation.

There are many different aspects of the term 'value', depending upon the perspective of the individual or group evaluating a new product and the needs that are met by the product itself. When developing new medical technologies it is useful to look to the market to determine the aspects of a product that could create and capture the greatest amount of value. Two products that have entered the market in recent years provide good examples of the different ways in which value is assessed.

Activase (tPA) from Genentech entered the market priced at nearly ten times the price level of streptokinase, its nearest competitor. This product, which is used solely in the hospital setting, significantly increased the cost of medical treatment of patients suffering myocardial infarctions. But the problems associated with streptokinase, and the great urgency of need for treatments for acute infarctions, was such that many cardiologists believed that any product that proved useful in this area would be worth the added cost. The hospitals, which in the US are reimbursed on a capitated basis for the bulk of such procedures, were essentially forced to subsidize the use of the agent, as they were unable to pass the added cost of tPA to many of their patients' insurers. The pricing of the product created a significant controversy, but the sales of Activase have been growing consistently since its launch. The key driver of value for tPA has been, and continues to be, the urgency of the underlying condition. The ability of the product to reduce the rate of immediate mortality is what drives its value.

A product that delivers a different type of value is the colony stimulating factor from Amgen (G-CSF, Neupogen). Neupogen was priced well below its economic value. The product's primary benefit is in the reduction of serious infections in cancer patients, who often suffer significant decreases in white blood cells due to chemotherapy. By bolstering the white count, Neupogen allows oncologists to use more efficacious doses of cytotoxic oncology agents while decreasing the rate of infection and subsequent hospitalizations for cancer patients. It has been estimated that the use of Neupogen reduces the expected cost of treating infections by roughly $6,000 per cancer patient per course of therapy. At a price of roughly $1,400 per course of therapy, Neupogen not only provides better clinical care, but also offers savings of approximately $4,600 per patient. The economic benefits of the product have helped it to rapidly gain use, with significantly fewer restrictions than products such as tPA, whose economic value is not as readily apparent.

These two very successful products provide clear clinical benefits, but their sources of value are quite different. The value of a new product may come from several sources, depending on the needs of clinicians and their perceptions of the situations in which they treat patients. Some current treatments bring risk, either because of the uncertainty of their effects on the patient (positive or negative) or because of the effort or cost required to use or understand a treatment. A new product that reduces this risk will be perceived as bringing new value to the market. In such cases, the new product removes or reduces some negative aspects of treatment. Neupogen, by reducing the chance of infection and reducing the average cost of treatment brought new value to the marketplace in this manner.

Value can come from the enhancement of the positive aspects of treatment, as well. A product that has a higher rate of efficacy than current therapies is the most obvious example of such a case. But any product that provides benefits in an area of critical need, where few or no current treatments are available, will be seen as providing immediate value. This was, and remains, the case for tPA.

Any new product under development should be evaluated with these aspects of value in mind. A generalized model of value, presented in Figure 19.1 below, can be used to determine the areas of greatest need in the marketplace for a new agent, and to provide guidance in product development. By talking with clinicians, patients, and others involved in current treatments, and keeping this model in mind, the shortcomings of those approaches can be evaluated and the sources of new incremental value can be determined.

Understanding the source of the value brought to the market by a new product is crucial to the development of the eventual marketing strategy. Using Figure 19.1 as a guide, the potential sources of value can be determined for a product candidate and appropriate studies, both clinical and economic, can be designed to measure and demonstrate that value.

An Overview of Economic Analysis for new Technologies

A thorough economic analysis should be used to guide the clinical research protocol, to be sure the endpoints measured are commercially relevant and useful. It should describe important elements of the market to the firm, helping

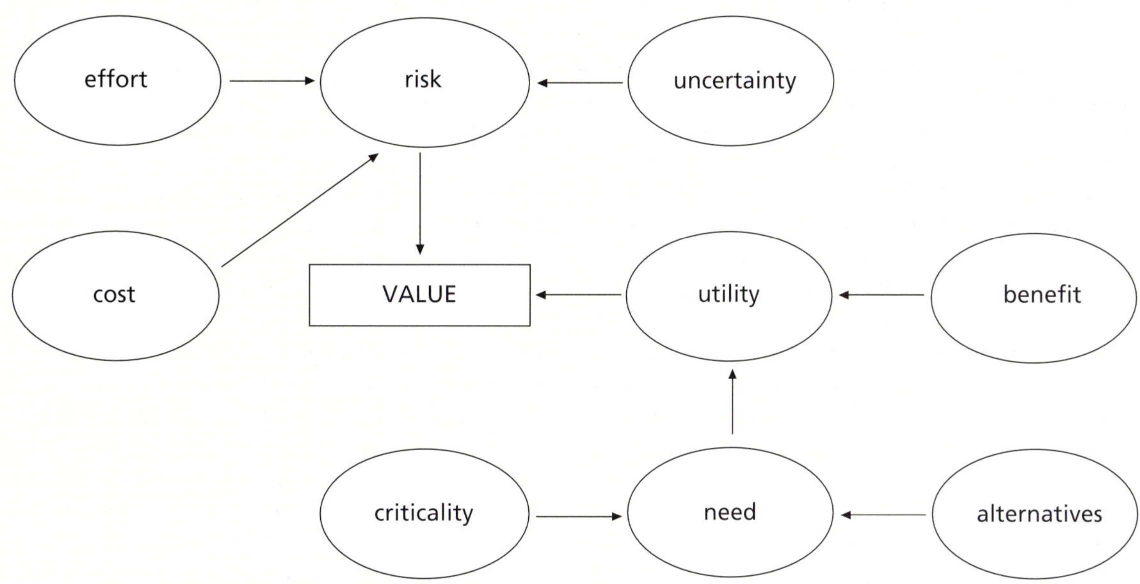

Figure 19.1. Generalized model of value.

decision-makers to understand the way decisions are made and to provide guidance in affecting those decisions. Later, the results of economic analyses should inform and guide marketing and pricing decisions as the product is prepared for launch, as well as help customers to use products efficiently and effectively.

To prepare a thorough economic analysis, the researchers must first seek to have a comprehensive understanding of the flow of patients, services, goods, and money through the various healthcare systems. This process should begin as soon as the likely indications for a new product have been identified, and continue throughout the development process. The first step is to create basic economic models of the current treatment for the disorder(s) for which the product is likely to be indicated. This step will be used to provide better information to fine-tune financial assumptions and to provide critical input into the clinical development process to assure that the clinical protocols are designed to extract the greatest commercial potential from the product. If the product is likely to be used for more than one indication, and/or if there is the potential that several different levels of the same indication (e.g. mild, moderate, and severe) would be treated by the same product, separate models should be prepared for each indication and level.

The purpose of the basic model is to provide a greater understanding of the costs associated with the disorder and to identify areas and types of cost that provide the greatest potential for the product to generate cost savings. For example, the cost of a disorder that currently requires a significant amount of laboratory testing offers the potential for savings, and thus better pricing, if the new product can reduce or eliminate the need for tests. Similarly, some indications, such as prophylaxis for deep vein thrombosis (DVT) in hip replacement surgeries, are well treated, but the incidence of side-effects is sufficiently high to warrant special attention. In the case of DVT prophylaxis, presented in Tables 19.1 through 19.3, the introduction of low molecular weight heparin significantly reduced the incidence and cost of DVT and pulmonary emboli, but did little to affect the rate of bleeding episodes. In this case, any new drug for DVT prophylaxis must reduce the episodes of bleeding in order to deliver economic savings, and be able to command a premium over current choices. A new agent that delivers equal rates of reduction of thromboembolic events without a reduction in bleeding will bring no new value to the market, whereas one that is equally efficacious and provides a reduction in bleeding episodes also brings new value.

These figures are based on work performed by Alan Bakst, Pharm.D., at the Cleveland Clinic (Bakst, 1995). The resultant article provides very useful background on the performance and use of economic analysis.

The starting point for the analysis is to consider the incidence of complications from hip replacement surgery. As can be seen in Table 19.1, enoxaparin renders significant reductions in thrombosis and emboli, when compared with warfarin and standard heparin. Moving to Table 19.2, which lists the costs of treating these complications, enoxaparin significantly reduces the incidence of some of

	low dose Warfarin	Heparin 5K u TID	Enoxaparin 30 mg BID
proximal deep vein thrombosis	5%	4.8%	2%
distal deep vein thrombosis	19%	5.3%	2%
non-fatal pulmonary embolism	2.7%	1.9%	0.1%
major bleeding episode	3.6%	6.2%	4.1%
minor bleeding episode	6.9%	5.7%	8.2%

Table 19.1. Incidence of complications in hip replacements.

	cost of treatment
major bleeding episode	$ 2,791
minor bleeding episode	$ 189
non-fatal pulmonary embolism	$ 6,510
proximal deep vein thrombosis	$ 1,394
distal deep vein thrombosis	$ 860

Table 19.2. Cost of treatment of complications of hip replacement.

the costly complications, but the cost of dealing with bleeding episodes is still high.

Combining the incidence and cost data it is possible to derive a set of expected costs for each treatment option. As Table 19.3 demonstrates, prophylaxis with enoxaparin results in significantly lower costs.

What is left unaddressed by these tables, however, is the next important source of value for new products used in this indication. Reductions in bleeding episodes with no loss of efficacy in the prevention of thrombo-embolic events would bring new value to the market.

From this basic model it can be determined that a primary endpoint of measurement for clinical trials, and a desirable feature of any new product, should be the reduction of bleeding episodes. Success on this measure will determine whether a new biotechnology-produced product can command a premium over current therapies or must compete on price with those already on the market.

Pharmacoeconomics

The field of economic evaluation of medical technologies goes by several names, depending on the discipline of the researchers undertaking the study and the type of technology being measured. For pharmaceutical and biotechnology products, the field has settled in on the name of pharmacoeconomics, and an entire discipline has emerged

	Warfarin	Heparin	Enoxaparin
major bleeding episode	$ 100,476	$ 173,042	$ 114,431
minor bleeding episode	$ 13,041	$ 10,773	$ 15,498
non-fatal pulmonary embolism	$ 175,770	$ 123,690	$ 6,510
proximal deep vein thrombosis	$ 69,700	$ 66,912	$ 27,880
distal deep vein thrombosis	$ 163,400	$ 45,580	$ 17,200
total/1000 pts (complications only)	$ 522,387	$ 419,997	$ 181,519

Table 19.3. Expected cost of treating 1000 patients for the complications of hip surgery by method of prophylaxis.

to fill the needs of the area. Contributions to the development of the field have come from several disciplines, including economics, pharmacy administration, and many of the behavioral sciences.

In recent years a set of pharmacoeconomic standards, or guidelines, has been generally accepted by researchers and health system authorities. These standards have helped to establish a common set of techniques and a general preference for the type of analysis used. The predominant analytical techniques are Cost-Effectiveness Analysis (CEA) and Cost-Utility Analysis (CUA), which is derived from CEA and is often much more useful and meaningful. In a CEA of a product such as tissue plasminogen activator (tPA) for use in myocardial infarction, typical measures used for the analysis would be the cost of saving an additional life (or preventing a death). This measure would be extended using life expectancy tables to determine the cost of providing a patient with an additional year of life. This measure is called the "Cost per Life Year Saved."

As patients are often left with less than ideal functional status and quality of life after a serious medical event, it is desirable to consider the outcome from the perspective of the patient and to factor in any reductions in quality of life. CUA allows researchers to factor in such differences, called patient preferences, by applying different weights to the value of additional years of life gained, depending on the functional status of the patient. In the case of myocardial infarction, a significant proportion of patients who survive will find their abilities to participate in strenuous recreational activities impaired, which would reduce the quality of life for many patients, compared with those in a more ideal health state. CUA reduces the value of the additional years of life gained through the specific treatment under evaluation. The resultant revised figure is called a Quality-Adjusted Life Year, or "QALY." The cost of achieving a QALY has become such a common measure in pharmacoeconomic evaluations that the Canadian Government uses this figure to determine the appropriateness of the reimbursement of new agents.

Under the Canadian system, a product that renders a cost per QALY gained of $50,000 (Canadian) or less will be generally accepted into the system an reimbursed without difficulty. Products delivering an additional QALY for $100,000 or more will not be reimbursed, while those with costs between $50,000 and $100,000 will be subjected to more study, scrutiny, and negotiation. The Canadian Coordination Office for Health Technology Assessment conducts many of its own studies to determine the value of new products, and these studies are routinely made available to the public. Copies of the studies can be downloaded from the Internet at www.ccohta.ca.

It has been estimated that each year over 600 health economics studies are published, and that each pharmaceutical company, on average, begins 23 new studies (Boston Consulting Group, 1993). The basic goal of such studies is to determine the value of pharmaceutical products.

It is important for a company to conduct and support research that determines or establishes the value of a product it is about to introduce, but it is important to understand that the value upon which a price should be based is the value to the customer – not the marketer. As such, one must look to a conservative and rather narrow definition of value as a starting point.

The first, and perhaps most important measure of value to determine after the economic studies have been completed is the break even or "zero-based" value. This value is derived by modeling the new product into the treatment process, as determined through a burden of illness study, and measuring the difference with and without the new product, which has been assigned a cost of $0. The "economic value" of the new product is the difference between the two treatment approaches: the cost of the original treatment minus the cost of treatment with the new product. Ideally, the treatment with the new product results in lower costs than treatment without it. The alternative, that treatment with the new product is more costly than treatment without, requires serious decisions as to the launch of the product.

The economic value of the product may have elements besides the basic economic efficiency implied by the break even level just discussed. Quality differences, in terms of reduced side-effects, greater efficacy, or other substantive factors can result in increases in value beyond the break-even point calculated in a simple cost comparison. Should these factors be present, it is crucial to capture that value in the price of the product – but how much value should be captured?

It is important to recognize that a product can provide a significant economic benefit in one indication but none in another. Therefore it is prudent to perform these studies on all indications considered for a new product. A case in point is that of erythropoietin α (EPO). Initially developed and approved for use in dialysis patients, where its principle benefit is to reduce, or even eliminate, the need for transfusion, studies have shown that EPO doses that drive hematocrit levels to between 33% and 36% result in significantly lower total patient care costs than when used at lower doses or not at all (Collins *et al.*, 2000). The same product, when used to reduce the need for transfusion in elective surgery, however, has been shown not to be cost effective (Coyle *et al.*, 1999). Although EPO was shown to reduce the need for transfusion in this study, the cost of the drug far outweighed the savings from reduced transfusions, as well as reductions in the transmission and reatment of blood-born pathogens. Economic efficiency is not automatically transferred from one indication to another.

The lack of economic savings in the surgical indication does not necessarily mean that the product should not be used in that manner, only that users recognize that this use results in substantially higher costs where EPO use in dialysis actually reduces the total cost of care.

In the pharmaceutical marketing environment of the foreseeable future, it is wise to consider surrendering some value to the market – pricing the product at some point below the full economic value of the product. This is appealing for several reasons:

- the measurement of economics is imprecise, and the margin for error can be large;
- if the market is looking for lower costs, filling that need enhances the market potential of the product;
- from a public relations and public policy perspective, launching a new product with the message that it provides savings to the system can also provide positive press and greater awareness.

As society continues to focus on the cost of healthcare interventions we must all be concerned about the economic and clinical implications of the products we bring into the system. Delivering value, in the form of improved outcomes, economic savings, or both, is an important part of pharmaceutical science. Understanding the value that is delivered should be the responsibility of everyone involved with new product development. ■

Further Reading on pharmacoeconomic methods

- **Bootman JL, Townsend JT, McGhan WF.** (1991). *Principles of Pharmacoeconomics*, Harvey Whitney Books.
- **Bonk RJ.** (1999). *Pharmacoeconomics in Perspective*, Haworth Press.
- **Drummond, O'Brien, Stoddart, Torrance** (1997). *Methods for the Economic Evaluation of Health Care Programmes*, 2nd Edition, Oxford: Oxford University Press.

Further Reading on pharmacoeconomics of biotechnology drugs

- **Hui JW, Yee GC.** (1998). Pharmacoeconomics of Biotechnology Drugs (Part 1 of 2). *Journal of the American Pharmaceutical Association*, **38(1)**, 97–98.
- **Hui JW, Yee GC.** (1998). Pharmacoeconomics of Biotechnology Drugs (Part 2 of 2). *Journal of the American Pharmaceutical Association*, **38(2)**, 231–233.
- **Reeder CE.** (1995). Pharmacoeconomics and health care outcomes management: Focus on biotechnology (special supplement). *American Journal of Health-System Pharmacy*, **52**(19,S4), S1–S28.

References

- **Bakst A.** (1995). Pharmacoeconomics and the Formulary Decision-making Process, *Hospital Formulary*, **30** (January), 42–50.
- **Blaker D, Detsky A, Hubbard E, Kennedy W, Konchak R, Menon D, Schubert F, Torrence G, Tugwell P.** (1994). Guidelines for Economic Evaluation of Pharmaceuticals: Canada, *Draft of Report of the Steering Committee*, February 1.
- **Boston Consulting Group.** (1993). *The Changing Environment For U.S. Pharmaceuticals*, Boston: Boston Consulting Group, April.
- **Collins-AJ, Li-S, Ebben-J, Ma-JZ, Manning-W.** (2000). Hematocrit levels and associated Medicare expenditures. *American Journal of Kidney Diseases*, **36/2**. 282–93.
- **Coyle D, Lee K, Laupacis A, Fergusson D.** (1999). Economic Analysis of Erythopoietin in Surgery, Canadian Coordinating Office of Health Technology Assessment, 3/9/99.
- **Drummond M.** (1992). Australian Guidelines for Cost-Effectiveness Studies of Pharmaceuticals: The Thin Edge of the Boomerang?, *PharmacoEconomics*, **1** (suppl. 1), 61–69.

20 Biotechnology Products in the Pipeline

Ronald P. Evens and Robert D. Sindelar

Introduction

The information assembled in preceding chapters of this book provides ample evidence to support the statement that biotechnology represents an enormous resource for drug discovery and development. Pharmaceutical biotechnology contributes to substantial advances in health care. These contributions include, (1) a greater understanding of the cause and progression of diseases, (2) the development of novel pharmacological screening methods to identify new pharmaceuticals, (3) the production of biopharmaceuticals being tested for the first time against several diseases, (4) the creation of innovative technologies for optimizing drug development, (5) improvements in the methods used to manufacture protein and peptide-based biopharmaceuticals, and finally (6) identification of new disease targets and therapeutic agents through genomics. With the advances in genomics and proteomics, biotechnology and various related techniques will continue to expand their influence in all areas of the drug discovery process and play a pivotal role in shaping the pharmaceuticals that will be dispensed in the future.

Drug Development and Biotechnology

Over the past 25 years, from the mid-1970s, when the first human gene was cloned, to the present, molecular biological technologies have assumed an important position along with established disciplines, such as organic chemistry and medicinal chemistry, in the field of drug discovery and development. Biotechnology has been responsible for developing and marketing over 75 products for therapeutic use, comprised of 65 different molecules, in the United States, Europe and Japan from 1982 to 2000 (Table 20.1). Most of the molecules are glycosylated proteins and include biological response modifiers (BRMs), hematopoietic growth factors (HGFs), enzymes, hormones, monoclonal antibodies (MAbs), and vaccines. About 35 different companies are responsible for these 75 products; however, over 1200 biotechnology companies in the US and 400 in Europe are conducting basic research, and over 100 companies had more than 360 molecules in human clinical trials in 1999 in the USA alone (Lee Jr. and Burrill, 1995; Evens *et al.*, 1995a; Evens *et al.*, 1995b; Pharmaceutical Research and Manufacturers of America, 2000).

Time and Cost of Modern Drug Discovery

Modern drug development is still a slow and expensive process. The time from discovery of a drug to market availability for a product is quite lengthy, ranging from 8 years to 20 years, as suggested by the New York Times (New York Times, 1995) (Figure 20.1). Research investment is substantial and risky, about $10 billion in 1998 by biotechnology companies, along with about $20 billion by traditional drug manufacturers, of which a significant percentage is devoted to biotechnology as well. The cost to bring a conventional, small molecule drug to market was estimated to be about $800 to $880 million, according to two recent independent studies in 2002 (DiMasi JA, 2002). A study of drug development by Merck and Co. found a marketing success rate of only 5% for 140 leading drug candidates: all 140 drugs made it through preclinical animal testing, 65 made it through Phase I trials (human safety), 27 made it through Phase II trials (efficacy), 9 made it through Phase III trials (large-scale safety and efficacy), and 7 were approved for marketing (Shapiro, 1995). An approximate time frame for each phase of these trials in Phase I – up to 1 year, II – up to 2 years, and III – 1–4 years with a FDA review time of 2 months-7 years (New York Times, 1995). Biotechnology products experience a similar complex process in success rates and time frames. For 1993 and 1996, clinical research was terminated in over 30 biologicals during Phase III, after successful Phase II trials, while product approvals numbered only four. The time frame for clinical trials with biologicals was calculated to be 3.4 years. Review times have been reduced in the US to about 12 months or less, due to user fees being paid by companies to the FDA for drug submissions, permitting the FDA to hire more staff and expedite the review process. Also, fast track status for these regulatory reviews is available for new treatments for life-threatening or catastrophic diseases, reducing FDA review times further to 3–6 months. (Bienz-Tadmor, 1993; Struck, 1994).

Product	Class [a]	Product	Class [a]
Abciximab	MAb	Insulin (3)	hormone
Acelluvax	vaccine	Interferon alfa (5)	BRM
Aldesleukin	BRM	Interferon alfa con	BRM
Alteplase	enzyme	Interferon beta (2)	BRM
Antihemophilic Factor VIII (2)[b]	enzyme	Interferon gamma	BRM
Basiliximab	MAb	Lenograstim	HGF
Capromab pentetate	MAb/Dx	Liposomal agents (5)	Liposome
Daclizumab	MAb	Lyme disease	vaccine
Denileukin diftitox	BRM	Molgramostim	HGF
DNase	enzyme	Muromonab-CD3	MAb
Entanercept	BRM	Nartograstim	HGF
Epoetin alfa (6)	HGF	Nefotumomab	MAb/Dx
Eptifibatide	enzyme	Oprelvekin	BRM
Filgrastim	HGF	Panorex	MAb
Factor VII	enzyme	Palivizumab	MAb
Factor IX	enzyme	Peg-Interferon (2)	BRM
Follitropin (2)	hormone	Polymer-BCNU	Drug delivery
Ganirelix	peptide	Rituximab	MAb
Gemtuzumab	MAb	Reteplase	enzyme
Glatiramer	BRM	Sargramostim	HGF
Glucagon	hormone	Somatropin (6)	hormone
Growth hormone releasing hormone	hormone	Satumomab Pendetide	MAb/Dx
Hepatitis B Vaccine (2)	vaccine	Tenecteplase	enzyme
Hyaluronate acid materials	Surgical adjuncts	Tirobifan	enzyme
Imiglucerase	enzyme	Trastuzumab	MAb
Imiciromab pentetate	MAb/dx	Vitravene	NA
Infliximab	MAb		

Table 20.1. Marketed biotechnology-produced pharmaceuticals.
a. Abbreviations include: MAb = monoclonal antibody; MAb/dx = MAb for diagnosis, HGF = hematopoietic growth factor; BRM = biological response modifier, NA = nucleic acid molecule.
b. The numbers in parentheses indicate the approximate number of products of the same molecule manufactured by different companies.

Techniques of Biotech Drug Discovery

Drug research (including discovery, lead optimization, preclinical, formulation efforts, etc.) and drug development (including safety studies, proof of efficacy, etc.) in the biotechnology era are evolving rapidly with the development of many new technologies and the production of novel types of molecules. Technology platforms are an exciting area of rapid evolution. There has been a significant paradigm shift in the types of technology platforms commonly utilized for drug discovery, optimization and lead development resulting from rapid biotechnology advances coupled with the exponential growth in computer capabilities. (Table 20.2). Before 1990, various molecular biological techniques such as rDNA, hybridoma technology and PCR were the cornerstones of biotechnology and as such, were making a significant impact on the drug discovery and development process. However, several new technologies are now available and advancing drug development with greater variety and sophistication.

During the 1970s and 1980s, organs, tissues, and cells were studied successfully to find proteins responsible for physiological responses in animals. For example, erythropoietin (Epoetin alpha) is produced by kidney cells, is secreted into the blood, and stimulates bone marrow to produce red blood cells. This conventional technique of drug discovery still accounts for many biologicals in clinical research to date, and biotechnology has made major

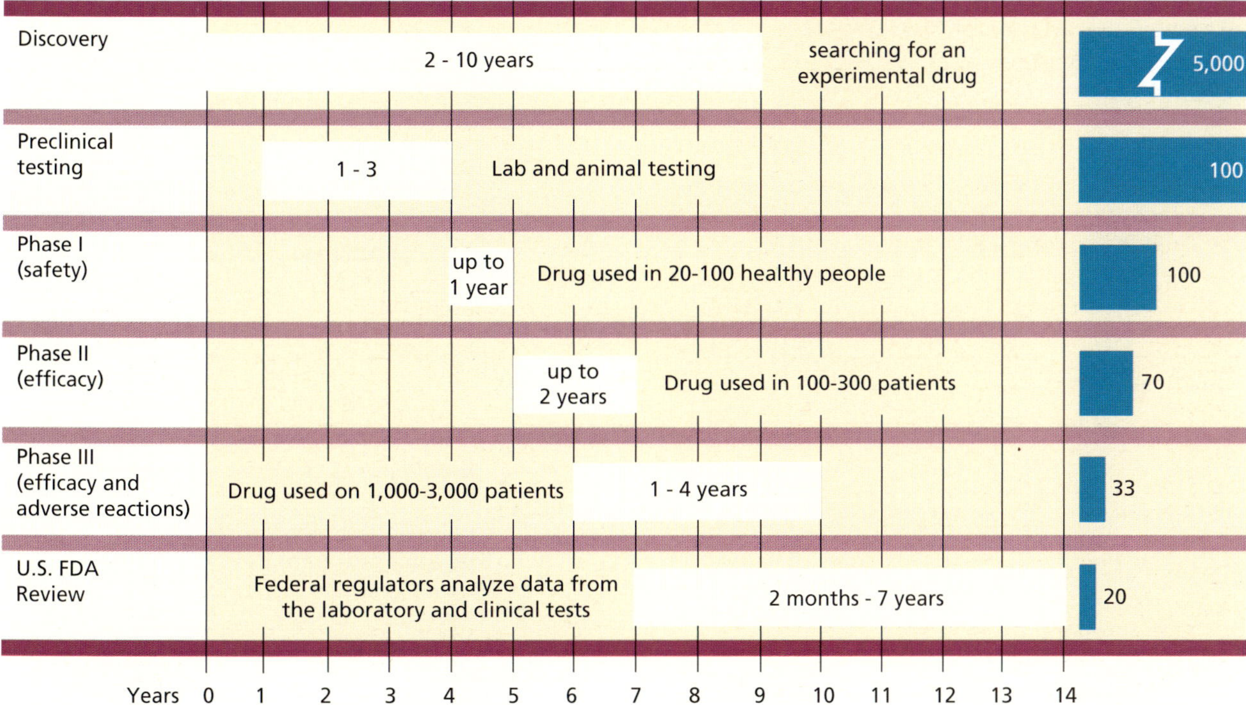

Figure 20.1. The drug development process from discovery to marketing (Modified from the New York Times, September 1995).

contributions to such discoveries. Innovations in small molecule drug-development technology, however, are providing unique ways of narrowing down choices and screening likely drug candidates. As described in detail in Chapter 6, one of the most powerful tools in the 1990s is combinatorial chemistry (Figure 20.2), a mix-and-match process in which a simple subunit (e.g. a six-membered-heterocycle with an ethylene substituent, a modified peptide, etc.) is joined to one or more other simple subunits (e.g. a four carbon olefin, a modified amino acid, etc.) in every possible combination (Maulik and Patel, 1997). Assigning the task to automated synthesizing equipment results in the rapid creation of large collections or "libraries" of diverse molecules, which can be quickly screened pharmacologically via high throughput screening (see Chapter 6) to identify the most active compound for a given therapeutic target. Combinatorial approaches to parallel synthesis may have an even greater impact on drug lead optimization studies. In most cases today, biotechnology contributes directly to the understanding, identification an/or the generation of the drug targets used in high-throughput screens (e.g. radioligand-binding displacement from a cloned protein receptor). Thus, thousands of novel chemical structures can be generated, screened and evaluated for further development in a matter of weeks rather than months or years as previously was the case. Advances in molecular medicine may now occur in a more rapid, less costly process.

Biotechnology contributes to another major resource for drug development; the identification and localization of gene sequence databases generated by the Human Genome Project (HGP) and other large-scale genome-sequencing programs associated with private genomic companies such as Celera, Incyte, Millenium, Myriad, Affymetrix, and Human Genome Sciences. An international venture, the Human Genome Project (HGP) was to construct detailed genetic and physical maps of each of the 23 different human chromosomes. Identifying the exact location and identity of all the human genes increases significantly the possibility of being able to predict the occurrence of thousands of known, and as of yet unknown, diseases with a strong genetic component. In 1999, the Human Genome Project and Celera Company both announced completion of the full sequencing of the human genome, a major landmark of scientific achievement to start the 21st Century [with publications appearing in 2001 (Vinter *et al.*, 2001; The Genome International Sequencing Consortium, 2001)]. Early disease detection and increased options for prevention and treatment are likely to be products of these efforts. Daily discoveries generated by these genomic companies and the Human Genome Project have resulted in critically important, novel molecular target databases for drug design. Automated sequencing equipment, sequencing by hybridization and "DNA on chip" methods ensure that these already large databases will continue to grow rapidly.

Technology Platforms for Drug Discovery and Development

1970s and 1980s

- Recombinant DNA (Cloning and Expression)
- Hybridoma technology (monoclonal antibodies)
- Polymerase chain reaction
- Drug lead optimization via new synthetic methodology (one molecule at a time)
- Electrophoretic analysis
- Gene sequencing

1990s and 2000 +

- Antisense technology
- Bioinformatics
- Cloning of animals
- Combinatorial chemistry (for drug lead optimization and discovery)
- Gene therapy
- Genomics
- High throughput screening
- Peptidomimetics
- Proteomics
- Macromolecular X-ray crystallography (routine)
- Transgenic animals

Table 20.2. The paradigm shift in types of technology platforms commonly utilized for drug discovery, optimization and lead development resulting from advances in biotechnology and computers over time are outlined.

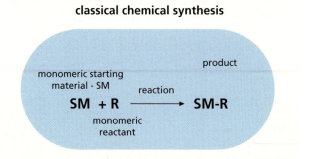

classical chemical synthesis

In classical chemical synthesis, a coupling reaction of one monomeric starting material with one monomeric reactant would yield just one product, SM-R.

combinatorial chemical synthesis

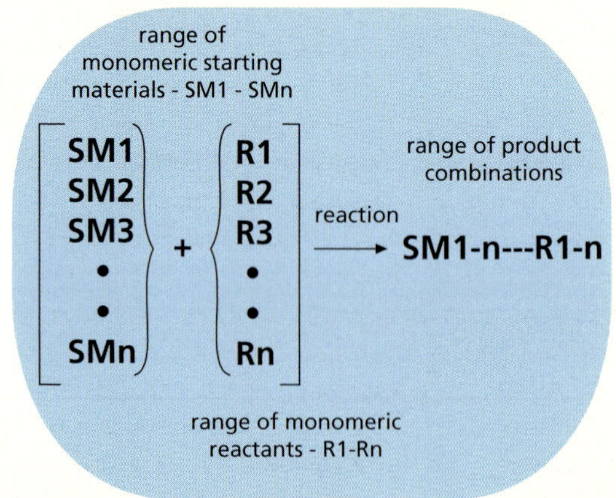

In combinatorial chemical synthesis, a coupling reaction of a range of monomeric starting materials with a range of monomeric reactants would yield any or all product combinations, SM1-n---R1-n.

Figure 20.2. Representation of the process of combinatorial chemistry (Cf. chapter 6, figure 17).

Major social, ethical and legal concerns, however, can accompany the use of any new technology. The unprecedented insights into human genetics and disease resulting from the sequencing of the human genome and efforts to realize its full potential raise societal questions concerning an individual's right to privacy versus who should have access to this rapidly increasing bank of knowledge. An informed society must initiate discussion and consider all these issues that are of critical importance.

Other information, including drug target structural data generated by X-ray crystallography and nuclear magnetic resonance techniques, also continue to accrue rapidly. Fast computers with cheap memory, massive storage, and 3-D simulation redrawing programs have made possible the large scale accessing and manipulation of this biological information for drug development. Large-scale gene-transfer techniques, perfected by Jaenisch and others in the early 1990s, enable the creation of transgenic rats and mice in which human diseases can be mimicked (see Chapter 6 for details). Also important is the use of rodents with one gene turned off, or "knocked out". These knockout animals provide insights into the causes of disease and "how missing genes and/or proteins function", and make accelerated development of new drugs possible. Transgenic mouse models now exist for hyperglyceridemia, Lesch-Nynan syndrome, hypertension, liver cancer, rheumatoid arthritis, cystic fibrosis, brain cancer, kidney cancer, scrapie/prion disease, and many others. This tremendous explosion of biological, product, and genomic data from all these technologies, e.g. combinatorial chemistry, genomics, proteomics, X-ray crystallography, and transgenics, needs to be stored and integrated to optimize the drug development process, which has created a whole new science of bioinformatics.

Classes of Molecules Being Discovered and Studied Through Biotechnology

The types of molecules being discovered and studied through biotechnology have broadened substantially over the past decade (Table 20.3). Proteins remain a major emphasis of research with active classes including additional hematopoietic growth factors (HGFs), biological response modifiers (BRMs) and other cytokines, enzymes and hormones (e.g. clotting factors, tissue plasminogen activators, etc.), vaccines (for cancer, AIDS, rheumatoid arthritis and multiple sclerosis, to list a few), and monoclonal antibodies (Table 20.3). Other novel classes of drug protein molecules are now being discovered including tissue/bone and nerve growth factors, soluble receptors and fusion molecules. Peptide drugs and peptidomimetics (see Chapter 6) are important adjuncts to typical biotechnology strategies. Nucleic acid based therapies, e.g. gene therapies (see Chapter 7), therapies using antisense molecules (see Chapter 6), and ribozymes (see Chapter 6), are being tested. Gene therapy is a rapidly growing category of biotechnology products under development (Pharmaceutical Research and Manufacturers of America, 2000). We also have carbohydrate-based pharmaceuticals and other products of glycobiology (see Chapter 6) being examined. Exciting technologies are developing using whole cells such as stem cells in autologous transplant therapy of cancer and in allogenic transplants in utero for bloodborne genetic diseases.

In Chapter 4, attention is paid to the issue of protein delivery by microencapsulated, secretory cells. The first clinical trials are now in progress to further evaluate the potentials and limitations of this exciting concept of microencapsulated protein secreting cells designed to self-regulate protein-drug release. The bottom line of Table 20.3 speaks about delivery systems for biotechnology drugs. In Chapters 3 and 4, the problems regarding the delivery of protein drugs are extensively discussed. Finding alternative routes of administration to the parenteral route, such as through a safe absorption enhancing system, would be highly desirable as it would make the administration of biotech products more patient friendly. Significant effort is being made to improve drug efficiency and reduce toxicity through the development of systems for release rate control (e.g. implants), or for site specific delivery including drug targeting with liposomes.

Structural manipulation of proteins serves to change the pharmacokinetics and perhaps the pharmacologic activities of the biological molecules. Pegylation employs the polyethyleneglycol molecule attached to a protein to prolong the half life of the protein (see Chapter 5). Interferons are being pegylated, as well as filgrastim, to produce whole new molecules with such unique properties. The benefit can be less frequent administration with at least equivalent biologic responses. Also, the epoetin alfa molecule has been altered by site-directed mutagenesis changing 5 amino acids, permitting hyperglycosylation of the protein. Hyperglycosylation adds several sialic acid carbohydrate moieties to the protein backbone, creating a novel molecule with extended duration of activity. The new erythropoietic molecule, darbepoietin, has a half life that is about three times longer than the parent drug. Studies in anemia of kidney disease show that a dose once or every other week was as effective as standard 2–3 times a week dosing in dialysis patients with anemia (Macdougall *et al.*, 1999).

Protein pharmaceuticals
Biological response modifiers and other cytokines Interferons Interleukins Enzymes Clotting factors Dismutases Tissue plasminogen activators Hormones Growth factors Hematopoietic growth factors Tissue/bone growth factors Neurotropic factors Recombinant protein vaccines Monoclonal antibodies Diagnostic antibodies Therapeutic antibodies Recombinant soluble receptors Fusion molecules
Peptides and peptidomimetics
Nucleic acid therapies with:
Genes Oncogenes Ribozymes Antisense molecules Telomeres and telomerase
Carbohydrate-based pharmaceuticals and other products of glycobiology
Whole cells
Blood Cells Epidermal Cells
Delivery systems for biotechnology drugs

Table 20.3. Types of biotechnology pharmaceuticals, adjunct pharmaceuticals and technologies in development today.

It is always difficult to predict which new products might be approved by regulatory agencies worldwide in any given year and what their impact on pharmaceutical care will be. For instance, several monoclonal antibodies and a soluble receptor protein were hailed as major advances in therapy for the treatment of septic shock, but the US Food and Drug Administration, however, has denied approval of these products because Phase III pivotal trials failed to demonstrate efficacy. Monoclonal antibodies (MAbs) were suggested as the panaceas to treat many diseases in the 1970s, but by 1990 only one product was approved for use. However, in the 1990s, eight MAbs have been approved due to major advances in MAb product development, that is, humanization of the original murine MAb molecules. MAbs have four primary protein components, all of which are murine in origin, and the new molecules have most of these murine components changed to human components, which decreases side effects and may increase activity of the molecules (see Chapter 13).

For the remainder of this section, we present a selection of some potential biotechnology pharmaceuticals that are in the development pipeline. Figure 20.3 and Tables 20.4–20.11 provide a breakdown by class of the biotech drugs in development in the US. The tables are not intended to be definitive or all-inclusive and will be somewhat dated due to the rapid changes occurring each day in the pharmaceutical and biotech industries. Brief explanatory notes are provided for some, but not all of the products.

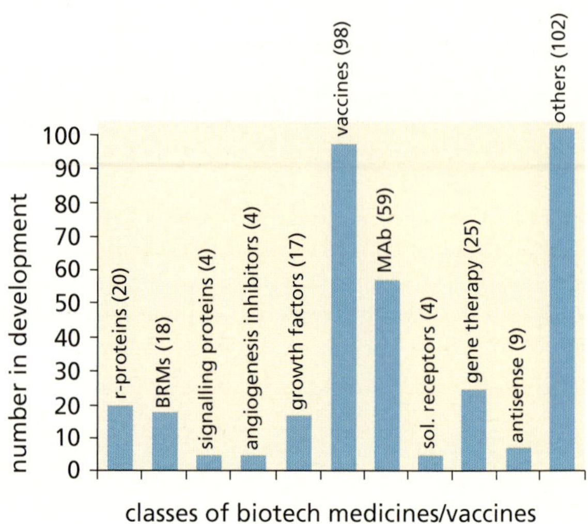

Figure 20.3. Biotech drugs in development in the U.S. Data taken from Pharmaceutical Manufacturers Association 2000

Some Protein Pharmaceuticals in Development

The "early" period of biotechnology (1970s and 1980s) was defined by the development of proteins of known source and function. Recombinant insulin, tissue plasminogen activator, Factor VIII, granulocyte colony-stimulating factor (G-CSF), and interferons all derive from this style of biotechnology drug development, and the trend continues as many new native proteins with therapeutic value are discovered. Protein products in clinical trials as of 2000 include at least nine categories of proteins and over 200 molecules (Pharmaceuticals Research and Manufacturers of America, 2000).

Hematopoietic Growth Factors, Interferons and Interleukins

A list of some biotechnology-derived colony-stimulating factors, interferons and interleukins in various stages of clinical trials (Pharmaceuticals Research and Manufacturers of America, 2000) can be found in Table 20.4a,b. Some examples are described below.

Hematopoietic Growth Factors

Many times, clinical trials examine currently approved protein products for additional therapeutic indications. Examples include the use of filgrastim (recombinant granulocyte colony stimulating factor, rG-CSF) in allogeneic progenitor cell transplants and Crohn's disease and sargramostim (granulocyte macrophage-colony stimulating factor, GM-CSF) for the prophylaxis and treatment of chemotherapy-induced neutropenia, and the prevention of infection in very low birth weight infants.

Interferons

Interferons in each sub class (α, β, or γ) are available, and clinical research primarily focuses on new indications with only a few new products, principally of second generation nature, e.g. pegylated interferons. These molecules are longer acting, and thus, may be administered once weekly instead of three times a week.

Interleukins

Interleukins, as intercellular communication proteins, continue to be targets for drug development. As described earlier in this text, they bind to receptors on the surface of target cells and stimulate cellular activity including proliferation and cytotoxicity. Many different cells display interleukin receptors on their surface, including monocytes, megakaryocytes, neutrophils, myeloma cells and blast cells. Because of their proliferative effect on hematopoietic stem cells, several ILs currently are in clinical trials for treatment

Hematopoietic Growth Factors (HGFs)		
Product	**Company**	**Indication**
Sargramostim (GM-CSF)	Immunex	prophylaxis and treatment of chemotherapy-induced neutropenia
		reduction of post-operative infections, neonatal sepsis, prevention of infection in very low birth weight infants
Darbepoietin (ARANESP)	Amgen	anemia related to kidney disease, cancer, and chronic disease
Filgrastim (rG-CSF)	Amgen	allogeneic blood cell transplants, Crohn's disease
Filgrastim SD-01	Amgen	prophylaxis and treatment of chemotherapy-induced neutropenia
Progenipoietin	Searle	treatment of chemotherapy-induced neutropenia
Ancestim (Stem cell factor)	Amgen	adjunct to chemotherapy, improving blood cell transplantation
Platelet Factors		
Product	**Company**	**Indication**
Thrombopoietin	Pharmacia	treatment of chemotherapy-induced thrombocytopenia
Interferons (INFs)		
Product	**Company**	**Indication**
Recombinant interferon beta	Serono Laboratories	malignant diseases unresponsive to standard therapies, hepatitis C, relapsing, remitting and secondary progressive multiple sclerosis

Table 20.4a. Some biotechnology-derived protein products in various stages of clinical trials: CSFs and INFs (Source: Pharmaceutical Research and Manufacturers of America, 2000).

of thrombocytopenia or acceleration of platelet engraftment following bone marrow transplantation or peripheral blood progenitor cell transplantation. These include IL-3, and IL-6 (see Chapter 9). Several ILs are also under development for cancer indications and for the treatment of HIV infection, e.g. IL-4, IL-10 and IL-12.

Liposomal IL-2

Liposomal IL-2 is an example of attempts to improve drug delivery of proteins (see Chapter 4 and Table 20.4b of this section). While Proleukin (aldesleukin, IL-2) is already used for the treatment of renal cell carcinoma and melanoma, satisfactory drug delivery of this protein product is lacking. Now liposomal IL-2 is used to improve therapeutic efficacy in renal cell carcinoma, and also to enhance IL-2 induced adjuvant effects in anti-tumor vaccines.

Fusion Molecules

Using ligation chemistry, researchers have created biologically active molecules that combine the activities of two individual proteins into fusion molecules. Fusion molecules contain portions or the entire amino acid sequences of both parent proteins. Fusion technologies hold promise for developing "custom" molecules expressing a variety of activities. An example of a fusion product in clinical trials is IL-2 fusion protein, DAB389 IL-2 (Denileukin diftitox)

Interleukins (ILs) – Agonists and Antagonists		
Product	Company	Indication
Recombinant human interleukin-2	Chiron	HIV infection
Recombinant human interleukin-3 (rhIL-3)	Sandoz Pharmaceuticals	acceleration of engraftment of blood cells following bone marrow transplantation of peripheral blood stem cell transplantation in patients receiving myeloablative chemotherapy
Recombinant human interleukin-4	Schering-Plough	non-small-cell lung cancer
Recombinant human interleukin-6 (rhIL-6)	Sandoz Pharmaceuticals	acceleration of engraftment of platelets following myelosuppressive chemotherapy for various cancers
Interleukin-1 receptor antagonist	Amgen	rheumatoid arthritis
Interleukin-6 mutein	Imclone Systems	thrombocytopenia secondary to chemotherapy
Recombinant human interleukin-10	Schering	rheumatoid arthritis, Crohn's disease
Recombinant human interleukin-12 (rhIL-12)	Genetics Institute and Wyeth-Ayerst Laboratories	HIV infection, cancer
Liposomal interleukin-2	Blomira USA	renal cell carcinoma
Interleukin-2 fusion protein, Denileukin diftitox	Seragen	psoriasis HIV infection, lymphomas, severe rheumatoid arthritis, recent onset type 1 diabetes

Table 20.4b. Some biotechnology-derived protein products in various stages of clinical trials: ILs (Source: Pharmaceutical Research and Manufacturers of America, 2000).

is approved for the treatment of cutaneous T-cell lymphoma (Ajinomoto, Seragen, 1994). Denileukin diftitox (also called IL-2 fusion toxin) is a recombinant protein consisting of the first 389 amino acids of diphtheria toxin "fused" to amino acid residues 2–133 of human IL-2 (the IL-2 residues replace the amino acids of the receptor binding domain of the native diphtheria toxin).

Enzymes

A selection of biotechnology-derived enzymes in clinical development (Pharmaceutical Research and Manufacturers of America, 2000) including clotting factors, dismutases, tissue plasminogen activators and others can be found in Table 20.5. Two examples are described to illustrate the importance of this group.

Protein (Enzyme) Deficit Diseases

Several enzymes have been identified as missing or deficient in some rare, but catastrophic diseases, such as Fabry's Disease. Fabry's disease is a deficiency of galactosidase. Also, the enzyme, glucosidase, is deficient in Pompe's Disease. These enzymes offer the hope of providing a new protein therapeutic to correct these diseases, where no therapy exists today.

Enzymes (Dismutases, Tissue Plasminogen Activators and Others)		
Product	Company	Indication
Alpha-glucosidase	Genzyme	Pompe's disease
Alpha-galactosidase	Genzyme	Fabry's disease
Alronidase	BioMarin	mucopolysaccharidase-1 disease
Argatroban	Texas Biotech	Heparin-induced idiopathic thrombocytopenic purpura
Superoxide dismutase (oxsodrol)	Bio-Technology I Genera	oxygen toxicity in premature infants
tPA (tissue-type plasminogen activator)	Bristol-Myers Squibb	acute myocardial infarction
X-galactosidase	Transkaryotic Therapy	Fabry's disease
Carboxypeptidase G-2	National Cancer Institute	methotrexate overdose following intrathecal administration
PEG – glucocerebrosidase	Enzon	Gaucher's disease
Platelet activating factor – acetylhydrolase	ICOS	adult respiratory distress syndrome (ARDS)
		pancreatitis
		asthma
DNase (dornase alpha)	Genentech	lupus nephritis
Urate oxidase (recombinantly-produced enzyme)	Sanofi	prophylaxis for chemotherapy-related hyperuricemia treatment of cancer-related hyperuricemia

Table 20.5. Some biotechnology-derived protein products in various stages of clinical trials: Enzymes (Source: Pharmaceutical Research and Manufacturers of America, 2000).

SUPEROXIDE DISMUTASE

Superoxide dismutase (SOD) is a ubiquitous copper-and zinc-containing enzyme which destroys oxygen free radicals (see mechanistic scheme below). A familial variant of amyotrophic lateral sclerosis (ALS, Lou Gehrig's disease) has been linked to deficits in human cytosolic SOD. Recombinant SOD is in clinical trials for the treatment of oxygen toxicity in premature infants and has the potential to be useful in patients with myocardial infarction, organ transplantation and stroke.

$$O_2^- + O_2^- + 2H^+ \text{ —— SOD } \longrightarrow O_2 + H_2O_2$$

Hormones and Growth Factors

A list of some biotechnology-derived hormones and growth factors in various stages of clinical trials (Pharmaceutical Research and Manufacturers of America, 2000) can be found in Table 20.6a,b. Some examples are described below.

NEUROTROPHIC FACTORS

Growth factors (GFs) are cytokines responsible for regulating the production, maturation and function of cells in specific tissues and organs. Each cell type's response will be specific for each particular growth factor and will differ from growth factor to growth factor. Families of GFs and

Hormones		
Product	**Company**	**Indication**
Human corticotropin-releasing hormone (hCRH)	Neurobiological Technologies	rheumatoid arthritis, brain tumor edema, post-surgical edema
Human chorionic gonadotropin	Serono	breast cancer
Human insulin in powder form	Inhale	diabetes mellitus (by inhalation route of administration)
Leptin	Amgen	obesity control and treatment of diabetes mellitus
Recombinant human parathyroid hormone (rhPTH)	Allelix Biopharmaceuticals	post-menopausal osteoporosis
Recombinant human thyroid stimulating hormone	Genzyme	adjunct in procedures used for detection and treatment of recurrent thyroid cancer
Symlyn (pramlintide)	Amylin	metabolic control in diabetes mellitus
Proteins		
Product	**Company**	**Indication**
ConXn (relaxin)	Connetics	scleroderma, infertility
Antide (GhRHA, gonadotropin hormone-releasing hormone antagonist)	Ares-Serono	female fertiltity
Abarelix	Amgen / Praecis	prostate cancer
FLT 3 ligand	NCI	melanoma, renal cancer
Osteoprotogerin	Amgen	osteoporosis, metastatic cancer
Bactericidal/permeability factor (Neurex)	Xoma	cystic fibrosis, meningococcemia
Natrecor BNP (brain naturiuretic peptide)	Scios	congestive heart failure
Ovidrel	Serono	female fertility
Trecetilide	Pharmacia	atrial arrhythmia

Table 20.6a. Some biotechnology-derived protein products in various stages of clinical trials: Hormones and Other Proteins (Source: Pharmaceutical Research and Manufacturers of America, 2000).

their receptors include many of the CSFs, ILs, erythropoietins, and other cytokines already mentioned (see Chapters 8 and 9). Additional classes of GFs are neurotrophic factors and various tissue specific growth factors. Several rDNA-produced growth factors are now undergoing clinical trials.

Neurotrophic factors (NFs or nerve growth factors) have emerged in the 1990s into a significant class of molecules to treat various serious neurological diseases, such as amyotrophic lateral sclerosis (ALS) and Parkinson's disease; the molecules include brain-derived neurotrophic factor (BDNF), ciliary neurotrophic factor, glial-derived

Growth Factors		
Product	Company	Indication
Transforming growth factor-beta 2	Genzyme	chronic skin ulcers
		multiple sclerosis
Brain derived neurotrophic factor (BDNF)	Amgen	amyotrophic lateral sclerosis (ALS)
FIBLAST trafermin	Scios	stroke
Insulin-like growth factor (IGF-1)	Celtrix	diabetes, burns, hip fracture
Insulin-like growth factor binding protein 3	Somatokine	diabetes, burns
Recombinant Keratinocyte growth factor	Amgen	mucositis in cancer chemotherapy
Recombinant Keratinocyte growth factor	Human Genome Sciences	wound healing
Myotrophin, rhIGF-1	Amgen-Regeneron Partners	peripheral neuropathies, ALS
Recombinant human platelet-derived growth factor-BB (PDGF)	Chiron and Johnson & Johnson	wound healing
Vascular endothelial growth factor (VEGF)	GenVec	cardiovascular disorders

Table 20.6b. Some biotechnology-derived protein products in various stages of clinical trials: Growth Factors (Source: Pharmaceutical Research and Manufacturers of America, 2000).

neurotrophic factor (GDNF), nerve growth factor and neurotrophin-3. Neurotrophic factors exert the ability to regenerate damaged or partially severed nerve cells. With the identification of these nerve growth factors, a long-sought means of repairing neurological trauma appears to be within reach (Hotzman and Mobley, 1994). The dream of repairing nerve damage became a reality in 1991 with a report in the *New England Journal of Medicine* describing the effects of the lipid "GM-I ganglioside" (Geisler *et al.*, 1991). This material is present in high concentrations in the outer portion of nerve sheath cells, and it stimulates production of nerve growth factor, which in turn both protects and restores nerve function and growth. The search for protein growth factors that can produce the same effects continues. A neurotrophic factor in trials include neurotrophin-3 and nerve growth factor (NGF) for peripheral neuropathies.

A non-neurotrophic cytokine with a nerve specific effect is insulin-like growth factor-I (IGF-I, Myotrophin). First viewed as a candidate for growth disorders and diabetes, it was then discovered that nerve cells also have receptors for this cytokine. Myotrophin exhibited highly positive results in a Phase III clinical study involving 266 ALS patients (Piascik, 1996). A second Phase III clinical study in Europe in 183 patients for ALS, and a Phase II study for other indication including peripheral neuropathies caused by chemotherapy, diabetes, and polio are ongoing. Since it causes new nerves to sprout and strengthen interactions between muscle and nerve connections, IGF-I could possible be used to repair neurologic damage caused by these conditions.

OTHER GROWTH FACTORS

Tissue growth factors are being discovered and tested for tissue repair. Growth factors regulating bone development have also been identified. They belong to the tissue growth factor β (TGF-β) superfamily of growth-regulating cytokines. They guide bone stem cells through their various differentiation pathways and very specifically regulate skeletal development. Bone growth factor research is of great interest to develop a bone-mending putty for repairing severe fractures, in treating osteoporosis and connective tissue damage, and for dental reconstruction. Other growth factors such as β Kine (transforming growth factor β) and platelet-derived growth factor (PDGF) are in clinical trials to promote healing of wounds and skin ulcers.

Keratinocyte growth factor and fibroblast growth factor are other tissue growth factors with potential therapeutic use. Keratinocyte growth factor (KGF) stimulates epithelial cell proliferation. Fibroblast growth factor (FGF) is a member of a family of heparin-binding growth factors. Indications for FGF being explored include tissue repair in corneal and cataract surgeries, angiogenesis (new capillary formation), and improvement in wound healing including burns and tendon repair. The indication for KGF is the treatment of mucositis associated with cancer chemotherapy.

Another exciting growth factor being studied by the pharmaceutical industry is stem cell factor (SCF; also known as c-kit ligand and steel factor). A protein on the surface of bone marrow stromal cells, SCF stimulates early pluripotent and committed stem cells, acts synergistically with various other cytokines, increases B-cell formation and stimulates mast cells and melanocytes (Huang *et al.*, 1990). SCF is being studied as an adjunct to cancer chemotherapy to facilitate hematopoiesis in patients unable to mobilize blood progenitor cells to be used in blood cell transplants.

Vaccines

Some biotechnology-derived vaccines in clinical development (Pharmaceutical Research and Manufacturers of America, 2000) are listed in Table 20.7. Thanks to molecular techniques, vaccines are undergoing a renaissance (see Chapter 12 and references contained therein). Live attenuated vaccines made non-pathogenic by a gene deletion may elicit a greater immune response. With the availability of entire bacterial genomic sequences such as that of Haemophilus influenzae, this method is likely to be improved by engineering "out" (or in) specific genes to create non-pathogenic live vaccines. Genetic engineering also makes it possible to express combinations of elements that would never occur in natural selection. Recombinant methods have given us new types of vaccines including the subunit vaccine or DNA vaccines that deliver a code to the host to produce subunits endogenously, such as "naked DNA."

An anti-hormone vaccine is under development directed against gastrin, a peptide hormone that regulates digestion and is present at elevated levels in cancers of the gut, stomach, pancreas and other organs. This vaccine may also be useful in gastroesophageal reflux disease (GERD), peptic ulcers and ulcers induced by non-steroidal anti-inflammatory drugs (NSAIDs). Another target is gonadotropin-releasing hormone, which regulates testosterone and estrogen levels and is involved in prostate, breast and endometrial cancers.

Vaccines for herpes simplex infections, HIV disease (AIDS) and cytomegalovirus infection (CMV) are now in clinical trials. An acellular subunit vaccine for diphtheria-pertussis tetanus successfully completed a large trial. Another vaccine in late-stage trials is Melacine, a therapeutic vaccine based on interferon α to treat stage IV melanoma. Another late clinical trial of Melacine for stage II melanoma with no evidence of disseminated disease, to prevent recurrence after surgery to remove primary disease is underway.

A new class of vaccine, the fusion vaccine is an extenuation of the idea of mobilizing the immune system against undesirable entities. One example of a fusion vaccine is a contraceptive vaccine that is directed against chorionic gonadotropin, a hormone essential to implantation of the embryo. Chorionic gonadotropin is normally not recognized as a foreign protein, for obvious reasons. A strong antigenic response to the vaccine is elicited by attaching the β chain of the hormone to a bacterial toxoid. The effects of the vaccine are said to be reversible, and the vaccine lacks the burdensome side effects of steroid contraceptives. Eighty per cent of the women in early clinical trials produced large amounts of antibody in response to it. The vaccine holds great promise for population control especially in developing countries (Aldous, 1994). The fusion vaccine concept has considerable potential and many be extended to many new indications.

Recombinant Soluble Receptors

Receptors are macromolecules (generally, but not always proteins) which specifically recognize a binding ligand. Receptor-ligand binding initiates a specific biological response directly or causes an intracellular signal transduction resulting in the observed biological effect. Natural protein receptors may be soluble, circulating proteins (such as enzymes and released cell surface proteins), cell surface proteins, proteins found embedded in and spanning a cellular membrane (transmembrane receptors), or entirely intracellular proteins. Many small molecule drugs act as specific receptors. With the advent of DNA cloning and other recombinant DNA techniques, it is possible to produce receptor proteins found on the surface of cells and portions of transmembrane proteins in soluble forms. A recombinant soluble receptor may be the entire cellular receptor amino acid sequence, or a portion of the sequence, i.e. the rDNA-produced extracellular portion of a transmembrane receptor lacking the membrane spanning and intracellular amino acids. A selection of recombinant soluble receptors in clinical development (Pharmaceutical Research and Manufacturers in America, 2000) can be found in Table 20.8. Examples of soluble receptor molecules in clinical development include tumor necrosis factor receptor, IL-I receptor, IL-4 receptor and a human complement cascade receptor. The therapeutic aim of these receptor molecules is to bind to their normal ligands, preventing the ligands from binding to the cellular receptors, thus interrupting the expected specific biological response or signal transduction event.

Vaccines		
Product	Company	Indication
APC 8015/8020	Dendreon	cancers, prostate and multiple myeloma
Anerva X.RA	Corixa	rheumatoid arthritis
Neutralizing G-17 hormone	Aphton	various cancers and gastrointestinal disorders
Cholera	AVANT	cholera
E. coli	MedImmune	urinary tract infections
Genital herpes	GlaxoWellcome	genital herpes
Glioma	Immune Response	glioblastoma multiforme
Gamma vaccinia muc1	NCI	breast cancer
Gp 120 vaccine	GenenVax	AIDS
Herpes simplex vaccine (recombinant)	SmithKline Beecham	prevention of herpes simplex infection
Herpes vaccine	The Biocine Company Chiron	treatment of herpes simplex infection
HIV vaccine (gp 120)	The Biocine Company Chiron	AIDS
HPV vaccine	MedImmune	cervical cancer
Her2/neu	Corixa	breast and ovarian cancers
Melanoma theraccine	RIBI ImmunoChem	melanoma
GVAX	Cell Gensys	prostate and lung cancers
Neutralizing hCG hormone vaccine	Aphton	female contraception
RCEA Vaccine (recombinant carcinoembryonic antigen)	MicroGeneSys	colon and breast cancer
Recombinant canarypox-CEA (human) vaccine (carcinoembryonic antigen)	National Cancer Institute	advanced cancers expressing CEA
Recombinant vaccine-CEA (70kDa) vaccine (carcinoembryonic antigen)	National Cancer Institute	adenocarcinoma of the colon and rectum
RSV subunit vaccine	Wyeth-Ayerst Laboratories	respiratory syncytial virus-mediated lower respiratory disease for at-risk children and elderly
Prostvac	Therion	prostate cancer
P53 tumor suppressor	Genzyme Molecular	solid tumors
Theratope	Biomira	breast cancer
RSV	AVANT	respiratory syncytial virus
Rpg120	VaxGen	HIV infection prevention

Table 20.7. Some biotechnology-derived protein products in various stages of clinical trials: Vaccines (Source: Pharmaceutical Research and Manufacturers of America, 2000).

Recombinant Soluble Receptors		
Product	**Company**	**Indication**
Interleukin-1 receptor (dry powder inhalant)	Immunex and Inhale Therapeutic Systems	asthma
Interleukin-4 receptor	Immunex	asthma
rhTNF binding protein	Serono	rheumatoid arthritis
Soluble TNF receptor inhibitor	Amgen	rheumatoid arthritis
TNF-receptor fusion protein	Hoffmann-La Roche	septic shock, severe sepsis, rheumatoid arthritis, multiple sclerosis
TP10 (Soluble complement receptor CR1)	AVANT	heart attacks, adult respiratory injury following first-time myocardial infarction
Tumor necrosis factor (TNF) receptor	Immunex Wyeth-Ayerst Laboratories	rheumatoid arthritis
Angiogenesis Inhibitors		
Product	**Company**	**Indications**
CA4P	Oxigene	advanced solid tumors
Endostatin	NCI	advanced solid tumors
SU6668	Sugen	advanced solid tumors
TNP-470	Tap	advanced solid tumors
Vitaxin	MedImmune	leiomyosarcoma

Table 20.8. Some recombinant soluble receptors and angiogenesis inhibitors in clinical development (Source: Pharmaceutical Research and Manufacturers of America, 2000).

Monoclonal Antibodies

Indications for some of the therapeutic and diagnostic MAbs that are in development (Pharmaceutical Research and Manufacturers in America, 2000) are listed in Table 20.9. A brief discussion of some areas of current development follows.

Therapeutic Monoclonal Antibodies

Therapeutic MAbs as potential products from drug development helped propel the early biotechnology industry, but thus far diagnostic MAbs have proved to be more useful. Some of biotechnology's biggest disappointments have been therapeutic MAb products, such as several high-profile products for septic shock that failed to show efficacy in large-scale trials in 1994: Centoxin®, E-5, T-88 and Bradycor®. A MAb that received FDA marketing approval in 1995 was ReoPro®, a human/murine chimeric antibody aimed at blocking the aggregation of platelets and fibrin in angioplasty patients, in order to prevent cardiovascular complications (see Chapter 13 and appendices).

Technology advances (see Chapter 13) are addressing some of the challenges encountered in developing MAbs and have increased their therapeutic potential (Holliger and Hoogenboom, 1998; Adair, 2000). Earlier versions of MAbs possessed mouse-constant regions which could lead to possible immune recognition. This murine structure limited them to one time only therapeutic uses and rendered repeated uses, as in chronic disease states, inappropriate. "Humanized" mice now can be created by transferring the

Monoclonal Antibody Indications	
Indication	Indication (continued)
Acute kidney rejection	Inflammatory bowel disease
Acute myeloid leukemia	Leukemia and metastatic melanoma
Graft vs host disease	Multiple sclerosis
Acute myocardial infarction	Neuroblastoma (pediatric)
Allergic rhinitis	Non-Hodgkin's B-cell lymphoma
Asthma	Pancreatic cancer
Atherosclerotic plague imaging agent	Poison ivy, poison oak
Blood clot imaging agent	Prevention of respiratory syncytial virus (RSV) disease
Breast cancer	Prevention of secondary cataract
Cardiac imaging agent	Nephritis
CMV infections in AIDS patients	Refractory unstable angina
Colorectal cancer	Relapsed AML
Diagnosis of osteomyelitis, infected prosthesis, appendicitis	Renal prophylaxis
Epidermal growth factor receptor positive cancers	Rheumatoid arthritis
Idiopathic thrombocytopenic purpura	Sepsis syndrome
Extent of disease staging of liver and germ cell cancers	Stroke
Psorasis	Systemic lupus erythematosus
Extent of disease staging of lung cancer	Targeted radiotherapy for prostrate malignancies
Gram-negative sepsis	T-cell lymphoma
Hemorrhagic shock	Thermal injury
HIV-infection, AIDS	Thrombolytic complications of PTCA

Table 20.9. Indications of some of the many therapeutic and diagnostic monoclonal antibodies in development. For most indications, there are several monoclonal antibodies in development by various companies. (Source: Pharmaceutical Research and Manufacturers of America, 2000).

complete segment of the human heavy-chain antibody gene into mouse blastocysts generating completely human MAbs for treating rheumatoid arthritis, transplant rejection, chronic inflammation, and other conditions. Also novel MAbs conjugated to toxins or radioisotopes are being developed as therapeutic agents.

Diagnostic Monoclonal Antibodies

Diagnostic MAbs are in wide use in the familiar enzyme-linked immunosorbent assay (ELISA) for detecting food contaminants and environmental toxins. In human medicine, they are most typically utilized in the form of conjugates composed of a recognition site that is specific to a tumor antigen or another pathological marker and an imaging moiety like technetium Tc99m (a gamma-emitter) or gadolinium that emits a detectable signal when excited by an appropriate impulse during magnetic resonance imaging or other scanning procedures.

Some Nucleic Acid Therapies in Development

Early development of nucleic acid therapy concentrated on the use of gene therapy aimed at genetic deficiency diseases amenable to gene replacement (see Chapter 7). Research in the use of antisense oligonucleotides (see Chapter 6) which suppress or block selected protein expression by interacting with genes or mRNA has increased significantly (Crooke, 1995). Success was demonstrated with the FDA approval of forniversen sodium injectable (Vitravene; Ciba Vision/Isis) the first therapeutic antisense drug on the market. It is indicated for the treatment of CMV retinitis in AIDS patients. The potential use of oligonucleotides in therapy now goes well beyond their ability to interact with nucleic acid receptors (genes or mRNA). Oligonucleotides targeted toward non-nucleic acid receptors such as proteins in "aptamer technology" are also under intense investigation (see Chapter 6). There is little doubt that the rapidly developing area of nucleic acid therapy will provide interesting therapeutics for clinical development.

Gene Therapy

Chapter 7 provides an excellent overview of the development of gene therapies. It is to be expected that the list of clinical studies will continue to grow rapidly. Altogether, over 3000 patients have been treated, and the preliminary conclusions that can be drawn from these studies are that gene transfer to humans is possible, although the levels are still low in most cases. The quadruple major challenge in gene therapy is: (1) identification and reproduction of the required gene; (2) creation of a vector for carrying the gene into human cells that offers no genetic contamination, high cell delivery, high expression and persistence; (3) use of the best human host cell for the gene insertion that can be manipulated *in vitro*, inserted into the body, and remain alive and functional over an extended period of time; and (4) clinical testing of this gene-vector product for safety and efficacy (Mulligan, 1993; Smith, 1999). Table 20.10 provides a list of indications for the gene therapy protocols currently approved (Pharmaceutical Research and Manufacturers of America, 2000).

Gene Therapy Trials
Indications
Angina pectoris, exertional
Asymptomatic HIV-1-infection
Brain cancer
Breast cancer
Colon cancer
Coronary artery disease
Cystic fibrosis, sinusitis
Disseminated malignant melanoma
Factor VIII – Hemophilia A
Gaucher's disease
Hematopoietic stem cell protection in chemotherapy
HIV infection
Metastatic renal cell carcinoma
Neuroblastoma
Non-small cell lung cancer
Ovarian cancer

Table 20.10. Gene therapy trials (Source: Pharmaceutical Research and Manufacturers of America, 2000).

Antisense Oligonucleotides

Antisense technology (anti-RNA or anti-DNA) is highly sequence-specific to nucleic acid chains, disrupting the translation process of specific messenger RNA molecules, thus preventing the production of potentially damaging proteins (Table 20.11). They are expected to have few side effects due to their specificity. Also, antisense molecules have the additional advantages of morphologic simplicity and of being easy to synthesize. As discussed in Chapter 6, native antisense molecules are subject to rapid degradation by endogenous RNAses. The half lives and binding affinity of antisense constructs can be increased by chemically modifying their phosphodiester backbones

Antisense Molecules		
Product	Company	Indication
GEM 92	Hybridon	HIV infection, AIDS
G 3139	Genta	various cancers
ISIS 2503 / 3521	Isis	various cancers
ISIS 2302	Isis	ulcerative colitis, psoriasis, transplant rejection
Resten-NG	AVI BioPharma	cardiovascular restenosis

Table 20.11. Some biotechnology products in development from antisense technology (Source: Pharmaceutical Manufacturers and Research Association, 2000)

by substituting moieties such as methylphosphonate or methylphosphorothionate. Also, drug delivery of the antisense drug is a major challenge, similar to gene therapy, since the targeted RNA to be turned off resides inside cells. Thus, future developments will address these issues. While early in clinical trials, antisense molecules are being examined for their use in HIV infection, CMV retinitis in AIDS patients, various cancers and inflammatory diseases (Pharmaceutical Research and Manufacturers of America, 2000).

Development of Adhesion Molecules, Glycoproteins, Carbohydrate-Based Pharmaceuticals and Other Products of Glycobiology

Glycobiology

As described in Chapter 6, glycobiology is an emerging field that has opened up a whole new realm of possibilities for drug development. Carbohydrate recognition and adhesion by molecules, viruses, and cells to various cells are mediated by transmembrane proteins called selectins (E-selectin and P-selectin are expressed on endothelium and platelets; L-selectin is expressed on some leukocytes) and other cell surface carbohydrate-binding proteins. The structure of the oligosaccharides present of glycoproteins, glycolipids and these component's presentation on cell surfaces may dramatically alter cell biological function. Because of the immense number of combinations possible in rearranging a small number of carbohydrate subunits, complex specificities are possible. Highly specific drug/target interactions at the cell surface involving carbohydrates of adhesion molecules are thus attractive points for intervention (Varki, *et al.*, 1999).

Fibronectin and Fibronectin Receptor Antagonists

Fibronectin is a type of adhesion glycoprotein. It is a component of the extracellular matrix, the fibrous scaffolding that surrounds the exteriors of cells (Nichols *et al.*, 1994). It holds the cells in their proper positions, and also helps them to move from place to place during normal transport and turnover processes such as would healing. Fibronectin binds integrins, and in a wound cavity provides a temporary scaffolding whereby fibroblasts can more easily commute to the wound site. Other fibronectin receptors (integrins) are located on platelets, which produce fibrinogen, which in turn clogs the area, slows down the migration of fibroblasts, and retards wound healing.

By preventing or reducing the action of platelets, wound healing can be promoted. Non-healing wounds plague persons with diabetes, bedridden patients, and others with circulatory problems. Conversely, blocking the binding of fibronectin to integrins could slow down the clotting process in heart attacks or could retard the build-up of excess scar tissue in the corneal disease known as dry eye (Sjögren's syndrome) or in the glomerular membrane of the kidney, another threat to persons with diabetes. One drug is marketed that is aimed at carbohydrate moieties, Integrelin for arterial thrombosis. Integrelin prevents platelet binding to the fibronectin receptor, GPIIb-IIIa (also called α_{IIB}/β_3 or CD 41/CD61) (Nichols *et al.*, 1994). Integrelin is now in Phase III trials for coronary angioplasty and in Phase II trials for acute myocardial infarction and unstable angina.

Concluding Remarks

Pharmaceutical biotechnology and its various related techniques will continue to expand its influence in all areas of the drug discovery process. The development of novel pharmacological screening methods to identify new pharmaceuticals, the production of biopharmaceuticals being tested for the first time against several diseases, and the creation of innovative technologies for optimizing drug development will play defining roles in the genesis of pharmaceuticals that will serve as the foundation of modern pharmaceutical care. With the number of biotechnology-derived products in clinical development increasing each year, the prospects for continued innovation of our therapeutic arsenal look bright. ■

Further Reading

- **Biotechnology Update Column**. In *Journal of the American Pharmaceutical Association*, edited by P. Piascik. The column usually appears each month and frequently contains information about biotech products in development.
- **Pharmaceutical Research and Manufacturers of America.** (2000). *Biotechnology Medicines in Development.* Washington, DC. This publication appears approximately once each year. It can be obtained on line along with other biotechnology-related information at: http://www.pharma.org.

References

- **Adair F.** (2000). Immunogenicity: The last hurdle for clinically successful therapeutic antibodies. *Pharmaceut Technol*, 24, 50–56.
- **Aldous P.** (1994). A booster for contraceptive vaccines. *Science*, 266, 1484.
- **Bienz-Tadmor B.** (1993). Biopharmaceuticals go to market: patterns of worldwide development. *Bio/technology*, 11 168–172.
- **Crooke ST.** (1995). Oligonucleotide Therapeutics. In *Burger's Medicinal Chemistry, Fifth Edition*, edited by ME Wolff, Vol. 1 New York, New York: John Wiley & Sons, Inc., pp. 863–900.
- **Evens RP, Dinarello GA, Browne J, Fenton D.** (1995a). Biotechnology and clinical medicine, Part 1. *Hospital Physician*, 31, (11), 27–36.
- **Evens RP, Dinarello GA, Browne J, Fenton D.** (1995b). Biotechnology and clinical medicine, Part 2. *Hospital Physician*, 31, (12), 26–31.
- **The Genome International Sequencing Consortium.** (2001). Initial sequencing and analysis of the human genome. *Nature*, 409, 860–921.
- **Geisler FH, Dorsey FC, Coleman WP.** (1991). Recovery of motor function after spinal-cord injury – a randomized, placebo-controlled trial with GM-1 ganglioside. *N Eng J Med*, 324, 1829–1838.
- **Holliger P, Hoogenboom H.** (1998). Antibodies come back from the brink. *Nature Biotech*, 16, 1015–1016.
- **Hotzman DM, Mobley WC.** (1994). Neurotrophic factors and neurological disease. *West J Med*, 161, 246–254.
- **Haung E, Nocka K, Beier DR, Chu TY, Buck J, Lahm HW,. Wellner D, Leder P, Besmer P.** (1990). The hematopoietic growth factor K1 is encoded at the S1 locus and it is the ligand of the c-kit receptor, gene product of the W locus. *Cell*, 63, 225–233..
- **Lee Jr KB, Burrill GS.** (1995). Biotech 96: The Industry Annual Report. Ernst and Young LLP.
- **Maulik S, Patel SD.** (1997). *Molecular Biotechnology, Therapeutic Applications and Strategies.* Wiley-Liss, New York, New York, 72–83.
- **Macdougall IC, *et al.*** (1999). Pharmacokinetics of novel erythropoiesis stimulating protein compared with epoetin alfa in dialysis patients. *J Am Soc Nephrol*, 10, 2392–2395.
- **Mulligan RC.** (1993). The basic science of gene therapy. *Science*, 260, 926–932.
- **Nichols AJ, Vasko JA, Koster PF, Valocik RE, Samanen JM.** (1994). GPIIb/IIIa Antagonists as novel antithrombic drugs. In *Cellular Adhesion – Molecular Definition to Therapeutic Potential*, edited by BW Metcalf, BJ Dalton, G Poste. New York, New York: Plenum Press, pp 213–237.
- **Pharmaceutical Research and Manufacturers of America.** (2000). *Biotechnology Medicines in Development.* Washington, DC.
- **Piascik P.** (1996). New hope for treatment of Lou Gehrig's disease. *Amer Pharm*, NS36, (6), 355–356.
- **Sharpiro B, Merck and Co.** (1995). The impact of biotechnology on drug discovery. *9th International Congress of Immunology*. San Francisco, California..
- **Smith AE.** (1999). Gene therapy: where are we? *Lancet*, 354 (suppl. 1), 1–4.
- **Struck MM.** (1994). Biopharmaceutical R&D success rates and development times. *Bio/technology*, 12 674–677.
- **Varki A, Cummings R, Esko J, Freeze H, Hart G, Marth J. (Eds).** (1999). *Essentials of Glycobiology*, Cold Spring Harbor Press, Cold Spring Harbor, New York.
- **Venter JC, *et al.*** (2001). The sequence of the Human Genome. *Science*, 291, 1304–1351.

Index

Note: page numbers in *italics* refer to figures and tables.